The Suicidal

Clinical Guide to the Ass_____ _____ment Suicide ____

Second Edition

IGOR GALYNKER

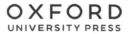

OXFORD
UNIVERSITY PRESS

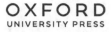

Oxford University Press is a department of the University of Oxford. It furthers the University's objective of excellence in research, scholarship, and education by publishing worldwide. Oxford is a registered trade mark of Oxford University Press in the UK and certain other countries.

Published in the United States of America by Oxford University Press
198 Madison Avenue, New York, NY 10016, United States of America.

© Oxford University Press 2023

All rights reserved. No part of this publication may be reproduced, stored in a retrieval system, or transmitted, in any form or by any means, without the prior permission in writing of Oxford University Press, or as expressly permitted by law, by license, or under terms agreed with the appropriate reproduction rights organization. Inquiries concerning reproduction outside the scope of the above should be sent to the Rights Department, Oxford University Press, at the address above.

You must not circulate this work in any other form and you must impose this same condition on any acquirer.

Library of Congress Cataloging-in-Publication Data
Names: Galynker, Igor I., 1954– author.
Title: The suicidal crisis : clinical guide to the assessment of imminent suicide risk / Igor Galynker.
Description: 2. | New York : Oxford University Press, [2023] |
Includes bibliographical references and index.
Identifiers: LCCN 2022044627 (print) | LCCN 2022044628 (ebook) |
ISBN 9780197582718 (paperback) | ISBN 9780197582732 (epub) |
ISBN 9780197582749 (online)
Subjects: MESH: Suicide—psychology | Suicide—prevention & control |
Risk Factors | Risk Assessment—methods | Models, Psychological
Classification: LCC RC569 (print) | LCC RC569 (ebook) | NLM WM 165 |
DDC 362.28—dc23/eng/20230120
LC record available at https://lccn.loc.gov/2022044627
LC ebook record available at https://lccn.loc.gov/2022044628

DOI: 10.1093/med/9780197582718.001.0001

This material is not intended to be, and should not be considered, a substitute for medical or other professional advice. Treatment for the conditions described in this material is highly dependent on the individual circumstances. And, while this material is designed to offer accurate information with respect to the subject matter covered and to be current as of the time it was written, research and knowledge about medical and health issues is constantly evolving and dose schedules for medications are being revised continually, with new side effects recognized and accounted for regularly. Readers must therefore always check the product information and clinical procedures with the most up-to-date published product information and data sheets provided by the manufacturers and the most recent codes of conduct and safety regulation. The publisher and the authors make no representations or warranties to readers, express or implied, as to the accuracy or completeness of this material. Without limiting the foregoing, the publisher and the authors make no representations or warranties as to the accuracy or efficacy of the drug dosages mentioned in the material. The authors and the publisher do not accept, and expressly disclaim, any responsibility for any liability, loss, or risk that may be claimed or incurred as a consequence of the use and/or application of any of the contents of this material.

Printed by Marquis Book Printing, Canada

To the American Foundation for Suicide Prevention

Contents

Acknowledgments

I am thankful to Oxford University Press for believing that The Suicidal Crisis is an important book worthy of a second edition. I am equally thankful to my editors, Andrea Knobloch and Katie Lakina, for their expertise and support throughout the writing process.

I thank the American Foundation for Suicide Prevention for its support of research in acute suicidal states and in predicting short-term suicide risk. In particular, I thank Dr. Jill Harkavy-Friedman for her dedication to the cause of suicide prevention; for her generosity with her time and her ideas; for her brilliant knowledge of suicidology; for her unparalleled scientific rigor; for her belief in the importance of developing clinical approaches to suicide prevention; and for her grace, wit, and good humor. I am deeply grateful to Rob and Kathy Masinter for their visionary and inspirational trust in our work and gratefully acknowledge the Eric Masinter Memorial Fund for its generous support of the Mount Sinai Beth Israel Suicide Prevention Research Laboratory.

This book would not have been possible without the work of my long-time collaborator, Dr. Lisa Cohen. During our many years of trying to solve the puzzle of the psychological processes that make suicide possible, I benefited greatly from Lisa's intellectual voracity, unparalleled commitment to both clinical work and science, and unwavering moral compass. She has been invaluable in providing scientific evidence for the Narrative Crisis Model of Suicide, which is the backbone of this book.

I also thank my other collaborators from the Mount Sinai Suicide Prevention Research Laboratory. Their contribution to *The Suicidal Crisis* lies in many stimulating and lively discussions we have had during our research meetings and clinical work rounds. For this I am particularly grateful to Drs. Megan Rogers, Shira Barzilay, Sarah Bloch-Elkouby, and Benedetta Imbastaro. I am indebted to Inna Goncearenco and Olivia Lawrence for their editing work on the book as a whole and for their co-authorship of several book chapters, and to Inna Goncearenco alone for her development of the second edition's wonderful cover design. I am most grateful to my other chapter co-authors—Lakshmi Chennapragada and Kimia Ziafat.

I consider working in the field of suicide prevention a great privilege, and the decision to change my research focus to suicidology was the best career decision I have ever made. Writing the second edition of this book gave me an opportunity to add experimental evidence to 30 years of clinical experience as an inpatient and outpatient psychiatrist. With increasing specialization in both research and clinical work, this essential blend of research and clinical expertise is becoming increasingly rare, and yet it is critically important for keeping psychiatric research clinically relevant. In this book, the names and identifiers of individual patients and their family members have been changed to protect their privacy. I remember all of them, and I am deeply grateful for their trust in my skill and judgment.

Finally, I thank my wife Asya for her love, kindness, and patience. The second edition of *The Suicidal Crisis* was written after hours (as was the first edition) and the Guide would not be possible without her support.

1

Introduction and Overview

The Ticking Time Bomb of the American Suicide Health Crisis

In June of 2019, the summer before the COVID-19 pandemic, three Navy sailors assigned to the USS *George H.W. Bush* aircraft carrier died by suicide in three separate incidents. These deaths marked the third, fourth, and fifth crew members of the carrier to take their own lives in two years. The military suicide problem is echoed by a similar problem in the medical field. Every day, one U.S. doctor ends his or her own life—one of the highest suicide rates in any profession (Peterson et al., 2020). In another demographic subgroup, American Indians have the highest rate of suicide of any racial or ethnic group in the United States (Curtin et al., 2021). The suicide epidemic has reached all of us.

The U.S. suicide statistics are sobering, and the scope of the suicide epidemic represents a major public health crisis. In 2020, 45,979 people in the United States died by suicide (Centers for Disease Control and Prevention [CDC], 2020) and it is estimated that 1,200,000 attempted suicide. To put this in perspective, among individuals under the age of 45, suicide accounts for more annual deaths than homicide, AIDS, car accidents, and war (Heron, 2021). More teenagers and young adults will die from suicide than from cancer, heart disease, AIDS, birth defects, stroke, pneumonia, influenza, and chronic lung disease combined. While the first year of the COVID-19 pandemic coincided with a drop in overall suicide rates in the United States, there was an increase in suicide rates in children and adolescents and young adults 10 to 34 years old. Remarkably, in 2020, deaths among Black girls and women between ages 10 and 24 increased more than 30%, from 1.6 to 2.1 per 100,000 people. Black boys and men of the same age had a 23% increase, from 3 to 3.7 per 100,000 (Curtin et al., 2021). According to the CDC, in the summer of 2020, 11% of surveyed adults over 18 years old reported having seriously considered suicide since the beginning of the pandemic. This translates into an astounding 22,000,000 Americans who should be evaluated for suicide risk (Czeisler et al., 2020).

While the suicide rates in the United States have been steadily increasing over the past two decades, in other industrialized countries, such as Great Britain, pre-COVID suicide rates have been steadier, while the rates have decreased worldwide, from their peak at 1,000,000 in 1995 to the estimated 703,000 in 2019 (World Health Organization, 2021). In the United States, however, in 2017 alone, suicide rates increased by 10% in adolescents and young adults age 15 to 24 and rose by a staggering 50% in children age 10 to 14. Despite a 3% decrease in U.S. suicide rates in 2019, suicide is currently the tenth leading cause of death overall and the second leading cause of death in adolescents and young adults 10 to 34 years old (Heron, 2021).

Although somewhat obscured by the COVID-19 pandemic, the U.S. suicide epidemic continues unabated, and it is time to confront it with the same determination that we confronted the epidemic of HIV/AIDS. We can start the battle by understanding that the mental state leading to suicide is an independent medical condition, one that can be diagnosed and treated with medications and psychotherapy.

As doctors and therapists have learned from decades of experience, a suicidal person cannot be expected to volunteer the truth about suicide plans. This is partly because the suicidal crisis may be very short-lived, and partly because the mind of a suicidal person is critically afflicted and therefore cannot be relied upon to adequately assess its own dangerous state. Recent research shows that the pre-suicidal state of mind is an illness in itself, a mental state characterized by five recognizable criteria, including entrapment, affective dysregulation, loss of cognitive control, hyperarousal, and acute social withdrawal (Bloch-Elkouby et al., 2020; Calati et al., 2020; Rogers et al., 2019; Schuck et al., 2019). This condition is called the Suicide Crisis Syndrome (SCS), and SCS can and should be treated.

Because our understanding of the pre-suicidal mental state is relatively new and has yet to be incorporated into the *Diagnostic and Statistical Manual of Mental Disorders* (DSM), contemporary clinical practice largely sees suicide as a manifestation of other mental disorders, such as depression or schizophrenia. Clinicians try to prevent suicide by treating the underlying condition, while relying on individuals to develop insight into, and to report, their mental processes that may lead to suicide. Specifically, mental health professionals rely on patients to honestly and accurately disclose their suicidal ideation (SI) by answering questions like "Have you ever thought of harming yourself?" or "Are you planning to harm yourself?"

The success rate of this method is low, performing slightly above chance. That is not surprising, given that about 75% of people who die by suicide never reveal their suicidal thoughts to anyone, according to the CDC (Stone et al., 2018). Indeed, some of them may not have a conscious suicidal plan until the very last moment of their life, or even not at all.

Such was the case of Kathy (name changed), the mother of a 12-year-old boy, who was in the throes of a hostile divorce and who, at the last second, did not move away from an oncoming van. Somehow, Kathy survived. When her many fractures healed, she said, pensively, "I never thought I was suicidal, but I guess I was, because otherwise I would have moved away." Kathy would not have reported being suicidal, but she met all the SCS criteria.

In the inpatient and outpatient facilities at Mount Sinai Beth Israel, in New York, the attending staff and psychiatry residents were trained to recognize SCS and to use it as the centerpiece of suicide risk assessment. Through training and practice, they were able to confidently identify high-risk individuals and help them recover, without relying on the patients' self-diagnosis via admission of their suicidal intent. Furthermore, after SCS assessment was implemented in the NorthShore University Health System in Chicago, the emergency department clinicians started using SCS diagnosis as a tool to inform their admission and discharge decision-making related to SI. Over the first two years, there were no completed suicides, and the readmission rate for suicide risk went down by 40% (Figure 1.1).

While doctors would never dream of basing a diagnosis solely on a patient's declaring "I am schizophrenic" or "I am bipolar," the pre-suicidal mind is more distorted and acutely life-threatening than either schizophrenia or bipolar disorder. Still, for decades, risk assessment has been based

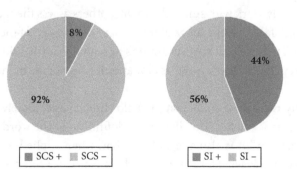

Figure 1.1 Clinical utility of abbreviated SCS assessment versus suicidal ideation (admission).

on the suicidal patient's accurate answer to the question, "Are you planning to kill yourself?"

Today, most professionals remain wedded to this conventional wisdom. The problem with this practice, and with the administrative and clinical tools using similar approaches for predicting suicides, is that they fail to identify the majority of those who go on to take their lives. If we want to save lives, we must get smarter and more efficient at addressing this issue and stop making critical life-saving treatment decisions based on the clouded judgment of a person suffering from the unbearable pain that precedes suicide.

The pre-suicidal mental state of SCS is a life-threatening illness that can be diagnosed by mental health professionals, after they have been appropriately trained. Anybody who is concerned that his or her loved one may be suicidal could, with proper education, recognize the signs of SCS. For this approach to enter the mainstream of psychiatry, SCS symptomatology should be taught in medical schools and other training programs for clinicians, alongside the symptoms of schizophrenia and other psychiatric disorders. Education about SCS should be available to all concerned, both in person and online.

By training doctors and the public at large to understand SCS, we can save thousands of lives. Like a heart attack, SCS can be treated; it does not have to be fatal.

What Is Imminent Suicide?

One of the most difficult determinations a psychiatrist makes is whether the chronically suicidal patient is at risk for imminent suicide. Although some clinicians rarely work with suicidal patients, others assess them daily, and all clinicians will face this challenge at least once. Hence, one of the goals of the National Alliance for Suicide Prevention's Research Prioritization Task Force is to find ways to assess who is at risk for attempting suicide in the immediate future.

Currently, there is no guide that can help clinicians accurately evaluate the risk of imminent suicide. The dictionary definition of the word *imminent* is "about to happen." It is also a legal term that, when applied to suicide risk, implies that suicide will happen so soon that immediate clinical intervention is required to prevent it. The phrase "risk for suicide in the immediate future" was chosen by the task force instead of "imminent risk" because the latter may imply (incorrectly) that mental health professionals have the ability to predict precisely when an impending suicidal act is going to take place (Claassen et al., 2014). The more accurate terms *near-term* and *short-term* suicide risk refer to a defined time period, such as one month, that could be used in suicide research studies. However, these terms may obscure the urgency of the life-and-death decisions made daily by frontline clinicians.

To underscore the pressure experienced by psychiatrists in their daily risk assessments, this guide retains the term *imminent suicide risk*, and this term is used interchangeably with the more research-oriented terms and with the intuitive clinical term *acute risk*. In this guide, the term *imminent suicide* designates the time interval from the moment the patient parts from the psychiatrist until the next appointment. Defined in this manner, imminent suicide implies that unless action is taken, the patient will attempt suicide prior to his or her next clinical visit. The length of the "imminent" time period can vary from hours for the same-day postdischarge outpatient appointment to months, as is the case for a regular outpatient visit for medication management.

Most often, however, "imminent" or "immediate future" means several days, reflecting the regular interval between care appointments after hospital discharge or while in weekly or biweekly therapy. Regardless of the duration of the interval, however, in the eyes of the patient's loved ones, the medical profession, and the law, during this time, it is the clinician who last saw the patient alive who bears the responsibility for the suicide, should it occur.

Long-Term versus Imminent Suicide Risk: Who versus When

Unfortunately, at present, despite substantial research efforts, our ability to identify those at risk for suicide in emergency departments, outpatient offices, and inpatient units has not changed in the last 50 years and remains close to chance (Franklin et al., 2017; Large et al., 2011). However, although the current clinical reality may be disheartening, recent advances in the field of suicidology have resulted in new, promising approaches to assessing short-term suicide risk. One such development is the recent attention toward the distinction between long- and short-term risk for suicide. This distinction lies in the difference between identifying who is at risk of dying by suicide at some point and when such individuals would actually take their lives.

The long-term risk factors for suicide (the "who") are well known. The most widely assessed factors are the history of mental illness (Backmann, 2018; Brådvik, 2018) and past suicide attempt (Probert-Lindström et al., 2020; Suokas et al., 2001), which increase the odds for eventual suicide 30-fold each. These two factors, however, have two major shortcomings in the context of assessing imminent suicide risk. The first shortcoming is that nearly every person evaluated by psychiatrists for suicide risk has either a mental illness or a history of suicide attempt, or both, which makes these aspects of little relevance in the clinical setting. In other words, for those diagnosed with a mental health condition, we know who is at risk. What we do not know is whether the "when" factor for imminent risk for suicide is within days, hours, or minutes. Recent machine learning (ML) analyses of electronic health records have started to narrow the "when" window and to succeed in identifying those who were seven times more likely to die by suicide in the next three months (Simon et al., 2018). However, the main risk factors identified with ML methods are the same: diagnoses of mental illness and history of suicide attempts. Hence, the second shortcoming of the mental illness/past attempt risk factors is that over 50% of those who have died by suicide never received a mental health diagnosis (Stone et al., 2018) and over 50% of those dying by suicide have succeeded in their first attempt (Bostwick et al., 2016).

The difference between the long-term and short-term risk factors for suicide was first described by Fawcett, Scheftner, and Clark (1987), who, in a prospective study, discovered that risk factors for suicide attempts differed, depending on the time elapsed since the initial assessment. In that pioneering study, "short-term" was relatively long and was defined as one year, while "long-term" was the period between two and ten years. The authors discovered that the short-term and the long-term risk factors were different (Table 1.1).

Surprisingly, in the Fawcett study, the well-known risk factors for suicide—depression, hopelessness, helplessness, and SI—were associated only with eventual risk for suicide. The short-term risk factors were the anxiety-related factors: anxiety, panic attacks, insomnia, agitation, and anhedonia. The latter finding has since been supported by multiple epidemiological and clinical studies (Black et al., 2019; Galynker et al., 2017; Goldblatt et al., 2016; Katz et al., 2011; Lim et al., 2015; Nam et al., 2016; Pilowsky et al., 1999; Rappaport et al., 2014; Scheer et al., 2020; Weissman et al., 1989; Yaseen et al., 2013). Moreover, the predictive value of panic, insomnia, and agitation

Table 1.1 Long-Term Versus Short-Term Risk Factors for Suicide

Short Term (< 1 Year)	Long Term (1–5 Years)
Anhedonia	Hopelessness
Panic attacks	Helplessness
Psychic anxiety	Suicidal ideation
Insomnia	Past suicide attempts
Moderate alcohol abuse	

as symptoms of an acute pre-suicidal mental state was supported in several prospective studies in the United States and abroad (Galynker et al., 2017; Otte et al., 2020).

Another important development in imminent risk assessment is the growing appreciation that a unique and acute negative affective state of short duration may precede suicide attempts (Bagge et al., 2014, Bagge & Borges, 2017; Diesenhammer et al., 2009). Initially, this state was called the suicide trigger state (Yaseen et al., 2010), but later it was called the suicide crisis syndrome (SCS) in homage to Dr. Herbert Hendin, a pioneering suicidologist, who was one of the first to hypothesize the existence of an acute pre-suicidal mental state, which he called the suicidal crisis. Thomas Joiner and colleagues later proposed a related syndrome called the acute suicidal affective disturbance (ASAD), which is characterized by a rapid onset of interrelated symptoms associated with acute suicide risk (Tucker et al., 2016).

Conceptually, the difference between long-term risk factors for suicide and the short-term factors comprising SCS is similar to the difference between long-term risk factors for cardiovascular disease and unstable angina. The ongoing Framingham study has shown that cardiovascular long-term risk factors include hypertension, obesity, diabetes, lack of exercise, and high cholesterol (Hajar, 2016). These factors identify who may have a myocardial infarction during the next decades (the "who"). An imminent heart attack is predicted by unstable angina, which is the syndrome reflecting lack of myocardial perfusion or ischemia and manifesting with chest pain, shortness of breath, and diaphoresis. These symptoms identify the time that the heart attack may occur (the "when"). In suicidology, the long-term risk factors identifying "who" include the history of mental illness, past suicide attempts, and others (see Chapter 4), while SCS is the unstable angina equivalent identifying "when." Unstable angina, if untreated, may lead to near-term

myocardial infarction, while SCS, if untreated, may lead to near-term suicide. One of the main aims of both suicide research and the suicide prevention effort is the appreciation of the difference between long-term risk factors
and SCS, and the need to identify and treat the latter. Although the suicide
crisis–myocardial infarction analogy is not literal, it is a useful parallel to
keep in mind when assessing imminent suicide risk. Assessing the long-term
risk factors will identify "who," but SCS intensity will predict "when."

Lack of Tests for Suicide Prediction

The suicide assessment instruments currently in use do not distinguish between long-term risk factors for eventual suicide and short-term risk factors
for imminent suicide. Moreover, most of these scales rely on consensus
opinion, or on psychological autopsies and past suicide attempts, which may
not be predictive of future suicidal behavior. Indeed, when tested for prediction of completed suicide and suicide attempt, these instruments were not
predictive of short-term events.

A well-known example of a consensus-derived, widely used scale that was
never validated is the SAD PERSONS scale (see Chapter 9). In a large-scale
retrospective study, the SAD PERSONS scale was not predictive of suicide
attempts and suicides in the immediate future (six months; Bolton et al.,
2012). Another large study showed that 60% of persons who completed suicide within one year after psychiatric discharge were judged "low suicide
risk" by this scale (Large et al., 2011). Finally, a recent series of British studies
prospectively investigated the predictive validity of the SAD PERSONS scale,
the Modified SAD PERSONS Scale, ReACT Self-Harm Rule, Manchester
Self-Harm Rule, and Barratt Impulsivity Scale (McClatchey et al., 2019;
Quinlivan et al., 2019; Steeg et al., 2018; Runeson et al., 2017; Taylor et al.,
2021). None of the scales showed prospective predictive validity for near-
term (six months) suicidal behavior, and none has achieved widespread use
(Quinlivan et al., 2017).

In contrast to the above-mentioned instruments, the Columbia Suicide
Severity Rating Scale (C-SSRS; Posner, 2011), an evidence-based questionnaire developed in the last decade, has had widespread use. Although initially developed as the first tool for the comprehensive descriptive assessment
of both SI and suicidal behavior, C-SSRS has been increasingly used for prediction of suicidal behavior and risk assessment stratification. The results of

Table 1.2 Prospective Studies Examining Suicidal Outcomes

Predictor	Studies	Attempt	Completion	Time of Follow-Up
Beck Depression Inventory (BDI)	Oquendo et al. (2004)	X	X	2 years
Beck Hopelessness Scale (BHS)	Beck et al. (1985, 1989)		X	5–10 years
Barratt Impulsivity Scale	Steeg et al. (2018)	X	X	0.5 years
Suicide Intent Scale (SIS)	Harriss & Hawton (2005)		X	5 years
Physical Anhedonia Scale (PAS)	Loas (2007)		X	6.5 years
Implicit Association Task (IAT)	Nock et al. (2010)	X		0.5 years
Manchester Self-Harm Rule	Quinlivan et al. (2017); Steeg et al. (2018)	X	X	0.5 years
ReACT Self-Harm Rule	Steeg et al. (2018); Runeson et al. (2017)	X		0.5 years
SKA-2	Guintivano et al. (2014)	X		0.5 years
Suicide Trigger Scale (STS)	Yaseen et al. (2014)	X		0.5 years
Suicide Stroop	Cha et al. (2010)	X		0.5 years
Columbia Suicide Severity Rating Scale (C-SSRS)	Pmosner et al. (2011); Horwitz et al., (2015)	X		4 months; 9 months

short-term prospective suicidal outcome studies, along with other prospective prediction studies' outcomes, are listed in Table 1.2. The C-SSRS showed modest predictive validity for those who disclose SI. However, because over 75% of those who die by suicide do not reveal their suicidal thoughts to anyone (Stone et al., 2018), the C-SSRS may fail to detect a large portion of the population who go on to attempt suicide.

The Problem of "Non-Disclosure"

As previously discussed, imminent suicide risk assessment remains difficult, with no reliable predictive methods available. This conceptual and diagnostic void requires a clinician to organize disparate bits of information into a subjective and actionable clinical opinion. In the absence of diagnostic tests in formulating this opinion, clinicians overwhelmingly rely on the patient's truthful answers to explicit questions about their suicidal history and intent. However, this overreliance on the patient's self-report (SI) in assessing imminent suicide risk may be misguided.

Early research showed that only one-third of patients seen in the emergency department for a serious suicide attempt had persistent SI, whereas the rest had either fleeting thoughts about suicide or none at all (Paykel et al., 1974). Thus, patients may not have SI or a plan until immediately before their attempt. On the other hand, those who are determined to end their lives often hide their intent (Horesh & Apter, 2006; Horesh et al., 2004) and may specifically hide it from their clinicians, while disclosing their SI to others, such as research assistants (B Bloch-Elkouby et al., 2022; Rogers et al., 2022). The most frequent reason for deliberately hiding SI is fear of involuntary hospitalization (Blanchard & Farber, 2020). Therefore, posing the question, "Have you been thinking about killing yourself?" to somebody who will attempt suicide imminently is often likely to provoke a negative response.

Nevertheless, contemporary practices and established guidelines for suicide risk assessment emphasize assessing the presence and severity of SI as a crucial first step in determining who may be at risk for suicidal behavior (Chu et al., 2015; National Suicide Prevention Lifeline, 2007; Posner et al., 2011). However, because of the fleeting nature of suicidal intent, along with patients' deliberate concealment of SI from their clinicians, there are several notable limitations associated with relying on SI for the prediction of future suicidal behavior. For one, SI alone is a poor predictor of suicidal behavior (Borges et al., 2008; Ribeiro et al., 2016). The past-year and lifetime prevalence of SI is consistently several times higher than that of suicide attempts (Borges et al., 2012; Kessler et al., 1999; Nock et al., 2008), indicating that few who have SI go on to make a suicide attempt. Additionally, many individuals opt not to disclose SI when it is present. In several studies, only a minority (approximately 25%) of suicide decedents reported SI in the final communications with healthcare providers prior to their deaths (Berman, 2018; Busch et al., 2003; Smith et al., 2013; Stone et al., 2018), and many decedents were viewed to be at low or no immediate risk for suicide (Appleby et al., 1999). Finally, additional evidence suggests that SI fluctuates substantially over short periods of time (Harris et al., 2010; Kleiman et al., 2017) and that retrospective ratings may be discordant from real-time ratings of SI (Gratch et al., 2020).

Altogether, these findings indicate that many instances of SI may go undetected and that, even if identified, these thoughts do not indicate who is at risk for suicidal behavior. Moreover, since SI may not appear until minutes before suicide, making self-reported SI the centerpiece and the gateway item for suicide risk assessment is an unsound practice both scientifically and conceptually. Scientifically, there is no experimental evidence to support the claim that SI is the single most important predictor of imminent suicide (Franklin et al., 2017), with abundant evidence to the contrary. Conceptually, just as we would never rely on those with schizophrenia or bipolar disorder to self-diagnose their illness, neither should we rely on those with an acutely life-threatening pre-suicidal mental state to self-diagnose their suicidal risk. Thus, the role of self-reported SI in risk assessment must be reconsidered.

Suicide Crisis Syndrome

SCS is conceptualized as an acute transdiagnostic pre-suicidal mental state that develops within days, hours, and minutes before suicide (Yaseen et al., 2010). Given the prevalence of patients' concealment of SI and the lack of scientific evidence supporting the validity of self-reported SI, the presence of SI is not required for the diagnosis of SCS, although it may have been present (Schuck et al., 2019). Given the urgent need to predict suicide, and the fact that there has never been a suicide-specific diagnosis in the DSM (American Psychiatric Association, 2013), the eventual goal for SCS, should it prove to be a valid and clinically useful syndrome, is its inclusion in the DSM to aid and improve suicide prevention. Since the DSM is a widely used tool for diagnosis of mental disorders, and up to 22% of suicide decedents have contact with a mental health professional within one week of their attempt (Stene-Larsen & Reneflot, 2019), a suicide-specific SCS diagnosis could be crucial in identifying those at risk for imminent suicide.

Two main arguments can be made for the use of SCS as a suicide-specific diagnosis. First, suicide has been included only as a symptom of other disorders in the DSM. For example, one possible criterion of major depressive disorder is thoughts of suicide (American Psychiatric Association, 2013), and SI also appears in other diagnoses, such as bipolar disorder and borderline personality disorder. Recommended treatment for those presenting with suicidal thoughts includes treating the underlying disorder, so suicide may be treated as a symptom of a broader disorder. Second, some individuals do not meet the criteria for any existing mental disorders and still go on to attempt suicide. In fact, a recent CDC report found that more than half of individuals who died by suicide did not have a psychiatric diagnosis at the time of their death (Stone et al., 2018).

SCS initially had two components (Yaseen et al., 2010). The first factor was the loss of cognitive control over one's thoughts and was termed "ruminative flooding." The second factor was the affective state of "frantic hopelessness," which is also referred to as entrapment (Galynker et al., 2014). These initial findings were replicated and extended in many research studies in diverse clinical and cultural settings (Galynker et al., 2017; Otte et al., 2020). In its current form, which is under consideration for inclusion in the DSM as a suicide-specific diagnosis, SCS has five components, separated into two criteria. Both criteria must be met to receive a diagnosis of SCS. Criterion A is entrapment/frantic hopelessness, or the urgent feeling of needing to escape a perceived inescapable life situation. Frantic hopelessness/entrapment has been found to be the strongest predictor of near-term suicidal behavior, as well as a mediator of the relationship between some of the other SCS components and near-term suicidal behavior (Li et al., 2017, 2018). Criterion B has four components, each enhancing the predictive validity of Criterion A: affective disturbance, loss of cognitive control, hyperarousal, and acute social withdrawal. Each of the four must be present for Criterion B to be met. Individuals meeting both Criterion A and Criterion B, as compared with those meeting partial criteria, are at higher risk for a near-term suicide attempt (Yaseen et al., 2019). It is important to note that although the diagnosis of SCS may identify those at risk for suicide, it is not intended to be a "diagnosis of risk." Rather, SCS describes the acute mental state that is associated with near-term suicidal behavior (for in-depth review and case examples, see Chapter 6).

Recent research assessing the predictive validity of SCS for imminent (within one month) suicidal behavior showed the syndrome to be prevalent in the general population as a specific response to some of the stressors of the COVID-19 pandemic (Park et al., 2021; Richards et al., 2021) SCS has also shown to be a more specific predictor for near-term suicide attempts than SI(. Moreover, a machine-learning analysis of the data from a large prospective study showed that adding SI to the SCS did not materially add to the SCC predictive validity (McMullen et al., 2021). Nevertheless, patients with both

SCS and SI are likely to be at higher risk for imminent suicidal behavior than patients with either SCS or SI alone. This finding supports the long-term goal of appropriate evidence-based integration of SI into the SCS. The recently proposed ASAD (Tucker et al., 2016) is a syndrome conceptually similar to the SCS, but it includes the crescendo of SI as its central component. One possible solution to the inclusion of SI in the SCS is to use both SI and ASAD as SCS modifiers, so that SCS can be diagnosed with and without SI/ASAD. The work on testing this framework is ongoing.

The Narrative-Crisis Model of Suicide

SCS is the centerpiece of the narrative-crisis model of suicide (NCM), developed by our research group (Bloch-Elkouby et al., 2020; Cohen et al., 2022). Multiple models of suicidal behaviors have been proposed in the past (and are reviewed in detail in Chapter 2). Why, then, is there a need to propose another model? Just as the conceptualization of the SCS and the research that defined its phenomenology was initiated because of the urgent need to fill a large gap in knowledge about the acute pre-suicidal mental state (or states), the formulation of, and research into, NCM was brought on by the urgent need to describe the mental processes leading to the emergence of the SCS in a way that would serve as a framework for comprehensive suicide prevention. Another reason for proposing and experimentally testing NCM is that empirical support for previously published models has been modest at best. Ultimately, NCM has the potential to be an evidence-based guide to suicide prevention for frontline clinicians.

SCS is an acute syndrome that is shorter in its duration than acute (state) anxiety (Galynker et al., 2017). It may last hours or days, and it lasts longer than the suicidal urge, which may appear within minutes before suicide, when it is too late to intervene. SCS is therefore treatable if detected in time. However, the subacute mental states that lead to SCS emergence in response to life stresses that may befall anyone—romantic rejections, financial setbacks, or world catastrophes, such as the COVID-19 pandemic—remain to be determined. What makes some of us vulnerable to experiencing these states, while others seem to be resilient and impervious to them? Finally, how can we integrate disparate risk and protective factors, reported to date, into one coherent framework for suicide prevention?

NCM is the organizing structure for this book. The model is described in detail in Chapter 3, while most of the subsequent chapters are devoted to its components, their use for the assessment of imminent risk, and how the model can function as a framework for suicide prevention. Some of NCM's distinguishing features, however, are noted here. NCM is empirically based and builds on the elements of other models that have had some experimental support. Specifically, NCM has a diathesis-stress framework, not unlike Beck's and Mann's stress-diathesis models (see Chapter 2). It also uses elements of Joiner's interpersonal theory of suicide (Joiner, 2009), such as thwarted belongingness and perceived burdensomeness, as well the concepts of psychache and emotional pain, as proposed by Shneidman (1993) and O'Connor (2011), respectively.

Several critical features distinguish NCM from other models. First, NCM does not include SI as a risk factor. As is shown in Chapter 9, self-reported SI is included in the suicide risk assessment but is not essential for the assessment of risk and for clinical decision-making. Second, the model distinguishes between chronic long-term factors or trait vulnerabilities, which are associated with lifetime suicide risk, and acute SCS, which give rise to imminent risk for suicide. Third, the model includes and relies on a new concept, the suicidal narrative (SN). SN is a subacute cognitive state that may emerge in response to stressful life events and that allows an emotional crescendo of several different but interrelated symptoms to develop and take the form of the suicidal crisis (Galynker et al., 2017). SN has been developed based on previous reports of the life narrative, whereby individuals integrate their experiences into a story of self (McLean et al., 2007). SN is one such story of self, wherein individuals begin to perceive themselves as having no future, and, consequently, begin to view suicide as both an imaginable and an acceptable alternative. It is at this point that SN develops into SCS (Cohen et al., 2018; Galynker et al., 2017).

Thus, NCM distinguishes among three components of the mental process that makes suicide possible. The chronic long-term risk component is associated with many genetic and environmental vulnerabilities, examples being perfectionism and childhood trauma, respectively. These are lifetime risk factors. The second component is the subacute SN, which emerges in those with lifetime risk when they experience life stressors. The duration of SN is weeks and days. Finally, the third component is the acute SCS, lasting days to hours, which may lead to imminent suicide.

Each component contributes differentially to the risk of suicide, and each of the components requires specific treatments to be differentiated accordingly. The most urgent treatments must target the most acute component, SCS, followed by those for restructuring SN, and finally those addressing the chronic risk. This differentiated and comprehensive suicide prevention approach, as well as the suggested treatment approaches, are described in Chapter 10.

One-Informant versus Multi-Informant Suicide Risk Assessments

Patients suffering acute psychosis or mania are often not able to provide a reliable account of their symptoms or the history of their illness. Consequently, obtaining collateral information from relatives or friends has become an essential component of any emergency department evaluation. Given that many suicidal patients do not disclose their suicidal intent to anyone, collateral information, particularly about SCS, a multi-informant assessment, can be as important for suicide prevention as for accurate diagnosis of serious psychiatric illnesses. Moreover, only recently have researchers realized that multi-informant psychiatric assessment also opens a completely new dimension of clinical evaluation. The opinions of other, independent informants not only may be less subjective than the patient's opinion, but also are subject to informative systematic biases of their own (Reyes et al., 2009).

For example, in a multi-informant study of depression and suicidality in adolescents (Lewis et al., 2014), parents' proxy reporting of adolescent depression and suicidal indices were only weakly correlated with their children's reports. Parents tended to overreport their adolescents depressive symptoms, while underreporting both their suicidal thoughts and behavior. In our own research work, suicidal inpatients gave dramatically different accounts of their SI and intent to the research assistants than they gave to their clinicians (Bloch-Elkouby et al., 2022). Moreover, the risk ratings obtained by the assistants were better predictors of postdischarge suicidal behavior than were clinician ratings.

Obtaining collateral information, however, does have its challenges, the most frequent one being obtaining the patient's consent to speak to other informants. The Health Insurance Portability and Accountability Act (HIPAA), although essential for protection of private information, requires separate consents for each informant. An acutely suicidal patient who on the surface has the capacity to make decisions may be unwilling or unable to sign the HIPAA form(s). Although the law may be bypassed if the clinician believes that the collateral information would be lifesaving, this subjective clinical judgment may open the clinician up to potential legal action. Legal considerations frequently present a barrier to a multi-informant patient assessment, even for assessing something as important as acute suicidal risk.

Unfortunately, even a multi-informant assessment does not guarantee accuracy in the diagnosis of SCS. Suicide risk assessment is difficult even for trained professionals, and laypeople often miss or misinterpret signs of impending suicide. Survivors of those who commit suicide often state that they had no idea that their loved one was acutely suicidal. Newspaper coverage of suicides by celebrities is full of statements like "I saw him the day before and he was laughing as usual." A close friend of model Ruslana Korshunova described their last meeting several hours before Korshunova leaped to her death off the roof of her apartment building in Manhattan as follows:

> We had dined in Manhattan, at our favorite bistro. We were planning for her to maybe come to Paris in a few days' time. Later that night, I took a plane to Paris for a shoot. She texted me when I landed—to see if I had arrived OK . . . and then a few hours later . . . a few hours later I saw on the news she was dead. (Pomerantsev, 2014, p. 144)

Yet, despite the seeming inability of significant others to decipher the suicidal state of mind, family involvement in psychiatric evaluation and treatment is critical both for suicide risk assessment and for suicide prevention. One reason is that the stigma of psychiatric illness starts inside the family. Andrew Salomon (2001) recounted how spouses, embarrassed or fearful of being labeled "mentally ill," hid their depression diagnoses and antidepressants (sometimes the same antidepressant) from each other. Helping patients and their significant others talk openly about their mental health issues makes the discussion of suicidality much more acceptable, and therefore more likely.

Another reason for family involvement in psychiatric assessment and treatment is that suicidal intent often pertains to interpersonal issues, such as unrequited love, being trapped in a painful marriage, or feeling railroaded into a hateful job or career by family obligations. Addressing those potential contributors to SN may start discussions of possible solutions that would bring suicide to the surface or find solutions to seemingly unsolvable life problems. Finally, by bringing the family into suicide risk discussion, it is often possible to create and maintain a connection between the suicidal patient, the significant other, and the clinician, a trusted and safe alliance that reduces the intensity of SCS and the seeming coherence of SN.

In short, in most cases, family members not only are additional informants who can either clarify or uncover suicide risk, but also are critically important suicide-prevention partners. Other possible informants may include clinicians, teachers, administrators, and community members. However, patient confidentiality and HIPAA make clinical use of information from these sources exceedingly difficult. The only automatic exception to HIPAA is clinicians who directly provide patient care and keep the medical records. The emotions these clinicians experience when working with suicidal patients are indicative of imminent risk.

Using Clinicians' Emotions in Suicide Prevention

Research shows that the accuracy of multi-informant assessments of suicide risk can be improved when the independent informants are the evaluating clinicians themselves. Indeed, the work of Reyes and colleagues suggests that in addition to involving suicidal patients' significant others, the multi-informant approach should include their clinicians (Reyes et al., 2013). This statement may sound paradoxical: Aren't we, the assessing clinicians, already obtaining another informant's professional opinion on the patient's suicide risk? This is true, but clinicians' professional reports, in accordance with professional training guidelines, omit their opinions about the patient being evaluated. Such personal opinions are often driven by a "gut feeling," which is quite different from the clinician's objective, fact-based report of suicide risk.

Discrepancies between clinicians' objective assessments and their subjective feelings are often seen in the inpatient setting, prior to discharge of patients admitted for danger to self. In the United States, criteria for psychiatric admission are centered not on severity of psychiatric illness per se, but on the patient's dangerousness to self or to community. Therefore, to be discharged, the patient needs only to be deemed "not dangerous to self and/ or others."

For clinicians to feel safe discharging a recently suicidal patient, the patient must deny suicidal intent and must be in control of his or her behavior. This means that, during hospitalization, there must not be suicide attempts or aggressive behavior toward others, and the patient must participate in the unit activities at a level commensurate with his or her illness severity. In most cases, such objective signs of patient improvement are listed in institutional discharge polices, and they make clinicians and hospital administrators feel secure about their discharge plan. However, even when the criteria are met, a clinician may often feel deep unease and anxiety. These complex discharge-related emotions are further complicated by clinicians' well-known negative emotional responses (NER) to suicidal patients (Michaud et al., 2021).

Whatever may be the mechanism of clinicians' NER to suicidal patients, the emotions need to be identified, because they may be reflective of the patient's risk for imminent suicide (Barzilay et al., 2019, 2020; Yaseen et al., 2017; Ying et al., 2021). However, once identified, NER also need to be managed because of their potential impact on the therapeutic alliance and clinical decision-making (Barzilay et al., 2019, 2022). The multifaceted role of the clinicians' emotional responses to suicidal patients is discussed in detail in Chapter 8. With regard to the risk assessment, clinicians' emotional reactions to suicidal patients are indicative of imminent suicide risk and need to be considered as independent and valuable data to be included in a decision-making algorithm. The framework for the inclusion of clinicians' emotional responses to suicidal patients in imminent risk assessment is reviewed in Chapter 9.

Risk Stratification versus Clinical Judgment

SI occurs in more than 10% of the population during their lifetime (Nock et al., 2013). Suicide decedents who do not disclose their suicidal plans to anyone frequently make contact with health services in the months leading up to their attempt. There is a widely recognized clinical need to identify those at risk, for targeted interventions, and to stop suicide before it happens. There is also a real legal liability on the part of both hospitals and clinicians should suicide occur either in the hospital or after discharge, given that patient suicide is the most frequent reason for lawsuits in psychiatry (Reid & Simpson, 2020). This concern with potential suicide-related lawsuits is one motivator for developing an administrative risk stratification system to adhere to as a means for improving the clarity and consistency in risk assessment and management.

In response to these challenges and to the urgent need to respond to the rise in suicide in the United States, the National Alliance for Suicide Prevention has issued a broad list of goals and objectives, the first of which is to "Integrate and coordinate suicide prevention activities across multiple sectors and settings" (https://theactionalliance.org). Others include "Provide training to community and clinical service providers on the prevention of suicide and related behaviors" and "Promote suicide prevention as a core component of healthcare services."

The coordination of suicide prevention activities has been brought about by state offices of mental health, which have created uniform risk assessment strategies to be used by local health systems. Typically, these Electronic Medical Record (EMR) drop-down lists have a gateway item inquiring about the presence of SI. If the answer is No, the rest of the items are skipped. If the answer is Yes, the list items need to be checked to determine a risk score, which is used in an algorithm for clinical decision-making. However, the algorithms are not evidence-based and their predictions are not clinically useful (Fountoulakis et al., 2012; Waern et al., 2010). Recent attempts to use ML analyses of EMR to predict near-term suicide identified the same long-term risk factors: history of mental illness, past suicide attempts, SI, and treatment with psychotropic medications (Simon et al., 2018, 2019, 2021).

The unfortunate consequence of administrative algorithms is that their use deprives clinicians of the opportunity to exercise their clinical judgment, which is overruled by risk stratification verdicts. A systematic review of risk stratification and risk scales in clinical practice concluded that the use of risk scales and excessive reliance on them to uncover risk factors for suicide may lead to erroneous results and is potentially dangerous (Chan et al., 2016). For that reason, the U.K. national suicide prevention strategy explicitly recommends against using risk assessment tools and algorithms for clinical decision-making   (https://www.nice.org.uk/donotdo/do-not-use-risk-assessment-tools-and-scales-to-determine-who-should-and-should-not-be-offered-treatment-or-who-should-be-discharged; Taylor et al., 2021). Accordingly, Oquendo and Bernanke (2017) noted that risk assessment and management are best conceptualized as a process—not a single event—that includes structured evaluation, intervention, and re-assessment.

Our premise is that a comprehensive diagnostic clinical interview informed by the SCS diagnosis and used within the framework of NCM should be the foundation for clinical decision-making in suicide prevention. In formulating treatment plans, clinicians must use all of the available information, the clinical history, and the multi-informant assessment method, which includes clinicians' rational judgment and their emotional responses to suicidal patients (Barzilay et al., 2019). Administrative risk stratification should be one only of many factors empowering clinicians' judgment, rather than overruling it. This book proposes a framework for exercising this judgment when making risk assessments and deciding on the best suicide prevention strategy, which can be taught to all clinicians in the course of their education and training (Foster et al., 2021).

How To Use *The Suicidal Crisis*

The Suicidal Crisis and NCM describe a structured and systematic assessment of risk for imminent suicide and propose a conceptual framework for comprehensive suicide prevention. The book is designed as a textbook and as a reference guide to be used in clinical settings.

In an academic setting, *The Suicidal Crisis* can be used as a comprehensive textbook for a dedicated course on the recognition, prevention, and treatment of imminent suicidal behavior. It can also be used as one of the textbooks in broader courses on psychopathology or in specialized seminars on emergency medicine and suicidology. Finally, the guide can be used as a reference book for mental health professional trainees: psychiatry residents, psychology interns, social workers, and others.

Outside the classroom, the guide can be (and the first edition has been) an educational reader for any clinician wanting to learn how to assess imminent risk for suicide. Whether on the acute psychiatric inpatient unit, on a medical/surgical floor, in an outpatient clinic, or in a private psychiatrist's office, the guide provides interested clinicians with a framework for inquiry into a suicidal state. *The Suicidal Crisis* contains more than 50 concise or extended case vignettes, illustrating specific aspects of risk-related clinical material, which may be useful when encountering a new or difficult clinical situation.

The book includes detailed risk assessment interviews, which readers can use as templates for real-life evaluations. Each aspect of the NCM is discussed in a separate chapter, under a descriptive heading and/or subheading, making finding an answer to a specific clinical question relatively easy. Specifically, the book contains detailed discussions of each long-term risk factor, of many stressful life events that increase imminent risk, of each component of the SN, and of each SCS symptom.

The examples of the assessment interviews for each NCM component are provided in Chapters 5, 6, and 7. High-, moderate-, and low-risk case discussions conclude with summary risk assessment tables. These are intended to help the reader organize the clinical information obtained in the course of each interview and to gauge the degree of suicide risk. It is important to remember that the risk tables are not meant as categorical risk stratification instruments. Their purpose is educational, and they are meant to provide illustrations and real-life examples of divergent risk cases. To underscore this point, the complete assessment interviews in Chapter 9 do not include risk tables, encouraging readers to use their clinical judgment, as they would in real life.

Chapters 6 and 7 also include "test" interviews and the summary risk assessment table shells to be used for self-assessment; the answer keys are listed at the end of the guide. After reading each chapter and doing the test cases, the reader should have sufficient mastery of the material and a gestalt memory of representative cases to make confident clinical judgments in real life. In addition to the test cases, the reader can use the individual case vignettes to practice risk assessment and to examine his or her own emotional reaction to particular types of suicidal patients.

It cannot be emphasized enough that this book is a guide to clinical decision-making and not a risk stratification tool that absolves a clinician from using their clinical judgment. The book does not include a questionnaire to be scored and used to determine an objective level of suicide risk that should automatically trigger a particular action by a clinician (i.e., hospitalization), depriving the clinician of their use of clinical judgment. Several versions of the Suicide Crisis Inventory are currently being tested in clinical trials, and it is hoped that it will aid clinicians in their decision-making in the future.

A Roadmap for Comprehensive Assessment

Suicide is a very complex behavior that results from a dynamic interplay of long-term risk factors (personal, societal, and cultural), stressful life events, the propensity to view one's life as a SN, added to the acuity of the SCS. Studying this guide, understanding the NCM, and doing the test cases should give clinicians the framework for conducting imminent suicide risk assessments with confidence. Following the risk assessment outlines (Chapter 9) ensures that all relevant information that could be obtained during a clinical interview was indeed obtained and analyzed appropriately. Regardless of the clinician's risk assessment skills, some suicidal patients will not cooperate with an interview, leaving the clinician perplexed. Finding similarities between the vignettes and real-life cases and using NCM as the organizing framework could help connect the dots when assessing a patient's SN or SCS and clarify the case.

The use of the NCM as a practical framework for comprehensive suicide prevention treatment approaches is described in Chapter 10 (Block-Elkouby et al., 2020;Cohen et al., 2022). Because our published work to date has been focused on new methods of imminent risk assessment, rather than new suicide prevention treatments, *The Suicidal Crisis* does not yet include novel evidence-based treatment recommendations. The most recent work at the NorthShore University Health System suggests that implementation of SCS assessment alone may improve suicidal outcomes, as well as clinicians' confidence and competence when working with suicidal patients (Karsen et al., under review). This is an encouraging development, but more implementation studies are needed.

The existing interventions, designed and evaluated by other research teams, are reviewed in Chapter 10. Several excellent books are currently available that give detailed instructions on how to care for and treat a person experiencing an acute suicidal crisis, using some of these treatment modalities (Bryan & Rudd, 2018; Michel & Gysin-Maillart, 2015; Jobes & Linehan, 2016; Kapur & Goldney, 2016; Wenzel et al., 2008). Chapter 10 describes differential, targeted, and timely use of these treatments.

Treatment of acutely suicidal individuals is useful only insofar as clinicians are able to identify those who are at imminent suicide risk. Currently, with very recent and welcome exceptions (King et al., 2021), imminent risk determination is primarily based on the answer to the question, "Are you planning to kill yourself?" As discussed previously and in Chapter 7, the answer to this question is often either inaccurate or intentionally misleading. *The Suicidal Crisis* is intended to help clinicians identify persons who are at imminent suicide risk with accuracy and confidence in their own assessment skills.

References

American Psychiatric Association. (2013). *Diagnostic and statistical manual of mental disorders* (5th ed.). American Psychiatric Publishing.

Appleby, L., Shaw, J., Amos, T., McDonnell, R., Harris, C., McCann, K., Kiernan, K., Davies, S., Bickley, H., & Parsons, R. (1999). Suicide within 12 months of contact with mental health services: National clinical survey. *BMJ, 318*(7193), 1235–1239. https://doi.org/10.1136/bmj.318.7193.1235

Bachmann, S. (2018). Epidemiology of suicide and the psychiatric perspective. *International Journal of Environmental Research and Public Health, 15*(7), 1425. https://doi.org/10.3390/ijerph15071425

Bagge, C. L., & Borges, G. (2017). Acute substance use as a warning sign for suicide attempts: A case-crossover examination of the 48 hours prior to a recent suicide attempt. *The Journal of Clinical Psychiatry, 78*(6), 691–696. https://doi.org/10.4088/JCP.15m10541

Bagge, C. L., Littlefield, A. K., Conner, K. R., Schumacher, J. A., & Lee, H. J. (2014). Near-term predictors of the intensity of suicidal ideation: An examination of the 24h prior to a recent suicide attempt. *Journal of Affective Disorders, 165*, 53–58. https://doi.org/10.1016/j.jad.2014.04.010

Barzilay, S., Gagon, A., Yaseen, Z. S., Chennapragada, L., Lloveras, L., Bloch-Elkouby, S., & Galynker, I. (2022). Associations between clinicians' emotional regulation, treatment recommendations, and patient suicidal ideation. *Suicide and Life-Threatening Behavior, 52*(2), 329–340. https://doi.org/10.1111/sltb.12824

Barzilay, S., Schuck, A., Bloch-Elkouby, S., Yaseen, Z. S., Hawes, M., Rosenfield, P., Foster, A., & Galynker, I. (2020). Associations between clinicians' emotional responses, therapeutic alliance, and patient suicidal ideation. *Depression and Anxiety, 37*(3), 214–223. https://doi.org/10.1002/da.22973

Barzilay, S., Yaseen, Z. S., Hawes, M., Kopeykina, I., Ardalan, F., Rosenfield, P., Murrough, J., & Galynker, I. (2019). Determinants and predictive value of clinician assessment of short-term suicide risk. *Suicide and Life-Threatening Behavior, 49*(2), 614–626. https://doi.org/10.1111/sltb.1246

Beck, A. T., Brown, G., & Steer, R. A. (1989). Prediction of eventual suicide in psychiatric inpatients by clinical ratings of hopelessness. *Journal of Consulting and Clinical Psychology, 57*(2), 309–310. https://doi.org/10.1037/0022-006x.57.2.309

Beck, A. T., Steer, R. A., Kovacs, M., & Garrison, B. (1985). Hopelessness and eventual suicide: A 10-year prospective study of patients hospitalized with suicidal ideation. *American Journal of Psychiatry, 142*(5), 559–563. https://doi.org/10.1176/ajp.142.5.559

Berman, A. L. (2018). Risk factors proximate to suicide and suicide risk assessment in the context of denied suicide ideation. *Suicide and Life-Threatening Behavior, 48*(3), 340–352. https://doi.org/10.1111/sltb.12351

Black, J., Bond, M. A., Hawkins, R., & Black, E. (2019). Test of a clinical model of poor physical health and suicide: The role of depression, psychosocial stress, interpersonal conflict, and panic. *Journal of Affective Disorders, 257*, 404–411. https://doi.org/10.1016/j.jad.2019.05.079

Blanchard, M., & Farber, B. A. (2020). "It is never okay to talk about suicide": Patients' reasons for concealing suicidal ideation in psychotherapy. *Psychotherapy Research, 30*(1), 124–136. https://doi.org/10.1080/10503307.2018.1543977

Bloch-Elkouby, S., Gorman, B., Lloveras, L., Wilkerson, T., Schuck, A., Barzilay, S., Calati, R., Schnur, D., & Galynker, I. (2020). How do distal and proximal risk factors combine to predict suicidal ideation and behaviors? A prospective study of the narrative crisis model of suicide. *Journal of Affective Disorders, 277*, 914–926.

Bloch-Elkouby, S., Gorman, B., Schuck, A., Barzilay, S., Calati, R., Cohen, L. J., Begum, F., & Galynker, I. (2020). The Suicide Crisis Syndrome: A network analysis. *Journal of Counseling Psychology, 67*(5), 595–607. https://doi.org/10.1037/cou0000423

Bloch-Elkouby, S., Zilcha-Maro, S., Rogers, M. L., Park, J-Y., Krumerman, M., Manlogat, K., & Galynker, I. (2022). Who are the patients who deny suicidal intent? Exploring patients' characteristics associated with self-disclosure and denial of suicidal intent. *Acta Psychiatrica Scandinavica,* 10.1111/acps.13511. Advance online publication. https://doi.org/10.1111/acps.13511

Bolton, J. M., Spiwak, R., & Sareen, J. (2012). Predicting suicide attempts with the SAD PERSONS scale. *The Journal of Clinical Psychiatry, 73*(06), e735–e741. https://doi.org/10.4088/jcp.11m07362

Borges, G., Angst, J., Nock, M. K., Ruscio, A. M., & Kessler, R. C. (2008). Risk factors for the incidence and persistence of suicide-related outcomes: A 10-year follow-up study using the National Comorbidity Surveys. *Journal of Affective Disorders, 105*(1-3), 25–33. https://doi.org/10.1016/j.jad.2007.01.036

Bostwick, J. M., Pabbati, C., Geske, J. R., & McKean, A. J. (2016). Suicide attempt as a risk factor for completed suicide: Even more lethal than we knew. *American Journal of Psychiatry, 173*(11), 1094–1100. https://doi.org/10.1176/appi.ajp.2016.15070854

Brådvik, L. (2018). Suicide risk and mental disorders. *International Journal of Environmental Research and Public Health, 15*(9), 2028. https://doi.org/10.3390/ijerph15092028

Bryan, C. J., & Rudd, D. R. (2018) *Brief cognitive-behavioral therapy for suicide prevention.* Guildford Press.

Busch, K. A., Fawcett, J., & Jacobs, D. G. (2003). Clinical correlates of inpatient suicide. *Journal of Clinical Psychiatry, 64*(1), 14–19. http://dx.doi.org/10.4088/JCP.v64n0105

Calati, R., Cohen, L. J., Schuck, A., Levy, D., Bloch-Elkouby, S., Barzilay, S., Rosenfield, P. J., & Galynker, I. (2020). The Modular Assessment of Risk for Imminent Suicide (MARIS): A validation study of a novel tool for suicide risk assessment. *Journal of Affective Disorders, 263*, 121–128. https://doi.org/10.1016/j.jad.2019.12.001

Centers for Disease Control and Prevention. (2020, February 20). *Web-based Injury Statistics Query and Reporting System (WISQARS) fatal injury reports.* https://webappa.cdc.gov/sasweb/ncipc/mortrate.html

Cha, C. B., Najmi, S., Park, J. M., Finn, C. T., & Nock, M. K. (2010). Attentional bias toward suicide-related stimuli predicts suicidal behavior. *Journal of Abnormal Psychology, 119*(3), 616–622. https://doi.org/10.1037/a0019710

Chan, M. K. Y., Bhatti, H., Meader, N., Stockton, S., Evans, J., O'Connor, R. C., Kapur, N., & Kendall, T. (2016). Predicting suicide following self-harm: Systematic review of risk factors and risk scales. *British Journal of Psychiatry, 209*(4), 277–283. https://doi.org/10.1192/bjp.bp.115.170050

Chu, C., Klein, K. M., Buchman-Schmitt, J. M., Hom, M. A., Hagan, C. R., & Joiner, T. E. (2015). Routinized assessment of suicide risk in clinical practice: An empirically informed update. *Journal of Clinical Psychology, 71*(12), 1186–1200. https://doi.org/10.1002/jclp.22210

Claassen, C. A., Harvilchuck-Laurenson, J. D., & Fawcett, J. (2014). Prognostic models to detect and monitor the near-term risk of suicide. *American Journal of Preventive Medicine*, *47*(3 Suppl 2), S181–S185. https://doi.org/10.1016/j.amepre.2014.06.003

Cohen, L. J., Ardalan, F., Yaseen, Z., & Galynker, I. (2018). Suicide crisis syndrome mediates the relationship between long-term risk factors and lifetime suicidal phenomena. *Suicide and Life-Threatening Behavior*, *48*, 613–623. https://doi.org/10.1111/sltb.12387

Cohen, L. J., Mokhtar, R., Richards, J., Hernandez, M., Bloch-Elkouby, S., & Galynker, I. (2022). The narrative-crisis model of suicide and its prediction of near-term suicide risk. *Suicide and Life-Threatening Behavior, 52*(2), 231–243. https://doi.org/10.1111/sltb.12816

Curtin, S. C., Hedegaard, H., & Ahmad, F. B. (2021). *Provisional numbers and rates of suicide by month and demographic characteristics: United States, 2020*. National Center for Health Statistics (U.S.) NCHS. Vital Statistics Rapid Release; no 24 https://www.cdc.gov/nchs/data/vsrr/VSRR016.pdf

Czeisler, M. É., Lane, R. I., Petrosky, E., Wiley, J. F., Christensen, A., Njai, R., Weaver, M. D., Robbins, R., Facer-Childs, E. R., Barger, L. K., Czeisler, C. A., Howard, M. E., & Rajaratnam, S. M. W. (2020). Mental Health, Substance Use, and Suicidal Ideation During the COVID-19 Pandemic—United States, June 24–30, 2020. *MMWR. Morbidity and Mortality Weekly Report, 69*(32), 1049–1057. https://doi.org/10.15585/mmwr.mm6932a1

Deisenhammer, E. A., Ing, C. M., Strauss, R., Kemmler, G., Hinterhuber, H., & Weiss, E. M. (2009). The duration of the suicidal process: How much time is left for intervention between consideration and accomplishment of a suicide attempt? *Journal of Clinical Psychiatry, 70*, 19–24. https://doi.org/10.4088/jcp.07m03904

Fawcett, J., Scheftner, W. A., Clark, D. C., Hedeker, D., Gibbons, R., & Coryell, W. (1987). Clinical predictors of suicide in patients with major affective disorders: A controlled prospective study. *American Journal of Psychiatry, 144*(1), 35–40. https://doi.org/10.1176/ajp.144.1.35

Foster, A., Alderman, M., Safin, D., Aponte, X., McCoy, K., Caughey, M., & Galynker, I. (2021). Teaching suicide risk assessment: Spotlight on the therapeutic relationship. *Academic Psychiatry, 45*(3), 257–261. https://doi.org/10.1007/s40596-021-01421-2

Fountoulakis, K. N., Pantoula, E., Siamouli, M., Moutou, K., Gonda, X., Rihmer, Z., Iacovides, A., & Akiskal, H. (2012). Development of the Risk Assessment Suicidality Scale (RASS): A population-based study. *Journal of Affective Disorders, 138*(3), 449–457. https://doi.org/10.1016/j.jad.2011.12.045

Franklin, J. C., Ribeiro, J. D., Fox, K. R., Bentley, K. H., Kleiman, E. M., Huang, X., Musacchio, K. M., Jaroszewski, A. C., Chang, B. P., & Nock, M. K. (2017). Risk factors for suicidal thoughts and behaviors: A meta-analysis of 50 years of research. *Psychological Bulletin, 143*(2), 187–232. https://doi.org/10.1037/bul000008

Galynker, I., Yaseen, Z., & Briggs, J. (2014). Assessing risk for imminent suicide. *Psychiatric Annals, 44*(9), 431–436. https://doi.org/10.3928/00485713-20140908-07

Galynker, I., Yaseen, Z. S., Cohen, A., Benhamou, O., Hawes, M., & Briggs, J. (2017). Prediction of suicidal behavior in high risk psychiatric patients using an assessment of acute suicidal state: The Suicide Crisis Inventory. *Depression and Anxiety, 34*(2), 147–158. https://doi.org/10.1002/da.22559

Goldblatt, M. J., Ronningstam, E., Schechter, M., Herbstman, B., & Maltsberger, J. T. (2016). Suicide as escape from psychotic panic. *Bulletin of the Menninger Clinic, 80*(2), 131–145. https://doi.org/10.1521/bumc.2016.80.2.131

Gratch, I., Choo, T. H., Galfalvy, H., Keilp, J. G., Itzhaky, L., Mann, J. J., Oquendo, M. A., & Stanley, B. (2020). Detecting suicidal thoughts: The power of ecological momentary assessment. *Depression and Anxiety, 38*(1), 8–16. https://doi.org/10.1002/da.23043

Guintivano, J., Brown, T., & Newcomer, A. (2014). Identification and replication of a combined epigenetic and genetic biomarker predicting suicide and suicidal behaviors. *American Journal of Psychiatry, 171*(12), 1287–1296. https://doi.org/10.1176/appi.ajp.2014.14010008

Hajar, R. (2016). Framingham contribution to cardiovascular disease. *Heart Views, 17*(2), 78. https://doi.org/10.4103/1995-705x.185130

Harris, K. M., McLean, J. P., Sheffield, J., & Jobes, D. (2010). The internal suicide debate hypothesis: Exploring the life versus death struggle. *Suicide and Life-Threatening Behavior, 40*(2), 181–192. https://doi.org/10.1521/suli.2010.40.2.181

Harriss, L., & Hawton, K. (2005). Suicidal intent in deliberate self-harm and the risk of suicide: The predictive power of the Suicide Intent Scale. *Journal of Affective Disorders, 86*(2-3), 225–233. https://doi.org/10.1016/j.jad.2005.02.009

Heron, M. (2021). Deaths: Leading causes for 2019. *National Vital Statistics Reports, 70*(9), 1–17. https://www.cdc.gov/nchs/data/nvsr/nvsr70/nvsr70-09-508.pdf

Horesh, N., & Apter, A. (2006). Self-disclosure, depression, anxiety, and suicidal behavior in adolescent psychiatric inpatients. *Crisis, 27*(2), 66–71. https://doi.org/10.1027/0227-5910.27.2.66

Horesh, N., Zalsman, G., & Apter, A. (2004). Suicidal behavior and self-disclosure in adolescent psychiatric inpatients. *Journal of Nervous and Mental Disease, 192*(12), 837–842. https://doi.org/10.1097/01.nmd.0000146738.78222.e5

Horwitz, A. G., Czyz, E. K., & King, C. A. (2015). Predicting future suicide attempts among adolescent and emerging adult psychiatric emergency patients. *Journal of Clinical Child and Adolescent Psychology, 44*(5), 751–761. https://doi.org/10.1080/15374416.2014.910789

Jobes, D. A., & Liinehan, M. M. (2016). *Managing suicidal risk, Second edition: A collaborative approach.* Guildford Press.

Joiner, T. E., Jr., Van Orden, K. A., Witte, T. K., Selby, E. A., Ribeiro, J. D., Lewis, R., & Rudd, M. D. (2009). Main predictions of the interpersonal–psychological theory of suicidal behavior: Empirical tests in two samples of young adults. *Journal of Abnormal Psychology, 118*(3), 634–646. https://doi.org/10.1037/a0016500

Kapur, N., & Goldney, R. D. (2016). *Suicide prevention* (3rd ed.). Oxford University Press.

Karsen, E., Miller, F., & White, B. (under review). Implementation of abbreviated Suicide Crisis Syndrome Checklist reduces suicidal outcomes.

Katz, C., Yaseen, Z. S., Mojtabai, R., Cohen, L. J., & Galynker, I. I. (2011). Panic as an independent risk factor for suicide attempt in depressive illness: findings from the National Epidemiological Survey on Alcohol and Related Conditions (NESARC). *The Journal of Clinical Psychiatry, 72*(12), 1628–1635. https://doi.org/10.4088/JCP.10m06186blu

Kessler, R. C., Borges, G., & Walters, E. E. (1999). Prevalence of and risk factors for lifetime suicide attempts in the National Comorbidity Survey. *Archives of General Psychiatry, 56*(7), 617–626.

King, C. A., Brent, D., Grupp-Phelan, J., Casper, T. C., Dean, J. M., Chernick, L. S., Fein, J. A., Mahabee-Gittens, E. M., Patel, S. J., Mistry, R. D., Duffy, S., Melzer-Lange,

M., Rogers, A., Cohen, D. M., Keller, A., Shenoi, R., Hickey, R. W., Rea, M., Cwik, M., . . . Pediatric Emergency Care Applied Research Network. (2021). Prospective development and validation of the computerized adaptive screen for suicidal youth. *JAMA Psychiatry, 78*(5), 540–549. https://doi.org/10.1001/jamapsychiatry.2020.4576

Kleiman, E. M., Turner, B. J., Fedor, S., Beale, E. E., Huffman, J. C., & Nock, M. K. (2017). Examination of real-time fluctuations in suicidal ideation and its risk factors: Results from two ecological momentary assessment studies. *Journal of Abnormal Psychology, 126*(6), 726–738. https://doi.org/10.1037/abn0000273

Large, M., Sharma, S., Cannon, E., Ryan, C., & Nielssen, O. (2011). Risk factors for suicide within a year of discharge from psychiatric hospital: A systematic meta-analysis. *Australian and New Zealand Journal of Psychiatry, 45*(8), 619–628. https://doi.org/10.3109/00048674.2011.590465

Lewis, A. J., Bertino, M. D., Bailey, C. M., Skewes, J., Lubman, D. I., & Toumbourou, J. W. (2014). Depression and suicidal behavior in adolescents: A multi-informant and multi-methods approach to diagnostic classification. *Frontiers in Psychology, 5*, 766. https://doi.org/10.3389/fpsyg.2014.00766

Li, S., Galynker, I., Briggs, J., Duffy, M., Frechette-Hagan, A., Kim, H. J., Cohen, L., & Yaseen, Z. S. (2017). Attachment style and suicide behaviors in high risk psychiatric inpatients following hospital discharge: The mediating role of entrapment. *Psychiatry Research, 257*, 309–314. https://doi.org/10.1016/j.psychres.2017.07.072

Li, S., Yaseen, Z. S., Kim, H. J., Briggs, J., Duffy, M., Frechette-Hagan, A., Cohen, L. J., & Galynker, I. (2018). Entrapment as a mediator of suicide crises. *BMC Psychiatry, 18*(4), 4. https://doi.org/10.1186/s12888-018-1587-0

Lim, S. W., Ko, E. M., Shin, D. W., Shin, Y. C., & Oh, K. S. (2015). Clinical symptoms associated with suicidality in patients with panic disorder. *Psychopathology, 48*(3), 137-44. https://doi.org/10.1159/000368904

Loas, G. (2007). Anhedonia and suicide: A 6.5-yr. follow-up study of patients hospitalized for a suicide attempt. *Psychological Reports, 100*(1), 183–190. https://doi.org/10.2466/pr0.100.1.183-190

McClatchey, K., Murray, J., Chouliara, Z., Rowat, A., & Hauge, S. R. (2019). Suicide risk assessment in the emergency department: An investigation of current practice in Scotland. *International Journal of Clinical Practice, 73*(4), e13342. https://doi.org/10.1111/ijcp.13342

McLean, K. C., Pasupathi, M., & Pals, J. L. (2007). Selves creating stories creating selves: A process model of self development. *Personality and Social Psychological Review, 11*, 262–278. https://doi.org/10.1177/1088868307301034

McMullen, L., Parghi, N., Rogers, M. L., Yao, H., Bloch-Elkouby, S., & Galynker, I. (2021). The role of suicide ideation in assessing near-term suicide risk: A machine learning approach. *Psychiatry Research, 304*, 114118. https://doi.org/10.1016/j.psychres.2021.114118

Michaud, L., Greenway, K.T., Corbeil, S. Bourquin, C., & Richard-Devantoy, S. (2021). Countertransference towards suicidal patients: A systematic review. *Current Psychology.* https://doi.org/10.1007/s12144-021-01424-0

Michel, K., & Gysin-Maillart, A. (2015). *ASSIP—Attempted Suicide Short Intervention Program: A manual for clinicians.* Hogrefe Publishing.

Nam, Y. Y., Kim, C. H., & Roh, D. (2016). Comorbid panic disorder as an independent risk factor for suicide attempts in depressed outpatients. *Comprehensive Psychiatry, 67*, 13–18. https://doi.org/10.1016/j.comppsych.2016.02.011

National Action Alliance for Suicide Prevention (n.d.) *Our strategy*. https://theactionallia nce.org/our-strategy

National Suicide Prevention Lifeline. (2007.) *Recommendations for an approach to asking lifeline callers about suicidality*. https://suicidepreventionlifeline.org/wp-content/uplo ads/2016/08/Suicide-Risk-Assessment-Standards-1.pdf

Nock, M. K., Borges, G., Bromet, E. J., Alonso, J., Angermeyer, M., Beautrais, A., Bruffaerts, R., Chiu, W. T., de Girolamo, G., Gluzman, S., de Graaf, R., Gureje, O., Haro, J. M., Huang, Y., Karam, E., Kessler, R. C., Lepine, J. P., Levinson, D., Medina-Mora, M. E., . . . Williams, D. (2008). Cross-national prevalence and risk factors for suicidal ide-ation, plans and attempts. *The British Journal of Psychiatry*, *192*(2), 98–105. https://doi. org/10.1192/bjp.bp.107.040113

Nock, M. K., Green, J. G., Hwang, I., McLaughlin, K. A., Sampson, N. A., Zaslavsky, A. M., & Kessler, R. C. (2013). Prevalence, correlates, and treatment of lifetime suicidal beha-vior among adolescents: Results from the National Comorbidity Survey Replication Adolescent Supplement. *JAMA Psychiatry*, *70*(3), 300–310. https://doi.org/10.1001/ 2013.jamapsychiatry.55

Nock, M. K., Park, J. M., Finn, C. T., Deliberto, T. L., Dour, H. J., & Banaji, M. R. (2010). Measuring the suicidal mind: Implicit cognition predicts suicidal behavior. *Psychological Science*, *21*(4), 511–517. https://doi.org/10.1177/0956797610364762

O'Connor, R. C. (2011). The integrated motivational–volitional model of suicidal beha-vior. *Crisis*, *32*(6), 295–298. https://doi.org/10.1027/0227-5910/a000120

Oquendo, M. A., Barrera, A., Ellis, S. P., Li, S., Burke, A. K., Grunebaum, M., Endicott, J., & Mann, J. J. (2004). Instability of symptoms in recurrent major depression: a pro-spective study. *The American Journal of Psychiatry*, *161*(2), 255–261. https://doi.org/ 10.1176/appi.ajp.161.2.255

Oquendo, M. A., & Bernanke, J. A. (2017).Suicide risk assessment: Tools and challenges. *World Psychiatry*, *16*(1), 28–29. https://doi.org/10.1002/wps.20396

Otte, S., Lutz, M., Streb, J., Cohen, L. J., Galynker, I., Dudeck, M., & Büsselmann, M. (2020). Analyzing suicidality in German forensic patients by means of the German version of the Suicide Crisis Inventory (SCI-G). *The Journal of Forensic Psychiatry & Psychology*, *31*(5), 731–746. https://doi.org/10.1080/14789949.2020.1787487

Park, J. Y., Richards, J., You, S., & Galynker, I. (2021). *Age and gender differences in utilizing suicide prevention resources during COVID-19* [Poster presentation]. APA 2021 Annual Meeting, Los Angeles, CA.

Paykel, E. S., Myers, J. K., Lindenthal, J. J., & Tanner, J. (1974). Suicidal feelings in the ge-neral population: A prevalence study. *British Journal of Psychiatry*, *124*(5), 460–469. https://doi.org/10.1192/bjp.124.5.460

Peterson, C., Sussell, A., Li, J., Schumacher, P. K., Yeoman, K., & Stone, D. M. (2020). Suicide rates by industry and occupation—National Violent Death Reporting System, 32 states, 2016. *Morbidity and Mortality Weekly Report*, *69*(3), 57–62. http://dx.doi.org/ 10.15585/mmwr.mm6903a1

Pilowsky, D. J., Wu, L. T., & Anthony, J. C. (1999). Panic attacks and suicide attempts in mid adolescence. *American Journal of Psychiatry*, *156*(10), 1545–1549. https://doi.org/ 10.1176/ajp.156.10.1545

Pomerantsev, P. (2014). *Nothing is true and everything is possible: The surreal heart of the new Russia*. Public Affairs.

Posner, K., Brown, G. K., Stanley, B., Brent, D. A., Yerishova, K. V., & Oquendo, M. A. (2011). The Columbia-Suicide Severity Rating Scale: Initial validity and internal consistency from three multisite studies with adolescents and adults. *American Journal of Psychiatry, 168*(12), 1266–1277.

Probert-Lindström, S., Berge, J., Westrin, Å., Öjehagen, A., & Skogman Pavulans, K. (2020). Long-term risk factors for suicide in suicide attempters examined at a medical emergency in patient unit: Results from a 32-year follow-up study. *BMJ Open, 10*(10), e038794. https://doi.org/10.1136/bmjopen-2020-038794

Quinlivan, L., Cooper, J., Meehan, D., Longson, D., Potokar, J., Hulme, T., Marsden, J., Brand, F., Lange, K., Riseborough, E., Page, L., Metcalfe, C., Davies, L., O'Connor, R., Hawton, K., Gunnell, D., & Kapur, N. (2017). Predictive accuracy of risk scales following self-harm: Multicentre, prospective cohort study. *The British Journal of Psychiatry, 210*(6), 429–436. https://doi.org/10.1192/bjp.bp.116.189993

Quinlivan, L., Steeg, S., Elvidge, J., Nowland, R., Davies, L., Hawton, K., Gunnell, D., & Kapur, N. (2019). Risk assessment scales to predict risk of hospital treated repeat self-harm: A cost-effectiveness modelling analysis. *Journal of Affective Disorders, 249*, 208–215. https://doi.org/10.1016/j.jad.2019.02.036

Rappaport, L. M., Moskowitz, D. S., Galynker, I., & Yaseen, Z. S. (2014). Panic symptom clusters differentially predict suicide ideation and attempt. *Comprehensive Psychiatry, 55*(4), 762–769.

Reid, W. H., & Simpson, S. (2020). The right way to avoid malpractice lawsuits. *Psychiatric Times, 37*(9), 16–25. https://www.psychiatrictimes.com/view/false-allegations-of-abuse-can-be-a-strategy-in-child-custody-litigation

Reyes, A. D., Henry, D. B., Tolan, P. H., & Wakschlag, L. S. (2009). Linking informant discrepancies to observed variations in young children's disruptive behavior. *Journal of Abnormal Child Psychology, 37*(5), 637–652. https://doi.org/10.1007/s10 802-009-9307-3

Reyes, A. D., Thomas, S. A., Goodman, K. L., & Kundey, S. M. (2013). Principles underlying the use of multiple informants' reports. *Annual Review of Clinical Psychology, 9*(1), 123–149. https://doi.org/10.1146/annurev-clinpsy-050212-185617

Ribeiro, J. D., Franklin, J. C., Fox, K. R., Bentley, K. H., Kleiman, E. M., Chang, B. P., & Nock, M. K. (2016). Self-injurious thoughts and behaviors as risk factors for future suicide ideation, attempts, and death: A meta-analysis of longitudinal studies. *Psychological Medicine, 46*, 225–236. https://doi.org/10.1017/S0033291715001804

Richards, J., Park, J. Y., Rogers, M., & Galynker, I. (2021). *Seeking resources in a pandemic: Rates of those utilizing mental health and suicide prevention resources during COVID-19* [Conference presentation]. APA 2021 Annual Meeting, Los Angeles, CA.

Rogers, M. L., Bloch-Elkouby, S., & Galynker, I. (2022). Differential disclosure of suicidal intent to clinicians versus researchers: Associations with concurrent suicide crisis syndrome and prospective suicidal ideation and attempts. *Psychiatry Research, 312*, 114522. https://doi.org/10.1016/j.psychres.2022.114522

Rogers, M. L., Hom, M. A., Stanley, I. H., & Joiner, T. E. (2019). Brief measures of physical and psychological distance to suicide methods as correlates and predictors of suicide risk: A multi-study prospective investigation. *Behaviour and Research Therapies, 120*, 103330. https://doi.org/10.1016/j.brat.2018.11.001

Runeson, B., Odeberg, J., Pettersson, A., Edbom, T., Jildevik Adamsson, I., & Waern, M. (2017). Instruments for the assessment of suicide risk: A systematic review evaluating the certainty of the evidence. *PLOS One, 12*(7), e0180292. https://doi.org/10.1371/jour nal.pone.0180292

Scheer, V., Blanco, C., Olfson, M., Lemogne, C., Airagnes, G., Peyre, H., Limosin, F., & Hoertel, N. (2020). A comprehensive model of predictors of suicide attempt in individuals with panic disorder: Results from a national 3-year prospective study. *General Hospital Psychiatry, 67,* 127–135. https://doi.org/10.1016/j.genhosppsych.2020.09.006

Schuck, A., Calati, R., Barzilay, S., Bloch-Elkouby, S., & Galynker, I. (2019). Suicide crisis syndrome: A review of supporting evidence for a new suicide-specific diagnosis. *Behavioral Sciences and the Law, 37,* 223–239.

Shneidman, E. S. (1993). Suicide as psychache. *The Journal of Nervous and Mental Disease, 181*(3), 145–147. https://doi.org/10.1097/00005053-199303000-00001

Simon, G. E., Johnson, E., Lawrence, J. M., Rossom, R. C., Ahmedani, B., Lynch, F. L., Beck, A., Waitzfelder, B., Ziebell, R., Penfold, R. B., & Shortreed, S. M. (2018). Predicting suicide attempts and suicide deaths following outpatient visits using electronic health records. *The American Journal of Psychiatry, 175*(10), 951–960. https://doi.org/10.1176/appi.ajp.2018.17101167

Simon, G. E., Matarazzo, B. B., Walsh, C. G., Smoller, J. W., Boudreaux, E. D., Yarborough, B. J. H., Shortreed, S. M., Coley, R. Y., Ahmedani, B. K., Doshi, R. P., Harris, L. I., & Schoenbaum, M. (2021). Reconciling statistical and clinicians' predictions of suicide risk. *Psychiatric Services, 72*(5), 555–562. https://doi.org/10.1176/appi.ps.202000214

Simon, G. E., Yarborough, B. J., Rossom, R. C., Lawrence, J. M., Lynch, F. L., Waitzfelder, B. E., Ahmedani, B. K., & Shortreed, S. M. (2019). Self-reported suicidal ideation as a predictor of suicidal behavior among outpatients with diagnoses of psychotic disorders. *Psychiatric Services, 70*(3), 176–183. https://doi.org/10.1176/appi.ps.201800381

Smith, E. G., Kim, H. M., Ganoczy, D., Stano, C., Pfeiffer, P. N., & Valenstein, M. (2013). Suicide risk assessment received prior to suicide death by Veterans Health Administration patients with a history of depression. *The Journal of Clinical Psychiatry, 74*(3), 226–232. https://doi.org/10.4088/JCP.12m07853

Solomon, A. (2001). *The noonday demon: An atlas of depression.* Scribner.

Steeg, S., Quinlivan, L., Nowland, R., Carroll, R., Casey, D., Clements, C., Cooper, J., Davies, L., Knipe, D., Ness, J., O'Connor, R. C., Hawton, K., Gunnell, D., & Kapur, N. (2018). Accuracy of risk scales for predicting repeat self-harm and suicide: A multicentre, population-level cohort study using routine clinical data. *BMC Psychiatry, 18*(1), 113. https://doi.org/10.1186/s12888-018-1693-z

Stene-Larsen, K., & Reneflot, A. (2019). Contact with primary and mental health care prior to suicide: A systematic review of the literature from 2000 to 2017. *Scandinavian Journal of Public Health, 47*(1), 9–17. https://doi.org/10.1177/1403494817746274

Stone, D. M., Simon, T. R., Fowler, K.A., Kegler, S. R., Holland, K. M., Ivey-Stephenson, A. Z., & Crosby, A. E. (2018). Vital signs: Trends in state suicide rates—United States, 1999–2016 and circumstances contributing to suicide—27 states, 2015. *Morbidity and Mortality Weekly Report (MMWR), 67,* 617–624. https://doi.org/10.15585/mmwr.mm6722a1

Suokas, J., Suominen, K., Isometsä, E., Ostamo, A., & Lönnqvist, J. (2001). Long-term risk factors for suicide mortality after attempted suicide—Findings of a 14-year follow-up study. *Acta Psychiatrica Scandinavica, 104*(2), 117–121. https://doi.org/10.1034/j.1600-0447.2001.00243.x

Taylor, A. K., Steeg, S., Quinlivan, L., Gunnell, D., Hawton, K., & Kapur, N. (2021). Accuracy of individual and combined risk-scale items in the prediction of repetition of self-harm: multicentre prospective cohort study. *BJPsych Open, 7*(1), e2. https://doi.org/10.1192/bjo.2020.123

Tucker, R. P., Michaels, M. S., Rogers, M. L., Wingate, L. R., & Joiner, T. E. (2016). Construct validity of a proposed new diagnostic entity: Acute suicidal affective disturbance (ASAD). *Journal of Affective Disorders*, *189*, 365–378. https://doi.org/10.1016/j.jad.2015.07.049

Waern, M., Sjostrom, N., Marlow, T., & Hetta, J. (2010). Does the suicide assessment scale predict risk of repetition? A prospective study of suicide attempters at a hospital emergency department. *European Psychiatry*, *25*(7), 421–426. https://doi.org/10.1016/j.eurpsy.2010.03.014

Weissman, M. M., Klerman, G. L., Markowitz, J. S., & Ouellette, R. (1989). Suicidal ideation and suicide attempts in panic disorder and attacks. *The New England Journal of Medicine*, *321*(18), 1209–1214. https://doi.org/10.1056/nejm198911023211801

Wenzel, A., Brown, G. K., & Beck, A. T. (2008). *Cognitive therapy for suicidal patients: Scientific and clinical applications*. American Psychological Association.

World Health Organization. (2021). *Suicide worldwide in 2019*. https://www.who.int/publications/i/item/9789240026643

Yaseen, Z. S., Chartrand, H., Mojtabai, R., Bolton, J., & Galynker, I. I. (2013). Fear of dying in panic attacks predicts suicide attempt in comorbid depressive illness: Prospective evidence from the National Epidemiological Survey on Alcohol and Related Conditions. *Depression and Anxiety*, *30*(10), 930–939. https://doi.org/10.1002/da.22039

Yaseen, Z. S., Galynker, I., Cohen, L. J., & Briggs, J. (2017). Clinicians' conflicting emotional responses to high suicide-risk patients—Association with short-term suicide behaviors: A prospective pilot study. *Comprehensive Psychiatry*, *76*, 69–78. https://doi.org/10.1016/j.comppsych.2017.03.013

Yaseen, Z. S., Hawes, M., Barzilay, S., & Galynker, I. (2019). Predictive validity of proposed diagnostic criteria for the suicide crisis syndrome: An acute presuicidal state. *Suicide and Life-Threatening Behavior*, *49*, 1124–1135. https://doi.org/10.1111/sltb.12495

Yaseen, Z., Katz, C., Johnson, M. S., Eisenberg, D., Cohen, L. J., & Galynker, I. I. (2010). Construct development: The Suicide Trigger Scale (STS-2), a measure of a hypothesized suicide trigger state. *BMC Psychiatry*, *10*(1), 110. https://doi.org/10.1186/1471-244x-10-110

Yaseen, Z. S., Kopeykina, I., Gutkovich, Z., Bassirnia, A., Cohen, L. J., & Galynker, I. (2014). Predictive validity of the Suicide Trigger Scale (STS-3) for post-discharge suicide attempt in high-risk psychiatric inpatients. *PLOS One*, *9*(1), e86768. https://doi.org/10.1371/journal.pone.0086768

Ying, G., Chennapragada, L., Musser, E. D., & Galynker, I. (2021). Behind therapists' emotional responses to suicidal patients: A study of the narrative crisis model of suicide and clinicians' emotions. *Suicide and Life-Threatening Behavior*, *51*(4), 684–695. https://doi.org/10.1111/sltb.12730

2

Psychological Models of Suicide

With Shira Barzilay and Olivia C. Lawrence

Introduction

Suicide is a complex behavior or set of behaviors originating out of a multilevel interplay of biological, psychological, social, and other factors as yet unknown. Suicide is also an endpoint of mysterious psychological processes that evolve over time and are still poorly understood. Thus, a coherent and comprehensive model of suicidal mental processes and behavior is essential both for the assessment of imminent risk for suicide, particularly in high-risk individuals, and for the informed design of interventions to reduce this risk.

To this end, over the last several decades, psychologists and psychiatrists have formulated models of suicidal behavior. The early psychodynamic models (Baumeister & Leary, 1995; Shneidman, 1993) were based on clinicians' individual clinical experiences and their clinical judgment. More recent so-called first-generation models of suicide (Claassen et al., 2014) went a step further and were based on a consensus opinion and consensus clinical judgment, rather than individual judgment. These models had more credibility, but, although they were attractive conceptually, they were never tested experimentally in predicting suicide (Litman et al., 1963).

The second-generation models that followed were intended to be tested in clinical experiments. Most of these models hypothesized that suicide risk was determined by certain measurable biological and clinical risk factors established either at birth or in early human development. These factors were static and long-term, and included biomarkers (i.e., serotonin levels), demographic factors (sex, age, occupation), and clinical factors (diagnosis of mental illness, prior suicide attempt), as well as standardized measures of psychopathology (HAM-D scores). Second-generation models were tested for predictive value and were modestly successful in identifying individuals at long-term suicide risk over decades and their lifetime. As demonstrated by Pokorny (1983), these models were either never tested for their short-term prediction of suicide risk or were not predictive of imminent suicidal behavior (Goldstein et al., 1991; Pokorny, 1983).

Third-generation models of suicidal behavior focused on dynamic risk elements, which appear later in life, change over time, and are operational immediately proximal to suicide. Some of these factors may be social stressors, such as a relationship break-up, career failure, or access to firearms. Others may describe mental processes leading to suicidal behavior, or the state of mind of acutely suicidal persons. Some third-generation models incorporate the second-generation static risk factors (Klonsky & May, 2015; O'Connor, 2011). Aspects of the third-generation models have recently been tested experimentally, with encouraging results (Dhingra et al., 2016). The narrative-crisis model (NCM), which may be considered a third-generation or fourth-generation model, is described in Chapter 3. The present chapter contains descriptions of several of the most influential theories of suicidal behavior and a critical assessment of their strong points and shortcomings.

Historical Perspective

The first theories of suicide originated in psychoanalysis and were formulated by Freud (1922) in his influential work *Beyond the Pleasure Principle*. Freud posited that the life and death drives were opposing basic instincts. The aim of the life drive was to overcome the conflicts associated with survival; the purpose of the death drive was to eliminate the conflicts of life itself. Freud believed that the desire to kill oneself was derived from an earlier repressed desire to destroy others. According to Freud, suicide represented an internalization of anger originally directed at others and a transformation of the external death wish into an internal one, directed against one's own ego.

In 1938, Menninger took Freud's concept of the death wish a step further by claiming that every suicide is an inverted homicide, or "murder in the 180th degree." Menninger theorized the existence of a suicidal triad, comprised of the wish to kill (murder), the wish to be killed (guilt), and the wish to die (depression). Menninger believed that the wish to kill is originally oriented toward external objects, which may include objects not acceptable to the ego (i.e., loved ones), leading to feelings of guilt for wishing the loved ones dead. As a result of ego destruction by guilt and self-loathing, depression and hopelessness ensue, leading to the wish to die as punishment for thoughts of killing others. On a different level, Menninger (1938) also linked suicide and self-injurious behavior to castrating or mutilating fantasies aimed at one's parents and siblings. Klein (1935, 1946) further developed the role of guilt in the death instinct. According to her theory, suicide is the result of unbearable guilt over aggressive fantasies toward internalized objects of envy. As the guilt causes feelings of malice and destructiveness, suicidal self-destructiveness prevents one's directing destructiveness toward others.

The above psychoanalytic approaches were intuitive rather than experimental and viewed suicide as a philosophical and moral dilemma rather than psychopathology (i.e., psychosis or depression). At that time in history, society at large agreed with this view. However, the work of early psychoanalysts accumulated the fund of knowledge that created momentum for a transformation of how suicide was perceived, moving it from a spiritual problem to a manifestation of a psychiatric disorder (Ellis, 2001).

The most serious flaw of psychoanalytic theories is that they are difficult or impossible to test experimentally. The very few studies that attempted to do so brought very mixed results. Baumeister and Scher (1988) studied the concept of self-destructiveness as an essential biological human need. Their experimental paradigm defined the self-destructive drive as the intention to harm the self as punishment for tolerating the disliked part of the self. The authors found no experimental evidence for such self-destructive drives in humans.

Conceptually related to the inherent self-destructiveness concept are the ideas of Apter et al. (1993) and others who hypothesized that suicide is due to aggression turned inward (Maiuro et al., 1989; Rustein & Goldberg, 1973; Tatman et al., 1993). In support of this concept, Orbach (1996, 2003a, 2003b) demonstrated that the relationship between early insecure attachment and suicidal behavior was mediated by negative attitudes toward the body, and Maltsberger (2004) and others found some experimental evidence for a psychodynamic explanation of suicide in psychological autopsies of suicide decedents. However, their conclusions were based on descriptions rather than statistical analyses, and so far psychoanalytic theories of suicide lack solid experimental support.

Shneidman's Theory of Psychache

Shneidman's influential theory posited that suicide is caused by "psychache" (Shneidman, 1993, p. 51; Figure 2.1), an intense and intolerable emotional

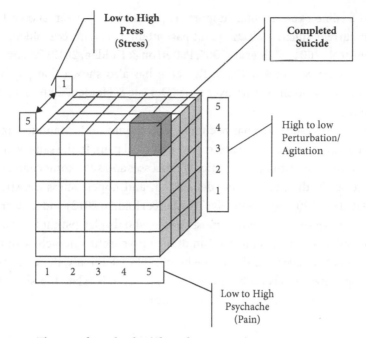

Figure 2.1 Theory of psychache (Shneidman, 1993).

pain that is different from depression and hopelessness. The tortured individuals seek, but cannot find, relief for their pain until there is no solution but death. Shneidman postulated two types of individual needs: primary or biological needs for survival, and secondary or psychological needs for fulfillment and, ultimately, also for survival. When the psychological needs that are essential for life, such as love and belonging, sense of control, positive self-image, and meaningful relationships, are frustrated by business or career failures, romantic rejections, and losses, psychache develops. Shneidman's connection with earlier psychoanalytic theories lay in his view of suicide as a means of fulfilling a specific psychodynamic need. According to Shneidman, although suicide stems from psychache, it is not only an escape from pain but also an attempt to achieve a goal or fulfill a need or fantasy, such as impressing a loved one, achieving fame or notoriety, or gaining love.

Shneidman's ideas are at the core of many contemporary psychological suicide models (Jobes & Nelson, 2006), and his conceptualization of suicide as a problem-solving behavior (Shneidman, 1993) influenced other psychological theories of suicide, most notably the escape theory (Baumeister, 1990) and the cry of pain model (Williams, 1997). The theory has also

received some experimental support, as psychache has been shown to relate to current suicidal ideation and past attempts (Flynn & Holden, 2007;
Holden et al., 2001; Mills et al., 2005; Patterson & Holden, 2012; Pereira et al.,
2010; Troister & Holden, 2010). Research has also shown that psychache
and suicidal ideation co-vary over time (DeLisle & Holden, 2009; Troister &
Holden, 2012).

However, to date there has been no research into understanding, and no
clear definition of, what constitutes psychological pain. In the same vein, it is
not clear what cognitive and emotional processes and symptoms characterize
psychache. Further, psychache, depression, and hopelessness are strongly
correlated ($r = .80$, approximately; Troister & Holden, 2012) and may or may
not be independent. Moreover, most people who display psychological pain
are not suicidal, and the mechanism of how psychache interacts with other
risk factors to trigger suicide has not been explored. Finally, there have been
no prospective studies probing whether psychache is related to short-term
suicide risk or to imminent suicidal behavior.

Suicide as Escape from Self

One of the earlier psychodynamic models that significantly influenced the
field of suicidology was Baumeister's concept of suicide as an escape from self
(Baumeister, 1990). Baumeister noted that escape from an aversive life situation and relief from unbearable mental anguish were the most common goals
reported by suicide attempters. He then suggested that there are six steps to
the suicidal process. The starting point is when unrealistically high expectations are created, in contrast to expectations based in reality, setting up an objective failure to meet those expectations. The second step is the individual's
interpretation of the objective failure as a personal defeat. Third, a negative
cognitive bias ensues, bringing on a distorted and unforgiving comparison of the self with an idealized and unrealizable success. The fourth step is
the resulting uncontrolled escalation of emotional pain, which, in the fifth
step, brings the state numbness and cognitive deconstruction. Baumeister
hypothesized that in the final step, cognitive deconstruction results in behavioral disinhibition, which allows one to overcome the fear of causing oneself
pain through death, and to actually end one's life by suicide.

Baumeister's theory did not consider suicide a sort of self-execution and
punishment, nor did it look for psychodynamic reasons for suicide; instead,

it viewed suicide as an escape from unbearable psychological pain through loss of consciousness. Baumeister's other unique assumption was that negative suicidal emotions are experienced as an acute state rather than a prolonged one, and it was consistent with Shneidman's conceptualization of suicide as an escape from mental pain. The two theories also shared the concept that self-destructive behaviors are rooted in cognitive distortion (Shneidman, 1993).

The theory of an escape from self found some indirect experimental support (Dean & Range, 1999; Hunter & O'Connor, 2003; O'Connor & O'Connor, 2003; Tassava & Ruderman, 1999), in that a major disappointment in oneself plays a major role in precipitating suicidal behavior (Chatard & Selimbegović, 2011; DeWall et al., 2008, 2011; Twenge et al., 2002, 2003). However, there has been no direct evidence linking Baumeister's theory of imminent suicidal behavior with short-term suicide risk. While the six-stage model is attractive, and the first four steps (prior to cognitive deconstruction) are intuitive, there have been no research data on when and how suicidal thoughts and behaviors emerge. No experimental data are available to support the cognitive and emotional processes that underlie the transition from one step to the next and culminate in suicide. Still, the escape theory is a compelling theory of suicidal behavior (O'Connor, 2003) and has influenced other theoreticians and researchers, including Williams (1997), O'Connor (2011), and the authors of this book.

The Cry of Pain/Arrested Flight Model

Williams (1997) posited that suicide results from a feeling of defeat in response to humiliation or rejection, leading to a perception of entrapment (Figure 2.2). When the latter is combined with a failure to find alternative ways to solve the problem (i.e., cognitive rigidity; Schotte & Clum, 1987), a suicidal person may see no exit out of the perceived entrapment but suicide. This model drew upon the concept of arrested flight reported in animal behavior literature and which has been suggested to account for depression in humans (Gilbert & Allan, 1998). Pollock and Williams (1998, 2001) suggested that when individuals perceive their attempts at solving problems to be unsuccessful, they feel powerless to escape the situation.

Specifically, Williams and Pollock's intuitively titled "cry of pain" or "arrested flight" model of suicidality posited that major alterations in the

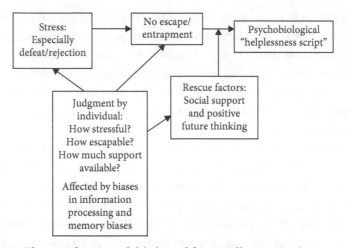

Figure 2.2 The cry of pain model (adapted from Williams, 2001).

domains of attention, memory, and judgment are related to three components of suicidal behavior: hypersensitivity to signals of defeat, the perception of being trapped, and the perception that there is no rescue from the situation, respectively. Their model was based on a sociobiological concept of depression as a phenomenon that predates human development, as described by Price and Sloman (1987).

With regard to hypersensitivity to signals of defeat, the authors argued that depression is a form of yielding behavior that is observed in animals, specifically birds, in the context of ritual agonistic behavior, or aggressive behavior among individuals in the group, which establishes a social hierarchy:

> Consider the behavior of birds establishing their territories. If birds meet within a single putative territory, they engage in aggressive displays. One wins, the other loses. The loser flies away to find another territory. It suffers little ill effects from its encounter. But if this meeting occurs in a limited territory, in a cage or other circumstance in which the defeated cannot escape, it is a different story. (Price & Sloman, 1987)

Birds pecking each other in fights over territory can be viewed as a simplified model of human struggles for power and control—with the assumption that in a struggle there will be a winner and a loser. Williams and Pollock hypothesized that once defeat or "loser status" is triggered, there is an attentional bias toward signals of defeat. They described the phenomenon of "perceptual pop-out," where stimuli of great interest seem to jump out at an individual. Using the emotional Stroop task, they showed that suicidal individuals had an attentional bias toward words associated with rejection or defeat and are thus hyperfocused on hyperattended these signals.

Much like Schotte and Clum, Williams and Pollock pointed out the impaired problem-solving in suicidal individuals but argued that the key feature was not the deficit in problem-solving itself but the feeling of being trapped, which arises as a result of this deficit. Specifically, they argued that suicidal individuals' problem-solving abilities are impaired due to alterations in their memory retrieval. Williams and Pollock observed that when asked to recall a happy time, suicidal patients responded with overgeneralized responses, such as "when people give me presents," rather than recalling a specific event. Williams and Pollock postulated that these patients "stopped short" of specific memory retrieval in an effort to regulate their emotional response to memories of traumatic events. The patients' strategy is problematic because specific memories provide associations that one can use in a given situation to explore different trains of thought and to create new solutions.

Finally, Williams and Pollock argued that a crucial factor in suicidality is the lack of rescue. They found that, in comparison to controls, suicidal individuals did not necessarily anticipate a greater number of negative lifetime events, but they anticipated significantly fewer positive events. Without the anticipation of positive events to rescue one from stressors, hopelessness sets in, which Williams and Pollock considered to be the final component of suicidality.

While this model incorporated empiric observations of the cognitive processes of suicidal individuals—specifically in terms of memory and attention—the model's basic premise is that social defeat flattens the human experience into simplistic antagonistic relationships where the ultimate outcome is a hierarchical pecking order. The model does not account for the possibility of social rescue factors, and modern models of animal behavior take into account the complexities of interactions within groups in maintaining cohesiveness and group survival (Warburton & Lazarus, 1991).

Cognitive Vulnerability Model

Based on studies of suicidal patients, Schotte and Clum (1987) proposed a stress-diathesis model of suicidality in which cognitive rigidity—inflexibility in both interpersonal and impersonal problem-solving—accounts for the association between stress and suicidal behavior. In lay terms, when faced with a difficult life problem, such patients tend to perceive it as impenetrable and are too rigid or perseverative in their thinking to imagine a viable alternative.

To test this hypothesis (i.e., the possible role of cognitive rigidity in suicidality), Schotte and Clum compared 50 psychiatric inpatients meeting the criteria for suicidality with 50 individuals who did not. Both groups were given an assessment of interpersonal problem-solving, where participants were presented with situations and desired outcomes and were asked to complete the middle of the story to achieve the stated goal (also known as the Alternative Uses Test). The participants were also asked to list problems that led to their hospitalization, to generate possible alternative solutions to the problems, and then to rate the probability of success of each alternative solution (also known as the Modified MEPS test).

The investigators found suicidality to positively correlate with life stress, hopelessness, and poor problem-solving skills, although not with depression. In the assessment of problem-solving, suicidal patients generated 60% fewer options on the Alternative Uses Test than nonsuicidal controls, and fewer than half as many potential solutions on the Modified MEPS. Additionally, suicidal patients anticipated more negative consequences from the possible solutions they generated, and generated more irrelevant solutions, than their nonsuicidal cohorts.

Schotte and Clum used their study to argue that cognitive rigidity, as manifested by inflexibility in interpersonal problem-solving, is a key moderator between life stress and suicidal ideation. The implication is that cognitive rigidity forms the diathesis of the stress-diathesis model, setting the stage for suicidal ideation when an individual has difficulty finding solutions to life's problems. Of note, the authors acknowledged that problem-solving deficits might be state dependent—activated by significant life stress, rather than an intrinsic trait—and proposed further study examining cognitive rigidity over time.

While this model is elegant in its simplicity and in drawing attention to the cognitive aspect of suicidal behavior, it is limited in its focus on problem-solving ability and does not look at other factors that may predict suicidal behavior, thus restricting possible interventions.

Fluid Vulnerability Model

To explain the suicidal process, Rudd (2006) proposed the fluid vulnerability theory, which is based on the assumption that suicidal episodes are time-limited and are triggered by factors that change over time and with the mental state of the individual, and are therefore fluid in nature. Rudd posited that each person has a set baseline vulnerability to suicide (Figure 2.3). The three main factors contributing to this vulnerability are cognitive susceptibility (attentional bias, inability to recall specific memories), biological susceptibility (physiological or major psychiatric symptoms, such as aberrant mood or psychosis), and behavioral susceptibility (deficient interpersonal skills and impaired affect regulation). According to the fluid vulnerability theory, long-term suicide risk is determined by the magnitude of the susceptibility factors.

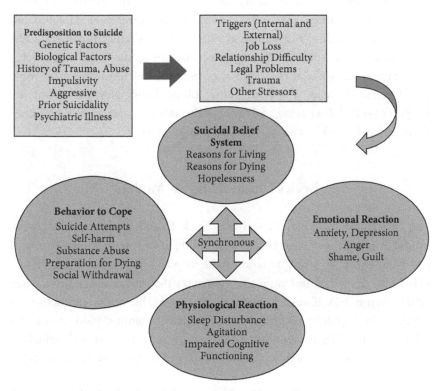

Figure 2.3 The fluid vulnerability model (Rudd, 2006).

The near-term risk is determined by the presence of constellations of in-ternal and external stimuli, interpreted by an individual through cognitive, emotional, behavioral, and other themes, forming a "suicide mode." The main cognitive themes that can activate the suicide mode are the notion of being unloved, the thought that one is a burden to others, feelings of help-lessness, and low distress tolerance. The constellation of unique themes that comprise a particular person's suicide mode recur and may define that person's vulnerability to a suicide crisis and the probable triggers of the crisis.

Repeated activation of a suicide mode lowers the threshold for its future activation, creating a unique vulnerability. Similar to Beck (1996), Rudd et al. (1994) suggested that the suicide mode is a combination of a suicidal belief system, physiological-affective symptoms, and associated behaviors and motivations. According to the fluid vulnerability theory, individuals with a sensitized suicidal belief system will have recurrent crises, with each crisis making them more vulnerable to future ones.

Like the cognitive vulnerability theory, the fluid vulnerability theory is supported by studies suggesting that rumination (Surrence et al., 2009) and cognitive inflexibility (Miranda et al., 2012) are predictive of suicidal idea-tion. Barzilay and Apter (2014) suggested that this model is the best at com-bining the acute risk factors, primarily current suicidal ideation, and chronic risk factors. However, the fluid vulnerability theory is vague about the triggers of suicidal behavior, and the hypothesis that cognitive vulnerabilities increase suicide risk has not been tested prospectively.

Beck's Diathesis-Stress Model

The behavioral theorists Wenzel and Beck (2008) proposed a cognitive model of suicidal behavior based on attempts to distinguish long-term and short-term suicide risk by separating the dispositional vulnerability factors (diathesis) and distorted cognitive processes that characterize the suicide crisis (Figure 2.4). If suicide diathesis is present, life stress can activate a maladaptive cognitive response, with increased attention paid to suicide-related stimuli. This distorted cognition narrows attention on the suicidal act and creates a scenario where suicide appears to be the only solution to life stressors.

The dispositional vulnerability factors postulated by Beck's model are long-standing stress vulnerability factors (traits), which are not specific for

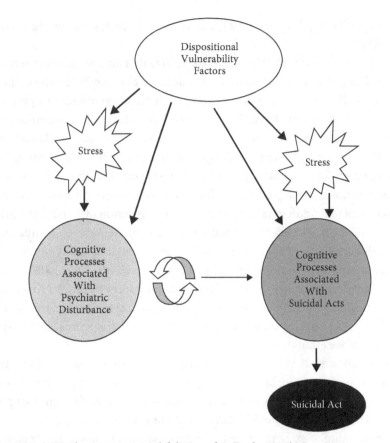

Figure 2.4 Diathesis-stress model (Wenzel & Beck, 2008).

suicide but make one susceptible to suicide crises even with low levels of stress. Beck defined five main dispositional vulnerability factors: impulsivity, deficits in problem-solving, an overgeneral memory style, a maladaptive cognitive style, and personality.

Beck distinguished between two types of impulsivity: lack of planning versus failure to inhibit responses, with the latter being more prominent in suicidal patients. Beck agreed with Brent and Mann (2005, 2006), whose model is described in the next section, and who reported that impulsive aggression is highly heritable, making it more likely that an individual will act on suicidal thoughts. While evidence is mixed regarding the way that problem-solving deficits may mediate suicidal behavior, Beck noted that suicidal patients generate fewer possible solutions to problems and posited that cognitive rigidity may prompt feelings of hopelessness in high-stress situations.

Beck also agreed with Williams et al. (2007) that an overgeneral memory and difficulty teasing apart memory details seem to exacerbate hopelessness, because individuals have difficulty judging specific situations and perceive that there is no escape from their distress. Beck also noted a traitlike maladaptive cognitive style, which is characterized by cognitive distortions, including "black and white" thinking, jumping to conclusions, and magnification, which form a chronic pattern of thought and exacerbate life stressors. Finally, he noted that a great deal of literature has examined personality traits among suicidal individuals, including, most prominently, perfectionism and particularly socially prescribed perfectionism, defined as "an interpersonal dimension involving perceptions of one's need and ability to meet the standards and expectations imposed by others" (Hewitt et al., 2006). Other personality traits related to suicidal risk were psychoticism, introversion, self-criticalness, novelty-seeking, harm avoidance, cynicism, sensitivity, dependency, and a decreased tendency to be warm and gregarious and to experience positive emotions.

In the context of vulnerability factors, stress then activates maladaptive cognitive processes, including more generalized cognitive processes associated with psychiatric disturbances as well as more specific cognitive processes associated with suicidal acts. According to Beck's cognitive model, "the processing of external events or internal stimuli is biased and therefore systematically distorts the individual's construction of his or her experiences, leading to a variety of cognitive errors" (Beck, 2005). Information is processed according to an individual's underlying schema, defined as "relatively enduring internal structures" used to organize new information, or the highly ingrained "lens" formed from early experiences that one uses to view the world.

For example, a depressive schema contains negative attitudes about loss and failure, and thus depressed individuals will place greater emphasis on processing negative information than on processing positive information. Beck asserted that hopelessness may form the core of a suicide schema, feeding back onto itself, reinforcing negative beliefs that things will never get better. He noted evidence that patients with recent suicide attempts showed attentional biases toward suicide-related stimuli (Becker et al., 1999). Beck posited that this additional attention to suicide-related stimuli feeds forward into a suicidal crisis when an individual is experiencing hopelessness, and this attention makes it difficult to disengage from these stimuli and thoughts.

Additionally, there is evidence that patients describe cognitive disorientation, racing thoughts, acute restlessness, and "tunnel vision" during a suicide crisis. Beck described these phenomena as part of a collective attentional fixation, or a narrowing of focus on suicide as a solution. He proposed that in the context of hopelessness, attentional fixation can lead to a downward spiral where suicide is identified as the only solution to one's problems.

One goal of Beck's model was to provide points for intervention. Beck suggested that cognitive behavioral therapy (CBT) can be used to modify dispositional factors, cognitive processes, and the very schema of suicide. Treatment is viewed as occurring in phases. In the early phase, the emphasis is placed on engaging patients in treatment and conveying a sense of hope, particularly since patients may be ambivalent about the perceived benefits of treatment in the context of hopelessness. Clinicians then perform a risk assessment and work with patients to create a safety plan, including identifying crisis signs, examining coping strategies, and creating a list of contacts the patient can turn to for support. One technique targets overgeneral memories by creating a "hope kit"—a memory aid, which includes texts and objects meaningful to the patient that can anchor them in times of crisis. In the intermediate phase, the clinician helps the patient develop cognitive and behavioral strategies to manage suicidal ideation. In the late phase, the clinician and patient prepare for termination of treatment, including defining a relapse prevention protocol where a patient is led through guided imagery to revisit the suicide crisis and the patient identifies coping strategies he or she has learned to reduce distress.

In summary, Beck's diathesis-stress model posits that long-standing chronic vulnerabilities can amplify the impact of life stressors. The stressors are then processed and distorted by a patient's maladaptive schema, leading to a fixation on suicide in which a patient's cognition is clouded and biased toward suicide-associated stimuli. In this context, wherein the patient is overwhelmed by suicidal thoughts, suicide appears to become an attractive solution to life stressors. The strengths of Beck's theory include its attention to how the patient's life story leads to the suicidal crisis and its suggested interventions through CBT. Its main drawbacks are its insufficient attention to the emotional side of the suicidal crisis and to its evolution in time.

Mann's Stress-Diathesis Model

The stress-diathesis clinical model suggested by Mann and others (Horesh et al., 1999; Mann et al., 2005) and most recently championed by Mann's group is similar to the Beck diathesis-stress model (Wenzel & Beck, 2008) in that it suggests that life stressors lead to suicide only when combined with vulnerability (Figure 2.5). Mann broadly defined stressors as either a psychiatric illness or psychosocial factors, while positing that the diathesis arises from low levels of serotonin and norepinephrine. The model is based on the clinical phenomenon of impulsive aggression, which is a propensity to react impulsively to frustrations with anger and aggression (Apter et al., 1991; Bridge et al., 2006).

The common feature of suicidal behavior, impulsive aggression, is a mediator between psychopathology and suicidal actions, and is subserved by low serotonergic activity. Brent and Mann (2006) proposed that the vulnerability to suicidal behavior is biological, with a strong familial component that is both genetic and environmental. The genetic component is rooted in parental mood disorder and/or impulsivity and aggression, while childhood abuse and neglect add the environmental component. Thus, an abused child with genetic loading develops impulsive-aggressive traits, which in the presence of life stressors may lead to suicidal behavior.

The stress-diathesis model has generated a voluminous body of research into neurochemical and neuroanatomical pathways underlying both the diathesis and the stress-activated susceptibility to suicidal behavior (Mann et al., 2009; Melhelm et al., 2007). Indeed, many studies have suggested a

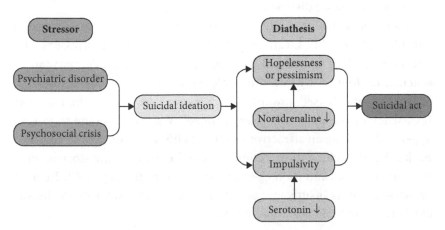

Figure 2.5 Stress-diathesis model (Mann, 2003).

link between impulsivity and suicide (Brodsky et al., 1997; Hawton et al., 1999; Mann et al., 1999; Nock & Kessler, 2006) as well as evidence that impulsive suicide is more common among young suicide attempters and suicide completers (Brent & Mann, 2005, 2006). Some familial suicidal behavior may indeed be mediated by serotonergic mechanisms (Mann, 2013).

However, the stress-diathesis model does not explain planned and deliberate suicidal behavior, and a number of studies did not find a significant association between impulsivity and suicidal behavior (Horesh, 2001; Keilp et al., 2006; Oquendo et al., 2000). Recently, Witte et al. (2008) reported that less than one-fourth of suicide attempters did so without planning, a finding consistent with the view that although impulsivity may be a risk factor for suicidal behavior, suicide is not necessarily an impulsive act. Furthermore, patients who made impulsive suicide attempts appeared to have the same level of impulsivity as patients who had planned their attempts (Baca-Garcia et al., 2005).

Although Mann and colleagues found a correlation between aggression and impulsivity, as well as between suicidal ideation and fewer reported reasons for living, the model was not useful in identifying those who are currently at risk for future suicidal behaviors. In retrospective studies, rates of lifetime aggression and impulsivity were higher in attempters, but so were the rates of borderline personality disorder, smoking, past substance use disorder or alcoholism, family history of suicidal acts, head injury, and childhood abuse. Thus, it is possible that the stress-diathesis model identifies a general psychopathological trait not specific enough to distinguish those at risk for near-term suicide.

Joiner's Interpersonal Model

Although relatively recent, Joiner's interpersonal theory of suicide has generated a substantial body of research work. The theory posits that suicidal behavior requires a combination of suicidal desire and the acquired capability to act on that desire (Figure 2.6). Suicidal desire is framed by two simultaneous interpersonal constructs, thwarted belongingness and perceived burdensomeness. As lethal means of suicide are typically fear-inducing and painful, the additional step of acquired capability must develop before an individual engages in suicidal behavior. This capability arises through habituation and opponent processes in response to physically painful and/or fear-inducing experiences.

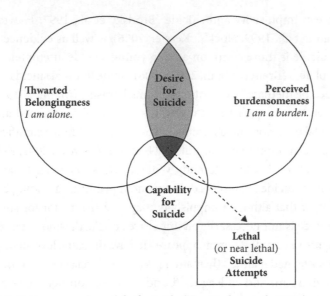

Figure 2.6 Interpersonal model of suicide (Van Orden et al., 2010).

Thwarted Belongingness

Joiner (2010) noted that social isolation is one of the strongest and most reli-able predictors of suicidal behavior and, as per Baumeister and Leary (1995), humans have a fundamental "need to belong." When this need is unmet, the state of thwarted belongingness emerges, and a desire for death or passive suicidal ideation develops. Furthermore, thwarted belongingness has two facets: loneliness—"an affectively laden cognition that one has too few social connections"—and the absence of reciprocally caring relationships. In a 2008 research study, Joiner's group found a linear relationship between thwarted belongingness and suicidal ideation, but only among participants who also reported high levels of perceived burdensomeness.

Perceived Burdensomeness

Suicidal individuals often perceive themselves as a burden to family and other loved ones and feel that people around them would be better off without them. Joiner cited Woznica and Shapiro's 1990 study, which found a positive corre-lation between adolescents' perceptions of their own expendability within their family structures and suicidal behavior. Joiner's own work (2010) examined suicide notes by individuals who made lethal and nonlethal attempts and found that the notes of those who died were characterized by a high degree of perceived burdensomeness. Additionally, among those who died, greater perceptions of burdensomeness predicted more lethal means of suicide. In Joiner's theory, perceived burdensomeness has two dimensions: a perception that the self is so flawed as to be a liability to others—"My death is worth more than my life to others"—and affectively laden self-loathing—"I hate myself."

Acquired Capability

Once thwarted belongingness and perceived burdensomeness have come together to promote suicidal ideation, an individual still must overcome the fear of pain and death. Joiner noted Ohman and Mineka's (2001) proposal that fear is evolutionarily protective because it signals potentially life-threatening situations that can then be avoided. Joiner posited that through repeated practice and repeated exposure, an individual can overcome this fear by habituating to the frightening and physically painful aspects of self-harm. To engage in suicidal behavior, an individual must have a degree of fearlessness. As many means of suicide are extremely painful, fear of pain provides another barrier to suicidal behavior. Joiner stipulated that to engage in such behavior, an individual must be convinced that the pain associated with a chosen means of suicide is tolerable.

Opponent Processing

Joiner posited that the capacity for suicide is acquired through habituation to the fear and pain involved in self-injury (typically through a pattern of self-injury). Additionally, Solomon and Corbit's 1974 model of opponent processing was used to explain how lethal actions can take on a positive emotional valence. In opponent processing, an individual engaged in a repeat behavior will have an initial emotional response that eventually becomes overtaken by an acquired opponent response. For example, the primary response to skydiving will likely be fear, but with repeated exposure, the opponent process of exhilaration will arise and become amplified. Eventually, the opponent process overtakes the initial response.

Orden and Joiner hypothesized that self-harm behaviors have a primary effect of fear and pain (2010) but acquire an opponent process of relief and analgesia. Through repeated practice, fear remains constant or diminishes, and as the opponent process becomes dominant, self-harm behaviors come to be primarily associated with emotional relief. The model of opponent processing provides a framework for viewing prior attempts (one of the strongest predictors of eventual suicide) as rehearsals, leading to pain desensitization and cultivation of positive emotional valence surrounding suicidal behavior and ultimately helping an individual acquire capability by overcoming their naturally protective fears of pain and death.

In summary, the advantages to Joiner's model are its elegance and intuitiveness, using only three proximal factors as the "danger zones" to predict suicidal behavior. Hypothetically, by evaluating for these factors, clinicians can screen for patients at high risk. A clinician can assess acquired capability by asking: "Do you think you have the courage or capability to kill yourself?" Any response other than a definitive No indicates a degree of fearlessness with regard to suicidal behavior. The drawback of this model is that in experiments, both perceived burdensomeness and thwarted belongingness have been associated with suicidal ideation but not suicidal behavior (Ma et al., 2016). Furthermore, the concepts of acquired capability and opponent processing have been contradicted by research on military suicide, which found no association between veterans' suicidal behavior and their exposure to weapons or combat (Griffith, 2012).

O'Connor's Integrated Motivational-Volitional Model of Suicide

Rory O'Connor's integrated motivational-volitional (IMV) model of suicide uses Ajzen's theory of planned behavior to examine suicide as a volitional rather than impulsive action (O'Connor et al., 2006). However, the model does incorporate elements of the stress-diathesis model of suicidality in the pre-motivational phase (Figure 2.7). The suicidal process is considered as moving along a simple timeline, starting with the biopsychosocial groundwork laid out by the stress-diathesis model, then following the arrested flight model (Pollock & Williams, 2001) before transitioning from ideation to action. The emphasis of the integrated model is on the proximal predictor of suicide—suicidal intention rather than simply ideation—and the

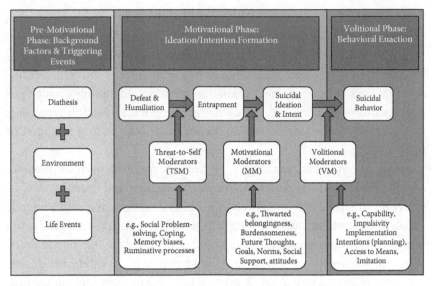

Figure 2.7 The integrated motivational-volitional model of suicide (O'Connor, 2011).

model explores the stages of suicidal ideation from background setting (pre-motivational phase) to ideation (motivational phase) through the crucial transition from ideation to intention and ultimately suicidal behavior (volitional phase).

The pre-motivational phase provides the groundwork for suicidal ideation and is based on the diathesis-stress model (Schotte & Clum, 1987). Combining nature and nurture, the pre-motivational phase explores how environmental factors or negative life events can activate biological vulnerabilities. Personality traits, such as perfectionism, particularly socially prescribed perfectionism, can provide vulnerability, so that a stressful life event can push an individual forward toward the motivational phase of suicidality. In his research, O'Connor showed that for adolescents with high levels of socially prescribed perfectionism, even low-level life stress could lead to a dramatically increased probability of self-harm.

Once the groundwork is laid, suicidal ideation and intention formation can occur. The motivational phase is based on the arrested flight model (Pollock & Williams, 2001), where feelings of defeat and humiliation lead to a feeling of entrapment. Once the individual feels entrapped, if there is little hope for rescue through social support and positive thinking is absent, suicidal ideation may arise as a possible solution to the seemingly hopeless situation. Feelings of defeat and humiliation can be compounded by what are termed threat-to-self moderators, including overgeneralized memory and rumination (particularly brooding rumination), and can help the feeling of defeat escalate to a feeling of entrapment. Once an individual feels entrapped, motivational moderators, including a paucity of positive future thinking, influence whether the suicidal ideation progresses to intent. O'Connor considered all moderators to be targets for possible interventions.

Finally, the volitional phase provides the key transition from suicidal ideation to action. This transition from suicidal ideation and intent to suicidal behavior is marked and influenced by volitional moderators, which include access to means of suicide, knowing others who have engaged in suicide, and impulsivity. Interventions in this final phase of suicidality are highly desirable, and studies are underway looking at psychosocial interventions, including a volitional help sheet, to prevent individuals from making the final leap from intention to action.

The IMV model is important because it combines aspects of several different psychological theories in a way that provides a theoretical framework for how early vulnerability may progress to suicidal behavior. A recent prospective cohort study of the IMV model showed that its components could be somewhat predictive of future suicidal ideation, providing some support of its assumptions (O'Connor, O'Carroll, et al., 2012; O'Connor, Rasmussen, & Hawton, 2009, 2012). Further research in other settings is needed to confirm these findings and to establish whether the model is predictive of behavior rather than ideation. Experimental evidence for specificity of the moderators of each step is also lacking.

Klonsky's Three-Step Theory of Suicide

The three-step theory (3ST; Klonsky & May, 2015) is the newest theory in the ideation-to-action framework (Klonsky et al., 2018). The 3ST postulates three consecutive steps: (1) mental pain (but also physical pain) and hopelessness interaction leads to suicidal ideation; (2) disrupted connectedness (defined as any sense of perceived purpose or meaning) fails to protect against, progression from passive to active suicidal ideation; and (3) capability for suicide, defined as dispositional (i.e., genetic variations in pain tolerance), acquired (i.e., develops through experience), and practical capability (i.e.,

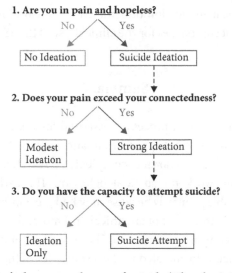

1. Are you in pain <u>and</u> hopeless?
No / \ Yes

No Ideation   Suicide Ideation

2. Does your pain exceed your connectedness?
No / \ Yes

Modest   Strong Ideation
Ideation

3. Do you have the capacity to attempt suicide?
No / \ Yes

Ideation   Suicide Attempt
Only

Figure 2.8 Klonsky's three-step theory of suicide (Klonsky & May, 2015).

access to, and familiarity with, lethal means), will predict the transition from suicidal ideation to suicidal acts (Klonsky & May, 2015, p. 119; Figure 2.8).

The 3ST was tested in, and supported by, a growing body of research. Cross-sectional studies within community adults and undergraduate students in the United States (Klonsky & May, 2015) and China (Yang et al., 2019) supported its main predictions. Several additional studies supported specific hypotheses of the 3ST in adolescents (Arango et al., 2016; Czyz et al., 2019; Gunn et al., 2018; King et al., 2019). Tsai et al. (2021) aimed to address the existing gaps in examining the 3ST prospectively in adult psychiatric patients. Findings among 190 psychiatric patients supported the validity of the 3ST, particularly steps 1 and 2, in predicting suicidal ideation and suicide attempts. Future work should further replicate and extend these findings and evaluate the 3ST in comparison to alternative theories, including the NCM.

The 3ST is valuable because it provides an alternative theoretical framework for describing how early vulnerability may progress to suicidal behavior. The early experimental evidence supporting its construct validity and predictive validity for suicide attempts is encouraging. However, as is true for all ideation-to-action theories, the clinical use of 3ST will have to rely on self-reported suicidal ideation, an approach that would miss 75% of those at imminent risk at the outset. Furthermore, like most of the suicide models, the 3ST does not have a syndromic approach for the pre-suicidal mental state, making its practical application difficult. More research may be needed to determine the best approaches for the clinical use of the 3ST.

Summary

Understanding the suicidal process is essential for research and the development of methods of suicide prevention, and over the last decades several psychological theories of varying complexity have attempted to provide a theoretical framework for suicidal behavior. The early psychoanalytic models were valuable primarily because they had great influence in changing the view on suicide from that of an ethical and moral dilemma to a psychopathological and clinical phenomenon. The second generation of psychological models of suicide, formulated in the last quarter of the 20th century and backed by a modest degree of experimental evidence, fell primarily into four domains: affective, cognitive, diathesis-stress, and suicidal crisis.

The key concepts emerging from the affective theories, which are exemplified by the cry of pain/arrested flight model, are the unbearable state of entrapment and Joiner's concepts of perceived burdensomeness and thwarted belongingness. The central concepts promulgated by the cognitive-behavioral theories—Schotte and Clum's (1987) cognitive vulnerability model and Rudd's fluid vulnerability model—are impulsivity, cognitive rigidity, and maladaptive cognitive style.

Of the two diathesis-stress models based on the concept of a biological trait vulnerability to stress, Beck's model is also based on cognitive-behavioral theories, adding the trait vulnerabilities of maladaptive cognitive style, personality, and impulsivity. On the other hand, Mann's model, in which the trait vulnerabilities are impulsive aggression and pessimism, modulated by low serotonin and low norepinephrine, respectively, emphasizes neurochemistry. The key feature of both models is separation of the long-term trait factors from dynamic precipitating stressors.

While the above models have advanced the field of suicide research substantially, they also have significant limitations. The main flaw of these theories is that, despite the complexity of suicidal behavior, they are narrow in focus and are not sufficiently comprehensive to integrate the cognitive, affective, and trait vulnerability factors for suicide into one coherent construct.

In the words of Fawcett, the second-generation suicide risk models "have identified an almost overwhelming number of nonspecific, static risk factors, producing a body of research that has been described as both 'daunting' and conceptually 'imprecise.'" Further, these models do not address the evolution of the suicidal process over time whereby stressful life events interact with trait vulnerabilities to form causal pathways making suicide possible. Finally, no theory has been clinically useful in identifying patients at high risk for imminent or near-term suicide, which is essential if we are to slow the rise in suicide rates in the United States and many countries worldwide (Bertolote & Fleischmann, 2015; Bustamante et al., 2016).

O'Connor's third-generation IMV theory of suicidal behavior attempts to overcome these limitations by considering the suicidal process in stages over time. The IMV model attempts to incorporate disparate static and dynamic factors into one comprehensive whole by including Beck's and Mann's stress-diathesis models in the pre-motivational phase of the IMV to serve as the basis for Williams' entrapment-based psychological schema of the evolution of the suicidal process, which takes place over the motivational phase. The main limitations of the IMV are the lack of a framework for the multiplicity of suicidal behaviors and for the diverse pathways subserving both impulsive and deliberate attempts, the lack of a clear definition of suicidal crisis, and its lack of applicability to assessing actual risk of near-term suicidal behavior.

Thus, significant progress in the theoretical understanding of the suicidal process and suicide has not yet translated into an ability to identify those at imminent risk for suicidal behavior and to prevent suicide. Therefore, there is a need for a fourth-generation model that integrates the stress-diathesis vulnerability construct with both affective and cognitive aspects of the suicidal process, clearly differentiates the trait and imminent suicide risks, provides a satisfactory narrative connecting these two clinical concepts, and explains both impulsive and planned suicides. The comprehensive narrative-crisis model, which meets these criteria, is described in the next chapter.

References

Apter, A., Kotler, M., Sevy, S., Plutchik, R., Brown, S.-L., Foster, H., Hillbrand, M., Korn, M. L., & Van Praag, H. M. (1991). Correlates of risk of suicide in violent and nonviolent psychiatric patients. *The American Journal of Psychiatry, 148*(7), 883–887. https://doi.org/10.1176/ajp.148.7.883

Apter, A., Plutchik, R., & van Praag, H. M. (1993). Anxiety, impulsivity and depressed mood in relation to suicidal and violent behavior. *Acta Psychiatrica Scandinavica, 87*(1), 1–5. https://doi.org/10.1111/j.1600-0447.1993.tb03321.x

Arango, A., Opperman, K. J., Gipson, P. Y., & King, C. A. (2016). Suicidal ideation and suicide attempts among youth who report bully victimization, bully perpetration and/or low social connectedness. *Journal of Adolescence*, *51*, 19–29. https://doi.org/10.1016/j.adolescence.2016.05.003

Baca-Garcia, E., Diaz-Sastre, C., García Resa, E., Blasco, H., Braquehais Conesa, D., Oquendo, M. A., Saiz-Ruiz, J., & de Leon, J. (2005). Suicide attempts and impulsivity. *European Archives of Psychiatry and Clinical Neuroscience*, *255*(2), 152–156. https://doi.org/10.1007/s00406-004-0549-3

Barzilay, S., & Apter, A. (2014). Psychological models of suicide. *Archives of Suicide Research*, *18*(4), 295–312. https://doi.org/10.1080/13811118.2013.824825

Baumeister, R. F. (1990). Suicide as escape from self. *Psychological Review*, *97*(1), 90–113. https://doi.org/10.1037/0033-295x.97.1.90

Baumeister, R. F., & Leary, M. R. (1995). The need to belong: Desire for interpersonal attachments as a fundamental human motivation. *Psychological Bulletin*, *117*(3), 497.

Baumeister, R. F., & Scher, S. J. (1988). Self-defeating behavior patterns among normal individuals: Review and analysis of common self-destructive tendencies. *Psychological Bulletin*, *104*(1), 3–22. https://doi.org/10.1037/0033-2909.104.1.3

Beck, A. T. (1996). Beyond belief: A theory of modes, personality and psychopathology. In P. M. Salkovaskis (Ed.), *Frontiers of cognitive therapy* (pp. 1–25). Guilford.

Beck, A. T. (2005). The current state of cognitive therapy. *Archives of General Psychiatry*, *62*(9), 953. https://doi.org/10.1001/archpsyc.62.9.953

Becker, E. S., Strohbach, D., & Rinck, M. (1999). A specific attentional bias in suicide attempters. *Journal of Nervous and Mental Disease*, *187*, 730–735.

Bertolote, J., & Fleischmann, A. (2015). A global perspective in the epidemiology of suicide. *Suicidologi*, *7*, 6–8. https://doi.org/10.5617/suicidologi.2330

Brent, D. A., & Mann, J. J. (2005). Family genetic studies, suicide, and suicidal behavior. *American Journal of Medical Genetics Part C: Seminars in Medical Genetics*, *133C*(1), 13–24. https://doi.org/10.1002/ajmg.c.30042

Brent, D. A., & Mann, J. J. (2006). Familial pathways to suicidal behavior—Understanding and preventing suicide among adolescents. *The New England Journal of Medicine*, *355*, 2719–2721.

Bridge, J. A., Goldstein, T. R., & Brent, D. A. (2006). Adolescent suicide and suicidal behavior. *Journal of Child Psychology and Psychiatry, and Allied Disciplines*, *47*(3–4), 372–394. https://doi.org/10.1111/j.1469-7610.2006.01615.x

Brodsky, B. S., Malone, K. M., Ellis, S. P., Dulit, R. A., & Mann, J. J. (1997). Characteristics of borderline personality disorder associated with suicidal behavior. *The American Journal of Psychiatry*, *154*(12), 1715–1719. https://doi.org/10.1176/ajp.154.12.1715

Bustamante, F., Ramirez, V., Urquidi, C., Bustos, V., Yaseen, Z., & Galynker, I. (2016). Trends and most frequent methods of suicide in Chile between 2001 and 2010. *Crisis*, *37*(1), 21–30. https://doi.org/10.1027/0227-5910/a000357

Chatard, A., & Selimbegović, L. (2011). When self-destructive thoughts flash through the mind: Failure to meet standards affects the accessibility of suicide-related thoughts. *Journal of Personality and Social Psychology*, *100*(4), 587–605. https://doi.org/10.1037/a0022461

Claassen, C. A., Harvilchuck-Laurenson, J. D., & Fawcett, J. (2014). Prognostic models to detect and monitor the near-term risk of suicide. *American Journal of Preventive Medicine*, *47*(3), S181–S185. https://doi.org/10.1016/j.amepre.2014.06.003

Czyz, E. K., Horwitz, A. G., Arango, A., & King, C. A. (2019). Short-term change and pre-diction of suicidal ideation among adolescents: A daily diary study following psychi-atric hospitalization. *Journal of Child Psychology and Psychiatry, and Allied Disciplines*, 60(7), 732–741. https://doi.org/10.1111/jcpp.12974

Dean, P. J., & Range, L. M. (1999). Testing the escape theory of suicide in an outpatient clinical population. *Cognitive Therapy and Research*, 23, 561–572.

DeLisle, M. M., & Holden, R. R. (2009). Differentiating between depression, hopeless-ness, and psychache in university undergraduates. *Measurement and Evaluation in Counseling and Development*, 42(1), 46–63. https://doi.org/10.1177/074817560 9333562

DeWall, C. N., Baumeister, R. F., & Vohs, K. D. (2008). Satiated with belongingness? Effects of acceptance, rejection, and task framing on self-regulatory performance. *Journal of Personality and Social Psychology*, 95(6), 1367–1382. https://doi.org/10.1037/a0012632

DeWall, C. N., Twenge, J. M., Koole, S. L., Baumeister, R. F., Marquez, A., & Reid, M. W. (2011). Automatic emotion regulation after social exclusion: Tuning to positivity. *Emotion*, 11(3), 623–636. https://doi.org/10.1037/a0023534

Dhingra, K., Boduszek, D., & O'Connor, R. C. (2016). A structural test of the integrated motivational–volitional model of suicidal behavior. *Psychiatry Research*, 239, 169–178. https://doi.org/10.1016/j.psychres.2016.03.023

Ellis, T. (2001). Psychotherapy with suicidal patients. In D. Lester (Ed.), *Suicide preven-tion: Resources for the millennium* (pp. 129–151). Brunner-Routledge.

Flynn, J. J., & Holden, R. R. (2007). Predictors of suicidality in a sample of suicide attempters. *Canadian Psychology*, 48(2a), 317.

Freud, S. (1922). *Beyond the pleasure principle*. International Psycho-Analytical Press.

Gilbert, P., & Allan, S. (1998). The role of defeat and entrapment (arrested flight) in de-pression: An exploration of an evolutionary view. *Psychological Medicine*, 28(3), 585–598. https://doi.org/10.1017/s0033291798006710

Goldstein, R. B., Black, D. W., Nasrallah, A., & Winokur, G. (1991). The prediction of sui-cide: Sensitivity, specificity, and predictive value of a multivariate model applied to sui-cide among 1906 patients with affective disorders. *Archives of General Psychiatry*, 48(5), 418–422. https://doi.org/10.1001/archpsyc.1991.01810290030004

Griffith, J. (2012). Suicide and war: The mediating effects of negative mood, posttraumatic stress disorder symptoms, and social support among Army National Guard soldiers. *Suicide and Life-Threatening Behavior*, 42(4), 453–469. https://doi.org/10.1111/ j.1943-278x.2012.00104.x

Gunn, J. F., Goldstein, S. E., & Gager, C. T. (2018). A longitudinal examination of social connectedness and suicidal thoughts and behaviors among adolescents. *Child and Adolescent Mental Health*, 341–350. https://doi.org/10.1111/camh.12281

Hawton, K., Kingsbury, S., Steinhardt, K., James, A., & Fagg, J. (1999). Repetition of delib-erate self-harm by adolescents: The role of psychological factors. *Journal of adolescence*, 22(3), 369–378. https://doi.org/10.1006/jado.1999.0228

Hewitt, P. L., Flett, G. L., Sherry, S. B., & Caelian, C. (2006). Trait perfectionism and sui-cide behavior. In T. Ellis (Ed.), *Cognition and suicide: Theory, research, and practice* (pp. 215–235). American Psychological Association.

Holden, R. R., Mehta, K., Cunningham, E. J., & McLeod, L. D. (2001). Development and preliminary validation of a scale of psychache. *Canadian Journal of Behavioural Science/Revue canadienne des sciences du comportement*, 33(4), 224–232. https://doi.org/10.1037/h0087144

Horesh, N. (2001). Self-report vs. computerized measures of impulsivity as a correlate of suicidal behavior. *Crisis, 22*, 27–31.

Horesh, N., Gothelf, D., Ofek, H., Weizman, T., & Apter, A. (1999). Impulsivity as a correlate of suicidal behavior in adolescent psychiatric inpatients. *Crisis, 20*(1), 8–14. https://doi.org/10.1027//0227-5910.20.1.8

Hunter, E. C., & O'Connor, R. C. (2003), Hopelessness and future thinking in parasuicide: The role of perfectionism. *British Journal of Clinical Psychology, 42*, 355–365. https://doi.org/10.1348/014466503322528900

Jobes, D. A., & Nelson, K. N. (2006). Shneidman's contributions to the understanding of suicidal thinking. In T. E. Ellis (Ed.), *Cognition and suicide: Theory, research, and therapy* (pp. 29–49). American Psychological Association.

Joiner, T. E., Jr., Van Orden, K. A., Witte, T. K., Cukrowicz, K. C., Braithwaite, S. R., & Selby, E. A. (2010). The interpersonal theory of suicide. *Psychological Review, 117*(2), 575–600. https://doi.org/10.1037/a0018697

Keilp, J. G., Gorlyn, M., Oquendo, M. A., Brodsky, B., Ellis. P., Stanley B., & Mann, J. (2006). Aggressiveness, not impulsiveness or hostility, distinguishes suicide attempters with major depression. *Psychological Medicine, 36*, 1779–1788.

King, C. A., Arango, A., Kramer, A., Busby, D., Czyz, E., Foster, C. E., Gillespie, B. W., & YST Study Team. (2019). Association of the youth-nominated support team intervention for suicidal adolescents with 11- to 14-year mortality outcomes: Secondary analysis of a randomized clinical trial. *JAMA Psychiatry, 76*(5), 492–498. https://doi.org/10.1001/jamapsychiatry.2018.4358

Klein, M. (1935). A contribution to the psychogenesis of manic–depressive states. *International Journal of Psychoanalysis, 16*, 145–174.

Klein, M. (1946). Notes on some schizoid mechanisms. *International Journal of Psychoanalysis, 27*, 99–110.

Klonsky, E. D., & May, A. M. (2015). The three-step theory (3ST): A new theory of suicide rooted in the "ideation-to-action" framework. *International Journal of Cognitive Therapy, 8*(2), 114–129.

Klonsky, E. D., Saffer, B. Y., & Bryan, C. J. (2018). Ideation-to-action theories of suicide: A conceptual and empirical update. *Current Opinion in Psychology, 22*, 38–43.

Litman, R. E., Curphey, T., Shneidman, E. S., Farberow, N. L., & Tabachnik, N. (1963). Investigations of equivocal suicides. *Journal of the American Medical Association, 184*, 924–929. https://doi.org/10.1001/jama.1963.03700250060008

Ma, J., Batterham, P. J., Calear, A. L., & Han, J. (2016). A systematic review of the predictions of the interpersonal–psychological theory of suicidal behavior. *Clinical Psychology Review, 46*, 34–45. https://doi.org/10.1016/j.cpr.2016.04.008

Maiuro, R. D., O'Sullivan, M. J., Michael, M. C., & Vitaliano, P. P. (1989). Anger, hostility, and depression in assaultive vs. suicide-attempting males. *Journal of Clinical Psychology, 45*(4), 531–541. https://doi.org/10.1002/1097-4679(198907)45:43.0.co;2-k

Maltsberger, J. (2004). Descent into suicide. *The International Journal of Psychoanalysis, 85*, 653–667. https://doi.org/10.1516/002075704774200799

Mann, J. J. (2003). Neurobiology of suicidal behaviour. *Nature Reviews Neuroscience, 4*(10), 819–828. https://doi.org/10.1038/nrn1220

Mann, J. J. (2013). The serotonergic system in mood disorders and suicidal behaviour. *Philosophical Transactions of the Royal Society of London. Series B, Biological Sciences, 368*(1615), 20120537. https://doi.org/10.1098/rstb.2012.0537

Mann, J. J., Apter, A., Bertolote, J., Beautrais, A., Currier, D., Haas, A., Hegerl, U., Lonnqvist, J., Malone, K., Marusic, A., Mehlum, L., Patton, G., Phillips, M., Rutz, W., Rihmer, Z., Schmidtke, A., Shaffer, D., Silverman, M., Takahashi, Y., Varnik, A., . . . Hendin, H. (2005). Suicide prevention strategies: A systematic review. *JAMA*, *294*(16), 2064–2074. https://doi.org/10.1001/jama.294.16.2064

Mann, J. J., Arango, V. A., Avenevoli, S., Brent, D. A., Champagne, F. A., Clayton, P., Currier, D., Dougherty, D. M., Haghighi, F., Hodge, S. E., Kleinman, J., Lehner, T., McMahon, F., Mościcki, E. K., Oquendo, M. A., Pandey, G. N., Pearson, J., Stanley, B., Terwilliger, J., & Wenzel, A. (2009). Candidate endophenotypes for genetic studies of suicidal behavior. *Biological Psychiatry*, *65*(7), 556–563. https://doi.org/10.1016/j.biopsych.2008.11.021

Mann, J. J., Waternaux, C., Haas, G. L., & Malone, K. M. (1999). Toward a clinical model of suicidal behavior in psychiatric patients. *The American Journal of Psychiatry*, *156*(2), 181–189. https://doi.org/10.1176/ajp.156.2.181

Melhem, N. M., Brent, D. A., Ziegler, M., Iyengar, S., Kolko, D., Oquendo, M., Birmaher, B., Burke, A., Zelazny, J., Stanley, B., & Mann, J. J. (2007). Familial pathways to early-onset suicidal behavior: Familial and individual antecedents of suicidal behavior. *The American Journal of Psychiatry*, *164*(9), 1364–1370. https://doi.org/10.1176/appi.ajp.2007.06091522

Menninger, K. A. (1938). *Man against himself*. Harcourt, Brace.

Mills, J. F., Green, K., & Reddon, J. R. (2005). An evaluation of the Psychache Scale on an offender population. *Suicide and Life-Threatening Behavior*, *35*(5), 570–580. https://doi.org/10.1521/suli.2005.35.5.570

Miranda, R., Gallagher, M., Bauchner, B., Vaysman, R., & Marroquín, B. (2012). Cognitive inflexibility as a prospective predictor of suicidal ideation among young adults with a suicide attempt history. *Depression and Anxiety*, *29*, 180–186.

Nock, M. K., & Kessler, R. C. (2006). Prevalence of and risk factors for suicide attempts versus suicide gestures: Analysis of the National Comorbidity Survey. *Journal of Abnormal Psychology*, *115*(3), 616–623. https://doi.org/10.1037/0021-843X.115.3.616

Orbach, I. (1996). The role of the body experience in self-destruction. *Clinical Child Psychology and Psychiatry*, *1*(4), 607–619. https://doi.org/10.1177/1359104596014012

Orbach, I. (2003a). Suicide and the suicidal body. Suicide and Life-Threatening *Behavior*, *33*(1), 1–8. https://doi.org/10.1521/suli.33.1.1.22786

Orbach, I. (2003b). Mental pain and suicide. *Israeli Journal of Psychiatry and Related Science*, *40*(3), 191–201.

O'Connor, R. C. (2003). Suicidal behavior as a cry of pain: Test of a psychological model. *Archives of Suicide Research*, *7*(4), 297–308. https://doi.org/10.1080/713848941

O'Connor, R. C. (2011). The integrated motivational–volitional model of suicidal behavior. *Crisis*, *32*(6), 295–298. https://doi.org/10.1027/0227-5910/a000120

O'Connor, R. C., Armitage, C. J., & Gray, L. (2006). The role of clinical and social cognitive variables in parasuicide. *British Journal of Clinical Psychology*, *45*, 465–481

O'Connor, R. C., O'Carroll, R. E., Ryan, C., & Smyth, R. (2012). Self-regulation of unattainable goals in suicide attempters: A two year prospective study. *Journal of Affective Disorders*, *142*, 248–255.

O'Connor, R. C., & O'Connor, D. B. (2003). Predicting hopelessness and psychological distress: The role of perfectionism and coping. *Journal of Counseling Psychology*, *50*(3), 362–372. https://doi.org/10.1037/0022-0167.50.3.362

O'Connor, R. C., Rasmussen, S., & Hawton, K. (2009). Predicting deliberate self-harm in adolescents: A six month prospective study. *Suicide and Life-Threatening Behavior, 39,* 364–375.

O'Connor, R. C., Rasmussen, S., & Hawton, K. (2012). Distinguishing adolescents who think about self-harm from those who engage in self-harm. *British Journal of Psychiatry, 200*(4), 330–335. https://doi.org/10.1192/bjp.bp.111.097808

Öhman, A., & Mineka, S. (2001). Fears, phobias, and preparedness: Toward an evolved module of fear and fear learning. *Psychological Review, 108*(3), 483–522. https://doi.org/10.1037/0033-295X.108.3.483

Oquendo, M. A., Waternaux, C., Brodsky, B., Parsons, B., Haas, G. L., Malone, K. M., & Mann, J. J. (2000). Suicidal behavior in bipolar mood disorder: Clinical characteristics of attempters and nonattempters. *Journal of Affective Disorders, 59*(2), 107–117. https://doi.org/10.1016/s0165-0327(99)00129-9

Patterson, A. A., & Holden, R. R. (2012). Psychache and suicide ideation among men who are homeless: A test of Shneidman's model. *Suicide and Life-Threatening Behavior, 42*(2), 147–156. https://doi.org/10.1111/j.1943-278X.2011.00078.x

Pereira, E. J., Kroner, D. G., Holden, R. R., & Flamenbaum, R. (2010). Testing Shneidman's model of suicidality in incarcerated offenders and in undergraduates. *Personality and Individual Differences, 49*(8), 912–917. https://doi.org/10.1016/j.paid.2010.07.029

Pokorny, A. D. (1983). Prediction of suicide in psychiatric patients. *Archives of General Psychiatry, 40*(3), 249. https://doi.org/10.1001/archpsyc.1983.01790030019002

Pollock, L. R., & Williams, J. M. G. (1998). Problem solving and suicidal behavior. *Suicide and Life-Threatening Behavior, 28,* 375–387.

Pollock, L. R., & Williams, J. M. G. (2001). Effective problem solving in suicide attempters depends on specific autobiographical recall. *Suicide and Life-Threatening Behavior, 31,* 386–396.

Price, J. S., & Sloman, L. (1987). Depression as yielding behavior: An animal model based on Schjelderup-Ebbe's pecking order. *Ethology & Sociobiology, 8*(3 Suppl.), 85–98. https://doi.org/10.1016/0162-3095(87)90021-5

Rudd, M. D. (2006). Fluid vulnerability theory: A cognitive approach to understanding the process of acute and chronic suicide risk. In T. E. Ellis (Ed.), *Cognition and suicide: Theory, research, and therapy* (pp. 355–368). American Psychological Association.

Rudd, M. D., Rajab, M. H., & Dahm, P. F. (1994). Problem-solving appraisal in suicide ideators and attempters. *American Journal of Orthopsychiatry, 64*(1), 136–149. https://doi.org/10.1037/h0079492

Rustein, E. H., & Goldberg, L. (1973). The effects of aggressive stimulation on suicidal patients: An experimental study of the psychoanalytic theory of suicide. In I. Rubinstein (Ed.), *Psychoanalysis and contemporary sciences (vol. 2)* (pp 157–174). Macmillan.

Schotte, D. E., & Clum, G. A. (1987). Problem-solving skills in suicidal psychiatric patients. *Journal of Consulting and Clinical Psychology, 55*(1), 49–54. https://doi.org/10.1037/0022-006x.55.1.49

Shneidman, E. (1993). Suicide as psychache. *Journal of Nervous and Mental Disease, 181,* 147–149.

Solomon, R. L., & Corbit, J. D. (1974). An opponent-process theory of motivation: Temporal dynamics of affect. *Psychological Review, 81*(2), 119–145. https://doi.org/10.1037/h0036128

Surrence, K., Miranda, R., Marroquín, B. M., & Chan, S. (2009). Brooding and reflective rumination among suicide attempters: Cognitive vulnerability to suicidal ideation. *Behaviour Research and Therapy, 47,* 803–808.

Tassava, S. H., & Ruderman, A. J. (1999). Application of escape theory to binge eating and suicidality in college women. *Journal of Social and Clinical Psychology, 18*(4), 450–466. https://doi.org/10.1521/jscp.1999.18.4.450

Tatman, S. M., Greene, A. L., & Karr, L. C. (1993). Use of the Suicide Probability Scale (SPS) with adolescents. *Suicide and Life-Threatening Behavior, 23*(3), 188–203.

Troister, T., & Holden, R. R. (2010). Comparing psychache, depression, and hopelessness in their associations with suicidality: A test of Shneidman's theory of suicide. *Personality and Individual Differences, 49*, 689–693. doi:10.1016/j.paid.2010.06.006

Troister, T., & Holden, R. R. (2012). A two-year prospective study of psychache and its relationship to suicidality among high-risk undergraduates. *Journal of Clinical Psychology, 68*(9), 1019–1027. https://doi.org/10.1002/jclp.21869

Tsai, M., Lari, H., Saffy, S., & Klonsky, E. D. (2021). Examining the three-step theory (3ST) of suicide in a prospective study of adult psychiatric inpatients. *Behavior Therapy, 52*(3), 673–685. https://doi.org/10.1016/j.beth.2020.08.007

Twenge, J. M., Catanese, K. R., & Baumeister, R. F. (2002). Social exclusion causes self-defeating behavior. *Journal of Personality and Social Psychology, 83*(3), 606–615. https://doi.org/10.1037/0022-3514.83.3.606

Twenge, J. M., Catanese, K. R., & Baumeister, R. F. (2003). Social exclusion and the deconstructed state: Time perception, meaninglessness, lethargy, lack of emotion, and self-awareness. *Journal of Personality and Social Psychology, 85*(3), 409–423. https://doi.org/10.1037/0022-3514.85.3.409

Van Orden, K. A., Witte, T. K., Cukrowicz, K. C., Braithwaite, S. R., Selby, E. A., & Joiner, T. E., Jr. (2010). The interpersonal theory of suicide. *Psychological Review, 117*(2), 575–600. https://doi.org/10.1037/a0018697

Warburton, K., & Lazarus, J. (1991). Tendency-distance models of social cohesion in animal groups. *Journal of Theoretical Biology, 150*(4), 473–488. https://doi.org/10.1016/s0022-5193(05)80441-2

Wenzel, A., & Beck, A. T. (2008). A cognitive model of suicidal behavior: Theory and treatment. *Applied and Preventive Psychology, 12*, 189–201.

Williams, J. M. G. (1997). *Cry of pain: Understanding suicide and self-harm.* Penguin.

Williams, J. M. G., Barnhofer, T., Crane, C., Herman, D., Raes, F., Watkins, E., & Dalgleish, T. (2007). Autobiographical memory specificity and emotional disorder. *Psychological Bulletin, 133*(1), 122–148. https://doi.org/10.1037/0033-2909.133.1.122

Witte, T. K., Merrill, K. A., Stellrecht, N. E., Bernert, R. A., Hollar, D. L., Schatschneider, C., & Joiner, T. E., Jr. (2008). "Impulsive" youth suicide attempters are not necessarily all that impulsive. *Journal of Affective Disorders, 107*, 107–116.

Woznica, J. G., & Shapiro, J. R. (1990). An analysis of adolescent suicide attempts: The expendable child. *Journal of Pediatric Psychology, 15*, 789–796. https://doi.org/10.1093/jpepsy/15.6.789

Yang, L., Liu, X., Chen, W., & Li, L. (2019). A test of the three-step theory of suicide among Chinese people: A study based on the ideation-to-action framework. *Archives of Suicide Research, 23*, 648–661. https://doi.org/10.1080/13811118.2018.1497563

3

The Narrative-Crisis Model of Suicide

Introduction

The narrative-crisis model of suicide (NCM), developed by our research group, provides a conceptual framework for imminent suicide risk evaluation. The NCM is a multistage diathesis-stress model of suicide that integrates empirically validated chronic, subacute, and acute risk factors for suicidal behavior. In the NCM, suicide is considered a self-destructive act taken in the context of highly pathological affective-cognitive mental state called the suicide crisis syndrome (SCS). SCS represents the final stage of the NCM, preceded by a culmination of mental processes in the presence of stressful life events (SLEs) and trait vulnerabilities.

The NCM is not a theoretical model of suicide; it is a practical model. The NCM was formulated based on decades of the author's clinical experience working with acutely suicidal patients and was later supported by rigorous experimental evidence (Bloch-Elkouby et al., 2020; Cohen et al., 2018). The NCM is considered a fourth-generation model of suicide because it reconceptualizes the third-generation models' mental processes that make suicide possible and conceives of the processes as preventable and treatable psychiatric syndromes.

The NCM uniquely adds to the previous models of suicide by formulating criteria for suicide-specific psychiatric diagnoses, such as SCS, to be included in the *Diagnostic and Statistical Manual of Psychiatric Disorders* (DSM) and to be used as targets for psychopharmacological and psychotherapeutic interventions. The construct validity, predictive validity, and clinical utility of the diagnoses are being tested experimentally.

In order to develop a more comprehensive understanding of the NCM, it is important to appreciate two key contrasts: trait versus state risk factors and static versus dynamic risk factors. The interplay of these factors critically shapes the development of the mental process that lead to suicide.

Trait versus State Risk Factors

When assessing for risk of imminent suicide, it is important to appreciate the difference between trait (long-term) and state (short-term) markers of suicide risk. Although there is no universally accepted definition of trait factors, the term generally refers to enduring and stable characteristics of the individual's interaction with the world, which may include genetic predisposition, temperament, and personality (Goldston et al., 2006). For example, some people may have persistently high levels of hopelessness and anxiety, regardless of life circumstances, while others may remain hopeful and calm even in times of extreme stress.

In contrast, state factors are considered transient and generally fluctuate with time. In the context of suicide risk assessment, state characteristics typically refer to mood, anxiety, thought content, and thought process, all of which may change either spontaneously or as a reaction to SLEs over periods of time ranging from minutes to weeks.

Some SLEs, such as childhood adversity, can result in both state and trait changes in suicide risk. Victims of childhood emotional, physical, and/or sexual abuse often suffer severe episodic "state" anxiety and depression coinciding with the abuse. Later on in life, the same childhood adversities carry the risk of significant long-lasting increases in suicidal behavior in adults (Bruwer et al., 2014). It has been suggested that these stress-related state factors can cause epigenetic changes and are therefore trait risk factors that may even be heritable (Labonte & Turecki, 2012).

The NCM considers the immediate psychological effects of childhood adversity to be state (short-term) phenomena and views the distal, lifelong consequences as trait (long-term) risk. In the same vein, the NCM views a person's societal and religious values, typically established in childhood, as trait phenomena with regard to suicidal behavior.

Overall, in the NCM, long-term risk factors for suicide comprise enduring and stable characteristics of the individual's interaction with the world that make them susceptible to suicide. This broad construct includes the cognitive dispositional vulnerability factors postulated by Beck's diathesis-stress model, the biological diathesis of low levels of serotonin/norepinephrine and impulsive aggression of Mann's model, the epigenetic factors related to childhood trauma, and entrenched societal, cultural, and religious norms.

Static versus Dynamic Risk Factors

The newer construct of static versus dynamic risk factors for suicide resembles and partly overlaps with the older construct of state versus trait risk factors, although the two are not identical. While both dichotomies contrast long-term and short-term clinical phenomena, the trait factors of the state–trait dichotomy refer to personality and neurobiology, whereas the static factors of the static–dynamic dichotomy pertain to demographic characteristics and elements of past psychiatric history that are known to be associated with increased long-term suicide risk. According to this new framework, the demographic static vulnerability factors include age, sex, race, ethnicity, socioeconomic status, and geographic location. The most significant static risks are a history of psychiatric illness and a remote history of suicide by the patient, family member, or a close friend. Childhood trauma, abuse, and neglect, as well as maladaptive parenting styles, are both static and trait risk factors for suicidal behavior (Bouch & Marshall, 2005).

On the other hand, dynamic risk factors are variables that encompass life stressors and/or an individual's psychological or behavioral responses to those stressors. Unlike most static risk factors, dynamic risk factors are modifiable and may fluctuate in both duration and intensity (Bouch & Marshall, 2005). Common dynamic life event risk factors are socioeconomic, such as job loss or eviction, and interpersonal stressors, usually involving either romantic rejection or control with peers or family. While the life stressors themselves are considered dynamic risk factors, the responses associated with these stressors also fall under the umbrella of dynamic risk. Examples of dynamic response risk factors include substance abuse, exacerbation of a psychiatric illness, neglected friendships, and/or abandoned hobbies, as well as preparatory actions and suicide attempts (Claassen et al., 2014).

Static and trait factors for suicide are so distal to suicidal behavior that they have become enduring personal characteristics and are referred to as trait vulnerabilities. Trait vulnerabilities remain stable over time and are associated with long-term suicide risk. In the NCM, they are most often referred to as long-term or chronic risk factors. In contrast, the state and dynamic risk factors are transient psychological and physiologic phenomena that are very proximal to suicidal behavior. The state risk factors are acute characteristics that last days, hours, or minutes, and are therefore discussed and assessed as part of the acute SCS. Dynamic risk factors, on the other hand, are somewhat longer in duration and may form the foundation of the narrative identity;

consequently, they are discussed in relation to the subacute suicidal narrative (SN).

The Narrative-Crisis Model: Overview

The NCM posits that when individuals with trait vulnerabilities for suicide (i.e., long-term or chronic risk factors) encounter SLEs, they may develop maladaptive views of themselves and the world around them. These views, collectively characterizing a SN, culminate in a perception of having no future and increase the likelihood of reaching a suicidal crisis. Thus, the model has three components: long-term risk factors, the SN, and SCS (see Figure 3.1).

Long-Term Risk Factors

The NCM posits that people who transition through the mental states that precede a suicide attempt likely have a heightened baseline vulnerability for suicide. This heightened vulnerability is defined by the presence of long-term or chronic risk factors for suicidal behavior. These include static historical

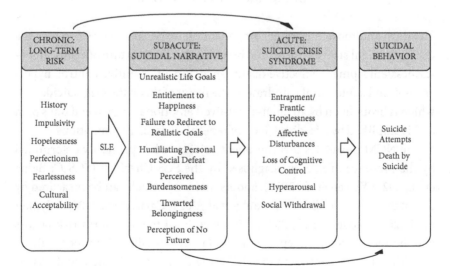

Figure 3.1 Narrative-crisis model of suicide (NCM).

risk factors, such as genetics and family history, childhood adversity, history of suicide in the family, or history of mental illness, which are both relatively stable over time and distal to the acute suicidal behavior. In addition, the long-term risk factor construct included in the NCM incorporates temperamentally related trait factors, such as perfectionism, fearlessness, and pessimism, as well as cultural and social factors, such as societal acceptability or approval of suicide as a solution to life's problems.

The Suicidal Narrative

The second component of the NCM is derived from the theory of narrative identity, which postulates that individuals "form their identity by integrating their life experiences into an internalized evolving story of self, which gives people the sense of wholeness and purpose in life" (McAdams, 2001, p. 100). The NCM posits that suicidal individuals feel entrapped in their life narrative, which they perceive as having a worthless past, intolerable present, and no acceptable future. Together, these perceptions characterize a SN, the subacute stage of the NCM. Although the content of the SN differs from person to person, the story arc remains relatively constant.

The Suicide Crisis Syndrome

The third and most important component of the NCM is the SCS, which is a distinct mental state characterized by an unbearable mixture of frantic hopelessness/entrapment, affective disturbance, loss of cognitive control, hyperarousal, and acute social withdrawal. The result of this state is the suicidal act, which is brought on by an often-short-lived emotional urge to end one's pain and is amplified by a feedback loop of repetitive circular ruminations.

The NCM postulates that imminent suicide risk is primarily determined by the presence of SCS, as diagnosed by the SCS Checklist (SCS-C; Bafna et al., 2022; Yaseen et al., 2019), and its intensity, which can be measured by one of the SCI scales (Bloch-Elkouby et al., 2021; Calati et al., 2020; Galynker et al., 2017; Rogers et al., 2021). However, both the long-term risk factors and the SN contribute independently and incrementally to imminent suicide risk. Therefore, according to the NCM, the overall imminent suicide risk is ultimately determined by the presence and intensity of all three components.

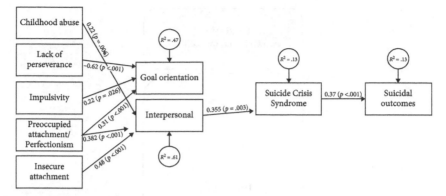

Figure 3.2 Structural equation modeling analysis of NCM in predicting near-term suicidal behavior (Bloch-Elkouby et al., 2020; Rogers et al., 2020).

To date, the components of the NCM have been supported by over 10 different studies, sampling from diverse patient populations and conducted using a variety of statistical approaches. Of note, three studies supported the validity of the NCM in predicting near-term suicidal behavior as a complete model. The most compelling of these is the structural equation modeling analysis by Bloch-Elkouby et al. (2020), further supported by the ruminative flooding analyses by Rogers et al. (2021; Figure 3.2). The data for these studies were collected at three different times, which made possible the analysis of the model components sequence.

Each NCM component has several elements, all of which have been shown in various research studies to correlate with different aspects of suicidal ideation (SI) and behavior. The specific elements of each component in the NCM are outlined in the sections that follow.

The Long-Term Risk Component

The long-term or chronic risk component of the NCM, as shown in Figure 3.3, draws conceptually from Beck and Mann's well-researched models of suicidal behavior, which show discriminant validity for past suicidal behavior and long-term suicide risk. Specifically, Beck's diathesis describes stress dispositional vulnerability factors that make one susceptible to SCS even under low levels of stress. He defined five main stress dispositional vulnerability factors: (1) impulsivity, (2) deficits in problem-solving, (3) an overgeneral memory style,

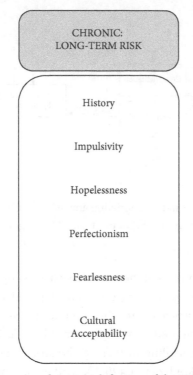

Figure 3.3 The long-term or chronic risk factors of the NCM.

(4) maladaptive cognitive style, and (5) personality (Wenzel & Beck, 2008). Two of these, impulsivity and personality, are biological temperament factors that are also the centerpieces of Mann's stress-diathesis model, as discussed in Chapter 2. The other three, deficits in problem-solving, an overgeneral memory style, and maladaptive cognitive style, are abnormalities in cognitive processes best considered within Beck's cognitive-behavioral approach.

Most of these vulnerability factors either have not been tested for predictive validity of near-term suicidal behavior or have only been predictive long term. However, their sensitivity to past behavior suggests that they could be used as auxiliary factors in making clinical decisions based on the intensity of the acute suicidal crisis. It seems intuitive that the trait vulnerability factors moderate the intensity of the SCS, but this relationship is yet to be tested experimentally.

As discussed in Chapter 2 long-term risk factors include static or trait factors, and the association between these factors and increased risk for imminent suicide was supported by credible experimental evidence.

Stressful Life Events

Because SLEs are external to the mental processes that contribute to suicide, they are not explicitly included as a core part of the NCM. However, SLEs are associated with both SCS and the SN (Cohen et al., 2022), and therefore they are included in this chapter and are discussed in more detail in Chapter 4. Moreover, this topic is of particular relevance in the context of the COVID-19 pandemic, during which SLEs have acutely intensified at a global level (Jean-Baptiste et al., 2020; Mousavi et al., 2020; Rossi et al., 2020). Prior to the pandemic, multiple studies found significant links between SLEs and suicide attempts (Farahbakhsh et al., 2020; McFeeters et al., 2015; Pompili et al., 2011) and death by suicide (Buchman-Schmitt et al., 2017; Coope et al., 2015; Fjeldsted et al., 2017).

The SLEs that correlate most with suicide deaths are financial problems (Coope et al., 2015; Farahbakhsh et al., 2020), family conflicts (Overholser et al., 2012), divorce, being a victim of violence, and imprisonment (Fjeldsted et al., 2017). Other commonly identified SLEs associated with suicide attempts are related to interpersonal conflict, specifically with spouses, romantic partners, family members, and friends (Bagge et al., 2013; Farahbakhsh et al., 2020; Liu et al., 2019).

During the COVID-19 pandemic, the association between SLEs and SCS was three times stronger than the relationship between SLEs and SI (Rogers et al., under review). In this study, relationship-related and role/identity-related stressors were consistently linked to SCS cross-nationally. Thus, SLEs before and during the COVID pandemic appear to have a strong association with imminent risk; this topic is reviewed in detail in Chapter 4.

The Suicidal Narrative: The Subacute Component

The SN component of the NCM describes the dynamic psychological processes of a subacute suicidal state (Figure 3.4). According to the NCM, these subacute psychological processes emerge when individuals with long-term trait vulnerabilities for suicide encounter SLEs. It is at this stage that a SN develops, evolving into the feelings, thoughts, and behaviors that bring on the acute suicidal crisis and the associated high imminent suicide risk. The SN is hypothesized as a subacute state, lasting days to weeks, and this hypothesis is currently being tested experimentally.

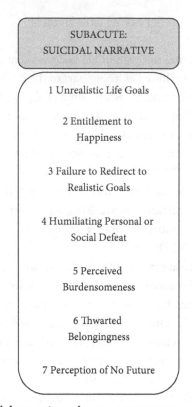

Figure 3.4 The suicidal narrative subacute component.

The SN construct focuses on the formation and power of the SN identity as a prerequisite for the development of SCS. The SN is also related to David Jobes' "drivers" approach to suicide risk. According to Jobes' theories, each suicidal person's story has to be examined for drivers, which are the uniquely meaningful events or thought patterns that "drive" the suicidal process of each suicidal individual. According to Jobes, the life stories of suicidal people are different, and so are the drivers (Jobes, 2012). The SN construct posits that all drivers have common elements, which form a characteristic life narrative arc applicable to most suicidal individuals. In fact, in the NCM, it is exactly the life narrative arc of suicidal individuals that is termed the SN.

The SN arc evolves through the following components:

Phase 1: Unrealistic life goals
Phase 2: Entitlement to happiness

Phase 3: Failure to redirect to more realistic goals
Phase 4: Humiliating personal or social defeat
Phase 5: Perceived burdensomeness
Phase 6: Thwarted belongingness
Phase 7: Perception of no future

The popular psychological theory of narrative identity, which inspired the term *suicidal narrative*, has received strong empirical support (Bauer et al., 2005; King & Hicks, 2007; Lodi-Smith et al., 2009; McLean et al., 2007; Pals, 2006; Pasupathi, 2001; Woike & Polo, 2001). The theory postulates that each person's identity is formed through the integration of their life experiences into an internalized, evolving story of the self that gives the individual a sense of wholeness and purpose in life (McAdams, 2001). This life narrative integrates one's reconstructed past, perceived present, and imagined future. The suicidal person's narrative evolves into one where the past narrative of one's life leads to a present that is so intolerable that the future becomes either irrelevant or unimaginable and suicide becomes a viable option.

While individual SNs are unique to particular suicidal individuals, many of the life plots and subplots that form SN arcs are variations of just a few themes, centered on general kinds of SLEs. The most common stressors are romantic rejection, threat to one's ego and identity, catastrophic financial losses, new-onset serious medical illness, intractable mental illness, and bullying (Cohen et al., 2022). Of note, SLEs may mediate the transition from a chronic to a subacute suicidal state (Figure 3.5). Research is underway to establish if certain types of SLEs may lead to specific components of SN, which may allow for future integration of distinct types of SLEs into the NCM.

At present, researchers believe that when individuals with trait vulnerability for suicide live through stressful experiences, they go through a progression of distinct affective states, some of which have been postulated in prior affective models of suicide. One of the most prominent frameworks to incorporate affective suicidal states is the arrested flight model (Williams, 2000), which emphasizes feelings of humiliation, defeat, and entrapment. Another notable example is the interpersonal model, which highlights perceived burdensomeness and thwarted belongingness as proximal mental states in suicidal individuals (Joiner et al., 2010).

According to the NCM, the central feature of the SN is that it views individual affective states and processes described in other models as a narrative

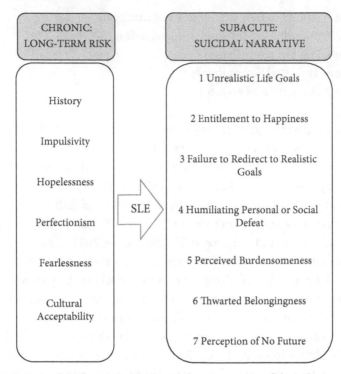

Figure 3.5 Stressful life events (SLE) and the emergence of the subacute suicidal state.

arc, culminating in the cognitive perception of a dead end and the emotional experience of entrapment. Most elements of the SN included in NCM have been shown to have some association with indices of suicidal behavior (Brown et al., 1995; Claassen et al., 2014; DeWall et al., 2008; Gilbert & Allan, 1998; Hendin et al., 2001; Morrison & O'Connor, 2008; O'Connor et al., 2012; Van Orden et al., 2012; Yaseen et al., 2012). Research establishing the cohesiveness of the SN construct, as well as its incremental predictive validity in determining imminent suicide risk, is currently underway, and early results lend support for SN as a cohesive construct (Chistopolskaya et al., 2020; Menon et al., 2022).

According to the NCM, the last phase of the SN, the feeling of being trapped in an intolerable dead-end life situation, from which the only escape is death, results in the emergence of the third component of the NCM: SCS.

The Suicide Crisis Syndrome: The Acute Component

In the NCM, suicidal behavior occurs when a person develops the distinct suicidal mental state called the SCS. SCS is a high-intensity negative mental state, characterized by symptoms of cognitive and affective dysregulation and an overwhelming sense of entrapment. The model further posits that both the diagnosable presence and the intensity of the suicide crisis is predictive of near-term suicidal behavior, and that SCS components are the most immediate indicators of imminent suicide risk.

The SCS component of the NCM stems from our earlier work on the acute suicide trigger state as well as our early positive-feedback model of suicide (Galynker et al., 2015; Katz et al., 2011; Rappaport et al., 2014; Yaseen et al., 2010, 2012a, 2012b, 2013, 2014, 2016).

Building on the "suicidal crisis" and "psychic pain" constructs of Shneidman, Baumeister, Fawcett, Hendin, and others, we have designed and tested several iterations of the Suicide Crisis Inventory (SCI), a self-report inventory developed to measure the emotions and cognitions constituting the SCS. Although some replication work is still ongoing, the most recent analyses of the data obtained in the United States, Europe, Asia, and Latin America suggest that the SCS consists of five distinct but correlated negative affective-cognitive states: frantic hopelessness/entrapment, affective disturbance, loss of cognitive control, hyperarousal, and acute social withdrawal (Bafna et al., 2022; Calati et al., 2020; Park et al., under review; Schuck et al., 2019).

SCS, defined by these five primarily affective factors, is a transient condition, and among high-risk psychiatric inpatients hospitalized for suicidal risk, its intensity may change significantly from admission to discharge. The SCS reflects the affective instability of the suicidal crisis more acutely than both trait and state anxiety, which remain constant throughout a hospital stay. Predictably, the SCS magnitude at admission correlates with suicidal behavior proximal to the admission. SCS intensity prior to discharge is less reflective of the proximal pre-admission suicidal behavior but correlates strongly with imminent suicidal behavior within a month after hospital discharge (Galynker et al., 2017). Thus, the SCS appears to be a true and sensitive marker of the suicidal crisis. Further research is needed to determine whether the NCM, the SCS-C, or the SCI short or long forms can be used to track suicidal risk over time.

Model Flexibility: Narrative-Driven versus Crisis-Driven Suicidal Behaviors

As discussed in this chapter thus far, the NCM posits that when people with trait vulnerability to suicide are faced with SLEs, they are likely to view their sense of identity as a dead-end SN, which in turn may bring on a suicidal crisis. Although this hypothesis has not been tested for the SN as a whole, it has been supported for the SN elements that the model shares with the integrated motivational-volitional (IMV) model and interpersonal theory of suicide (IPTS), such as burdensomeness and humiliating defeat (Buitron et al., 2016; Lockman & Servaty-Seib, 2015; Siddaway et al., 2015).

The relative contribution of the SN and SCS components to overall suicide risk depends on the coherence and power of an individual SN and on an individual's affective instability. For some individuals, their SN may be so compelling that it serves as the primary force in bringing on suicidal behavior, even in the presence of minimal affective instability. The result is meticulously planned, low-failure suicides. Suicides of individuals with unrelenting terminal illness or those facing certain torture and/or death in captivity are examples of such narrative-driven suicides (see Figure 3.1, bottom arrow).

Alternatively, a person with high affective lability could attempt, and die by, suicide after suffering a suicidal crisis, even if his or her SN is transient and reactive to an intense but short-lived life stressor. Examples of such crisis-driven suicides would be a response to business failure by somebody in a mixed manic state, or a response to romantic rejection by somebody with depression and borderline personality disorder (see Figure 3.1, top arrow), or a response to a seemingly trivial family conflict by an adolescent.

Thus, the NCM is flexible enough to explain several types of suicidal behaviors, from the premeditated narrative-driven to the impulsive and crisis-driven. Moreover, the model can accommodate several different kinds of narrative-driven suicides, depending on the relative intensity of different narrative components. All SNs conclude in a dead end, but the entry points into the narrative may differ from person to person depending on the nature of their life stressors.

For example, consider the narratives of two adolescents. The first is a first-generation immigrant student from a country where honor suicide is accepted culturally (for instance, Japan): the student's GPA is too low for a medical career, and he feels that he has disgraced his family. His narrative is different from that of the second adolescent, a high school student who is being bullied and ostracized for being "weird." The former may be described as a perfectionism-failure-burden narrative, while the latter is driven primarily by social defeat and thwarted belongingness. In both scenarios, individuals with trait vulnerability may feel that they have run out of options and develop an acute suicidal crisis.

Conclusion

This book is anchored in the comprehensive NCM.

Proposed as a fourth-generation model of suicidal behavior, the NCM integrates various well-established long-term and short-term risk factors into a coherent clinical diagnosis. The diagnostic criteria for SCS have been developed and tested over time, and the current formulation of SCS diagnosis is currently under consideration by the DSM steering committee for inclusion in DSM as a suicide-specific diagnosis. Both the diagnosis of SCS and SCS severity are directly predictive of imminent suicidal behavior and confer a short-term suicide risk. The SN provides a framework for the analysis of the psychological processes leading to the development of SCS in those with long-term vulnerability for suicide. The long-term risk component roughly corresponds to traditional chronic risk factors and therefore confers chronic suicide risk.

To date, solid experimental evidence supports the structure of the NCM and its components (Bloch-Elkouby et al., 2020; Cohen et al., 2018, 2022). This includes the association of long-term risk factors with chronic suicide risk and of the SCS with the imminent risk for suicide. The validity of the SN and its diagnostic components, as well as the related IMV and IPST models, in predicting suicidal behavior is under active investigation.

Overall, to the author's knowledge, the NCM is the only model of suicide that has gained empirical support in predicting near-term suicidal behavior, over other measures of traditional risk factors such as lifetime suicidal ideation (Bloch-Elkouby et al., 2020; Cohen et al., 2018, 2022). The NCM provides a coherent and clear framework for comprehensive assessment of critical aspects of suicidal behavior that have incremental input into imminent risk. Systematic use of the NCM for imminent risk assessment will ensure that no risk factor has been overlooked and at the same time will provide treatable targets for clinical intervention.

References

Bafna, A., Rogers, M. L., & Galynker, I. I. (2022). Predictive validity and symptom configuration of proposed diagnostic criteria for the Suicide Crisis Syndrome: A replication study. *Journal of Psychiatric Research*, *156*, 228–235. Advance online publication. https://doi.org/10.1016/j.jpsychires.2022.10.027

Bagge, C. L., Glenn, C. R., & Lee, H. J. (2013). Quantifying the impact of recent negative life events on suicide attempts. *Journal of Abnormal Psychology*, *122*(2), 359–368. https://doi.org/10.1037/a0030371

Bauer, J. J., McAdams, D. P., & Sakaeda, A. R. (2005). Interpreting the good life: Growth memories in the lives of mature, happy people. *Journal of Personality and Social Psychology*, *88*(1), 203–217. https://doi.org/10.1037/0022-3514.88.1.203

Bloch-Elkouby, S., Barzilay, S., Gorman, B., Lawrence, O. C., Rogers, M. L., Richards, J., Cohen, L., Johnson, B. N., & Galynker, I. (2021). The revised Suicide Crisis Inventory (SCI-2): Validation and assessment of near-term suicidal ideation and attempts. *Journal of Affective Disorders*, *295*, 1280–1291. https://doi.org/10.1016/j.jad.2021.08.048

Bloch-Elkouby, S., Gorman, B., Lloveras, L., Wilkerson, T., Schuck, A., Barzilay, S., Calati, R., Schnur, D., & Galynker, I. (2020). How do distal and proximal risk factors combine to predict suicidal ideation and behaviors? A prospective study of the narrative crisis model of suicide. *Journal of Affective Disorders*, *277*, 914–926.

Bouch, J., & Marshall, J. (2005). Suicide risk: Structured professional judgement. *Advances in Psychiatric Treatment*, *11*(2), 84–91. https://doi.org/10.1192/apt.11.2.84

Brown, G. W., Harris, T. O., & Hepworth, C. (1995). Loss, humiliation and entrapment among women developing depression: A patient and non-patient comparison. *Psychological Medicine*, *25*(1), 7–21.

Bruwer, B., Govender, R., Bishop, M., Williams, D. R., Stein, D. J., & Seedat, S. (2014). Association between childhood adversities and long-term suicidality among South Africans from the results of the South African Stress and Health study: A cross-sectional study. *BMJ Open*, *4*(6), e004644. https://doi.org/10.1136/bmjopen-2013-004644

Buchman-Schmitt, J. M., Chu, C., Michaels, M. S., Hames, J. L., Silva, C., Hagan, C. R., Ribeiro, J. D., Selby, E. A., & Joiner, T. E. (2017). The role of stressful life events preceding death by suicide: Evidence from two samples of suicide decedents. *Psychiatry Research*, *256*, 345–352. https://doi.org/10.1016/j.psychres.2017.06.078

Buitron, V., Hill, R. M., Pettit, J. W., Green, K. L., Hatkevich, C., & Sharp, C. (2016). Interpersonal stress and suicidal ideation in adolescence: An indirect association through perceived burdensomeness toward others. *Journal of Affective Disorders*, *190*, 143–149. https://doi.org/10.1016/j.jad.2015.09.077

Calati, R., Cohen, L. J., Schuck, A., Levy, D., Bloch-Elkouby, S., Barzilay, S., Rosenfield, P. J., & Galynker, I. (2020). The Modular Assessment of Risk for Imminent Suicide (MARIS): A validation study of a novel tool for suicide risk assessment. *Journal of Affective Disorders*, *263*, 121–128. https://doi.org/10.1016/j.jad.2019.12.001

Chistopolskaya, K. A., Rogers, M. L., Cao, E., Galynker, I., Richards, J., Enikolopov, S. N., Nikolaev, E. L., Sadovnichaya, V. S., & Drovosekov, S. E. (2020). Adaptation of the Suicidal Narrative Inventory in a Russian sample. *Suicidology*, *11*(4), 76–90. https://doi.org/10.32878/suiciderus.20-11-04(41)-76-90

Claassen, C. A., Harvilchuck-Laurenson, J. D., & Fawcett, J. (2014). Prognostic models to detect and monitor the near-term risk of suicide. *American Journal of Preventive Medicine*, *47*(3), S181–S185. https://doi.org/10.1016/j.amepre.2014.06.003

Cohen, L. J., Ardalan, F., Yaseen, Z., & Galynker, I. (2018). Suicide crisis syndrome mediates the relationship between long-term risk factors and lifetime suicidal phenomena. *Suicide and Life-Threatening Behavior, 48*, 613–623. https://doi.org/10.1111/sltb.12387

Cohen, L. J., Gorman, B., Briggs, J., Jeon, M., Ginsburg, T., & Galynker, I. (2019). The suicidal narrative and its relationship to the suicide crisis syndrome and recent suicidal behavior. *Suicide and Life-Threatening Behavior, 49*, 413–422. https://doi.org/10.1111/sltb.12439

Cohen, L. J., Mokhtar, R., Richards, J., Hernandez, M., Bloch-Elkouby, S., & Galynker, I. (2022). The narrative-crisis model of suicide and its prediction of near-term suicide risk. *Suicide and Life-Threatening Behavior, 52*(2), 231–243. https://doi.org/ 10.1111/sltb.12816

Coope, C., Donovan, J., Wilson, C., Barnes, M., Metcalfe, C., Hollingworth, W., Kapur, N., Hawton, K., & Gunnell, D. (2015). Characteristics of people dying by suicide after job loss, financial difficulties and other economic stressors during a period of recession (2010–2011): A review of coroners' records. *Journal of Affective Disorders, 183*, 98–105. https://doi.org/10.1016/j.jad.2015.04.045

DeWall, C. N., Baumeister, R. F., & Vohs, K. D. (2008). Satiated with belongingness? Effects of acceptance, rejection, and task framing on self-regulatory performance. *Journal of Personality and Social Psychology, 95*(6), 1367–1382. https://doi.org/10.1037/a0012632

Farahbakhsh, M., Fakhari, A., Davtalab Esmaeili, E., Azizi, H., Mizapour, M., Asl Rahimi, V., & Hashemi, L. (2020). The role and comparison of stressful life events in suicide and suicide attempt: A descriptive-analytical study. *Iranian Journal of Psychiatry and Behavioral Sciences, 14*(2), e96051. https://doi.org/10.5812/ijpbs.96051

Fjeldsted, R., Teasdale, T. W., Jensen, M., & Erlangsen, A. (2017). Suicide in relation to the experience of stressful life events: A population-based study. *Archives of Suicide Research, 21*(4), 544–555. https://doi.org/10.1080/13811118.2016.1259596

Galynker, I. I., Yaseen, Z. S., Briggs, J., & Hayashi, F. (2015). Attitudes of acceptability and lack of condemnation toward suicide may be predictive of post-discharge suicide attempts. *BMC Psychiatry, 15*(1), 87. https://doi.org/10.1186/s12888-015-0462-5

Galynker, I., Yaseen, Z. S., Cohen, A., Benhamou, O., Hawes, M., & Briggs, J. (2017). Prediction of suicidal behavior in high risk psychiatric patients using an assessment of acute suicidal state: The Suicide Crisis Inventory. *Depression and Anxiety, 34*(2), 147–158. https://doi.org/10.1002/da.22559

Gilbert, P., & Allan, S. (1998). The role of defeat and entrapment (arrested flight) in depression: An exploration of an evolutionary view. *Psychological Medicine, 28*(3), 585–598. https://doi.org/10.1017/s0033291798006710

Goldston, D. B., Reboussin, B. A., & Daniel, S. S. (2006). Predictors of suicide attempts: State and trait components. *Journal of Abnormal Psychology, 115*, 842–849.

Hendin, H., Maltsberger, J. T., Lipschitz, A., Haas, A. P., & Kyle, J. (2001). Recognizing and responding to a suicide crisis. *Suicide and Life-Threatening Behavior, 31*(2), 115–128. https://doi.org/10.1521/suli.31.2.115.21515

Jean-Baptiste, C. O., Herring, R. P., Beeson, W. L., Dos Santos, H., & Banta, J. E. (2020). Stressful life events and social capital during the early phase of COVID-19 in the U.S. *Social Sciences & Humanities Open, 2*(1), 100057. https://doi.org/10.1016/j.ssaho.2020.100057

Jobes D. A. (2012). The Collaborative Assessment and Management of Suicidality (CAMS): An evolving evidence-based clinical approach to suicidal risk. *Suicide and Life-Threatening Behavior, 42*(6), 640–653. https://doi.org/10.1111/j.1943-278X.2012.00119.x

Joiner, T. E., Jr., Van Orden, K. A., Witte, T. K., Cukrowicz, K. C., Braithwaite, S. R., & Selby, E. A. (2010). The interpersonal theory of suicide. *Psychological Review*, *117*(2), 575–600. https://doi.org/10.1037/a0018697

Katz, C., Yaseen, Z. S., Mojtabai, R., Cohen, L. J., & Galynker, I. I. (2011). Panic as an independent risk factor for suicide attempt in depressive illness. *Journal of Clinical Psychiatry*, *72*(12), 1628–1635. https://doi.org/10.4088/jcp.10m06186blu

King, L. A., & Hicks, J. A. (2007). Whatever happened to "What might have been"? Regrets, happiness, and maturity. *American Psychologist*, *62*(7), 625–636. https://doi.org/10.1037/0003-066X.62.7.625

Labonte, B., & Turecki, G. (2012). Epigenetic effects of childhood adversity in the brain and suicide risk. In Y. Dwivedi (Ed.), *The neurobiological basis of suicide* (pp. 275–296). Taylor & Francis/CRC Press.

Liu, B. P., Zhang, J., Chu, J., Qiu, H. M., Jia, C. X., & Hennessy, D. A. (2019). Negative life events as triggers on suicide attempt in rural China: A case-crossover study. *Psychiatry Research*, *276*, 100–106. https://doi.org/10.1016/j.psychres.2019.04.008

Lockman, J. D., & Servaty-Seib, H. L. (2016). College student suicidal ideation: Perceived burdensomeness, thwarted belongingness, and meaning made of stress. *Death Studies*, *40*(3), 154–164. https://doi.org/10.1080/07481187.2015.1105325

Lodi-Smith, J., Geise, A. C., Roberts, B. W., & Robins, R. W. (2009). Narrating personality change. *Journal of Personality and Social Psychology*, *96*(3), 679–689. https://doi.org/10.1037/a0014611

McAdams, D. P. (2001). The psychology of life stories. *Review of General Psychology*, *5*(2), 100.

McFeeters, D., Boyda, D., & O'Neill, S. (2015). Patterns of stressful life events: Distinguishing suicide ideators from suicide attempters. *Journal of Affective Disorders*, *175*, 192–198. https://doi.org/10.1016/j.jad.2014.12.034

McLean, K. C., Pasupathi, M., & Pals, J. L. (2007). Selves creating stories creating selves: A process model of self-development. *Personality and Social Psychology Review*, *11*(3), 262–278. https://doi.org/10.1177/1088868307301034

Menon, V., Bafna, A. R., Rogers, M. L., Richards, J., & Galynker, I. (2022). Factor structure and validity of the Revised Suicide Crisis Inventory (SCI-2) among Indian adults. *Asian Journal of Psychiatry*, *73*, 103119. https://doi.org/10.1016/j.ajp.2022.103119

Morrison, R., & O'Connor, R. C. (2008). A systematic review of the relationship between rumination and suicidality. *Suicide and Life-Threatening Behavior*, *38*(5), 523–538.

Mousavi, S. A. M., Hooshyari, Z., & Ahmadi, A. (2020). The most stressful events during the COVID-19 epidemic. *Iranian Journal of Psychiatry*, *15*(3), 220–227. https://doi.org/10.18502/ijps.v15i3.3814

O'Connor, R. C. (2007). The relations between perfectionism and suicidality: A systematic review. *Suicide and Life-Threatening Behavior*, *37*(6), 698–714.

O'Connor, R. C., O'Carroll, R. E., Ryan, C., & Smyth, R. (2012). Self-regulation of unattainable goals in suicide attempters: A two year prospective study. *Journal of Affective Disorders*, *142*, 248–255.

Overholser, J. C., Braden, A., & Dieter, L. (2012). Understanding suicide risk: Identification of high-risk groups during high-risk times. *Journal of Clinical Psychology*, *68*(3), 349–361. https://doi.org/10.1002/jclp.20859

Pals, J. L. (2006). Narrative identity processing of difficult life experiences: Pathways of personality development and positive self-transformation in adulthood. *Journal of Personality*, *74*(4), 1079–1110. https://doi.org/10.1111/j.1467-6494.2006.00403.x

Park, J., Rogers, M. L., Bloch-Elkouby, S., Richards, J. A., Lee, S., Galynker, I., & You, S. (under review). Factor structure and validation of the revised Suicide Crisis Inventory (SCI-2) in a Korean population. *Journal of Affective Disorders*.

Pasupathi, M. (2001). The social construction of the personal past and its implications for adult development. *Psychological Bulletin, 127*(5), 651–672. https://doi.org/10.1037/0033-2909.127.5.651

Pompili, M., Innamorati, M., Szanto, K., Di Vittorio, C., Conwell, Y., Lester, D., Tatarelli, R., Girardi, P., & Amore, M. (2011). Life events as precipitants of suicide attempts among first-time suicide attempters, repeaters, and non-attempters. *Psychiatry Research, 186*(2–3), 300–305. https://doi.org/10.1016/j.psychres.2010.09.003

Rappaport, L. M., Moskowitz, D. S., Galynker, I., & Yaseen, Z. S. (2014). Panic symptom clusters differentially predict suicide ideation and attempt. *Comprehensive Psychiatry, 55*(4), 762–769.

Rogers, M. L., Cao, E., Richards, J., Mitelman, S., Barzilay, S., Blum, Y., Chistopolskaya, K., Çinka, E., Dudeck, M., Husain, I., Kantas Yilmaz, E., Kuśmirek, O., Menon, V., Nikolaev, E., Pilecka, B., Titze, L., Valvassori, S., Luiz, T., You, S., & Galynker, I. (under review). Associations between long-term and near-term stressful life events, suicide crisis syndrome, and suicidal ideation. *International Journal of Stress Management*.

Rogers, M. L., Cao, E., Sinclair, C., & Galynker, I. (2021). Associations between goal orientation and suicidal thoughts and behaviors at one-month follow-up: Indirect effects through ruminative flooding. *Behaviour Research and Therapy, 145*, 103945. https://doi.org/10.1016/j.brat.2021.103945

Rogers, M. L., Vespa, A., Bloch-Elkouby, S., & Galynker, I. (2021). Validity of the Modular Assessment of Risk for Imminent Suicide in predicting short-term suicidality. *Acta Psychiatrica Scandinavica, 144*(6), 563–577. https://doi.org/10.1111/acps.13354

Rossi, R., Socci, V., Talevi, D., Mensi, S., Niolu, C., Pacitti, F., Di Marco, A., Rossi, A., Siracusano, A., & Di Lorenzo, G. (2020). COVID-19 pandemic and lockdown measures impact on mental health among the general population in Italy. *Frontiers in Psychiatry, 11*, 790. https://doi.org/10.3389/fpsyt.2020.00790

Schuck, A., Calati, R., Barzilay, S., Bloch-Elkouby, S., & Galynker, I. (2019). Suicide crisis syndrome: A review of supporting evidence for a new suicide-specific diagnosis. *Behavioral Sciences and the Law, 37*, 223–239.

Siddaway, A. P., Taylor, P. J., Wood, A. M., & Schulz, J. (2015). A meta-analysis of perceptions of defeat and entrapment in depression, anxiety problems, posttraumatic stress disorder, and suicidality. *Journal of Affective Disorders, 184*, 149–159.

Van Orden, K. A., Cukrowicz, K. C., Witte, T. K., & Joiner, T. E. (2012). Thwarted belongingness and perceived burdensomeness: Construct validity and psychometric properties of the Interpersonal Needs Questionnaire. *Psychological Assessment, 24*(1), 197–215. https://doi.org/10.1037/a0025358

Wenzel, A., & Beck, A. T. (2008). A cognitive model of suicidal behavior: Theory and treatment. *Applied and Preventive Psychology, 12*, 189–201.

Williams, J. M. G., & Pollock, L. R. (2000). The Psychology of Suicidal Behaviour. In K. Hawton & K. van Heeringen (Eds.), *The International Handbook of Suicide and Attempted Suicide* (pp. 79–93). John Wiley & Sons Ltd., Chichester. http://dx.doi.org/10.1002/9780470698976.ch5

Woike, B., & Polo, M. (2001). Motive-related memories: Content, structure, and affect. *Journal of Personality, 69*(3), 391–415. https://doi.org/10.1111/1467-6494.00150

Yaseen, Z. S., Chartrand, H., Mojtabai, R., Bolton, J., & Galynker, I. I. (2013). Fear of dying in panic attacks predicts suicide attempt in comorbid depressive illness: Prospective evidence from the National Epidemiological Survey on Alcohol and Related Conditions. *Depression and Anxiety, 30*(10), 930–939. https://doi.org/10.1002/da.22039

Yaseen, Z. S., Fisher, K., Morales, E., & Galynker, I. I. (2012b). Love and suicide: The structure of the Affective Intensity Rating Scale (AIRS) and its relation to suicidal behavior. *PLOS One, 7*(8), e0044069. https://doi.org/10.1371/journal.pone.0044069

Yaseen, Z. S., Galynker, I. I., Briggs, J., Freed, R. D., & Gabbay, V. (2016). Functional domains as correlates of suicidality among psychiatric inpatients. *Journal of Affective Disorders, 203,* 7–83. https://doi.org/10.1016/j.jad.2016.05.066

Yaseen, Z. S., Gilmer, E., Modi, J., Cohen, L. J., & Galynker, I. I. (2012a). Emergency room validation of the revised Suicide Trigger Scale (STS-3): A measure of a hypothesized suicide trigger state. *PLOS One, 7*(9), e45157. https://doi.org/10.1371/journal.pone.0045157

Yaseen, Z. S., Hawes, M., Barzilay, S., & Galynker, I. (2019). Predictive validity of proposed diagnostic criteria for the suicide crisis syndrome: An acute presuicidal state. *Suicide and Life-Threatening Behavior, 49,* 1124–1135. https://doi.org/10.1111/sltb.12495

Yaseen, Z., Katz, C., Johnson, M. S., Eisenberg, D., Cohen, L. J., & Galynker, I. I. (2010). Construct development: The Suicide Trigger Scale (STS-2), a measure of a hypothesized suicide trigger state. *BMC Psychiatry, 10*(1), 110. https://doi.org/10.1186/1471-244x-10-110

Yaseen, Z. S., Kopeykina, I., Gutkovich, Z., Bassirnia, A., Cohen, L. J., & Galynker, I. I. (2014). Predictive validity of the Suicide Trigger Scale (STS-3) for post-discharge suicide attempt in high-risk psychiatric inpatients. *PLOS One, 9*(1), e86768. https://doi.org/10.1371/journal.pone.0086768

Yaseen, Z. S., Fisher, K., Morales, E., & Galynker, I. I. (2012). Love and suicide: The structure of the Affective Intensity Rating Scale (AIRS) and its relation to suicidal behavior. *PloS One, 7*(8), e44069. https://doi.org/10.1371/journal.pone.0044069

4

Long-Term or Chronic Risk Factors

As discussed in the preceding chapter, the narrative-crisis model of suicide (NCM) posits that people attempting suicide have long-term (chronic) risk factors for suicidal behavior. Multiple research studies identified disparate demographic, biological, psychological, historical, and societal factors showing an association with increased lifetime risk for suicidal behavior and suicide. Well-researched demographic risk factors include age, sex, race, ethnicity, marital status, and employment status. The biological risk factors are not discussed here because currently their assessment is not included in routine clinical workflow. Psychological factors include temperament traits, such as perfectionism, fearlessness, and pessimism, as well as attachment style. Historical factors include family history, childhood adversity, history of suicide in the family, or history of mental illness, all of which are considered relatively stable over time and distal to acute suicidal behavior. Finally, the NCM long-term risk factor construct includes cultural and social factors, such as cultural acceptability of suicide as a solution to life's problems.

Demographics

Gender and Age

Suicide rates and patterns differ according to age group and gender. Overall, the suicide rate for men in the United States continues to be much higher than that for women, but the difference varies across age groups. Data from the Centers for Disease Control and Prevention (CDC) in 2018 showed that suicide rates among males in the United States started with 3.66 per 100,000 in the 10- to 14-year-old age group, rose to 17.32 in the 15- to 19-year-old age group, remained around 28 in the 20- to 44-year-old age group, peaked in the 55- to 59-year-old age group with 33.46, decreased to 28 in the 70- to 74-year-old age group, and sharply rose to a second peak in the 85-year-old and older age group with 47.17 per 100,000. Among females, suicide rates started with 2.02 per 100,000 in the 10- to 14-year-old age group, gradually and steadily rose to a peak of 10.84 in the 50- to 54-year-old age group, and gradually decreased to 3.58 in women 85 years old and older (CDC, 2018).

Women attempt suicide significantly more often than men, but men die by suicide almost three times more often than women (Freeman et al., 2017; Wang et al., 2020). This finding generally holds true for the United States and Western cultures as a whole; the pattern shifts dramatically in other areas of the world. In China, the most populous country in the world, women die by suicide more often than men (Zhang et al., 2011). Nevertheless, several studies show that men generally use methods that are much more lethal in their suicide attempts, such as firearms and hanging/suffocation. Given this trend, it makes sense that male suicide attempts tend to be more lethal than female attempts and that men are more likely to die from their attempts (CDC, 2020; Curtin et al., 2016).

Examining the data for the United States in more detail, the gender disparity in the lethality of suicide methods means that firearm decedents are more likely to be foreign-born, elderly, non-Hispanic, Caucasian, married men. Decedents from hanging and suffocation also tend to be male and foreign-born but never-married, young, and from racial/ethnic minorities. Regarding less lethal methods, such as using sharp objects, decedents are more likely to be foreign-born, older, non-Hispanic, African American, never-married women. Similarly, self-poisoned decedents are more likely to be unmarried females, middle-aged, and non-Hispanic Caucasian (Kleiman & Liu, 2013). These gender differences may suggest disparities in the intentionality of suicidal behavior between men and women, with men being more determined to die even when using less lethal methods (Mergl et al., 2015).

It is worth noting that events precipitating suicide in children are different from those in the elderly, and events precipitating suicide in both these groups are different from those in adults. Parent–child conflicts are the most common precipitant for suicide in children, and hanging is the most frequent method (Soole et al., 2014). In the elderly, the major factor leading to suicide is depression, followed by physical disability. The majority of elderly suicide victims are not seen by a psychiatrist prior to their suicide (Snowden et al., 2009).

Sexual Orientation and Identity

Data regarding suicide risk in sexual minorities remains mainly limited to suicide attempts rather than completed suicide rates. Youth who identify as sexual minorities are at three times greater risk than their heterosexual peers for suicide attempts, and this risk persists even after controlling for other suicide risk factors (Johns et al., 2018). The increase in suicide risk is associated with negative familial response to an adolescent's "coming out" process, lack of acceptance, and discrimination (Green et al., 2020; Layland et al., 2020). Family rejection of an adolescent who is lesbian, gay, bisexual, or transgender (LGBT) is associated with an eightfold greater likelihood of attempted suicide compared to the likelihood among adolescents who experience minimal or no family rejection (Cash & Bridge, 2009).

Race, Ethnicity, and Geographic Region

In terms of race, ethnicity, and geographic region, worldwide frequencies of suicidal behavior vary from country to country. According to data from World Health Organization, in 2016, the highest suicide rates were reported in Lithuania, the Russian Federation, Guyana, Korea, Belarus, Suriname, Kazakhstan, and Ukraine. The United States ranked number 29 among 185 countries and many of the Western European countries fell between 15 and 30 on the ranking. Meanwhile, many of the countries in the Middle East and North Africa fell toward the end of the ranking. Lithuania's annual suicide rate of 31.9 per 100,000 was the highest in the world, whereas the lowest was in Antigua and Barbuda, which has an annual rate of 0.5 per 100,000.

In the United States, there are significant differences between individual states' suicide rates. States with the most suicides report rates that are almost two times higher than the national average and three times higher than the rates of states with the least suicides. Data from 2018 showed that the highest suicide rates were in the West, in Wyoming (25.2), New Mexico (25.0), Montana (24.9), and Alaska (24.6). The lowest rates were in the East, in the District of Columbia (7.5), New York and New Jersey (8.3), and Rhode Island (9.5; MMWR, 2020). According to the CDC, in 2016 the highest rates of suicide in the United States were observed in non-Hispanic Whites (~17), followed by American Indians/AK Natives (13.59), compared to relatively low rates in non-Hispanic Blacks (6.3), Hispanics (6.7), and Asians/Pacific Islanders (6.84; MMWR, 2018).

Even subtle differences in cultural attitudes result in significant differences in suicide rates. In the United States, western and southern states are sometimes classified as "honor states" due to their emphasis on self-sufficiency and their negative view of federal entitlement programs.

These states have higher suicide rates, particularly among Caucasians living in rural areas (Stark et al., 2011). Of note, in rural communities, suicides are more often associated with social isolation, and youth suicide rates are two to ten times higher than the national average (Hirsch, 2006). Furthermore, levels of antidepressant prescriptions (an indicator of mental health help-seeking) are lower in honor states, despite levels of major depression being higher.

Combining the previous demographic data on age, gender, and ethnicity creates clinically meaningful contrasts between higher and lower suicide risk groups. Although demographics alone are not predictive of imminent risk, they provide a valuable reference point.

Psychological Factors

Impulsivity

The complex relationship of impulsivity with suicide has been extensively studied. Beck's impulsivity vulnerability factor overlaps with the biological diathesis for suicidal behavior from Mann's stress-diathesis model (Mann et al., 2005). According to Mann, biological vulnerability is associated with genetically or epigenetically encoded low levels of norepinephrine and serotonin. The link between low levels of serotonin, past suicide attempts, and completed suicides is supported by numerous well-designed studies (Mann et al., 1999). These studies show that the link is mediated by impulsivity, hopelessness, and depression, which in turn have been shown to be associated with past suicidality and may be related to long-term suicide risk. More recently, and in the context of the interpersonal theory of suicide (IPTS), only the attention subdomain of trait impulsivity has been weakly linked with thwarted belongingness but not with other constructs of the ITPS (Hadzic et al., 2019). The same study also demonstrated an association of trait impulsivity with suicidal behavior and fluctuations in suicidal ideation but not with suicidal ideation itself. Deficits in conscientiousness, as a domain of impulsivity, were linked with high likelihood of suicide attempt (Cole et al., 2019). Thus, it appears that impulsivity increases the risk of suicide more distally through facilitating the action of suicide rather than precipitating suicidal ideation.

Hopelessness and Pessimism

Although hopelessness is usually considered a state factor, it also has a strong trait component that remains stable over time. Some research suggests that trait hopelessness, also defined as pessimism about the future, may be a strong predictor for all indices of suicidal ideation and behavior (Burr et al., 2018; O'Connor et al., 2013). In one classic long-term prospective study, hopelessness scores at baseline predicted more than 90% of all suicides in high-risk psychiatric inpatients during a 10-year follow-up period. Other studies showed that hopelessness was not predictive of suicidal behavior during short periods of time, suggesting that it is indeed a trait rather than an acute state condition (Goldston et al., 2006).

Perfectionism

Perfectionism was defined by Beck as a maladaptive cognitive style, and it refers to unrealistically high expectations that some individuals have for themselves, which set them up for failure. The concept of perfectionism is surprisingly complex and multifaceted, with research suggesting that many of its features are associated with suicidal behavior and ideation (reviewed by O'Connor, 2007). The aspects of perfectionism most consistently associated with suicidality are self-criticism, concern over mistakes, doubts about one's actions, and socially prescribed perfectionism, which is defined as the belief that others hold unrealistically high expectations for one's behavior and will only be satisfied if those expectations are met. It particular, it is shown that the effect of perfectionism on suicidal thoughts and behaviors is mediated through fear of humiliation and precipitation of the suicide crisis syndrome (Pia et al., 2020). It also appears that the relationship between thwarted belongingness, perceived burdensomeness, and suicidal ideation is moderated by perfectionism (Sommerfeld & Malek, 2019). Prospective studies of the predictive value of perfectionism for future suicidal behavior seem to suggest that this association exists. In short, perfectionism is a powerful motivating trait that forms the core of many suicidal narratives. It can be easily assessed both with psychometric scales and with direct questions, making it a useful target for imminent suicide risk assessment.

Fearlessness and Pain Insensitivity

Fearlessness is predictor of suicide attempt (Ferm et al., 2020) irrespective of the method of suicide (Bauer et al., 2020). A capability for suicide is theorized to be a key ingredient in making it possible for someone to end their life (Joiner, 2005; Ohman & Mineka, 2001). With adequate support, this theory would provide a framework for why most people who have suicidal intent never attempt suicide. If true, the acquired capability for suicide would help explain the relatively high suicide rates in physicians (Cornette et al., 2009) and military personnel (Selby et al., 2010), which may be due to repeated exposure and habituation to death and dying.

Joiner's interpersonal model emphasizes the construct of acquired capability for suicide (see Chapter 2). However, it is important to note that this capacity could also be genetic. Some people are brave and fearless beginning in early childhood, whereas others are more timid and fearful. Research supports the notion that the former have externalizing personality traits, whereas the latter have internalizing ones. Psychopaths, for example, who are the most extreme externalizers, exhibit reduced anxiety and fear reactions—a phenomenon that has been shown to have a prominent genetic component.

Several studies reported that higher levels of fearlessness of death were associated with a higher number of suicide attempts (Anestis & Joiner, 2011). In the military, thwarted belongingness and perceived burdensomeness were associated with suicidal behavior only in those with high levels of fearlessness with regard to suicide. Clinically, however, the connection between capability for suicide and suicide intent or imminent suicidal behavior cannot be easily discerned.

Much more evident is the function of fear as a barrier to suicide, even when desire for suicide is palpable. For some patients, the fear of the physical pain associated with most methods of suicide is visceral. This is usually expressed by the suicidal individual as some variation of "I am not afraid to die, but I am afraid of the pain." For others, the fear of pain is more vague and undifferentiated. In such cases, patients typically make statements like "I will never do it; I do not have the courage." Such a statement could indicate fear of pain, of nothingness, of the unknown, or of all of these.

Attachment Style

Attachment theory, pioneered by Bowlby (1969, 1980), hypothesizes that early experiences with caregivers translate into internal representations of relationships that influence an individual's ability to navigate social situations (Crowell et al., 2009). Some researchers suggest a strong association between attachment styles and long-term (and possible short-term) risk of suicidal behavior (Levi-Belz et al., 2013; Stepp et al., 2008), while a recent review has found substantial heterogeneity among previous findings and has called for more longitudinal evidence (Green et al., 2020). The researchers also suggested that the association between attachment security and suicidality is probably mediated by a range of predisposing, precipitating, and crisis-state factors.

Griffin and Bartholomew's (1994) four-category model of "self" and "other" describes four attachment styles: secure, fearful, preoccupied, and dismissing. The attachment styles are defined by one's view of the self and the other. The secure attachment style is defined by a positive view of self and others (which translates behaviorally into low anxiety and low avoidance, correspondingly). Securely attached individuals have an internalized sense of self-worth and are comfortable with intimacy in close relationships. The three other attachment styles are described as insecure. The fearful attachment style is defined by a negative view of self and others. Fearful individuals are highly dependent on others for the validation of their self-worth; however, because of their negative expectations of others, they shun intimacy to avoid the pain of potential loss or rejection. The preoccupied attachment style is defined by a negative view of self and a positive view of others. Preoccupied individuals, like fearful individuals, have a deep-seated sense of unworthiness. However, their positive view of others motivates them to validate their precarious self-worth through excessive closeness in personal relationships, leaving them vulnerable to extreme distress when their intimacy needs are not met. Finally, the dismissing attachment style is defined by a positive view of self and a negative view of others. Dismissing individuals also avoid closeness with others because of negative expectations; however, they maintain their high sense of self-worth by defensively denying the value of close relationships and stressing the importance of independence.

It has been suggested that the likelihood of engaging in suicidal behavior could be related to how negative early attachment experiences are structured into internal adult working models of attachment (Adam et al., 1982). Indeed, research has identified impairment of parental attachment and bonding as one key risk factor for suicidal behavior later in life (Fergusson et al., 2000).

It appears that early insecure attachment may operate as a general vulnerability factor, increasing the risk of poor work functioning and suicide attempts. Individuals with an insecure attachment style may exhibit impaired social and collaborative behaviors and thus lack the interpersonal skills required to be successful in a work environment (e.g., balancing teamwork with functioning independently, good communication skills, etc.). This may result in impaired self-esteem and depressed mood, thereby increasing suicide risk (Levi-Belz et al., 2013; Stepp et al., 2008).

However, depending on the patient population, there may be other mechanisms linking specific insecure attachment styles with suicidal behaviors (Green et al., 2020). For example, in high-risk psychiatric inpatients, the relationship between the fearful attachment style and future suicidal behaviors is strong but indirect, and it is mediated entirely by entrapment (Clark et al., 2016). Clark et al. found that the secure attachment style had a protective effect against future suicidal behaviors, also fully mediated by entrapment, whereas dismissing and preoccupied attachment had no significant relationship with future behaviors.

Historical Factors

History of Mental Illness

Having a diagnosis of a psychiatric disorder, with the exception of dementia, is a well-known risk factor for suicide, and the risk of suicide among patients with psychiatric disorders is about eight times higher than the risk among patients without psychiatric disorders (Too et al., 2019). The differences in suicide rates for each disorder are modulated by other factors, such as comorbidity, history of previous attempts, and gender differences in mental disorders.

Approximately 90% of individuals who die by suicide have a mental illness, although the percentage varies globally (Chang et al., 2011). The most common diagnoses are affective disorders, followed by schizophrenia, substance use disorders, personality disorders, and anxiety disorders (Gianatsi et al., 2020; Thibodeau et al., 2013; Varnik, 2012).

In the United Kingdom, approximately 25% of suicide decedents with a psychiatric disorder did not receive any relevant treatment prior to their suicide (Gianatsi et al., 2020). Similarly, suicide risk is thought to be greatly increased following discharge from inpatient mental health wards, although inpatient suicides have declined significantly during the past 20 years (see the next section).

Thus, it appears that many psychiatric disorders may increase suicide risk. However, psychiatric disorders rarely occur in isolation and are too frequently comorbid to be a matter of chance (Kessler et al., 2005). This comorbidity can be explained through the manifestation and interaction of the two genetic vulnerability factors known as internalizing and externalizing behaviors or disorders. These two transdiagnostic factors may explain the links between individual disorders and suicidal behavior.

The term *internalizing behaviors* originated in child psychiatry and refers to mood dysregulation caused by difficulties in managing negative emotions. In children, internalizing behaviors may manifest as withdrawn behavior, frequent worrying, self-denigrating comments, and low self-confidence, and they typically do not result in disruptive behaviors. The term *externalizing behaviors* refers to problems that are manifested in disruptive behavior and reflect a child's negative reactions to his or her environment. The manifestations may include aggression, delinquency, and hyperactivity. In general terms, internalizers tend to blame themselves for their problems, and externalizers tend to blame everyone around them.

In adults, the Axis I internalizing disorders include major depressive disorder, generalized anxiety disorder (GAD), dysthymia, panic disorder, seasonal affective disorder, and social phobias. Axis I externalizing disorders are primarily addiction disorders, such as alcohol use disorder, drug use disorder, and pathological gambling. Internalizing Axis II disorders in adults are the avoidant-dependent, histrionic, schizoid, and schizotypal personality disorders, whereas the externalizing personality disorders include antisocial, narcissistic, and borderline personality disorders (Cosgrove et al., 2011). Although distinctly different, both dimensions arise from a general psychopathology factor, which makes people vulnerable to both dimensions and increases the risk of suicidal behavior (Hoertel et al., 2015).

The mechanism of a general psychopathology risk factor, rather than (or in addition to) the alternative mechanism of distinct disorder-specific risk factors, may explain suicides that occur after the worst symptoms of a disorder have improved or completely resolved. If the yet-to-be-defined generalized risk factor underlies most or even some suicidal behaviors, then treatments for specific symptoms typically associated with suicide risk may not eliminate it completely.

Many case histories describe suicides that took place after the person's depression either improved or turned into euthymia. Sudden brightening of mood has been suggested anecdotally to be a warning sign of imminent suicide. Similarly, patients with severe anxiety disorders or with psychotic disorders do not necessarily take their lives at the height of their anxiety or psychosis. Many suicides occur in individuals who in the eyes of a casual observer seemed normal and even happy.

In addition to the treatment of specific disorders and symptoms associated with increased suicide risk, interventions are needed for the underlying transdiagnostic factor that increases suicide risk regardless of the *Diagnostic and Statistical Manual of Mental Disorders* (American Psychiatric Association, 2013) diagnostic structure. In other words, increased suicide risk could be considered a transdiagnostic syndrome that presents both an important research domain and a valuable treatment target.

History of Suicide Attempts

One of the strongest risk factors for suicide is a history of suicide attempts or of previous deliberate self-harm (Bostwick et al., 2016; Sakinofsky, 2000). The distinction between the two is that *suicide attempt* implies a conscious intent to die, whereas *deliberate self-harm* is purely behavioral and includes intentional self-poisoning or self-injury, irrespective of motivation (Hawton et al., 2003). Because in most studies the intent to die cannot be established with certainty, a purely behavioral definition of deliberate self-harm, rather than suicide attempt, may be more accurate for describing past self-injurious behavior.

Regardless of definition, longitudinal studies of past self-injurious behavior as a risk factor for future suicide attempts and completed suicide show very similar results. In developed countries, a history of deliberate self-harm or suicide attempt is found in approximately half of all suicides (range, 40% to 60%; Nordentoft et al., 1993). One in 100 suicide attempters goes on to die by suicide in a subsequent attempt(s) within the first year (Hawton et al., 2003). Suicide death rates for previous attempters are on average 30 times higher than those for the general population. As many as 5% of suicide attempters will die by suicide within nine years (Owens et al., 2002).

The number of previous suicide attempts and advanced age further increase the risk of an upcoming fatal attempt, particularly in the elderly (300-fold increase in the group more than 85 years old, compared to the general population without a history of attempts). Those with histories of past suicide attempt in other age groups have suicide rates 30 to 50 times higher than the rate in the general population. Although this is a very high rate, it is an order of magnitude lower than that in the elderly (Hawton et al., 2003; Nordentoft et al., 1993).

The ratio of men to women who die by suicide after previous attempts is lower than that for all suicides. In contrast to the 3:1 men:women ratio among all suicides, some studies show only a 2:1 ratio among previous attempters, whereas other studies have shown that equal numbers of men and women die by subsequent suicide attempt. Considering that men tend to use more lethal means of suicide, one possible explanation for this discrepancy is that those who do not die in their first attempt are a self-selected group of men less prone to using lethal means of suicides (Nordentoft et al., 1993; Qin & Nordentoft, 2005).

The incremental increase in risk due to previous suicide attempts appears to be higher in the West than in the developing world and in developed Asian countries. For example, compared to 30% to 47% of patients in the West (Gunnell & Frankel, 1994), only 8% or 9% of patients in rural Sri Lanka and only 17% of patients in urban areas of this country report previous episodes of self-harm (Mohamed et al., 2010). In India, only 13% of those who died by suicide had previously self-harmed (Gururaj et al., 2004), whereas a figure of 25% was reported in a large study from China. Suicide attempts and the suicide rate in previous attempters in Taiwan (Weng et al., 2016) were also lower than those in the West (Phillips et al., 2002).

It is important to note that, whereas a suicide attempt in the remote past could be classified as a trait vulnerability for suicide, a recent suicide attempt (up to one year in the past) represents a short-term risk factor. It appears that the stress of an acute episode of psychiatric illness, recent hospitalization, or suicide attempt sharply increases short-term suicide risk. For that reason, all these factors are further discussed in Chapter 4.

Suicide in the Family

Independent of familial history of mental illness, family history of suicide increases suicide risk, suggesting a social transmission effect. A family history of mental illness increases suicide risk only in adults without a history of psychiatric illness, whereas a family history of suicide increases suicide risk two- or threefold equally, irrespective of psychiatric illness history (Qin et al., 2002). Therefore, family history of suicide should be established in the assessment of acute suicide risk.

In adolescents, exposure to suicidal behavior of family or friends is associated with a threefold increase in the risk of future suicidal behaviors. In fact, exposure to a friend's or a family member's suicidal behavior significantly increased risk in adolescents (Nanayakkara et al., 2013). Maternal suicidal behavior is more strongly associated with suicidal behavior in children compared to paternal suicidal behavior (Geulayov et al., 2012). Children are more likely to be affected by parental suicidal behavior than are adolescents or adults, and the effects of maternal suicide on boys and girls are the same. As in adults, there is no evidence of an interaction between exposure to a peer's or family member's suicide attempt and depression in children and adolescents.

Parental suicide weighs heavily on children throughout their lives, particularly when children approach the age at which their parent committed suicide. This is particularly pertinent for families with a genetic predisposition to a mental illness that causes deterioration later in life. As the suicide survivor's condition worsens, parallels with the deceased parent may become inevitable, thus increasing the sense of apprehension, hopelessness, and entrapment.

Suicide Exposure and Practicing

In contrast to genetic trait fearlessness, the acquired capability for suicide is developed largely through environmental exposure to painful events, bodily injury, and/or violent deaths. Although this theory of gradual inoculation to the fear of the physical pain of death is intuitive, it is not well supported by research. Suicide rates in the military, for example, are not strongly related to the duration or type of combat exposure (Reger et al., 2011). Likewise, there does not seem to be a relationship between exposure to violence and suicide among policemen (Miller, 2006). It has been shown that surviving genocide, abuse, and loss of a family member to genocide are also not significantly associated with suicide (Rubanzana et al., 2014).

Suicidal behavior is an unambiguous and ominous sign of an imminent attempt. Although 50% of completed suicides occur on the first attempt (Schaffer et al., 2016), some suicides may involve extensive preparation and remain undiscovered in the majority of cases. This preparatory behavior becomes known only in high-profile suicides or murder-suicides, as a result of considerable effort and resource expenditure. The clearest recent example of this is the German Wings copilot who crashed a plane into a mountain when the pilot left the cockpit to use the bathroom. The massive investigation that followed revealed that the copilot had been researching previous pilot suicides and that in the week preceding his murder-suicide, he practiced locking the cockpit door and initiating the accelerated descent that he ultimately used to bring down the plane.

The remaining 50% of unsuccessful initial suicide attempts differ greatly in their lethality. Statistically, the most common methods, in increasing order of lethality, are self-injurious cutting, drug overdose, poisoning, asphyxiation, drowning, hanging, jumping from heights, and firearms (Chang et al., 2011). Completed suicides are usually executed attempts via the same method used in the last attempt or attempts via a method of higher lethality. For example, a nonlethal overdose is followed by a lethal overdose with more pills or by jumping off the roof of a building. Failed attempts of high lethality are more likely to be followed by completed attempts compared to failed attempts of low lethality (Ajdacic-Gross, 2008).

In general, the lethality of the method used is significantly correlated with the intensity of the suicidal intent (Nishimura et al., 1999). Methods also differ regionally, depending on their availability. In the United States, most people die by suicide using a firearm (American Foundation for Suicide Prevention, 2016). Overdose by pesticides, which are highly toxic and readily available in developing countries (Ajdacic-Gross, 2008), is most common worldwide. The most successful method of suicide rate reduction to date is control of the means, rather than clinicians' improved ability to identify and treat suicidal patients.

Childhood Trauma

A massive body of literature indicates that childhood maltreatment, particularly sexual abuse, is associated with increased suicide risk in adulthood. The link between childhood sexual abuse and adult suicide is strongest when the abuse was long-lasting, the perpetrator knew the victim, and there was force and/or penetration. Adults with a history of childhood abuse may be four times more likely to engage in suicide attempts than non-abused individuals, especially if the abuse was sexual or physical (Zatti et al., 2017).

Parenting Style

Parental bonding is a construct developed by Parker and colleagues (Parker, 1981, 1989; Parker et al., 1979) that classifies parenting style into four categories based on the level of care afforded to children and the level of control or overprotection exercised by the parents. Optimal parental bonding is described as a combination of high care and low overprotective behaviors, whereas poor parental styles involve the three other combinations. Neglectful parenting involves both low care and low control, whereas authoritarian ("helicopter") parents provide high care but also a high level of control. Parents who are emotionally distant and controlling exercise the parental bonding style of affectionless control. Research suggests that there is a strong relationship between poor parental bonding and suicide (Gureje et al., 2010; McGarvey et al., 1999; Saffer et al., 2015).

All poor parental bonding, particularly low care, has a significant association with suicidal behavior. However, affectionless control, the combination of low care and overprotection, has a particularly strong association with suicidality. The data are less consistent with regard to overprotection alone because both parental gender and cultural factors appear to be pertinent (Goschin et al., 2013). Affectionless control is a significant risk factor for both suicidal ideation and behavior in adolescents and adults. All of the studies on adolescents reviewed by Goschin et al. (2013) showed that affectionless control is a risk factor for suicidality, and studies using adult populations were nearly as uniform. This suggests that poor parenting style has long-term and possibly lifelong consequences.

The association between affectionless control and increased suicidality is noted more often in relation to mothers than in relation to fathers. The difference could be related to a historically dominant role of mothers relative to fathers in the family environment (McKinney et al., 2008). The discrepancy also appears to be related to culture. In countries in which the mother is the primary figure in raising and educating children, perceived maternal affectionless control is likely more important than paternal bonding. Given the increasingly multicultural nature of societies, cultural characteristics are an increasingly important part of risk assessment.

It is unclear why affectionless control has a particularly strong association with suicidality. One hypothesis is that perceived overprotection can influence children's sense of their own identity and autonomy, which in turn can raise the risk of suicidal ideation. The literature shows that overcontrolling behaviors in mothers are associated with psychopathology in children and adolescents (Affrunti & Ginsburg, 2012) and that an overcontrolling style in both parents is associated with a variety of specific psychiatric disorders, including anxiety disorders (Spada et al., 2011), social phobia (Knappe et al., 2012), eating disorders (Lobera et al., 2011), and depression (Campos et al., 2010).

Social Factors

Cultural Attitudes and Immigration Status

Any person's suicide risk is significantly influenced by cultural attitudes. Historically, cultures that place a strong emphasis on personal honor tend to foster higher rates of suicide. For example, "honor suicides" (i.e., suicides in the face of defeat or capture) were common in Greek and Roman civilizations (Dublin, 1963). Japanese warriors who brought shame to their family voluntarily committed a ritualized form of suicide known as Seppuku to restore their honor. In Jodhpur, India, a wall by the fortress gate is full of 16th-century hand imprints left by women who fell to their death in response to the deaths of their husbands who died defending their city ("Sati Handprints," 2016). Thus, in many cultures, suicide has been (and, in some cases, still is) viewed as an appropriate response to certain types of perceived dishonor (Osterman & Brown, 2011).

In cultures in which family honor has historically been valued more than the wishes of the individual, people may feel unable to seek help for any distress caused by their cultural standards. In doing so, they would only amplify their shame, as well as impose additional dishonor on their families by revealing their distress. In such cultures, fear of reputational damage could create self-imposed barriers to seeking professional help, thus putting people at higher risk for suicide.

Finally, immigrant groups from "honor cultures" may exhibit high suicide rates under circumstances that would imply family dishonor in their
native countries. A frequent scenario encountered in a psychiatric emergency department (ED) is a suicide attempt by an Asian college student
after failing to earn the grades needed for acceptance into a prestigious
graduate program. In Asian families, failure to succeed can be a family disgrace (Chambers, 2010). College suicide attempts are not limited to Asian
students, but this scenario highlights the pivotal role that culture can play
in suicide risk.

Interestingly, compared to US-born citizens, immigrants to the United
States have lower suicide rates prior to their immigration. However, sui-
cide rates increase with acculturation and may exceed the rates of those who
are born in the United States (Borges et al., 2011). Immigrants of Asian and
African American ethnicity who migrated as children show higher lifetime
prevalence of attempts than U.S.-born individuals of the same ethnicity
(Borges et al., 2011). The same is true for Middle Eastern immigrants (Nasseri
& Moulton, 2009). The highest risk of suicide has been reported among non-
European immigrant women, including South Asian and Black African
women. Common reasons are language barriers, worrying about family back
home, and separation from family (Forte et al., 2018). Paradoxically, despite
high stress, recent immigration appears to be somewhat protective against
suicidal behavior.

Thus, when assessing imminent risk, clinicians must obtain a detailed cultural history. In summary, cultural and religious factors play a significant role
in moderating acute suicide risk. Aspects pertaining to personal and family
honor, religious or moral prohibition, and moral acceptability of suicide are
of particular importance. In the United States, attention should focus specifically on second-generation immigrants, who may believe they have not
met their parents' expectations and thus have failed to repay them for the
sacrifices made during immigration.

Moral, Philosophical, and Religious Objections

Religion generally disapproves of suicide, and having a religious affiliation
is considered to be a protective factor against suicide risk (Lawrence et al.,
2015). Whereas for atheists, suicide may signify the end of life and escape
from mental pain, for those with a religious affiliation, suicide is a sin and a

violation of the divine code of behavior (*Catechism of the Catholic Church*, n.d.; Holland, 1977; Roth, 2009). Thus, for many believers, religious affiliation is a protective factor against suicide.

Studies have confirmed the protective effect of moral and/or religious objections to suicide against suicidal behavior (Galynker et al., 2015; Lawrence et al., 2015). Patients with depression and bipolar disorder (Dervic et al., 2011), as well as those without a specific psychiatric diagnosis, have been shown to have lower rates of suicidal behavior if they endorsed a religious affiliation. Conversely, lack of moral objections to suicide predicts higher rates of postdischarge suicidal behavior in high-risk psychiatric inpatients (Galynker et al., 2015).

The discussion of religious aspects of suicidal behavior would be woefully incomplete without addressing the topics of suicide terrorism and mass suicides, two rare but conspicuous circumstances in which religious affiliation actually increases the risk of suicide. Scientific data on suicide terrorism are understandably lacking. The empirical data on suspected suicide terrorists suggest many discrepancies between suicide terrorists and other suicides (Townsend, 2007). This implies that such individuals are not truly suicidal and should not be viewed as a subgroup of the general suicidal population. Understanding suicide terrorism cannot be done outside of historical and cultural contexts, and it requires a multidisciplinary approach that includes not only psychological but also anthropological, economic, historical, and political factors.

The literature addressing mass suicides is even more sparse. Mass suicide is the simultaneous suicide of all members of a social group. The mass suicides of approximately the past 20 years are all related to the establishment of religious sects, which are defined as mystic, idiosyncratic, and often bizarre self-contained belief systems that may sometimes lead to the self-destruction of the sect under the guise of being an act of self-assertiveness (Mancinelli et al., 2002). People who join cults are often psychiatrically ill, have propensities toward dissociative states, have histories of severe child abuse/neglect, show tendencies to abuse controlled substances, have experienced debilitating situational stressors, and labor under intolerable socioeconomic conditions. They are vulnerable to mass suicide when incited by the cult's charismatic leader. Two prominent cases of mass suicide are the 900 deaths in Jonestown and the 39 members of the Heaven's Gate group who committed suicide because they believed they would reach an alien spacecraft following Comet Hale–Bopp (Lamberg, 1997).

Suicide Clusters

A suicide cluster is defined as an excessive number of suicides occurring in close temporal and geographic proximity (Larkin & Beautrais, 2012). In the United States, it has been estimated that at least 2% of teenage suicides occur in temporal–spatial clusters. Clustering is thought to be two to four times more common among adolescents and young adults (15 to 24 years old) than among other age groups (Gould et al., 1990). Suicide clusters tend to occur in those who have contact with mental health services (McKenzie, 2005) or are in psychiatric hospitals (Haw, 1994), prisons (McKenzie & Keane, 2007), and schools (Brent et al., 1989).

We have a limited understanding of what triggers a suicide cluster and what causes it to continue and to eventually subside. A psychological explanation for the phenomenon is that suicide clusters occur when already vulnerable individuals, who are socially connected through shared characteristics, experience the suicide of a peer (Joiner, 1999). Other psychological processes, such as suggestion, identification, social learning, and susceptibility, are also implicated in the development of suicide clusters (Haw et al., 2013). Most theories rely on the analogy of contagious illness, suggesting that clustering is a result of imitation of suicidal behavior. Novel channels of transmission for suicide contagion may include social networks (Mesoudi, 2009), media reporting (Niederkrotenthaler et al., 2010), and the Internet (Pirkis & Nordentoft, 2011).

COVID-19 Pandemic

Beginning in March 2020, the COVID-19 pandemic and response, which included physical distancing and stay-at-home orders, disrupted daily life in the United States and around the world. Compared with the rate in 2019, a 31% increase in the proportion of mental health-related ED visits occurred among adolescents 12 to 17 years old in 2020. In June 2020, 25% of surveyed adults 18 to 24 years old reported experiencing suicidal ideation related to the pandemic in the past 30 days. More recent patterns of ED visits for suspected suicide attempts among these age groups are unclear. Using data from the National Syndromic Surveillance Program (NSSP), the CDC examined trends in ED visits for suspected suicide attempts during January 1, 2019, to May 15, 2021, among persons 12 to 25 years old, by sex, and at three distinct

phases of the COVID-19 pandemic. In comparison to the corresponding period in 2019, during March 29 to April 25, 2020, persons 12 to 25 years old
made fewer ED visits for suspected suicide attempts. However, by early May
2020, ED visit counts for suspected suicide attempts began increasing among
adolescents 12 to 17 years old, especially among girls.

During July 26 to August 22, 2020, the mean weekly number of ED
visits for suspected suicide attempts among girls age 12 to 17 was 26.2%
higher than during the same period a year earlier; during February 21
to March 20, 2021, mean weekly ED visit counts for suspected suicide
attempts among girls age 12 to 17 were 50.6% higher than during the
same period in 2019. Suicide prevention measures focused on young persons call for a comprehensive approach that is adapted during times of
infrastructure disruption, that involves multisectoral partnerships (e.g.,
public health, mental health, schools, and families), and that implements
evidence-based strategies (3) addressing the range of factors influencing
suicide risk.

Case Examples

The first two parts of the imminent suicide risk assessment, the suicidal
narrative and the suicide crisis syndrome, intentionally do not contain any
questions about suicide. The purpose of this omission is to avoid openly revealing the true purpose of the interview, making it difficult for those with
high suicidal desire to hide the degree of their suicidal intent. The implicit
risk/attitude/capability assessment uses the word *suicide* and asks general
questions about suicide attitudes and exposure. Still, the module assesses suicide risk only indirectly, reducing the risk of the patient's becoming defensive
and giving misleading answers.

Interview Algorithm

1. Attitudes toward suicide
    a. Cultural
        i. General questions
            I am not sure about your exact cultural background, please tell
            me a little about your family.

In your culture, how important is it to be loyal to your family?

How far do people go in restoring family honor?

What is your culture's attitude toward suicide?

Is suicide sometimes the right thing to do?

What is your personal opinion?

 ii. Suicide questions

Do you think for some misdeeds suicide is the right solution?

The only solution?

 b. Religious

  i. General questions

Are you a religious person?

How does your religion regard human life?

How does it regard the human soul?

Is there life after death?

How does what you do in life affect what happens after death?

Are you spiritual?

Are we one with the Universe?

  ii. Suicide questions

Does suicide mean the end of one's immortal soul?

Does it mean you will go to Hell?

Make you one with the Universe?

2. Capability for suicide

 a. Trait fearlessness and pain insensitivity

  i. General questions

Are you more fearless than most people?

Are you less sensitive to pain than others?

Are you afraid of death?

Are you afraid of pain of death?

  ii. Suicide questions

Would you be scared to kill yourself?

Would you be afraid of the pain associated with suicide?

 b. Acquired capability: Exposure and practicing

  i. General questions

Can you train yourself to be brave?

To not be scared of death or pain?

How?

How do you think it should be done?

ii. Suicide questions

Have you tried to hurt yourself before? By what means?

Have you attempted suicide? By what means?

Did this make you less scared of suicide?

c. Suicide in the military

i. General questions

How was military service for you?

Did it provide purpose and self-respect?

How is it to be a civilian?

Was it a difficult transition?

Do you feel like a burden?

Do you feel a lack of understanding and respect?

Do you feel alone?

ii. Suicide questions

Can it be so bad, it would not be worthwhile (possible) to continue?

3. Contagion

a. Suicide of family and friends

i. Suicide questions

Has anybody among your family and friends died by suicide?

What happened?

Where were you?

How did this affect you?

b. Suicide clusters

i. Suicide questions

Has anybody among your friends died by suicide?

What happened?

Where were you at the time?

How did this affect you?

Have any of your favorite celebrities died by suicide?

What happened?

Where were you at the time?

How did this affect you?

Do you know anybody who posted suicide messages on social media?

Have you gone on suicide sites? Chats?

What would friends do if they became suicidal?

Case 1: High Risk for Imminent Suicide

Randy, a 22-year-old college student, was brought to the ED after he staggered into a lecture hall and passed out on the floor. Six months earlier, Randy was hospitalized after a suicide attempt via overdose. He was diagnosed with depression, treated with Wellbutrin, and discharged. He stopped Wellbutrin and did not follow up with his therapist.

1. Attitudes toward suicide
   a. Cultural
      i. General questions
         DR: Randy, please tell me a little about your family.
         RANDY: What do you want to know? They are stupid.
         DR: What do you mean?
         RANDY: They are wrapped up in their miserable lives, they have no idea what is going on.
      ii. Suicide questions
         DR: Let's say you were close to your parents. Could you do anything so shameful that the only way to redeem yourself would be suicide?
         RANDY: That's crazy. I can see many reasons why life may not be worth living, but failing to live up to parents' expectations is not one of them.
   b. Religious
      i. Suicide questions
         DR: Since you mentioned it, what would be such a reason?
         RANDY: The world is a miserable place.
         DR: Isn't suicide a morally wrong thing to do?
         RANDY: It's a choice. I see no intrinsic value to life.
2. Capability for suicide
   a. Trait fearlessness and pain insensitivity
      i. General questions
         DR: Are you a brave person?
         RANDY: I am not a coward.
         DR: Tell me something brave you have done.
         RANDY: I graduated from high school. I had to fight. I got beat up a lot.
         DR: Are you more or less sensitive to pain than others?

RANDY: See this? (Proceeds to show scars on forearms from cutting.) I am not afraid of pain.

DR: Are you afraid of death?

RANDY: No.

ii. Suicide questions

DR: Suicide can be a violent and painful, particularly when you are young and healthy.

RANDY: If you do it right you should not feel anything.

DR: Like how?

RANDY: With a gun

DR: Do you have a gun?

RANDY: I can get one if I need to.

b. Acquired capability: Exposure and practicing

i. General questions

DR: Have you seen a lot of violence in your life?

RANDY: No more than anybody else.

ii. Suicide questions

DR: When you tried to kill yourself, what did you overdose on?

RANDY: Valium and vodka.

DR: Did you mean to die?

RANDY: Not sure. I kind of wanted to see what would happen.

DR: And?

RANDY: I wouldn't do that again. Too unreliable.

3. Contagion

a. Suicide in family

i. Suicide questions

DR: Has anybody in your family committed suicide?

RANDY: My cousin shot himself when he was 18.

DR: Were you close with him?

RANDY: Pretty close.

DR: Did he kill himself on the first try?

RANDY: Yeah with a shotgun.

DR: Where were you at the time?

RANDY: Sleeping.

DR: How did this affect you?

RANDY: It seemed sudden. . . . He was not happy. It seemed like a solution.

b. Suicide clusters

Table 4.1 Suicide implicit factors assessment, Case 1

Component	Risk Level				
	Minimal	Low	Moderate	High	Severe
Attitudes		X			
Moral religious prohibition/ permissiveness					X
Capability—trait					X
Capability—practicing					X
Family suicide					X
Suicide clusters					X
Total					X

    i. Suicide questions
       DR: How long ago did your cousin kill himself?
       RANDY: Six months now.
       DR: Didn't you overdose at about the same time? (Silence)
       DR: Did you plan on it together?
       RANDY: I don't want to talk about it.
       DR: Did you research your overdose method?
       RANDY: You don't need to research much. It's right out there.

Randy's risk for imminent suicide is very high (Table 4.1). He does not value human life, has no moral or religious prohibitions, and has a philosophical position justifying suicide. He is fearless and had a practice attempt. Finally, he had a suicide in the family, may have had a suicide pact with his cousin, and has access to a gun.

Case 2: Moderate Risk for Imminent Suicide

A 20-year-old Asian, Christian female with a previous suicide attempt by overdose was admitted to an inpatient unit. When asked about her mental state, she said she was fine other than she could not control her crying and screaming. During interviews, she would interrupt her answers with loud wailing.

1. Attitudes toward suicide
    a. Cultural
        i. General questions
            DR: I am not sure about your exact cultural background; please tell me a little about your culture.

            A: I am Korean, my parents are Korean.

            DR: I do not know much about Korean culture or about Korean values. How important is family honor in Korea?

            A: Very important.

            DR: What does a young person need to do to be honorable?

            A: Study hard and get good grades.

            DR: What if they try and can't? Can they live with that?

            A: That would be shame on the family! They just need to study harder.

            DR: In your culture, would one rather die than bring shame on the family?

            A: Yes, sometimes, but I am a Christian—it's a sin. Your soul only goes to Heaven if you are not a sinner.
        ii. Suicide questions
            DR: If you were not Christian, would you think suicide the right solution?

            A: Yes, if your family is ashamed of you (crying).

            DR: The only solution?

            A: I don't know.
    b. Religious
        i. General questions
            DR: You said you are a Christian. What denomination are your parents, and you, as a matter of fact?

            A: We go to the same church; it is Korean.

            DR: For Christians, suicide is a sin, isn't it?

            A: Yes.

            DR: What happens to your soul when you die?

            A: It goes to Heaven if you are not a sinner.
        ii. Suicide questions
            DR: And if you kill yourself?

            A: Hell.

            DR: You tried to kill yourself before . . .

A: I don't want to go to Hell, I will never do that again, it was a mistake (wailing).

2. Capability for suicide
   a. Trait fearlessness and pain insensitivity
      i. General questions
         DR: Are you a brave person?
         A: No.
         DR: Are you scared of pain?
         A: No, pain makes me feel good sometimes.
         DR: Are you scared of death?
         A: Yes.
         DR: Are you scared of the pain you would feel when you die?
         A: Yes.
      ii. Suicide questions
         DR: Would you be scared to kill yourself?
         A: Yes.
         DR: But you tried to overdose.
         A: (Wailing) It was not serious . . .
         DR: Was it painful?
         A: When they pumped my stomach.
   b. Acquired capability: Exposure and practicing
      i. Suicide questions
         DR: Now that you have tried overdosing once and it was not painful, would it be easier a second time?
         A: I am not going to. . . . I already told you—I am a Christian.
         DR: What about the last time? You took a whole bottle.
         A: I don't know what happened, I could not think straight.

3. Contagion
   a. Suicide in family
      i. Suicide questions
         DR: Has anybody in your family committed suicide?
         A: Yes, my grandfather jumped off a bridge
         DR: Where?
         A: Home in Korea. I was in the US.
   b. Suicide clusters
      i. Suicide questions
         DR: Has anybody among your friends recently died by suicide?
         A: No.

Table 4.2 Suicide implicit factors assessment, Case 2

Component	Minimal	Low	Moderate	High	Severe
			Risk Level		
Attitudes				X	
Moral religious prohibitions/ permissiveness		X			
Capability—trait			X		
Capability—practicing				X	
Family suicide			X		
Suicide clusters	X				
Total			X		

DR: Do you know of anybody who did?
A: Yes, Robin Williams. I think he hanged himself.
DR: Have you visited any suicide websites? Taken part in chats?
A: No.

A's risk for suicide is moderate (Table 4.2). Her culture accepts honor suicide to avoid family disgrace, and she is aware of this. She is not intrinsically brave and is scared of pain, but she overcame that by finding a painless way to die. Her Christian faith still seems somewhat protective, the suicide in her family was remote, and she does not seem to care about the suicide of a public figure or want to be part of a "suicide community."

Case 3: Low Risk for Imminent Suicide

Mark is a 60-year-old married Jewish lawyer with a history of bipolar disorder who lost his practice while having a hypomanic episode. His depression was not improving despite his medications, and he was getting desperate. He felt like he had become useless and a burden to his family.

1. Attitudes toward suicide
   a. Cultural
      i. General questions
         DR: I know you are Jewish, what denomination are you?

MARK: I am Orthodox.

DR: How important is it in the Orthodox community to be loyal to your family?

MARK: Our whole culture is about community, family, and tradition.

DR: How does the community react to someone who brings shame on their family?

MARK: We help the family, and we have rabbis who try to help the person, too.

   ii. Suicide questions

DR: What is your community's attitude toward suicide?

MARK: Suicide means desertion of your family and religion.

DR: Do you think for some misdeeds suicide is the right solution?

MARK: It is never the right solution.

b. Religious and moral attitudes
   i. General questions

DR: Are you a religious person?

MARK: Yes, I am very active in my synagogue.

DR: How does Judaism regard the human soul?

MARK: We have one.

DR: And what happens to it when you die? Does it depend on how you live your life?

MARK: It must. But we don't know.

   ii. Suicide questions

DR: What if one dies by suicide?

MARK: Nothing good—how can you do that to your family?

2. Capability for suicide
   a. Trait fearlessness and pain insensitivity
      i. General questions

DR: Would you call yourself a brave person?

MARK: I guess so.

DR: Would you say that you are fearless?

MARK: I am not fearless, everybody has fears. I am average.

      ii. Suicide questions

DR: Would killing yourself be a scary act?

MARK: Of course it would.

3. Contagion
   a. Suicide in family

      i. Suicide questions

DR: Has anybody in your family died by suicide?

MARK: Yes, my mother. She was bipolar. She overdosed when she was depressed.

DR: That must have been awful. How old were you?

MARK: I was 40. I was at work. I got a call from her home attendant who found her dead when she came to work in the morning.

DR: How did this affect you?

MARK: I am scared that I will end up the same way.

DR: What has prevented you so far?

MARK: It's just the wrong thing to do. And my family.

  b. Suicide clusters

      i. Suicide questions

DR: Besides your mother, did anybody else you know attempt suicide?

MARK: Not personally. Just celebrities. Robin Williams.

DR: How did this affect you?

MARK: It was scary. They say he was depressed, but he was clearly bipolar. He was so manic when he was young.

DR: Do you know of any online suicide sites?

MARK: No.

Although the acuity of Mark's suicidal state may be high, his capability for suicide is low (Table 4.3). Mark has negative attitudes toward suicide both

Table 4.3 Suicide implicit factors assessment, Case 3

Component	Risk Level				
	Minimal	Low	Moderate	High	Severe
Attitudes	X				
Moral religious prohibitions/permissiveness	X				
Capability—trait	X				
Capability—practicing	X				
Family suicide			X		
Suicide clusters	X				
Total		X			

culturally and from a moral and religious perspective. However, his mother did kill herself, which elevates his suicide risk from minimal to low.

Test Case 1

Lenny is a 60-year-old man, never married, with bipolar disorder. When he was 57 years old, he was hospitalized with a manic episode after being promoted at work and losing sleep due to stress. He subsequently lost his job and has been depressed for three years, with daily suicidal thoughts.

1. Attitudes toward suicide
   a. Cultural
      i. General questions
         DR: Tell me a little about your family.
         LENNY: My sister is a social worker, and my brother is a sound technician. My father is dead. My mother is in a nursing home with Alzheimer's disease.
         DR: Are you a close family?
         LENNY: No. I have not spoken to my brother in months. I talk to my sister once a week, but she does not want to talk to me right now because I am making her depressed. I am not even sure if they would miss me if I died.
         DR: I am sorry to hear that you feel alone in your family. When you have your thoughts about suicide, is your family holding you back?
         LENNY: No, just my fear of actually doing it.
      ii. Suicide questions
         DR: Do you think that there are situations when suicide is a legitimate option?
         LENNY: Yes, if the pain is unbearable
   b. Religious
      i. General questions
         DR: Are you religious?
         LENNY: I am Jewish, but I am not observant.
         DR: How does Judaism regard suicide?
         LENNY: I would imagine negatively.
         DR: What does this mean to you?

LENNY: Not much.

DR: Do you believe in God? In the human soul?

LENNY: Maybe there is God—somebody had to create the Universe. I don't think there is an eternal soul or life after death.

    ii. Suicide questions

    DR: Should the fate of your eternal soul be a consideration when someone contemplates suicide?

    LENNY: For somebody like me? No.

2. Capability for suicide

    a. Trait fearlessness and pain insensitivity

        i. General questions

        DR: You said that it is the fear of actually doing it that would prevent you from killing yourself. Are you a brave person?

        LENNY: No.

        DR: Are you less sensitive to pain than other people?

        LENNY: About the same.

        ii. Suicide questions

        DR: A few minutes ago, you said that fear is holding you back. You mean that you would be scared to kill yourself?

        LENNY: Yes.

        DR: What is it you are afraid of? Pain?

        LENNY: Yes. The whole thing is so violent. Even "humane" lethal injection executions are violent—people die for hours. What if you miscalculate?

    b. Exposure and practicing

        i. General questions

        DR: Can you train yourself to not be scared of death?

        LENNY: Isn't that what military training is about?

        ii. Suicide questions

        DR: Do you think it is possible to train yourself not to be scared of suicide?

        LENNY: Maybe.

3. Contagion

    a. Suicide in family

        i. Suicide questions

        DR: Has anybody in your family died by suicide?

        LENNY: No.

Table 4.4 Suicide implicit factors assessment, Test Case 1

	Risk Level				
Component	Minimal	Low	Moderate	High	Severe
Attitudes					
Moral religious prohibitions/ permissiveness					
Capability—trait					
Capability—practicing					
Family or friend suicide					
Suicide clusters					
Total					

    b. Suicide clusters

        i. Suicide questions

            DR: Have any of your friends died by suicide?

            LENNY: Yes. One of my friends. He hanged himself.

            DR: How did this affect you?

            LENNY: It was very upsetting. I wished I were dead instead.

            DR: How long ago was that?

            LENNY: Two years.

            DR: Are you aware of any celebrities who died by suicide?

            LENNY: Robin Williams. He also hanged himself. He was depressed.

            DR: Do you know of any suicide sites?

            LENNY: Yes, I went to some.

            DR: Did you post messages?

            LENNY: No, just read.

Lenny is alienated from his family and has no moral objections to suicide. He believes that suicide is justifiable if one is in too much pain. These two factors put him at high risk (Table 4.4). He is fearful of pain and timid, factors that decrease his risk. However, he had a strong and personal reaction to his friend's suicide, increasing his risk. Overall, Lenny is at high risk for imminent suicide.

References

Adam, K. S., Lohrenz, J. G., Harper, D., & Streiner, D. (1982). Early parental loss and suicidal ideation in university students. *Canadian Journal of Psychiatry, 27*(4), 275–281.

Affrunti, N. W., & Ginsburg, G. S. (2012). Maternal overcontrol and child anxiety: The mediating role of perceived competence. *Child Psychiatry & Human Development, 43*(1), 102–112.

Ajdacic-Gross, V. (2008). Methods of suicide: International suicide patterns derived from the WHO mortality database. *Bulletin of the World Health Organization, 86*(9), 726–732.

American Foundation for Suicide Prevention. (2016). *Suicide statistics.* https://afsp.org/about-suicide/suicide-statistics

American Psychiatric Association. (2013). *Diagnostic and statistical manual of mental disorders* (5th ed.). American Psychiatric Association Publishing.

Anestis, M. D., & Joiner, T. E. (2011). Examining the role of emotion in suicidality: Negative urgency as an amplifier of the relationship between components of the interpersonal-psychological theory of suicidal behavior and lifetime number of suicide attempts. *Journal of Affective Disorders, 129*(1-3), 261–269.

Bauer, B. W., Gai, A. R., Duffy, M. E., Rogers, M. L., Khazem, L. R., Martin, R. L., Joiner, T. E., & Capron, D. W. (2020). Fearlessness about death does not differ by suicide attempt method. *Journal of Psychiatric Research, 124*, 42–49.

Borges, G., Orozco, R., Rafful, C., Miller, E., & Breslau, J. (2011). Suicidality, ethnicity and immigration in the USA. *Psychological Medicine, 42*(06), 1175–1184.

Bostwick, J. M., Pabbati, C., Geske, J. R., & McKean, A. J. (2016). Suicide attempt as a risk factor for completed suicide: Even more lethal than we knew. *American Journal of Psychiatry, 173*(11), 1094–1100.

Bowlby, J. (1969). *Attachment and loss: Vol. 1. Attachment.* Basic Books.

Bowlby, J. (1980). *Attachment and loss: Vol. 3. Loss: Sadness and depression.* Hogarth.

Brent, D. A., Kerr, M. M., Goldstein, C., Bozigar, J., Wartella, M., & Allan, M. J. (1989). An outbreak of suicide and suicidal behavior in a high school. *Journal of the American Academy of Child & Adolescent Psychiatry, 28*(6), 918–924.

Burr, E. M., Rahm-Knigge, R. L., & Conner, B. T. (2018). The differentiating role of state and trait hopelessness in suicidal ideation and suicide attempt. *Archives of Suicide Research, 22*(3), 510–517.

Campos, R. C., Besser, A., & Blatt, S. J. (2010). The mediating role of self-criticism and dependency in the association between perceptions of maternal caring and depressive symptoms. *Depression and Anxiety, 27*(12), 1149–1157.

Cash, S. J., & Bridge, J. A. (2009). Epidemiology of youth suicide and suicidal behavior. *Current Opinion in Pediatrics, 21*(5), 613–619.

Catechism of the Catholic Church. (n.d.). http://www.scborromeo.org/ccc/p3s2c2a5.htm

Centers for Disease Control and Prevention. (2018, April 13). *QuickStats: Age-adjusted suicide rates, by race/ethnicity—National Vital Statistics System, United States, 2015–2016.* http://dx.doi.org/10.15585/mmwr.mm6714a6

Centers for Disease Control and Prevention. (2020, March 6) *QuickStats: Age-adjusted suicide rates, by sex and three most common methods—United States, 2000–2018.* http://dx.doi.org/10.15585/mmwr.mm6909a7external%20icon

Centers for Disease Control and Prevention. (2020, May 1). *QuickStats: Age-adjusted suicide rates, by state—National Vital Statistics System, United States, 2018.* http://dx.doi.org/10.15585/mmwr.mm6917a4

Centers for Disease Control and Prevention. (2021, December 2). *WISQARS™ —Web-based Injury Statistics Query and Reporting System.* https://webappa.cdc.gov/sasweb/ncipc/mortrate.html

Chambers, A. (2010, August 3). Japan: Ending the culture of the "honourable" suicide. *The Guardian.*

Chang, B., Gitlin, D., & Patel, R. (2011). The depressed patient and suicidal patient in the emergency department: Evidence-based management and treatment strategies. *Emergency Medicine Practice, 13*(9), 1–23.

Clark, C. B., Li, Y., & Cropsey, K. L. (2016). Family dysfunction and suicide risk in a community corrections sample. *Crisis, 37*(6), 454–460.

Cole, A. B., Littlefield, A. K., Gauthier, J. M., & Bagge, C. L. (2019). Impulsivity facets and perceived likelihood of future suicide attempt among patients who recently attempted suicide. *Journal of Affective Disorders, 257,* 195–199.

Cornette, M. M., deRoon-Cassini, T. A., Fosco, G. M., Holloway, R. L., Clark, D. C., & Joiner, T. E. (2009). Application of an interpersonal-psychological model of suicidal behavior to physicians and medical trainees. *Archives of Suicide Research, 13*(1), 1–14.

Cosgrove, V. E., Rhee, S. H., Gelhorn, H. L., Boeldt, D., Corley, R. C., Ehringer, M. A., Young, S. E., & Hewitt, J. K. (2011). Structure and etiology of co-occurring internalizing and externalizing disorders in adolescents. *Journal of Abnormal Child Psychology, 39*(1), 109–123.

Crowell, S. E., Beauchaine, T. P., & Linehan, M. M. (2009). A biosocial developmental model of borderline personality: Elaborating and extending Linehan's theory. *Psychological Bulletin, 135*(3), 495–510

Curtin, S. C., Warner, M., & Hedegaard, H. (2016). *Increase in suicide in the United States, 1999-2014* (No. 241). National Center for Health Statistics.

Dervic, K., Carballo, J. J., Baca-Garcia, E., Galfalvy, H. C., Mann, J. J., Brent, D. A., & Oquendo, M. A. (2011). Moral or religious objections to suicide may protect against suicidal behavior in bipolar disorder. *Journal of Clinical Psychiatry, 72*(10), 1390–1396.

Dublin, L. I. (1963). *Suicide: A sociological and statistical study.* Ronald.

Fergusson, D. M., Woodward, L. J., & Horwood, L. J. (2000). Risk factors and life processes associated with the onset of suicidal behavior during adolescence and early adulthood. *Psychological Medicine, 30*(1), 23–39.

Ferm, M. S., Frazee, L. A., Kennard, B. D., King, J. D., Emslie, G. J., & Stewart, S. M. (2020). Fearlessness about death predicts adolescent suicide attempt: A preliminary analysis. *Suicide and Life-Threatening Behavior, 50*(6), 1288–1295.

Forte, A., Trobia, F., Gualtieri, F., Lamis, D. A., Cardamone, G., Giallonardo, V., Fiorillo, A., Girardi, P., & Pompili, M. (2018). Suicide risk among immigrants and ethnic minorities: A literature overview. *International Journal of Environmental Research and Public Health, 15*(7), 1438.

Freeman, A., Mergl, R., Kohls, E., Székely, A., Gusmao, R., Arensman, E. & Rummel-Kluge, C. (2017). A cross-national study on gender differences in suicide intent. *BMC Psychiatry, 17*(1), 234.

Galynker, I. I., Yaseen, Z. S., Briggs, J., & Hayashi, F. (2015). Attitudes of acceptability and lack of condemnation toward suicide may be predictive of post-discharge suicide attempts. *BMC Psychiatry, 15*(1), 87.

Geulayov, G., Gunnell, D., Holmen, T. L., & Metcalfe, C. (2012). The association of parental fatal and non-fatal suicidal behaviour with offspring suicidal behaviour and depression: A systematic review and meta-analysis. *Psychological Medicine, 42*, 1567–1580.

Gianatsi, M., Burns, H., Hunt, I. M., Ibrahim, S., Windfuhr, K., While, D., Appleby, L., & Kapur, N. (2020). Treatment of mental illness prior to suicide: A national investigation of 12,909 patients, 2001–2016. *Psychiatric Services, 71*(8), 772–778.

Goldston, D. B., Reboussin, B. A., & Daniel, S. S. (2006). Predictors of suicide attempts: State and trait components. *Journal of Abnormal Psychology, 115*, 842–849.

Goschin, S., Briggs, J., Blanco-Luten, S., Cohen, L. J., & Galynker, I. (2013). Parental affectionless control and suicidality. *Journal of Affective Disorders, 151*(1), 1–6.

Gould, M. S., Wallenstein, S., Kleinman, M. H., O'Carroll, P., & Mercy, J. (1990). Suicide clusters: An examination of age-specific effects. *American Journal of Public Health, 80*(2), 211–212.

Green, J., Berry, K., Danquah, A., & Pratt, D. (2020a). The role of psychological and social factors in the relationship between attachment and suicide: A systematic review. *Clinical Psychology & Psychotherapy, 27*(4), 463–488.

Green, A. E., Price-Feeney, M., & Dorison, S. H. (2020b). Association of sexual orientation acceptance with reduced suicide attempts among lesbian, gay, bisexual, transgender, queer, and questioning youth. *LGBT Health, 8*(1), 26–31.

Griffin, D., & Bartholomew, K. (1994). Models of the self and other: Fundamental dimensions underlying measures of adult attachment. *Journal of Personality and Social Psychology, 67*, 430–445.

Gunnell, D., & Frankel, S. (1994). Prevention of suicide: Aspirations and evidence. *BMJ, 308*(6938), 1227–1233.

Gureje, O., Oladeji, B., Hwang, I., Chiu, W. T., Kessler, R. C., Sampson, N. A., Alonso, J., Andrade, L. H., Beautrais, A., Borges, G., Bromet, E., Bruffaerts, R., de Girolamo, G., de Graaf, R., Gal, G., He, Y., Hu, C., Iwata, N., Karam, E. G., . . . Nock, M. K. (2010). Parental psychopathology and the risk of suicidal behavior in their offspring: Results from the World Mental Health surveys. *Molecular Psychiatry, 16*(12), 1221–1233.

Gururaj, G., Isaac, M. K., Subbakrishna, D. K., & Ranjani, R. (2004). Risk factors for completed suicides: A case-control study from Bangalore, India. *Injury Control and Safety Promotion, 11*(3), 183–191.

Hadzic, A., Spangenberg, L., Hallensleben, N., Forkmann, T., Rath, D., Strauss, M., Kersting, A., & Glaesmer, H. (2019). The association of trait impulsivity and suicidal ideation and its fluctuation in the context of the interpersonal theory of suicide. *Comprehensive Psychiatry, 98*, 152158.

Haw, C. (1994). A cluster of suicides at a London psychiatric unit. *Suicide and Life-Threatening Behavior, 24*, 256–266.

Haw, C., Hawton, K., Niedzwiedz, C., & Platt, S. (2013). Suicide clusters: A review of risk factors and mechanisms. *Suicide and Life-Threatening Behavior, 43*(1), 97–108.

Hawton, K., Zahl, D., & Weatherall, R. (2003). Suicide following deliberate self-harm: Long-term follow-up of patients who presented to a general hospital. *British Journal of Psychiatry, 182*(6), 537–542.

Hirsch, J. K. (2006). A review of the literature on rural suicide. *Crisis, 27*(4), 189–199.

Hoertel, N., Franco, S., Wall, M. M., Oquendo, M. A., Kerridge, B. T., Limosin, F., & Blanco, C. (2015). Mental disorders and risk of suicide attempt: A national prospective study. *Molecular Psychiatry, 20*(6), 718–726.

Holland, N. (1977). *Literary suicide: A question of style.* http://users.clas.ufl.edu/nholland/suicide.htm

Joiner, J. T. (1999). The clustering and contagion of suicide. *Current Directions in Psychological Science, 8*(3), 89–92.

Joiner, T. E. (2005). *Why people die by suicide.* Harvard University Press.

Johns, M. M., Lowry, R., Rasberry, C. N., Dunville, R., Robin, L., Pampati, S., Stone, D. M., & Kollar, L. M. M. (2018). Violence victimization, substance use, and suicide risk among sexual minority high school students—United States, 2015–2017. *Morbidity and Mortality Weekly Report, 67*(43), 1211–1215.

Kessler, R. C., Chiu, W. T., Demler, O., & Walters, E. E. (2005). Prevalence, severity, and comorbidity of 12-month DSM-IV disorders in the National Comorbidity Survey replication. *Archives of General Psychiatry, 62*(6), 617.

Kleiman, E. M., & Liu, R. T. (2013). Social support as a protective factor in suicide: Findings from two nationally representative samples. *Journal of Affective Disorders, 150*(2), 540–545.

Knappe, S., Beesdo-Baum, K., Fehm, L., Lieb, R., & Wittchen, H. (2012). Characterizing the association between parenting and adolescent social phobia. *Journal of Anxiety Disorders, 26*(5), 608–616.

Lamberg, L. (1997). Psychiatrist explores apocalyptic violence in Heaven's Gate and Aum Shinrikyo cults. *JAMA, 278*(3), 191–193.

Larkin, G. L., & Beautrais, A. (2012). Geospatial mapping of suicide clusters. *Te Pou o Te Whakaaro Nui.*

Lawrence, R. E., Oquendo, M. A., & Stanley, B. (2015). Religion and suicide risk: A systematic review. *Archives of Suicide Research, 20*(1), 1–21.

Layland, E. K., Exten, C., Mallory, A. B., Williams, N. D., & Fish, J. N. (2020). Suicide attempt rates and associations with discrimination are greatest in early adulthood for sexual minority adults across diverse racial and ethnic groups. *LGBT Health, 7*(8), 439–447.

Levi-Belz, Y., Gvion, Y., Horesh, N., & Apter, A. (2013). Attachment patterns in medically serious suicide attempts: The mediating role of self-disclosure and loneliness. *Suicide and Life-Threatening Behavior, 43*(5), 511–522.

Lobera, I. J., Ríos, P. B., & Casals, O. G. (2011). Parenting styles and eating disorders. *Journal of Psychiatric and Mental Health Nursing, 18*(8), 728–735.

Mancinelli, I., Comparelli, A., Girardi, P., & Tatarelli, R. (2002). Mass suicide: Historical and psychodynamic considerations. *Suicide and Life-Threatening Behavior, 32*(1), 91–100.

Mann, J. J., Apter, A., Bertolote, J., Beautrais, A., Currier, D., Haas, A., Hegerl, U., Lonnqvist, J., Malone, K., Marusic, A., Mehlum, L., Patton, G., Phillips, M., Rutz, W., Rihmer, Z., Schmidtke, A., Shaffer, D., Silverman, M., Takahashi, Y., . . . Hendin, H. (2005). Suicide prevention strategies: A systematic review. *JAMA Psychiatry, 294*, 2064–2074.

Mann, J. J., Waternaux, C., Haas, G. L., & Malone, K. M. (1999). Toward a clinical model of suicidal behavior in psychiatric patients. *American Journal of Psychiatry, 156*(2), 181–189.

McGarvey, E. L., Kryzhanovskaya, L. A., Koopman, C., Waite, D., & Canterbury, R. J. (1999). Incarcerated adolescents' distress and suicidality in relation to parental bonding styles. *Crisis, 20*(4), 164–170.

McKenzie, N. (2005). Clustering of suicides among people with mental illness. *British Journal of Psychiatry, 187*(5), 476–480.

McKenzie, N., & Keane, M. (2007). Contribution of imitative suicide to the suicide rate in prisons. *Suicide and Life-Threatening Behavior, 37*(5), 538–542.

McKinney, C., Donnelly, R., & Renk, K. (2008). Perceived parenting, positive and negative perceptions of parents, and late adolescent emotional adjustment. *Child and Adolescent Mental Health, 13*(2), 66–73.

Mergl, R., Koburger, N., Heinrichs, K., Székely, A., Tóth, M. D., Coyne, J., Quintão, S., Arensman, E., Coffey, C., Maxwell, M., Värnik, A., van Audenhove, C., McDaid, D., Sarchiapone, M., Schmidtke, A., Genz, A., Gusmão, R., & Hegerl, U. (2015). What are reasons for the large gender differences in the lethality of suicidal acts? An epidemiological analysis in four European countries. *PLOS One, 10*(7), e0129062.

Mcsoudi, A. (2009). The cultural dynamics of copycat suicide. *PLOS One, 4*(9), e7252.

Miller, L. (2006). Suicide by cop: Causes, reactions, and practical intervention strategies. *International Journal of Emergency Mental Health, 8*(3), 165–174.

Mohamed, F., Perera, A., Wijayaweera, K., Kularatne, K., Jayamanne, S., Eddleston, M., Dawson, A., Konradsen, F., & Gunnell, D. (2010). The prevalence of previous self-harm amongst self-poisoning patients in Sri Lanka. *Social Psychiatry and Psychiatric Epidemiology, 46*(6), 517–520.

Nanayakkara, S., Misch, D., Chang, L., & Henry, D. (2013). Depression and exposure to suicide predict suicide attempt. *Depression and Anxiety, 30*(10), 991–996.

Nasseri, K., & Moulton, L. H. (2009). Patterns of death in the first and second generation immigrants from selected Middle Eastern countries in California. *Journal of Immigrant and Minority Health, 13*(2), 361–370.

Niederkrotenthaler, T., Voracek, M., Herberth, A., Till, B., Strauss, M., Etzersdorfer, E., Eisenwort, B., & Sonneck, G. (2010). Role of media reports in completed and prevented suicide: *Werther v. Papageno* effects. *British Journal of Psychiatry, 197*(3), 234–243.

Nishimura, A., Shioiri, T., Nushida, H., Ueno, Y., Ushiyama, I., Tanegashima, A., Someya, T., & Nishi, K. (1999). Changes in choice of method and lethality between last attempted and completed suicides: How did suicide attempters carry out their desire? *Legal Medicine, 1*(3), 150–158.

Nordentoft, M., Breum, L., Munck, L. K., Nordestgaard, A. G., Hunding, A., & Laursen-Bjaeldager, P. A. (1993). High mortality by natural and unnatural causes: A 10 year follow up study of patients admitted to a poisoning treatment centre after suicide attempts. *BMJ, 306*(6893), 1637–1641.

O'Connor, R. C. (2007). The relations between perfectionism and suicidality: A systematic review. *Suicide and Life-Threatening Behavior, 37*(6), 698–714.

O'Connor, R. C., Smyth, R., Ferguson, E., Ryan, C., & Williams, J. M. G. (2013). Psychological processes and repeat suicidal behavior: a four-year prospective study. *Journal of Consulting and Clinical Psychology, 81*(6), 1137–1143.

Öhman, A., & Mineka, S. (2001). Fear, phobias and preparedness: Toward an evolved module of fear and fear learning. *Psychological Review, 108*, 483–522.

Osterman, L. L., & Brown, R. P. (2011). Culture of honor and violence against the self. *Personality and Social Psychology Bulletin, 37*(12), 1611–1623.

Owens, D., Horrocks, J., & House, A. (2002). Fatal and non-fatal repetition of self harm: Systematic review. *British Journal of Psychiatry, 181*, 193–199.

Parker, G. (1981). Parental reports of depressives. *Journal of Affective Disorders, 3*(2), 131–140.

Parker, G. (1989). The Parental Bonding Instrument: Psychometric properties reviewed. *Psychiatric Development, 7*(4), 317–335.

Parker, G., Tupling, H., & Brown, L. B. (1979). A parental bonding instrument. *British Journal of Medical Psychology, 52*, 1–10.

Phillips, M. R., Yang, G., Zhang, Y., Wang, L., Ji, H., & Zhou, M. (2002). Risk factors for suicide in China: A national case-control psychological autopsy study. *Lancet, 360*(9347), 1728–1736.

Pia, T., Galynker, I., Schuck, A., Sinclair, C., Ying, G., & Calati, R. (2020). Perfectionism and prospective near-term suicidal thoughts and behaviors: The mediation of fear of humiliation and suicide crisis syndrome. *International Journal of Environmental Research and Public Health, 17*(4), 1424.

Pirkis, J., & Nordentoft, M. (2011). Media influences on suicide and attempted suicide. In R. C. O'Connor, S. Platt, & J Gordon (Eds.), *International handbook of suicide prevention: Research, policy and practice* (pp. 531–544). Wiley Blackwell.

Qin, P., Agerbo, E., & Mortensen, P. B. (2002). Suicide risk in relation to family history of completed suicide and psychiatric disorders: A nested case-control study based on longitudinal registers. *Lancet, 360*(9340), 1126–1130.

Qin, P., & Nordentoft, M. (2005). Suicide risk in relation to psychiatric hospitalization: Evidence based on longitudinal registers. *Archives of General Psychiatry, 62*(4), 427–432.

Reger, M. A., Gahm, G. A., Kinn, J. T., Luxton, D. D., Skopp, N. A., & Bush, N. E. (2011). *Department of Defense Suicide Event Report (DoDSER) calendar year 2010 annual report*. National Center for Telehealth and Technology.

Roth, R. (2009). *Suicide and euthanasia—A biblical perspective*. http://www.acu-cell.com/suicide.htm

Rubanzana, W., Hedt-Gauthier, B. L., Ntaganira, J., & Freeman, M. D. (2014). Exposure to genocide and risk of suicide in Rwanda: A population-based case-control study. *Journal of Epidemiology and Community Health, 69*(2), 117–122.

Saffer, B. Y., Glenn, C. R., & David Klonsky, E. (2015). Clarifying the relationship of parental bonding to suicide ideation and attempts. *Suicide and Life-Threatening Behavior, 45*(4), 518–528.

Sakinofsky, I. (2000). Repetition of suicidal behaviour. In K. Hawton & K. Van Heeringen (Eds.), *The international handbook of suicide and attempted suicide* (pp. 385–404). Wiley.

Sati handprints. (2016). Retrieved on February 23 from http://www.atlasobscura.com/places/sati-handprints

Schaffer, A., Sinyor, M., Kurdyak, P., Vigod, S., Sareen, J., Reis, C., Green, D., Bolton, J., Rhodes, A., Grigoriadis, S., Cairney, J., & Cheung, A. (2016). Population-based analysis of health care contacts among suicide decedents: Identifying opportunities for more targeted suicide prevention strategies. *World Psychiatry, 15*(2), 135–145.

Selby, E. A., Anestis, M. D., Bender, T. W., Ribeiro, J. D., Nock, M. K., Rudd, M. D., Bryan, C. J., Lim, I. C., Baker, M. T., Gutierrez, P. M., & Joiner, T. E., Jr. (2010). Overcoming the fear of lethal injury: Evaluating suicidal behavior in the military through the lens of the interpersonal-psychological theory of suicide. *Clinical Psychology Review, 30*, 298–307.

Snowden, M., Steinman, L., Frederick, J., & Wilson, N. (2009). Screening for depression in older adults: Recommended instruments and considerations for community-based practice. *Clin Geriatr, 17*(9), 26–32.

Sommerfeld, E., & Malek, S. (2019). Perfectionism moderates the relationship between thwarted belongingness and perceived burdensomeness and suicide ideation in adolescents. *Psychiatric Quarterly, 90*(4), 671–681.

Soole, R., Kõlves, K., & De Leo, D. (2014). Factors related to childhood suicides. *Crisis, 35,* 292–300.

Spada, M. M., Caselli, G., Manfredi, C., Rebecchi, D., Rovetto, F., Ruggiero, G. M., Nikčević, A. V., & Sassaroli, S. (2011). Parental overprotection and metacognitions as predictors of worry and anxiety. *Behavioural and Cognitive Psychotherapy, 40*(3), 287 296.

Stark, C. R., Riordan, V., & O'Connor, R. (2011). A conceptual model of suicide in rural areas. *Rural and Remote Health, 11*(2), 1622.

Stepp, S. D., Morse, J. Q., Yaggi, K. E., Reynolds, S. K., Reed, L. I., & Pilkonis, P. A. (2008). The role of attachment styles and interpersonal problems in suicide-related behaviors. *Suicide and Life-Threatening Behavior, 38*(5), 592–607.

Thibodeau, M. A., Welch, P. G., Sareen, J., & Asmundson, G. J. (2013). Anxiety disorders are independently associated with suicide ideation and attempts: Propensity score matching in two epidemiological samples. *Depression and Anxiety, 30*(10), 947–954.

Too, L. S., Spittal, M. J., Bugeja, L., Reifels, L., Butterworth, P., & Pirkis, J. (2019). The association between mental disorders and suicide: A systematic review and meta-analysis of record linkage studies. *Journal of Affective Disorders, 259,* 302–313.

Townsend, E. (2007). Suicide terrorists: Are they suicidal? *Suicide and Life-Threatening Behavior, 37*(1), 35–49.

Värnik, P. (2012). Suicide in the world. *International Journal of Environmental Research and Public Health, 9*(3), 760–771.

Wang, J., Sumner, S. A., Simon, T. R., Crosby, A. E., Annor, F. B., Gaylor, E., Xu, L., & Holland, K. M. (2020). Trends in the incidence and lethality of suicidal acts in the United States, 2006 to 2015. *JAMA Psychiatry, 77*(7), 684–693.

Weng, S. C., Chang, J. C., Yeh, M. K., Wang, S. M., & Chen, Y. H. (2016). Factors influencing attempted and completed suicide in postnatal women: A population-based study in Taiwan. *Scientific Reports, 6,* 25770.

Zatti, C., Rosa, V., Barros, A., Valdivia, L., Calegaro, V. C., Freitas, L. H., Cereser, K. M. M., Rocha, N. S. D., Bastos, A. G., & Schuch, F. B. (2017). Childhood trauma and suicide attempt: A meta-analysis of longitudinal studies from the last decade. *Psychiatry Research, 256,* 353–358.

Zhang, J., Li, N., Tu, X. M., Xiao, S., & Jia, C. (2011). Risk factors for rural young suicide in China: A case-control study. *Journal of Affective Disorders, 129*(1-3), 244–251.

5

Stressful Life Events

With Olivia C. Lawrence, Inna Goncearenco, and Kimia Ziafat

Introduction

Stressful life events are some of the most critical factors precipitating suicidal behavior. They often occur during the week or month preceding suicide and are directly related to near-term suicide. Stressful life events dramatically increase the risk of suicidal ideation (SI) and behavior (Howarth et al., 2020), and up to 40% of suicide decedents experience a stressful event either on the day of a suicide attempt or on the day before. Commonly, the stressful life events leading up to the attempt are related to conflicts with family members or intimate partners (Heikkinen et al., 1994; Liu et al., 2019) and financial difficulties (Coope et al., 2015). Furthermore, although many features of psychiatric disorders (e.g., category, comorbidity) typically fall under the domain of long-term risk, recent onset of a psychiatric illness, as well as the immediate course of illness following initial onset or diagnosis, is considered an acute stressor that may heighten near-term suicide risk (Qin et al., 2014). Work- and career-related problems, serious medical illness, recent substance use, and Internet/social media use are among the other sources of stressful life events that can precipitate suicide.

The links between stressful events and suicide are undeniable but not straightforward. Taken as a whole, however, evidence supporting a direct causal and temporal relationship between life stressors, motives for suicide, and suicide attempts is not unequivocal. Although evidence for an association between negative life events and SI and suicidal behavior is fairly consistent (Howarth et al., 2020), there seems to be no direct relationship between stress severity and the lethality of SI and suicidal behavior. Thus, examining potential stressors related to imminent suicide risk is essential to our understanding of their impact on an individual's life, and it is just as important to understand the role of these stressors in the suicidal narrative.

Remarkably, there is often no apparent relationship between psychiatric illness and suicidal behavior. For example, among patients with major depressive disorder (MDD), there is a weak correlation between suicide attempts and recent stressful life events for patients with comorbid borderline personality disorder (Oquendo et al., 2014). Some researchers argue that the weak association between sources of stress and suicide attempts among individuals with psychiatric illnesses may be explained by a potential lack of individual awareness of the stressor as a worsening element of their illness leading to suicide (Lim et al., 2014).

Work and Financial Hardship

Economic Hardship

Although a positive relationship between economic hardship and suicide rate is intuitive, it has been studied relatively little. Research shows that financial strain, including debt/crisis, unemployment, past homelessness, and lower income, are strong predictors of suicide attempt and SI (Elbogen et al., 2020). It appears that even in stable economic climates, suicide rates are higher in lower socioeconomic classes (Rehkopf & Buka, 2006). Low savings rates and lack of leisure time also correlate with higher suicide risk (Machado et al., 2015). Moreover, lower family income (relative to local poverty thresholds) was found to increase risk for suicidal thoughts and behaviors within the next year, and this relationship was strengthened among those who had been diagnosed with a psychiatric disorder (Pan et al., 2013).

The relationship between financial hardship and suicidal behaviors is most evident during economic crises. For example, with a worsening economic climate, suicide rates in the United States started rising in the early 2000s, after decades of decline. Although changes in suicide rates tend to reflect complex social and economic conditions that are difficult to study in isolation, a likely explanation for the reversal in trend lies in deteriorating economic conditions, culminating in the sharp rise in unemployment in 2007 to 2009. Indeed, during this time, there was a strong positive association between unemployment and suicide rates in the United States (Harper et al., 2015), specifically in middle-aged individuals (Chang et al., 2013). Likewise, a large-scale time-analysis study found a clear rise in suicide rates following the 2008 global economic crisis: in 2009 alone, 27 European countries and 18 American countries saw excess numbers of suicide deaths, surpassing expected rates based on previous trends in each country. The trends were especially pronounced in men, as well as in countries with low unemployment levels before the 2008 recession (Chang et al., 2013).

Likewise, although there was an initial decline in suicide rates during the COVID-19 pandemic in the general U.S. population (Curtin et al., 2021), it is expected that suicide rates will ultimately rise amid the long-term effects of COVID-19, as mediated by a myriad of factors, including social isolation, heightened anxiety, and serious economic hardships and dramatic mental health status deterioration (Gunnell et al., 2020). In April 2020, shortly after the outbreak of COVID-19, the unemployment rate in the United States peaked at 14.7%—the highest number ever recorded by the Bureau of Labor Statistics (Smith et al., 2021). At the time this book is being edited, there are several studies underway to address the impact of the COVID-19 pandemic on mental health and suicide in the general population, and there are statistics suggesting a decrease in suicide rates (American Foundation for Suicide Prevention, 2022; Curtin et al., 2021), as well as concomitant increases in SI, suicide attempts, and mental health utilization (American Psychological Association, 2020; Ammerman et al., 2021; Dubé et al., 2021). Nevertheless, given the well-established link between past economic recessions and increased rates of suicide (Luo et al., 2011), it is critical to incorporate an individual's financial and vocational circumstance into imminent suicide risk assessment, both in the context of pandemic-related financial hardship and beyond the COVID-19 era.

Business or Work Failure

Losing a job may serve in a suicidal narrative as failure to achieve a life goal, humiliating social defeat, or a feeling of burdensomeness. Shame and alienation combined with financial hardship and failure to find another job may result in intense entrapment and desperation (discussed further in this chapter). Thus, job loss could markedly increase suicide risk, contributing to different phases of the suicidal narrative (Hawton et al., 2015).

Case 4

Paul was a 63-year-old lawyer with a history of bipolar disorder who died in the medical intensive care unit (MICU) of a large urban hospital after being admitted for overdosing on psychiatric medications. He overdosed impulsively after his wife left the apartment, saying that she was filing for divorce. Before this, he had not expressed suicidal intent to his wife, therapist, or psychopharmacologist. This was Paul's third marriage. He met his wife when he was 50 years old, and for him it was love at first sight. Despite fairly frequent fights about his wife's out-of-control spending, their marriage was generally happy. Yet, after Paul was unexpectedly let go by his law firm during the Great Recession, their relationship started to deteriorate. At first, Paul was sure he would get a job at another law firm. After years of an unsuccessful job search, Paul retired and began living on a fixed income. Due to the stock market crash and some unwise investment decisions, he soon became depressed. He told his therapist that each time he tried to tell his wife that they needed to budget their finances differently, she would threaten a divorce. He said that she made him feel like a failure. Paul was too ashamed to face his friends, so he stopped socializing and considered himself a failure, with no way out of the situation. Paul and his wife were scheduled to meet with his therapist two days after Paul took his life.

Paul's case illustrates the relationship between business failure, economic hardship, and suicide. Because Paul had enough savings for him and his wife to live comfortably but not lavishly for the rest of their lives, his economic hardship was exacerbated by his wife's unrealistic expectations. However, given his predisposition to emotional dysregulation due to his bipolar disorder, he became acutely suicidal, resulting in a completed suicide.

Loss of Home

Homelessness is arguably the most visible sign of social and economic failure; thus, there is a direct and strong relationship between foreclosure rates and suicide rates. From 2005 through 2010, increased foreclosure rates explained 18% of the variance in the suicide rate, suggesting that the foreclosure crisis likely contributed to increased suicides, specifically in middle-aged men, independent of other economic factors associated with the Great Recession (Houle & Light, 2014). The Great Recession in Western Europe and North America was associated with at least 10,000 additional economic-related suicides. signifying that 1,800 of the suicides were due to loss of home in foreclosure (Reeves et al., 2014).

Critically, for imminent suicide risk assessment, 79% of suicides occurred before an actual housing loss, and 37% of decedents experienced acute eviction or foreclosure crises within two weeks of the suicide. Thus, impending foreclosure signifies a very high suicide risk for middle-aged men, requiring quick and preventive intervention (Fowler et al., 2015). The overall increase in suicides due to foreclosure was five times higher than that due to eviction.

Particularly for those with mental illness, imminent eviction must be considered a significant risk factor for imminent suicide (Serby et al., 2006). Eviction or foreclosure is often considered a traumatic rejection, a denial of basic human needs, and a shameful experience, particularly for those of middle-class background. Given the much higher suicide rates related to foreclosure than for eviction, it is conceivable that higher socioeconomic status may contribute to psychological vulnerability to the loss of one's home.

Case 5

Joan was a 58-year-old Caucasian woman with bipolar disorder. Although she had attempted suicide several times in recent years, her level of functioning and treatment adherence had improved considerably in the months before her death. When it became apparent that she would be evicted, plans were made for her to move into the home of friends. Her case manager and sister both spoke with her in the evening and did not notice anything amiss. The next morning, she was found dead of a self-inflicted stab wound. (This case was taken from Serby et al., 2006.)

Case 6

Jose was a 48-year-old married White man. Six weeks before his suicide, he was hospitalized with mixed mania, SI, and compulsive gambling. He was nearly $250,000 in debt and facing eviction. He had petitioned to block the eviction and was optimistic that the judge would rule in his favor. On the day before his death, the court ruled that the landlord was entitled to evict him. Jose went missing and was found the next day, dead from a drug overdose. (This case was taken from Serby et al., 2006.)

Both cases describe completed suicides related to eviction in the high-risk group of 45- to 64-year-olds. Characteristically, both took place prior to eviction and after that this measure became official and inevitable. In Joan's case, the precipitating event was the meeting with the case manager, whereas in Jose's case it was the court decision.

Relationship Conflict

Together with economic hardship or financial difficulties, intimate relationship conflict accounts for close to 80% of stressful life events preceding suicide (Kõlves et al., 2006). In an ongoing international study of suicide crisis syndrome (SCS) prevalence, relationship stressors and threats to one's role or identity were the strongest contributors to both SCS and SI (Rogers et al., under review). *Intimate relationship conflict* is the term used to describe serious and emotionally charged disagreements with a current or former intimate partner, typically involving divorce, breakups, infidelity, jealousy, or other problems. In suicide notes, marital and intimate relationship conflict is the most frequent reason given (Ortega & Karch, 2010). In psychological autopsies, approximately one-third of suicides either are preceded by a serious relationship conflict in the past two weeks of life or precede the certainty of such conflict in the next two weeks. Furthermore, suicide attempt survivors frequently indicate that marital and intimate relationship conflict precipitated the attempt (Zhang & Ma, 2012).

Romantic Rejection

Among the many stresses inherent in relationships, romantic rejection leads most frequently to suicide attempts. Two-thirds of spouses who have survived their former partner's suicide perceive their recent separation (i.e., within three months of the suicide) as the most critical event leading to the suicide (Heikkinen et al., 1992). In serious suicide attempts, the three most common precipitants are, in order, the end of a romantic relationship, other interpersonal intimate relationship difficulties, and economic hardship (Beautrais et al., 1997). The numbers are similar for those in the military: Half of Air Force decedents experienced a failure in spousal or intimate relationships, one-third of which typically occurred within the month before the suicide (Reger et al., 2011).

Case 7

Gus was a 27-year-old genetics graduate student at a major university who overdosed two weeks after his girlfriend ended their relationship. His girlfriend Mary was a chemistry graduate student two years his senior. After several months, Mary felt that she was being used and that Gus was too ambitious and self-absorbed. She believed that she was getting nothing out of the relationship. She suggested that they have a closure dinner, which turned into a prolonged fight. Gus called several times to apologize and asked to meet again. Mary accepted the apology but said that she needed a break. Gus continued to text her, but Mary stopped answering. A week later, she received a call from Gus's PhD adviser saying that he was found dead in his lab. An e-mail from Gus with the heading "This is how I killed myself" arrived almost simultaneously.

Gus's is a typical case of suicide of a young person because of romantic rejection. He killed himself a week after his girlfriend stopped answering his texts, which was a message of irrevocable rejection. Furthermore, although he clearly understood that he was about to die, Gus's last e-mail about how he had died was meant to connect him to her for the last time by providing the details of his death. Perfectionism, failure to disengage, thwarted belongingness, and other elements of the suicidal narrative are clearly discernible.

Intimate Relationship Conflict

Despite findings that married individuals are at lower risk for suicide compared to unmarried individuals (Smith et al., 1988), relationship quality appears to supersede marital status. Marital dissolution and dissatisfaction have been associated with suicide risk (Prigerson et al., 1999; Stack & Wasserman, 1993). In adolescents, more than half of relationships' breakups and disappointments occur in the final 24 hours before suicide (Marttunen et al., 1993). In general, marriage appears to be a protective factor against suicide, particularly for men (Goldsmith et al., 2002), whereas for women, suicidal behavior does not depend on marital status.

Married or not, those who die by suicide are likely to have experienced recent intimate relationship conflict (Cheng et al., 2000; Phillips et al., 2002). In particular, sexual minorities and men with a recent history of separation are more vulnerable to intimate partner relationship problems (Kazan et al., 2016). Compared to married or cohabitating men, divorced and separated men are up to six times more likely to die by suicide. This is possibly due to the vulnerability associated with interpersonal stressors during the separation phase (Cantor & Slater, 1995). In fact, recently separated individuals may have more than a fourfold greater suicide risk than currently married, cohabiting, widowed, or single individuals, especially in men between 15 and 24 years old (Wyder et al., 2009).

In the United States, approximately one in four women and one in 10 men report experiencing sexual violence, physical violence, and/or stalking by an intimate partner during their lifetime (Smith et al., 2018), and recent population studies indicate that the association between reports of domestic violence and suicide attempts exists among both women and men, although it is better established for women. Moreover, the association between suicide attempts and intimate partner violence appears stronger for men. It is possible that men with SI go on to attempt suicide (Hawton & Van Heeringen, 2009) or that men are reluctant to seek help for domestic violence due to the shame and humiliation of appearing weak (Galdas et al., 2005). Thus, when assessing suicide risk, evaluation of intimate partner violence should not exclude either sex. Overall, compared to the risk for suicide attempts in families without domestic violence, the risk in families with domestic violence is six times higher for women and eight times higher for men (Dufort et al., 2015).

Case 8

Josh was a 60-year-old married accountant. He had a long history of bipolar II disorder with fairly predictable seasonal cycling. With age, his hypomanic episodes had become shorter, and his depressive episodes grew longer; thus, by age 60 years, he was depressed 10 months of the year and hypomanic for one month, with only one month of euthymia. As his disease progressed, he had an increasingly difficult time keeping his clients, and his relationship with his wife grew more strained. She had always been the main breadwinner in the family and was very critical of Josh, including when they were with friends. At home, she was hostile and disdainful, verbally abusive, and cast herself as both a saint and a victim for putting up with such a loser and wasting her life on him. These fights made Josh feel like a failure, and he often thought of suicide during his depressive episodes. During hypomanic periods, he was fairly successful in getting new clients, but he also overspent and had affairs. Josh's last depression was particularly severe, and after missing several deadlines at work, he lost his only major client. When he told his wife, she was furious; she slapped him, threw his books at him, and told him to get out of the house because she was filing for divorce. Josh begged to stay, but his wife physically pushed him out the door. He banged on the door several times, but she did not open it. He went to the roof of their apartment building, sent her a text stating "I am jumping off, you will be better off without me," and then jumped to his death.

As in Gus's case, Josh's suicide followed rejection, but it was primarily the result of ongoing domestic emotional abuse and the onset of physical abuse. His shame in telling others—their children, his friends, and relatives—about his failure and the feeling of entrapment are almost palpable.

Parents in Conflict with Children

Conflict with children is a less frequent stressful life event and suicide trigger than romantic rejection and economic hardship, but it can still be a significant contributor to suicidal behavior. Just as the meaning and the emotional significance of parent–child conflicts strongly depend on culture, religion, and ethnicity, so does the association between these factors and suicidal behavior. Some studies indicate that such conflicts are most damaging in Asian cultures that value close family ties, and they are of lesser importance in countries that value individualism and independence, such as the United States. Even from a sociocultural standpoint, the Asian view of the self is more dependent on correlations with others than it is in Western countries, and this is likely to affect the suicide narrative (Tanaka et al., 1998). In this respect, acute life stresses evoked by family conflicts and job and financial security issues should not be viewed as isolated stressors, but can be grouped as negative relationships with others. These relationships play more important roles for suicide in Asian countries than in Western countries (Chen et al., 2012). Thus, it is not surprising that in Japan, for example, conflicts with children, after depression and physical illness, are most strongly associated with long-term suicide risk, on par with severe economic hardship and ahead of romantic rejection and loneliness (Shiratori et al., 2014).

Case 9

Lin was a 58-year-old Chinese woman with a long history of schizophrenia who was admitted to an inpatient unit. Lin immigrated to the United States with her husband and two boys in her early 30s when she was already ill but fairly functional; at the time, she was able to take care of her household and also help out at her brother-in-law's grocery store. However, when Lin was in her mid-40s, she had several violent psychotic episodes requiring hospitalization. The patient's husband and sons, who described their mother as dysfunctional, were clearly tired of taking care of her, and there was much angry talk among them at the family meeting. The patient did not participate and just sat in her chair staring at the floor. The husband asked to place Lin in a nursing facility, but she had worked off the books and had no insurance. The social worker told them to apply for disability, and Lin was discharged home. Three hours later, she jumped to her death off the roof of her building.

Lin had many risk factors for suicide. She had a trait vulnerability of severe mental illness and cultural acceptability of suicide conferring chronic suicide risk. Her agitation, ruminations, and affective disturbance were part of severe SCS, indicating imminent risk, but it was primarily during her last admission that her life narrative took the shape of the suicidal narrative. Her family's behavior made it painfully obvious that she was a burden and that she had lost the respect of the entire family. Moreover, her medical team placed all control of her life in her family's hands, creating a dead end. Thus, according to the narrative-crisis model (NCM), Lin was at a very high risk of suicide. Tragically, Lin's culture added the final risk factor. Lin's language barrier made her isolated from her treatment team, which could not perform an objective mental status examination. If it had, team members might have realized that Lin's placement in a nursing facility by her family was rejection according to her culture.

Serious Medical Illness

Recent Diagnosis

Being diagnosed with a serious medical illness may bring on reassessment of one's life narrative. If the reconfigured life narrative involves significant narrowing of life's remaining options and perception of a looming end, a suicidal crisis may ensue.

Patients who have recently received a cancer diagnosis are at increased risk for imminent suicide in the first year after being diagnosed, with the highest increase occurring in the first week. Elderly patients, who may have a better understanding of the diagnosis and may have had friends or relatives die of cancer, are at particularly high risk. In contrast, younger patients who lack such experiences and who may be in denial of its meaning do not have as prominent an increase in risk (Fang et al., 2012). Moreover, the extent to which risk of suicide increases shortly after learning about one's cancer diagnosis appears to vary based on the type of cancer: within the first year of receiving a diagnosis, the highest rates of suicide deaths were found among those receiving a diagnosis of pancreatic, lung, or colorectal cancer, whereas a diagnosis of breast or prostate cancer did not coincide with an increase in suicide risk (Saad et al., 2019).

Of note, people with serious hereditary disorders, such as Huntington's disease, who choose to learn about their diagnosis and do so by consulting trained specialists are at no higher risk for imminent suicide than healthy individuals. Even knowing that they will develop a terminal neurological disorder in the future, such persons do not appear to have catastrophic reactions to learning about their fate and express satisfaction regarding their decision to be tested. Training medical staff in how to deliver appropriate support to these individuals in a timely manner is critical (Dufrasne et al., 2011).

Finally, people with psychiatric illness who are told of their diagnosis of a life-threatening medical illness are at much higher risk of attempting suicide than those do not have a psychiatric disorder. Of note, suicide risk in physically ill people varies substantially by the presence of psychiatric comorbidity, particularly the relative timing of onset of the two types of illness. Unexpectedly, the risk of suicide attempt is even higher in those who have developed a psychiatric disorder, primarily depression, soon after learning of their medical diagnosis. This means that patients who develop a major depressive or psychotic episode after being informed of a serious medical illness have increased suicide risk. Thus, closer collaboration between general and mental health services should be an essential component of suicide prevention strategies (Qin et al., 2014).

Case 10

Alonso was a 25-year-old man who was admitted to an intensive rehabilitation unit. At the time of his diagnosis, he was working and engaged to be married the following spring. His biopsy results showed that the disease had already metastasized. Alonso was told the biopsy results and researched his treatment options and his dismal life expectancy on the Internet. He told his oncology team that with such a poor prognosis, he "might as well kill my- self, because what is the point?" Psychiatry consultation was called to assess Alonso's suicide risk. When the psychiatrist came to see him, Alonso denied SI. During the interview, he was anxious but upbeat. He told the psychia- trist that after speaking to his fiancée and his family, he felt much better. His fiancée told him she loved him no matter what, that the wedding was still on, and that they had to finalize their guest list. His parents told him that he needed to take care of himself and not to worry and that they would help fi- nancially, if needed.

Alonso's case is a good example of how adaptive denial may help young people diagnosed with terminal illness and also how a family can reduce the risk. With their actions and words, Alonso's fiancée and his family quickly reminded Alonso that he is part of the family and that he is anything but a burden to them. Instead of feeling trapped by his diagnosis of terminal illness, Alonso was being asked to help make wedding choices with many options. This approach eliminates or weakens certain components of the su- icidal narrative (such as thwarted belongingness) and makes suicidal crisis less likely.

Prolonged and Debilitating Illness

The association of medical illness with suicide is not limited to instances of recent diagnosis. Having a prolonged, terminal illness also increases suicide risk. One-third of persons who died by suicide and left a suicide note gave health-related reasons for taking their lives, and two-thirds of those had un- derlying chronic medical conditions (Cheung et al., 2015a). Surprisingly, in only a small minority were the illnesses possibly terminal (Cheung et al., 2015b), and it appears that the type of illness may be more directly related to suicide than how life-threatening the illness may actually be. Psychological autopsies show that of medical illnesses, cancer, prostate disorders, and chronic obstructive pulmonary disease (COPD) may be associated with completed suicide, whereas ischemic heart disease, cerebrovascular disease, peptic ulcer, and diabetes mellitus may not (Quan et al., 2002). The elevated risk of suicide increases progressively with the number of comorbid illnesses.

Among the commonly reported diagnoses, cancer, stroke, and a group of illnesses comprising dementia, hemiplegia, and encephalopathy have a particularly strong incremental effect on risk for suicide (Jia et al., 2014).

It also appears that functional impairment due to illness, rather than illness severity per se, is associated with increased risk for suicide. Studies have shown that lung cancer, gastrointestinal cancer, breast cancer, genital cancer, bladder cancer, lymph node cancer, epilepsy, cerebrovascular disease, cataracts, heart disease, COPD, gastrointestinal disease, liver disease, arthritis, osteoporosis, prostate disorders, male genital disorders, and spinal fracture conferred higher risks for completed suicide even three years after the initial diagnosis (Erlangsen et al., 2015). Thus, evaluations of imminent suicide risk in patients with medical illness should include detailed assessments of their functional status. Furthermore, treatments aimed at reducing suicide risk in individuals with serious medical illness must also aim to improve the individuals' level of functioning and their satisfaction with it (Tanriverdi et al., 2014).

Healthcare and the ability of the healthcare system to address the functional needs of persons with medical illness differ between countries, as does suicide risk due to medical illness. Countries with superior healthcare, such as the United Kingdom, have lower incremental risks of suicide due to medical illness. In the United Kingdom, of the physical illnesses, modest increases in risk of self-harm are associated with epilepsy (risk ratio = 2.9), asthma (1.8), migraine (1.8), psoriasis (1.6), diabetes mellitus (1.6), eczema (1.4), and inflammatory polyarthropathies (1.4). On the other hand, compared to the general population, lower risks for suicide are associated with cancers (risk ratio = 0.95), congenital heart disease (0.9), ulcerative colitis (0.8), sickle cell anemia (0.7), and Down's syndrome (0.1; Singhal et al., 2014).

Case 11

Sheridan, an 80-year-old retired businessman, was brought to the emergency department (ED) by ambulance after he told his wife of 55 years that he had just taken an entire bottle of propranolol. For 14 years since his retirement, he had been teaching a business class in a local community college as a volunteer. He had congestive heart failure, which had increasingly limited his mobility, and he was considering ending his volunteer work after the spring semester. Sheridan told the team that the MICU scared him and that he was no longer suicidal. He believed he was strong enough and was discharged home with no physical therapy or psychiatric follow-up. A few months later, he was admitted with another overdose. The patient was very articulate about the fact that he did not want to live anymore because his disability prevented him from doing anything he enjoyed; he had nothing good to look forward to. His wife said that she tried many times to dissuade him but was not successful and that she doubted that the medical team would be either. His wife said that she did not believe in psychiatry and was doubtful that medications would succeed where she had failed.

Sheridan's case illustrates how functional disability due to chronic and debilitating medical illness may reach a threshold when it suddenly narrows one's options in life, creating a sense of entrapment with no good solutions and sharply increasing imminent suicide risk. Physical therapy, antidepressant treatment for Sheridan's depression, and couples' therapy focused on improving commutation between partners and helping Sheridan's wife be more supportive in words and deeds of her husband's teaching could be life-saving for Sheridan.

Acute and Chronic Pain

Chronic pain, which affects one-third of the U.S. population annually (Elman et al., 2013), is a highly debilitating manifestation of illness. Reviews of the available evidence indicate an increased risk of suicidal behavior in patients with chronic pain, particularly older adults (Hinze et al., 2019; Santos et al., 2020). In fact, there appear to be common psychological processes involved in both chronic pain and suicidal thoughts and behaviors (Kirtley et al., 2020).

Independent of psychiatric and medical comorbidities, the rate of suicide attempts among individuals with chronic pain is two to three times higher than that of the general population (Santos et al., 2020; Tang & Crane, 2006). The greatest increase in suicide risk occurs in the context of chronic back pain (9-fold risk of completed suicide; Penttinen, 1995), followed by severe headaches (6.5-fold), nonarthritic chronic pain (6.2-fold), and other generalized pain conditions, such as fibromyalgia and irritable bowel syndrome (4-fold; Spiegel et al., 2007). Poisoning by drugs is more common among suicide attempters with chronic pain compared to those without chronic pain (Campbell et al., 2020). Approximately 20% of poisoning deaths in pain patients are misidentified as accidental overdoses (Cheatle, 2011), so the actual suicide rates are probably 20% higher.

Case 12

Betty, a 55-year-old woman with a history of back trauma and multiple past surgeries, was admitted to the spine service with severe back pain. An infected rod was removed, and a psychiatric consult was called to assess the patient's suicide risk. Betty's postsurgical pain was 10/10, and she was told that the insertion of a new rod was not feasible. Betty was a thin, ill-appearing woman lying in an orthopedic bed equipped with complicated-looking hardware. She was in visible discomfort. Her husband, at her bedside, was very distraught and told the consultant that Betty was at the end of her rope and that he could understand why. He said that the painkillers were not working, the staff was inattentive to his wife's needs, and that something needed to change—quickly. The consultant tried to reassure the husband, who seemed to then feel better. The consultant diagnosed Betty with adjustment disorder and prescribed a stat dose of a benzodiazepine. That same evening, the patient had a respiratory arrest and was intubated. An empty bottle of oxycodone was found in her night table. The husband said that he brought it into the hospital because he could not watch his wife suffer.

This case describes a suicide attempt by a woman with chronic pain, brought on by new acute pain after surgery and a sense of entrapment and desperation due to both ineffective analgesic treatment and no clear path to relief in the future. Her husband unknowingly, or possibly even knowingly, helped his wife's overdose by bringing her the pills. He even indirectly alerted the team to a possible suicide attempt by telling them that she was "at the end of her rope." In cases like Betty's, rooms should be routinely searched for "contraband" painkillers, and imminent suicide risk should be assessed forcefully.

Serious Mental Illness

Recent Diagnosis

As discussed in Chapter 3, receiving a diagnosis of a psychiatric disorder, except dementia, is linked to increased risk of suicide (Nordentoft et al., 2012).

The suicide rates are different for different disorders. Whereas the type of psychiatric disorder, the comorbidities, and the demographics confer trait vulnerability to suicide and are more related to the long-term suicide risk, the timing of the diagnosis is significantly related to suicide risk in the near term.

For many psychiatric disorders, including depression, substance use disorders, and schizophrenia, the risk of dying by suicide is particularly high within the first 90 days after initial diagnosis. During this time, patients newly diagnosed with schizophrenia are 20 times more likely to die by suicide than those without a psychiatric diagnosis. The risk of completed suicide within three months after being diagnosed is 10 times higher for major depression and substance use disorders. The elevated risk for suicide attempts persists during the first year following a diagnosis of major depression and anxiety disorders, but not schizophrenia. Thus, clinicians should be aware of the heightened risk of suicide and suicidal behavior within the first three months after initial diagnosis (Randall et al., 2014).

Some of the elevated short-term suicide risk in newly diagnosed individuals may be due to their having just been hospitalized in an inpatient unit (discussed further in this chapter). However, high rates of suicide in the first three months after diagnosis are more related to self-awareness of mental illness and its implications for the future. Adolescents with psychotic symptoms who are aware of their mental illness and who do not seek help are 20 times more likely to be suicidal than those without psychotic symptoms who do seek help; for adolescents with psychotic symptoms who do seek help, the risk is 10 times higher. This suggests that insight into mental illness may increase risk for suicide (Kitagawa et al., 2014) and that lack of awareness or denial may actually be a very adaptive coping mechanism. Indeed, it appears that individuals with mental illness who do not use denial as a coping mechanism may be at higher risk for suicide, indicating that self-deception may be a coping response to stressful life events in general (Pompili et al., 2011).

Case 13

John, a 19-year-old man, was brought to the ED by his parents because he started putting newspapers over his windows out of fear that the drug dealers in his neighborhood were watching him. He had not washed himself in weeks and was malodorous. His parents said that he was always a quiet kid and mostly kept to himself, spending a lot of time online. He liked to follow stories about organized crime. He parents said that recently he had become even more withdrawn and only left his room to use the bathroom. In the ED, John sat quietly in his chair, avoiding eye contact, and staring at the floor. He was clearly psychotic, and the ED team told the parents that their son might have schizophrenia. The parents said they believed that John was stressed from spending so much time on the Internet and needed to rest more. They refused to hospitalize him but promised to watch him carefully for signs of worsening mental illness, to limit his time on the computer, and to have him read more books. John was discharged, but two weeks later he was brought, unconscious, to the ED by emergency medical services after he attempted to hang himself in his room. He later died in the MICU. His parents said that after his first ED visit, he stopped sleeping and obsessively read postings about schizophrenia on the Internet.

John's story is a classic case of suicide by a patient newly diagnosed with schizophrenia. His parents' lack of insight and denial of the diagnosis demonstrate a frequent contributing factor to increased risk conferred by recent diagnosis. Parents' naive assurances of safety are also common in such cases.

Recent Hospitalization

Psychiatric hospitalization is an intensive treatment modality reserved for those with severe mental illness, for whom outpatient care is insufficient. In the United States, inpatient psychiatric hospitalization is covered by health insurance only if patients present a danger to themselves or others. The unspoken assumption is that inpatient psychiatric hospitalization could be life-saving. However, the first psychiatric hospitalization, in particular, is a significant stressful life event that labels an individual as mentally ill and exposes him or her to others with severe mental illness (Cohen, 1994).

Paradoxically, but not unexpectedly, high-risk suicidal patients are at the highest risk for imminent suicide when either just admitted to a psychiatric unit for protection from self-harm or when just discharged from an inpatient psychiatric hospital stay (Lawrence et al., 1999; Mortensen & Juel, 1993). According to a review of completed suicides in Denmark during a period of 16 years from 1981 to 1997, the odds ratio for completing suicide during the first week after discharge from an inpatient unit was approximately 250:1 for women and 105:1 for men, compared to those who have not been hospitalized (Qin & Nordentoft, 2005). In a Swedish study, one-third of drowning suicide decedents were discharged from an inpatient facility in the preceding week (Ahlm et al., 2015). The reversed gender ratio, compared to a higher ratio of completed suicides for men versus women overall, is probably due to suicidal men not being hospitalized in the first place; men tend to use more lethal methods, increasing their likelihood of completing their initial attempt (Sue et al., 2013). This explanation is consistent with the well-known statistic that 10 times as many women as men attempt suicide, whereas three times as many men as women die by suicide (Chang et al., 2011).

The increased risk of death from suicide following a psychiatric admission, compared to that of the general population, decreases with time but remains elevated for at least one year. Not surprisingly, past history of self-harm and symptoms of depression present prior to hospital admission increase the risk of postdischarge suicide, as do, to a lesser degree, unplanned discharge and recent social difficulties (for review and meta-analysis, see Large et al., 2011). Postdischarge suicide risk depends somewhat on the day of the week the patient is discharged. Suicide and nonfatal suicide attempts have a 6% to 10% excess occurrence on Mondays and Tuesdays and are 5% to 13% less likely to occur on Saturdays (Miller et al., 2012).

Approximately 3% of patients categorized as being at high risk can be expected to commit suicide within one year of discharge from psychiatric hospitalization. In a Danish study, 60% of patients who went on to die by suicide were characterized at the time of their discharge as low risk for suicide using administratively approved scales (Qin & Nordentoft, 2005). Thus, as discussed in the Introduction, postdischarge suicide risk assessment methods based on long-term risk factors are of little or no value in assessing short-term risk following an inpatient psychiatric hospitalization.

Historically, the military has had lower suicide rates than the general population. However, due to a recent steady increase, the suicide rate in the military is 71.6 suicides per 100,000 people yearly, compared to 14.2 per 100,000 in the general population. Among the U.S. military, personnel released from a psychiatric hospitalization are five times more likely to die from suicide than those who were not hospitalized (Luxton et al., 2013). The risk of dying from suicide within the first 30 days after a psychiatric hospitalization is 8.2 times higher than the risk after the first year after discharge from hospitalization (Luxton et al., 2013). Thus, in the first weeks after discharge from an acute psychiatric facility, military personnel need even closer psychiatric follow-up than civilians (Luxton et al., 2013).

Of note, recent hospitalization in a general hospital ward may also increase short-term suicide risk. In the United Kingdom, two-thirds of individuals who die by suicide have hospital records within one year of the suicide, and the majority are discharged from general, rather than psychiatric, facilities (Dougall et al., 2014). Although this high ratio is likely an artifact of a 30:1 ratio of general to psychiatric admissions, there is an association between general hospital discharge and subsequent completed suicide. Diagnosis of psychiatric comorbidity at admission appears to be related to the time interval between hospital discharge and suicide: Those with psychiatric diagnoses are much more likely to die by suicide within three months after discharge compared to those without psychiatric diagnoses (Dougall et al., 2014).

Finally, among people receiving treatment for drug dependence, discharge from hospitalization marks the start of a period of heightened vulnerability to drug-related death. It is not possible to determine which of the deaths are suicides and which are unintentional overdoses (Merrall et al., 2010).

To date, the best predictor of imminent postdischarge suicidal behavior in high-risk psychiatric inpatients is the severity of SCS at the time of hospital discharge (Galynker et al., 2016; Yaseen et al., 2014). High scorers on the Suicide Crisis Inventory, a measure developed to assess the presence and severity of SCS symptoms, are 15 times more likely to attempt suicide within six weeks after discharge than those who do not meet the high score threshold (Galynker et al., 2016). These results were recently replicated in a much larger, more diverse sample of psychiatric inpatients and outpatients (Bloch-Elkouby et al., 2021; Rogers et al., 2021). However, the data still need to be replicated in other hospital settings.

High-risk psychiatric inpatients exhibiting no signs of SCS are also at a high risk for postdischarge suicidal behavior (Yaseen et al., 2014). Indeed, high-risk psychiatric inpatients not infrequently report and demonstrate an incongruous quick resolution of their intense emotional pain. Although it is difficult to imagine a patient who has just survived a serious suicide attempt not to have any residual symptoms or signs of SCS, there are at least two possible reasons for this unexpected phenomenon: (1) patients with dramatic improvement of SCS hide their suicidal intent (Bloch-Elkouby et al., 2022; Hoyen et al., 2021; Rogers et al., 2022), and (2) such patients are unable to identify their emotions due to their poor emotional differentiation skills.

Regardless of whether such patients hide their suicidal plans or are so out of touch with their emotions that they are not aware of their intent to die, they are at high risk for imminent suicide and are likely to make an attentive clinician intensely uncomfortable. Instead of relief at their patient's rapid improvement, such clinicians often experience an eerie mixture of anxiety, discomfort, mistrust, and apprehension regarding the candor of their patient's self-report. However, because on the surface these are often the "model patients," they give their doctors no overt reason to question the honesty of their self-report. Moreover, they strictly follow treatment plans, take their medications on time, and become leaders when participating in therapeutic activities. Such patients often express vocal remorse about their recent suicidal behavior and promise to comply with all recommended treatments upon discharge. And yet, these assurances often sound hollow.

Clinicians are often aware of their negative and seemingly irrational emotional responses and try to suppress them because, on paper and in the emergency medical records, the patients deny SI. Such denials force the clinicians to document the patients' low suicide risk and to cleari them to be discharged from the hospital. However, the clinicians' emotional responses are often correct, and some of these patients are the ones who die by suicide within weeks and sometimes within hours after being documented as having low suicide risk. The use of clinicians' emotional responses for imminent risk assessment is discussed in Chapter 8.

Case 14

Sean was a 60-year-old single man admitted to an inpatient psychiatric unit following a serious suicide attempt by hanging while in his apartment alone. Sean had recently lost his business, leaving him without income. He could not find a job, and after several weeks he became depressed and started drinking. Before hanging himself, he drank an entire bottle of bourbon. After Sean's admission, the team contacted Sean's best friend, who came to the unit and offered to help Sean financially until he could find a job. The patient suddenly brightened up and requested discharge so he could start looking for a job. He called his suicide attempt a sucker's mistake and said that he would accept his friend's offer and try again. He attended groups enthusiastically and requested to go to Alcoholics Anonymous meetings.

There was something unnatural about his turnaround, and the staff felt apprehensive discharging him. They questioned the patient repeatedly about his future suicidal intent and about his plans. Sean described elaborate future plans and repeatedly denied suicidal intent. On the day of discharge, the patient was cheerful and appeared motivated to use his second chance on life well. He had an appointment scheduled for the following day with his new outpatient therapist. Sean's friend took him home and safely brought Sean to his apartment. However, as soon as the friend left, Sean leaped off his 17th-floor balcony to his death.

Sean's case starkly illustrates imminent suicide by a high-risk patient following discharge from an inpatient psychiatric unit. The case also illustrates difficult challenges faced by inpatient psychiatrists when discharging patients at high risk for imminent suicide who vehemently deny their suicide intent. Sean's failed attempt by hanging confers a very high risk for future successful suicide (see the section "Attempt Lethality"). The clinicians' anxious emotional responses to Sean are typical of the responses to patients at ultra high risk (see Chapter 8). This case illustrates that the combination of a high-lethality failed recent attempt and a strong negative emotional response on the part of the staff, even in the presence of explicit denial of suicidal intent, indicates high risk for imminent suicide warranting extraordinary attempts at establishing the patient's real intent and setting up close follow-up mechanisms.

Illness Exacerbation and Acute Episodes

Most of the data on the relationship between exacerbations/acute episodes of mental illness and suicidal behavior derive from large-scale epidemiological studies (Kessler et al., 2005). It is well known that as many as 90% of individuals who attempt suicide meet criteria for one or more disorders in the *Diagnostic and Statistical Manual of Mental Disorders* (DSM; American Psychiatric Association, 2013) during the 12 months preceding the suicidal act (Kessler et al., 2005), with depressive disorders being the most common category of diagnosis (Mościcki, 2001). Vigilance for mood disorders and routine screening for the signs of acute suicidal crisis are therefore warranted.

In general, for relapsing-remitting psychiatric disorders, such as depression, time spent in high-risk major depressive episodes or mixed states is likely to be a dominant factor determining overall risk for suicidal behavior. The incidences of attempts during major depressive episodes and during partial remission are 21 and four times higher than in full remission, respectively (Isometsa, 2014).

Among patients with bipolar disorder (BD), the risk of suicide attempts is different for different phases of the illness; the highest (38-fold) risk involves mixed and depressive mixed phases, whereas the second highest (18-fold) risk occurs during major depressive episodes (Fiedorowicz et al., 2009; Valtonen et al., 2009). In patients with BD, 86% of all suicide attempts occur during major depressive episodes and mixed states (Valtonen et al., 2009). Thus, time spent in high-risk illness phases carries the highest risk for near-term suicide attempts.

The previously discussed findings demonstrate that risk of both completed suicide (Nordentoft et al., 2011) and attempted suicide (Valtonen et al., 2009) may be slightly higher in BD than in MDD (Novick et al., 2010). Moreover, both factors are seen more frequently in individuals with BD II than in those with BD I. This paradoxical association of higher suicide risk with the less severe form of the disorder may be accounted for by differences in the duration of depressive and mixed episodes relative to the overall illness duration, which is longer for BD II. The patient's spending more time in depressed or in mixed illness phases may explain why BD II is often associated with more frequent suicidal behavior than is BD I.

On a clinical level, the reasons for peaking suicidal behavior during acute episodes in people with chronic mental illness may be complex, including the changes of mental state and the person's inability to recognize their emotional and cognitive dysregulation. Even patients who were previously suicidal and who have already experienced several episodes of their illness may not have the insight to appreciate the onset and escalation of the SCS. Their caregivers and significant others, even if they have already lived through their loved ones' previous illness exacerbations, may still not recognize subtle early signs of the new episode and thus may not appreciate the increasing risk for imminent suicidal behavior.

Moreover, patients with schizophrenia or related illnesses having an exacerbation of their psychotic symptoms rarely express worsening SI. In schizophrenia, the signs of worsening psychosis often obscure signs of depression, anxiety, or even panic attacks. Even patients who experience severe distress due to worsening psychotic symptoms and depressive mood exhibit only a minimal or no increase in their help-seeking behaviors, which may not even be recognized as a change in the patient's mental condition (Yamaguchi et al., 2015).

Finally, of all the psychotic conditions (schizophrenia included), the highest risk for suicide and even infanticide is brought on by psychosis within four weeks after childbirth. Excluding acute postpartum exacerbations of known schizophrenia, puerperal BD, and schizoaffective disorder, the risk of completed suicide and of high-lethality suicide attempt within weeks of delivery was reported to be as high as 10% (Kapfhammer & Lange, 2012). Overwhelmingly, the suicides were committed when patients were both depressed and suffering from delusions. Although the majority occurred during the mood episode, which had started imminently after delivery, others took place weeks after a seemingly good symptomatic remission.

Case 15

Walt, a divorced musician with a history of BD II, hanged himself in his bathroom after dinner with friends one evening. Walt was a successful pianist and teacher in his early 60s who started having difficulty playing after he was diagnosed with Parkinson's disease. Walt had several episodes of depression in the past and was even hospitalized, but he always recovered. After his death, his children discovered that their father's business calendar was empty, and the executor of the estate discovered that Walt's finances were in disarray. His medicine cabinet had bottles of psychotropic medications.

Walt took his life during one of his many depressive episodes. As many depressed working people do, he found ways to keep his illness out of the public domain. Using his very public (in musical circles) hypomanic persona, he was able to keep his illness secret, even from his children. As often happens, he killed himself in the middle of a depressive episode.

Medication Changes: Initiation, Discontinuation, or Nonadherence

Initiation of a new psychopharmacological treatment regimen is a relatively perilous time for a patient, and during this time, the patient requires close monitoring by the prescribing psychiatrist. Even with ultimately successful treatment, during the first days and weeks of taking a new drug, the patient encounters new side effects, such as antipsychotic-induced akathisia and antidepressant- or stimulant-related insomnia, which may exacerbate the initial condition. In addition, the patient almost always continues to experience the residual target symptoms of depression, anxiety, or psychosis. Finally, during treatment initiation, troublesome transient mood symptoms, such as increased anxiety in the early stages of selective serotonin reuptake inhibitor (SSRI) treatment for depression (or anxiety), may often temporarily worsen the overall clinical picture and increase near-term suicide risk (Pompili et al., 2010).

In response to concerns about the suicide danger zone with treatment initiation, in 2007 the U.S. Food and Drug Administration (FDA) ordered that all antidepressant medications carry an expanded black box warning incorporating information about an increased risk of suicidality in young adults 18 to 24 years old, as well as in children and adolescents (FDA, 2007; Friedman & Leon, 2007). The FDA justified its decision by identifying a possible activation syndrome (AS), which at times emerges during the antidepressant therapy process as a possible SI and suicidal behavior precursor. AS is composed of 10 symptoms: anxiety, agitation, panic attack, insomnia, irritability, hostility, aggressiveness, impulsivity, akathisia (psychomotor restlessness), and hypomania/mania.

The AS anxiety, panic attacks, and, to some degree, akathisia overlap with the SCS components of entrapment, panic–dissociation, and fear of death. Hypomania/mania overlaps with the affective disturbance of the SCS and the mood swings and affective instability induced by anabolic/androgenic steroids. Finally, impulsivity and aggressiveness correspond to the NCM's trait suicidality as well as the stress-diathesis model's suicide diathesis and O'Connor's pre-motivational stage. In other words, AS empirically overlaps somewhat with the SCS, but this hypothesis needs to be tested experimentally.

AS can also be interpreted as symptoms of dysphoric mania/hypomania and is phenomenologically similar to the syndrome of depressive mixed state (DMX) or mixed depression (Benazzi, 2007; Benazzi & Akiskal, 2001). DMX is observed predominantly in patients with bipolar depression, particularly those with BP II (Akiskal & Benazzi, 2005; Takeshima & Oka, 2013), and could be one of the strongest risk factors for suicidality (Valtonen et al., 2009). In line with the phenomenological similarities between AS and DMX, Akiskal and Benazzi (2006) and Rihmer and Akiskal (2006) argued that AS could be understood as antidepressant-induced DMX. In this context, it can be inferred that antidepressant treatment-emergent AS can be understood as antidepressant-induced DMX, which could substantially increase risk of near-term suicide. Consequently, the FDA recommended that the prescriber consider changing the therapeutic regimen, including discontinuing the antidepressant, if the symptoms are severe, abrupt in onset, or were not part of the patient's presenting symptoms (Culpepper et al., 2004; FDA, 2007).

When patients a priori known to be at higher risk for developing treatment-emergent manic symptoms are excluded, antidepressant initiation is associated with increased rates of suicide attempts within 120 days only in children, whereas the rate is decreased in adult males (Olfson & Marcus, 2008).

Discontinuation of prescription psychotropic medication may be even more troublesome than initiation, because almost all, if not all, prescription psychoactive drugs have been associated with significant withdrawal syndromes. The syndromes have been well described for benzodiazepines (Voshaar et al., 2006), antidepressants (Warner et al., 2006), first- and second-generation antipsychotics (Viguera et al., 1997), and mood stabilizers (Howland, 2010), and they are often concomitant with the relapse of the initial target symptoms for which they were intended—anxiety, depression, psychosis, and affective dysregulation. To a lesser degree, these considerations also apply to instances of stopping and restarting medication due to nonadherence to treatment.

Consequently, suicidal risk and behaviors, which are core features of depression, anxiety, panic, and psychosis, wax and wane in intensity at the times of treatment initiation and adjustment, often reflecting not only the mood fluctuations intrinsic to a particular illness but also drug initiation and discontinuation phenomena. Thus, in assessing near-term suicide risk specifically, it is always important to assess and understand fluctuations of mood, agitation, insomnia, and cognitive disturbances due to possible initiation and withdrawal symptoms associated with licit and illicit drugs. Once such symptoms are identified, maintaining careful surveillance and vigorous treatment are equally essential (Zisook et al., 2009).

Some discontinuation signs and symptoms are drug-specific. Patients report significantly fewer discontinuation symptoms with bupropion compared to escitalopram, paroxetine, and venlafaxine XR. Accordingly, suicide risk may be higher with the latter three drugs and with newer antidepressants in general (Hengartner et al., 2021). The empirical findings on the association between antidepressant treatment and discontinuation are conflicting, however (Bielefeldt et al., 2016; Mills et al., 2020), and more research is needed to fully understand this phenomenon.

The discontinuation profiles for antidepressants remain the same regardless of whether they have been used for the target symptoms of anxiety,

panic, or depression. For each antidepressant, no differences in discontinuation symptoms were observed among the three indications, and surprisingly, there seemed to be no evidence of increased symptom incidence with
increased length of treatment (Baldwin et al., 2007). Thus, discontinuation
profiles differ between antidepressants of the same class and are broadly similar in different disorders.

Discontinuation syndromes also differ between different people, who may
experience similar symptoms with different drugs in the same class. A woman
who had developed a discontinuation syndrome with paroxetine tapered
from 10 to 5 mg/day may present the same syndrome when she occasionally misses her 75 mg q 12 h venlafaxine doses. The symptoms—agitation,
numbness, pricking sensations, sweating, difficulty concentrating, weakness,
derealization, and perceived xerophthalmia—immediately subside upon re-
institution of either drug (Montgomery, 2008). In short, clinicians need to
pay more attention to patients' antidepressant initiation and discontinuation
symptoms and how they may contribute to SCS.

Unlike the case with SSRIs and selective norepinephrine reuptake
inhibitors, the severity of benzodiazepine withdrawal symptoms does depend on treatment duration and is more severe in patients who have taken
a benzodiazepine for more than five years. Benzodiazepines are commonly prescribed in primary care for anxiety disorders and insomnia. The
withdrawal can be so severe that even a relatively slow dose taper over
four weeks on a scheduled 25% dose reduction per week may be associated with repeated high-lethality suicide attempts and completed suicide
(Murphy & Tyrer, 1991). Withdrawal symptoms are most marked in those
with personality disorders, predominantly dependent ones (Murphy &
Tyrer, 1991).

Benzodiazepines are prescription drugs that are frequently sold on
the street. As with all street drugs, their misuse is associated with severe
symptoms of intoxication and withdrawal. Although both intoxication
and withdrawal symptoms may be obvious in the ED setting, subclinical
symptoms of withdrawal may not be readily observable, and patients may
not be able to differentiate them from their non-drug-related anxiety, agitation, or depression. With a strong suicidal diatheses and a suitable suicidal
narrative, both intoxication and withdrawal symptoms would contribute
to the intensity of the acute suicidal crisis. Hence, an inquiry into possible
changes in licit or illicit drug use is an important part of the imminent risk
assessment.

Case 16

Marge was a 53-year-old lawyer who was brought to the ED by her husband for paranoid thinking and irrational behavior. His wife thought that her partners at work were trying to fire her from the company. Convinced that they hacked her home computer to collect incriminating evidence, Marge started staying up at night watching the computer screen for suspicious activity. Marge's husband believed that there was no truth to her suspicions. Marge was an ambitious and anxious woman who was highly regarded and respected at work. She had few interests outside her work and family. Three months earlier, after she lost an important client, resulting in lower income for her and the other partners, Marge was diagnosed with major depression and was started on an SSRI. On medical screening examination in the ED, Marge was guarded but cooperative and well related. Her affect was anxious but appropriate, and her thinking was organized. When her delusions were challenged during the interview, she conceded that she had no evidence for them and that she may just have been stressed from increasing pressure at work. Marge was given a stat dose of risperidone, and her anxiety and paranoia decreased. She was diagnosed with a BD II depressive episode, was kept overnight, and was discharged on a small dose of risperidone and lithium; the SSRI was continued. Marge's family was supportive and involved in treatment. Marge gained weight, and two weeks after discharge, her husband and daughter asked the outpatient psychiatrist to stop risperidone because Marge seemed to have improved, and they had read online that antipsychotics should not be used for maintenance treatment. Marge was still very anxious, had a difficult time sleeping and concentrating, but was now saying that she had overreacted and that her partners were fine. Risperidone was stopped, and Marge became more anxious and agitated. She stopped sleeping altogether but was refusing risperidone because of the weight gain. There was no reason to admit her to the hospital because she was not suicidal, and the family kept a close watch over her. The psychiatrist prescribed clonazepam, and the patient, with her family, left the office. Despite the clonazepam, Marge did not sleep at all. One day, she went to work early but never made it because she jumped to her death in front of a subway train.

Marge's case is an illustration of a preventable suicide brought on in part by diagnostic uncertainty and misguided medication management. Marge had undiagnosed BD II and was living in a state of productive hypomania. The first time she became depressed, she was misdiagnosed with unipolar depression rather than bipolar depression and was treated with an SSRI without a mood stabilizer. This treatment resulted in a gradual emergence of a mixed manic episode with psychotic features, which included insomnia and premonition of social defeat, alienation, and entrapment. Marge's mixed manic episode was also misdiagnosed as depression with psychotic features. As a result, her SSRI treatment, which had created the mixed state in the first place, was continued and resulted in continued worsening of her mania and psychosis. Both of the latter symptoms were partially treated with risperidone and, to a lesser degree, lithium. When, tragically, the risperidone was stopped due to the family's request, the psychosis quickly returned. Because the psychotic content of the mixed episode had the typical themes of humiliating defeat (revoked partnership) and the dead-end life narrative (failed career), in the context of insomnia and agitation, Marge's delusional entrapment in a delusional reality quickly evolved into a severe SCS, culminating in her suicide.

Recent Suicide Attempt

In those with histories of suicide attempt and nonsuicidal self-injury, the risk of death is highest in the first year after self-harm; in the United Kingdom, this risk is 66 times the annual risk of suicide in the general population. This risk is similar to the risk of dying by suicide in the first year after discharge from an inpatient psychiatric unit, to which many patients are admitted after a suicide attempt (discussed previously). Although risk of suicide is highest in the first year following self-harm, a significant risk remains five and even 10 years later. As many as 20% of those who have attempted suicide will make another attempt within the first year, and as many as 5% will die by suicide within nine years (Owens et al., 2002). Thus, it may be that self-harm confers an increased risk for suicide over a lifetime.

As mentioned in Chapter 4, the incremental increase in risk due to previous suicide attempts appears to be higher in the West than in the developing world and in developed Asian countries. One possible explanation for the comparatively lower levels of repeat self-harm in rural Asia compared to the West may be that the high fatality rates associated with the first episode of deliberate self-harm mean that high-risk patients are removed from the pool of patients at risk of repetition. Another explanation is the longer lengths of hospital stay in Asian hospitals (average of three or four days), in part due to the greater toxicity of the substances taken in episodes of self-poisoning. In these cases, decisions to observe patients on the medical ward may contribute to the reduced risk of repeated and more serious suicide attempts; patients are relatively protected from a new attempt while in hospital, which is critical considering that the risk of repeat self-harm is greatest in the days immediately following an original attempt. In contrast, in the West, many patients who present to a hospital after self-harm are not admitted (Gunnell et al., 1996) and may be returned within hours to their community and the circumstances that surrounded their original attempt.

Case 17

Prameet, a 24-year-old Indian Hindu man, was admitted to an inpatient unit after he confessed to his Internet girlfriend, an American-born Indian woman, that he had overdosed on Tylenol because he felt rejected by her. The ED assessment had established that he had bought two bottles of Tylenol to kill himself but took only 10 pills. Prameet had immigrated with his parents when he was three years old and did well in high school until the 11th grade, when he started failing his classes despite studying days and nights. He had been depressed since then, except for two brief periods of time when he was taking antidepressants. In the hospital, his diagnosis of depression was confirmed, and treatment with venlafaxine was initiated. He was discharged when his mood improved, and he committed to safety. Two months later, after his girlfriend unfriended him on Facebook, Prameet was readmitted after taking all the pills from one of the two bottles of Tylenol he bought before his prior admission.

   Prameet's case illustrates escalating deliberate self-injury in an immigrant from Asia, and how a history of deliberate self-harm may increase the risk for future deliberate self-harm. The vignette is also an example of increased suicide risk in child immigrants.

Attempt Lethality

Although history of a failed suicide attempt is one of the most serious long-term risk factors for eventual suicide, the risk differs based on the previous attempt's method and lethality. The connection between the lethality of the past attempt and suicide risk is twofold: The more lethal the means of the previous attempt, the higher the lifetime risk for the next attempt, and the next attempt will use either the same means as, or more lethal means than, the previous attempt.

In the United States, firearms are both the most lethal and the most frequently used means of suicide (CDC, 2015a). More than 50% of all American suicide decedents die by firearms, 25% by hanging and asphyxiation, and 20% by poisoning. Suffocation has a lethality rate similar to that of firearms, typically 69% to 84% (Miller et al., 2012). Recently in the United States, across all racial/ethnic groups and Census regions, increases of suicide by hanging have been outpacing those of other means.

In the industrialized West, in areas where firearms are not as available to the general public, the most frequent means of suicide are hanging and suffocation, followed by poisoning. In the East, the most widespread method of suicide is pesticide ingestion (Krug et al., 2002). Because Asia is the most populous continent, in numerical terms, more people in the world die by pesticide ingestion than by any other means (Gunnel et al., 2007). In the United States, poisoning includes primarily drug overdose and nondrug chemical ingestion, such as bleach (CDC, 2016).

Death rates for repeat suicide attempts differ depending on the method of the previous failed attempt. Compared to poisoning, those with a failed hanging suicide attempt are six times more likely to die by suicide, with the majority of suicides occurring in the first year after the initial attempt. The likelihood of completed suicide following a failed attempt by drowning is fourfold. Failed attempts by jumping off heights and using firearms are three times more likely to be followed by suicide deaths (Runeson et al., 2010).

In all cases except cutting, more than 50% of suicide decedents die by the same means they used in their unsuccessful previous attempt (Runeson et al., 2010). This persistence is most pronounced among those who used hanging in their initial attempt: 93% of men and 92% of women later died from suicide by the same method. High proportions also used the same method for the final successful attempt after previous attempts by drowning, by use of a firearm (men), or by jumping from a height.

In summary, although previous suicide attempt is one of the strongest single predictors for future suicide, there are differences in the subsequent suicide death rates depending on the method of the previous failed attempt. Pertinent to assessment of imminent suicide risk, the majority of suicide deaths occur within one year after an initial failed attempt, and up to one-third of all completed suicides may occur within one week after the previous attempt.

Case 18

Joe was a successful sculptor who was very attractive and was known as a womanizer. However, Joe was quite unhappy and lonely because nobody ever met his criteria for an ideal partner. Finally, when Joe was 40 years old, he met Irena. Irena was a 40-year-old painter. She was very beautiful, smart, and successful. She was also childless. They had a passionate romance, and Irena got pregnant. Joe married Irena, and they had a daughter. One day, Joe looked through his wife's e-mails and discovered that she was having an affair with her manager. Joe was crushed. The love of his life was lying to him, and he was not sure whether he was his daughter's father. Joe begged Irena to end the affair. She initially refused, saying that her manager was vindictive and stopping their affair would end her career.

Devastated, Joe implored her. Finally, Irena promised to stop seeing the manager. Things were quiet for about a month, but then Joe looked through Irena's phone bill and discovered that she continued to exchange multiple texts daily with her manager. The next day, while driving, Joe confronted her again. Angry, Irena had a fit in the car and told him that she never loved him and that she married him only to have a baby, and now that she had a child, she wanted a divorce. They stopped at a gas station. Irena said she was calling a lawyer and went inside. Joe took out a rope from the trunk of the car and tried to hang himself from a branch of a tree next to the gas station. Irene came outside just as he was jumping. The tree branch broke, and Joe fell to the ground.

A rope burn was visible on his neck. Scared, Irena brought him to the ED, and he was hospitalized on the psychiatric ward. While Joe was in the hospital, Irena came daily and apologized, saying that what she said was in anger because he was so possessive. At the family meeting, Irena told the team she wanted to start couples therapy. Joe was mistrustful but too ashamed to reveal Irena's betrayal to his friends and felt lonelier than ever. Instead of sharing his pain, he hired a private investigator, who discovered that Irena still spent time in her manager's apartment, had met with a lawyer, and was planning a divorce. Joe hanged himself using nylon cord on a cabinet handle in his apartment. The handle did not break.

This case is illustrative of high risk associated with failed previous attempt by hanging in men. Characteristically, the successful suicide followed the failed attempt within weeks. Joe's suicide crisis was precipitated by romantic betrayal and rejection. Joe's narrative identity became a perfect fit for a suicidal narrative: setting an unrealistic goal for his personal life, finding it, and then failing to achieve it with Irena, followed by a humiliating defeat, failure to disengage, alienation, and entrapment.

Recent Substance Misuse

Drug and Alcohol Use Disorder

Although the relationship is not straightforward, suicide has been linked to the use of alcohol and drugs. It is further complicated by recent changes in the nomenclature of alcohol-related disorders from DSM-IV to DSM-5.

DSM-IV described two distinct disorders, alcohol abuse and alcohol dependence, with specific criteria for each. DSM-5 integrates the two DSM-IV disorders into one disorder, called alcohol use disorder (AUD), with mild, moderate, and severe subclassifications. The number of criteria met determines the AUD severity.

According to psychological autopsies and other research studies worldwide, AUD and other substance use disorders are the second most common group of mental disorders among suicide decedents (Conner et al., 2014). On its own, AUD is a risk factor for suicide attempts and completion, and alcohol is the most prominent substance of use in this regard (Amiri & Behnezhad, 2020; Edwards et al., 2020). Compared to nonsuicidal individuals with AUD, those with AUD who attempt or die by suicide are more likely to have comorbid depressive disorder, drug use disorder, aggressive behaviors, and medical illness or complaints. Suicidal persons with AUD have lower social support and more interpersonal stressful life events, such as unemployment or other indications of economic adversity (Conner et al., 2003; Pavarin et al., 2021). Just like the two other commonly assessed risk factors, mental illness and previous history of attempts, AUD is associated with long-term suicide risk. Whether and how AUD confers risk for near-term suicide or suicide attempts is unclear. Much clearer is the association between imminent suicide risk and acute alcohol intoxication.

Acute Alcohol Intoxication and Recent Drug Use

Among substances of abuse, alcohol has robust evidence indicating that it confers the risk of suicide significantly more than other substances (Pavarin et al., 2021; Orri et al., 2020). Acute use of alcohol (AUA), describing alcohol intoxication, is related to, but distinct from, AUD. Although AUA is not a DSM diagnosis, it is a significant risk factor for suicidal behavior and is independent of drinking patterns or AUD (Borges & Loera, 2010). Acts of suicide among individuals with a history of AUD can occur either while intoxicated or outside periods of acute intoxication (Simon et al., 2002; Wojnar et al., 2008), and the phenomenology of suicides while intoxicated and while sober may be quite different.

A remarkable 37% of suicides and 40% of suicide attempts are preceded by AUA (Cherpitel et al., 2004). Many studies have consistently demonstrated that AUA confers a 5- to 10-fold increase in risk of suicide. There are also data indicating that risk for suicidal behavior is increased at high drinking levels (Borges et al., 1996) and that use of firearms and hanging, the two most deadly methods of suicide, are associated with high drinking levels (Conner et al., 2014). This underscores the importance of alcohol dose in the link between AUA and suicidal behavior. Most important, although the SAD PERSONS scale as a whole is not predictive of short-term suicidal behavior, a recent increase in alcohol use is one of the SAD PERSONS scale items that does indicate increased near-term suicide risk within six months.

Consequently, to best inform prevention and intervention efforts concerning the association between AUA and suicidal behavior, it is important to understand its specifics. According to some studies (Bagge et al., 2013), one-third of suicidal individuals drink before the attempt, and most suicidal persons who use alcohol (73%) do not do so to facilitate the attempt. The others, however, deliberately use alcohol prior to suicidal behavior in order to remove psychological barriers to suicide by increasing their courage, numbing their fears, and anesthetizing the pain of dying. Thus, suicide attempters may use alcohol as an additional drug to make death more likely (e.g., "I mixed alcohol with pills"). It may be that approximately one-fourth of suicide attempters with AUA fit this pattern (Hawton et al., 1989), suggesting it is common.

Paradoxically, the minority who deliberately use alcohol to facilitate suicide are more similar to suicide attempters who do not drink prior to their attempt than to those who drink for other reasons. The latter, on the other hand, differ from non-intoxicated attempters in that they are more impulsive and have lower suicide intent.

Thus, alcohol-involved suicide attempts are heterogeneous (Bagge et al., 2013). The attempters who become intoxicated without specific intent to reduce the pain of suicide appear to be more impulsive; for these individuals, suicide risk may decrease when they sober up. On the other hand, suicide attempters who drink for attempt facilitation will continue to be high risk even upon a decrease in blood alcohol level.

There may be other mechanisms by which AUA increases suicidal thoughts and behavior. These mechanisms may include, but are not limited to, alcohol-related psychological distress, disinhibition, depressed mood and anxiety, aggressiveness, impulsivity, and cognitive constriction (Bagge & Sher, 2008; Hufford, 2001). Through these and other mechanisms, AUA may also evoke or exacerbate acute interpersonal conflicts, thereby escalating stress levels and stress-reactive suicidal behavior (Conner et al., 2014). It is also possible that suicidal acts preceded by AUA are a distinct phenotype of suicidal behavior (Fudalej et al., 2009).

The data on the relationship between suicide attempt lethality and alcohol use are conflicting. Some reports indicate that alcohol use is associated with more lethal means of suicide (Sublette et al., 2009), whereas others find no such association and suggest that cannabis use may be related to more lethal means, such as jumping from heights (Lundholm et al., 2014). The highest blood alcohol levels at the moment of suicide were recorded with rare suicides by explosive device, with the average blood alcohol concentration of 1.71 g/kg. This especially drastic method of suicide (distinct from suicide bombing, which is a murder-suicide) was frequent in Croatia during the period after the Croatian Independence War (1991–1995), possibly as a consequence of a high incidence of war-related posttraumatic stress disorder (Čoklo et al., 2008).

Finally, the use of alcohol in suicide decedents prior to their deaths differs widely by ethnicity. Autopsy blood alcohol levels are consistently the highest for American Indians and Alaskan Natives and the lowest for Asian Americans and Pacific Islanders (Caetano et al., 2013). The frequencies of legal intoxication (i.e., blood alcohol concentration at or above the legal limit of 0.08 g/dL) follow the same pattern, ranging from 37% in American Indians and Alaskan Natives to 23% in Asian Americans. Hispanics had the second highest frequency, 29% (CDC, 2005b).

Case 19

Wendy was a 28-year-old woman diagnosed with BD. She was hospital-ized during a manic episode and treated with a second-generation antipsy-chotic that brought on an episode of treatment-resistant depression. She was discharged in her parents' care and was treated with increasingly compli-cated combinations of medications, but she did not improve. Despite all the treatment efforts, Wendy's depression kept getting worse, and after several months she told her family that she could no longer take the pain and that she would kill herself. The parents put her on a pharmaceutical trial waiting list that was several months long. Wendy was getting desperate and started drinking to control her emotional pain. Her comments to her psychiatrist were becoming hopeless and despondent. She came to several appointments intoxicated. The psychiatrist alerted Wendy's parents to her acute suicidality and instructed them to stay with her and to remove liquor from the house. Finally, Wendy was interviewed for the trial, but she did not meet the criteria. She made up a story and asked one of her friends to come over and sneak two bottles of vodka into the house, which he did. As soon as he left, Wendy drank one bottle. The parents noticed that Wendy was drunk, searched her room, and found both bottles. The parents made an appointment with Wendy's psy-chiatrist for the next day. However, they never made it to the appointment because the next morning they found her dead in her room with a plastic bag around her head.

This case shows an increase in alcohol use proximal to a suicide attempt, where Wendy's AUA was likely an attempt to self-medicate refractory de-pression, emotional pain, and anxiety. Given that Wendy suffocated herself hours after an impulsive episode of acute intoxication, her AUA was not a conscious attempt to minimize pain of death with alcohol, which is the case for 75% of suicide decedents who drink before their suicide. On the other hand, anxiety and depression from alcohol withdrawal (discussed next) may have also contributed to her death.

Alcohol and Drug Withdrawal

Whereas alcohol and drug intoxication may contribute to acute suicide risk due to disinhibition or intentional use to diminish fear of death or numb its pain, the negative affective states of anhedonia, depression, anxiety, and

panic intrinsic to drug and alcohol withdrawal may increase risk for suicide by intensifying the syndrome of the acute suicidal crisis. As demonstrated by Galynker and Yaseen in patients with depression, panic attacks
in general are associated with past attempts (Katz et al., 2011), and those
with panic attacks with fear of death are seven times more likely to attempt suicide in the future (Yaseen et al., 2013). Thus, the turmoil of negative mood symptoms, including depression, anxiety, panic, and affective
instability, which is a distinguishing feature of many drug withdrawal
symptoms, turns periods of alcohol and drug withdrawal into times of high
suicide risk.

The ethanol withdrawal syndrome specifically may be observed within
eight hours of the last drink in the ethanol-dependent patient with blood alcohol concentrations in excess of 200 mg%, and it can be life threatening.
Symptoms consist of tremor, nausea and vomiting, increased blood pressure
and heart rate, paroxysmal sweats, depression, and anxiety. Thus, alcohol
withdrawal in these patients may be a time of heightened vulnerability to
suicide, and these patients must be assessed carefully, particularly prior to
discharge from the ED (Terra et al., 2004).

Unlike alcohol and benzodiazepine withdrawal, opiate withdrawal per se
is not as life threatening. However, during both acute and protracted opiate
withdrawal, patients experience severe anxiety and dysphoria, which could
exacerbate and increase the intensity of the underlying suicidal crisis that
may have led to opiate misuse to begin with. Thus, opiate misuse can be dangerous to a person's life both through an overdose and through withdrawal
syndrome. In some patients, opiate withdrawal may cause panic, presum-
ably through possible opiate noradrenergic interaction. Clonidine decreases
the anxiety related to opiate withdrawal (Gold et al., 1980), and one uncontrolled case series showed its association with lower self-injurious behavior
(Philipsen et al., 2004).

Cocaine withdrawal was initially described using a triphasic model
(Kleber & Gawin, 1986). However, subsequent studies have failed to support the phasic nature of cocaine withdrawal. After cessation of cocaine use,
rather than being phasic, cocaine withdrawal symptoms reach their maximum in the first 24 hours and decrease rapidly, in a linear fashion, 48 hours
after the last dose. The withdrawal symptoms consist of a "crash," along with
a number of other symptoms, including paranoia, depression, anhedonia,
anxiety, mood swings, irritability, and insomnia (Walsh et al., 2009). Some
cocaine users also feel like they are losing their mind. All the previously

mentioned symptoms are part of the acute suicidal crisis, making the first 48 hours of cocaine withdrawal a high-risk period for suicide.

Cannabis withdrawal syndrome has been described only recently and consists of two domains—one characterized by weakness, hypersomnia, and psychomotor retardation and the other by anxiety, restlessness, depression, and insomnia. Both are associated with significant distress to the patient and with depression. Thus, cannabis withdrawal, like alcohol and heroin withdrawal, can increase the intensity of the acute suicidal crisis (Hasin et al., 2008).

Last, although barbiturate abuse peaked in the second half of the 20th century, it can still be encountered clinically. Someone who is addicted to barbiturates will begin to feel acute withdrawal symptoms in eight to 16 hours after the last dose. Symptoms can be very severe, particularly in the beginning of withdrawal, and they include anxiety, insomnia, weakness, dizziness, nausea, sweating, and anxiety. There may be tremors, seizures, hallucinations, and psychosis, and users may become hostile and violent. Without proper treatment, hyperthermia, circulatory failure, and death may result.

Case 20

James was a 19-year-old high school senior with antisocial and border-line personality disorder as well as alcohol and substance use disorder. His drugs of choice were antihistamines, which made him hallucinate, and benzodiazepines, which caused euphoria and sedation. On the day of his suicide, James was staggering and falling asleep in classes and was brought to the local ED at 9 a.m. Although his urine toxicology was positive for barbiturates and marijuana, James denied drug use. As a routine, he was asked about his suicidality, which he adamantly denied. His parents were not available, and after hours in the ED he was given his cell phone to pass time. When his father arrived at 6 p.m., he noticed that James was texting furiously. James barely acknowledged his father and refused to talk to him. The father told the ED staff that this behavior was uncharacteristic for James. Prior to being discharged from the ED, James denied suicidal intent and was released to his father. On the way home, James continued to use his cell phone nonstop. When they got to their house, James ignored his mother and his sister and went to his room, closing the door. Fifteen minutes later, the family heard a gunshot. James was found lying dead on his bed. He left a digital suicide note addressed to his girlfriend, who had just broken up with him, and to his parents. The note accused them of not caring about his life.

Although James had character pathology and substance use disorder, his suicide took place in the context of acute barbiturate withdrawal, manifested by his increased hostility and anxiety. Given that his behavior was described as out of character, the withdrawal had likely intensified his negative affect and contributed to his suicide.

Adolescents

In contrast to the suicide rates in adults, which declined somewhat in the United States in 2019 and 2020, suicide rates in adolescents and children continued to climb (Curtin et al., 2021). Remarkably, nearly 75% of U.S. high school students who attempt suicide may do so for reasons other than a desire to die, such as revenge, sending a message, or regulating emotions. As is true for adults, adolescents with stronger depressive symptoms and premeditation prior to the attempt were at a higher risk for suicide with death as a clear motive (Jacobson et al., 2013). Conflicts with parents and peers, bullying, and cyberbullying are among the most frequent stressful life events preceding adolescents' and children's suicides.

Children in Conflict with Parents

Despite recent increases in suicide rates among 10- to 14-year-old children (Curtin et al., 2021), suicides in preteen children are still relatively rare. However, when they do occur, parent–child conflicts are their most frequent precipitants. In identifying children at high risk for suicide, it is important to assess for the presence of such conflicts and to understand the incremental risk contribution due to other sociodemographic variables. According to one review, the neglectful yet controlling parenting style known as affectionless control is likely to contribute to the parent–child conflicts that play a role in suicide risk in children, adolescents, and adults (Goschin et al., 2013).

During the past two decades in the United States, the suicide rate for children 10 to 14 years old tripled from 0.5 to 1.5 per 100,000. However, when ethnic and racial differences are considered, during this time there has been a dramatic increase in suicide amongr Black children and a decrease in suicide among White children (Curtin et al., 2016). The reasons for this divergent trend are not yet clear, but these recent patterns must be considered when conducting risk assessments (Bridge et al., 2015).

With regard to parenting styles, some parenting features appear to be protective for suicide risk, whereas others increase it. Maternal and paternal warmth in childhood and maternal control in adolescence have protective influences on suicide risk. Surprisingly, authoritative parenting is protective as well. On the other hand, rejecting–neglecting parenting strongly increases the risk for suicide attempts. Seven other factors increase suicide risk in prepubescent children: attention deficit hyperactivity disorder, smoking, binge drinking, absenteeism/truancy, migration background, and parental separation (Donath et al., 2014; Goschin et al., 2013).

The relative importance of trait suicidality and stressful life events in the etiology of suicide in children appears to differ from that in adolescents and adults. Whereas 90% of suicide decedents in adults had a psychiatric diagnosis (Chang et al., 2011), for suicide decedents younger than age 12 years, only 25% met the criteria for a psychiatric diagnosis and 30% had depressive symptoms at the time of death. In contrast, 60% of the parents of these suicide victims reported that the child experienced some kind of stressful conflict prior to death, whereas only 12% of the parents of children who died in accidents during the same time period reported such conflicts (Freuchen et al., 2012).

In retrospect, the stressful conflicts preceding child suicides were considered unimportant or even trivial at the time (Groholt et al., 1998), but were likely to involve shame (Lester, 1997; Orth et al., 2010). The parents' descriptions revealed behaviors of which children typically are ashamed, such as being caught stealing, having done something wrong, having been humiliated, and having experienced hurtful comments. In general, shame is a difficult feeling to deal with, and in combination with the personality traits of vulnerability and impulsiveness, it may prove dangerous. From this perspective, suicide may represent a child's attempt to resolve a shameful situation perceived as unbearable (Freuchen et al., 2012).

With regard to adolescents, as discussed in Chapter 3, those who die by suicide are more likely to have a family history of suicide and/or significant psychopathology (Shaffer et al., 1994). Not surprisingly, childhood abuse, a history of parental separation or loss of a parent (by death or divorce), as well as physical and/or sexual violence in the family are also associated with adolescent suicide (Schilling et al., 2009). Adolescents with suicidal behaviors are more likely to be living in broken families (Afifi et al., 2008; Brent & Mann, 2006; Zayas et al., 2009) and in an atmosphere of problematic communication, poor attachment, and high levels of conflict (Afifi et al., 2008; Bridge, 2008; Gould, 1996; Libby et al., 2009; Martin, 2005; Qin et al., 2009). In depressed adolescents, poor family function and family conflict are predictive of suicide attempts within one year after initial assessment (Bridge, 2008). Independent of parental conflict, young persons age 11 to 17 years old who frequently moved during childhood were more likely to make suicide attempts during adolescence (Qin et al., 2009). There is a dose–response relationship between the number of moves and risk of attempted suicide: Youth who had moved 3 to 5 times were 2.3 times more likely to have attempted suicide compared to those who had never changed residences, whereas those who had moved more than 10 times were 3.3 times more likely to attempt suicide, controlling for birth order, birthplace, and paternal and maternal factors. The same is true of suicide completers (Cash & Bridge, 2009).

The new concept of emerging adulthood has been created to describe young people between the ages of 18 and 25 years old who are still not independent of their families. In *The New York Times* column "How Adulthood Happens," David Brooks (2015) discussed the widespread phenomenon of young people not reaching maturity until their 30s. Correspondingly, the most common proximal risk factor for completed suicide for individuals less than 30 years old was not financial distress, but conflict with family members, partners, or friends (Foster, 2011). For both men and women in this age group, a negative relationship with either or both parents or conflicts between parents are significantly associated with suicide risk (Consoli et al., 2013).

Case 21

The mother of an 11-year-old boy, Scott, came home and found that her son had hanged himself with her scarf from their second-floor stair balcony. Scott had exhibited behavioral and academic problems in the past, and his suicide followed his being sent home from school after an incident in which he hit another student in his class. The school principal told Scott's parents that if he became violent one more time, he would be expelled and have to attend a school for children with behavioral problems. When they were driving home after the conference, Scott's parents told him that if he got kicked out of school, they would send him to boarding school and never visit. Scott had been threatened with boarding school before and did not appear scared. Scott's mother later remembered that approximately one year earlier, Scott and his sister had play-acted hanging after watching a Western movie on TV in which men were hanged.

Scott's suicide illustrates most major points about suicides by small children. It took place as a result of a major conflict with his parents involving shame, although the stressful life events preceding the suicide were only a continuation of his life as usual. As is often the case, his parents did not realize the danger or actual suicide risk.

Ongoing Childhood and Adolescent Abuse and Neglect

Results from dozens of studies generally suggest that childhood sexual, physical, and emotional abuse and neglect are associated with childhood and adolescent suicide attempts. This relationship holds true for children from different cultures and ethnicities, from families with or without mental illness, and with different peer relationships. All four types of childhood abuse or neglect are associated with adolescent SI and suicide attempts, and their effects are additive. However, there is evidence that sexual abuse and emotional abuse may be relatively more important than physical abuse or neglect in explaining suicidal behavior (Miller et al., 2013).

The strongest and clearest evidence exists for a link between sexual abuse and childhood and adolescent suicide attempts. This link is significant regardless of the child or adolescent's age and grade level (Waldrop et al., 2007), sex (Esposito & Clum, 2002a), IQ (Fergusson et al., 2000), and race or ethnicity (Brown et al., 1999; Thompson et al., 2012). However, although the previously mentioned associations are generally true, most may be stronger for boys than for girls, in whom they are present only if comorbid with hopelessness and depression (Bagley et al., 1995).

The strong relationship between sexual abuse and suicide attempts in adolescents appear to be remarkably independent from family structure, pathology, and peer relationships. The link remains robust for any family structure regardless of parental separation, parental role changes, mother's level of education, family socioeconomic status, parental violence or imprisonment, adolescent's attachment, parenting style, family functioning (Fergusson et al.,

1996, 2000), parents' psychiatric symptoms and substance abuse (Johnson et al., 2002), parental suicide, or general feelings of social connectedness (Rew et al., 2001).

Of note, the associations between childhood sexual abuse and adolescent suicide appear to be invariant to categorical psychiatric diagnosis and persist whether or not an adolescent has been diagnosed with MDD, conduct disorder, adjustment disorder, or social phobia (Glowinski et al., 2001). Individual dimensions, such as depressive symptoms (Fergusson et al., 2003; Rew et al., 2001), hopelessness (Martin et al., 2004; Rew et al., 2001), dissociative symptoms (Kisiel & Lyons, 2001), personality factors (Fergusson et al., 2000), and previous suicide attempts (Johnson et al., 2002), also do not appear to affect the link between childhood sexual abuse and suicidal behavior.

Results from studies of physical abuse also reveal a clear association with suicide attempts in adolescents, regardless of whether they live at home or are psychiatric inpatients, delinquent youth, homeless youth, or runaways. Similar to sexual abuse, the associations of childhood physical abuse with adolescent suicide attempts do not depend on youth gender, age, race/ethnicity, family socioeconomic status, or caregiver education level (Brown et al., 1999; Esposito & Clum 2002b; Johnson et al., 2002; Rew et al., 2001; Thompson et al., 2012). The link between physical abuse and suicide attempts in adolescents persists regardless of their psychological distress in childhood and early adolescence; depression severity; disruptive and risky behavior; comorbid internalizing and externalizing symptoms; diagnoses of MDD, conduct disorder, adjustment disorder, or social phobia; and prior suicide attempts (Fergusson et al., 2003; Glowinski et al., 2001; Johnson et al., 2002; Rew et al., 2001).

As with sexual abuse, the association between physical abuse and youth suicidal behavior is not related to family factors, such as history of suicide in the family, family alcohol and drug problems, maternal care, parent attachment, family composition, and parent psychiatric symptoms (Johnson et al., 2002; Rew et al., 2001). Nor is it related to peer variables, such as social connectedness, suicide of a friend, and attachment to friends (Rew et al., 2001).

Emotional abuse, but not neglect, also appears to be associated with suicide, regardless of youth demographics, mental health problems, or family variables (Thompson et al., 2012). The influence of family and peer relationship variables on this link is unknown.

Physical abuse and sexual abuse often take place simultaneously; when they do, it is sexual rather than physical abuse that is associated with suicide attempts, regardless of family socioeconomic status, youth dissociative symptoms, negative life events, parental violence, mental health symptoms, separation, imprisonment, education, attachment, and changes in caregiver (Brent et al., 1993; Fergusson et al., 2000; Kisiel & Lyons, 2001). Somewhat unexpectedly, when all four forms of abuse co-occur, adolescent suicide attempts are primarily associated with sexual and emotional abuse (Locke & Newcomb, 2005); suicide has no link to physical abuse and neglect.

Childhood maltreatment affects boys and girls differently, and the differences are most pronounced for sexual abuse (Bagley et al., 1995), for which the risk of a suicide attempt is 15 times greater for male victims of sexual abuse than for female victims (Martin et al., 2004). Physically abused boys may also be at higher risk for suicide attempts compared to physically abused girls (Rosenberg et al., 2005).

Regardless of the victim's gender, sexual abuse experiences that involve contact (i.e., touching and intercourse) with the perpetrator are more likely to lead to a suicide attempt than is noncontact sexual abuse (i.e., verbal sexual harassment). Suicide attempt risk is higher with a later age of onset of sexual abuse, when the perpetrator is an acquaintance rather than a parent or caregiver, when a parent denies the abuse's occurrence, and when a parent expresses anger toward the child rather than the perpetrator (Plunkett et al., 2001).

In summary, childhood maltreatment, particularly sexual and emotional abuse, is associated with increased risk of suicide attempts in childhood, adolescence, and adulthood. The risk is much higher for males than for females and when abuse involves physical contact and is perpetrated repeatedly within the family. Because most suicide attempts are preceded by a stressful life event within one month, when assessing risk for imminent suicide, it is important to establish whether the abuse is recent or ongoing.

Bullying

Bullying is unwanted, aggressive behavior among school-age children that involves a real or perceived power imbalance. The behavior must be repeated or must have the potential to be repeated over time. It has been reported that both perpetrators and victims of bullying are at an increased risk of suicidal behaviors (Dilillo et al., 2015; Duan et al., 2020). Students who are bullied, threatened, or injured by someone with a weapon, physically hurt by their partner, or have ever been forced to have sex are twice as likely as students who have not experienced victimization to attempt suicide (Van Geel et al., 2014).

The relationship between bullying and suicide risk is gender dependent and affects the victims and the perpetrators differently. Female victim-perpetrators and their victims have the highest risk for suicide attempts (Cook et al., 2010). Bullying is rarely the only factor contributing to suicidal behavior. Suicide in youth usually arises from a complex interplay of various biological, psychological, and social factors, of which bullying is only one.

Late adolescent victims of bullying are less likely to seek help from school administration and mental health professionals if they are suicidal compared to victims who are not suicidal; for bullied adolescents, there seems to be an inverse relationship between the severity of SI and help-seeking. Even more remarkably, targets of bullying with the most severe SI tend to not seek help from peers and family members, who are the most frequent source of help for adolescents. Thus, for known victims of bullying, an abrupt and unexplained end to complaints about bullying or a sudden denial of previous distress may be a sign of increased risk for imminent suicide.

Bullying is not limited to children and adolescents, and it is surprisingly common in the workplace. Among 642 completed work-related suicides from 2000 to 2007, 55% had an association with work stressors, identified as business difficulties, work injury, or conflicts with supervisors/colleagues (including workplace bullying). Thus, bullying in the workplace should be assessed whenever difficulties at work are identified as stressors (Routley & Ozanne-Smith, 2012).

Case 22

Sergei, a 17-year-old high school senior, was admitted to the ED after he tried to stab himself in the chest in a suicide attempt after being raped at his school. Once he was stabilized, he was admitted to an acute psychiatric unit on constant observation for SI. Sergei was a student at an exclusive boarding high school for boys. He did not like the school from the beginning and begged his parents to take him home. Sergei was also overweight and awkward, and he was quickly given the nickname "the Oligarch Fag," which was used by everybody behind his back but not to his face. He completed ninth grade without making any friends but was not bullied or abused. At the beginning of tenth grade, however, he was jumped in the bathroom and his watch was stolen. Sergei complained to the principal's office, the dorms were searched, and the watch was found in a night table of one of the popular kids. The delinquent student was expelled from school, and from that moment on, Sergei's life became a living hell. His classmates beat him up at least one night a week, always putting a pillowcase over his head so he could not recognize the perpetrators. He was threatened that if he squealed one more time, he would be dead. The beatings continued until one night Sergei was dragged to the gym, gagged, and raped with a plastic beer bottle. He was left bleeding on the floor, where he was found by one of the cleaning staff.

Case 23

Yana, the 16-year-old daughter of Greek immigrants, was brought to the ED after her mother found her lying on her bed, unresponsive, with two empty bottles of her psychotropic medications by her side. There was no note. Yana was attending one of the small, elite private schools in New York on a scholarship and had trouble fitting in with the rest of the students. Yana's parents told the treatment team that Yana's only friend in her class was the other scholarship student, who was from Iran. Both girls were often teased for being overweight and wearing the wrong clothes and makeup. Yana begged her parents to transfer her to another school, but her parents were adamant that she should continue because of the high quality of the education and the high admission rates into Ivy League colleges. Yana had never threatened suicide before, and recently she had complained less about the school, which made the family think that the situation had improved. However, during the physical exam, the team saw multiple scarred cuts on Yana's forearms and thighs. Yana was admitted to the MICU with hypotension and bradycardia and was stabilized. When she woke up, she told the medical team that the girls were cruel, worse than in the movies, that they made her feel like she was trash, and that her parents did not listen. On the day of the attempt, her only friend told her that she needed some space because Yana was just "too weird." Yana said she gave up on talking to her parents because it was useless.

Sergei's case is a result of ongoing relentless bullying and heinous physical one-time sexual abuse, tacitly condoned by the school. Yana's case illustrates most aspects of bullying: a power imbalance between her wealthy classmates and the two second-generation immigrants from lower-income families, no help-seeking, and fewer complaints to the family before the suicide attempt because of the breakdown in communication and trust. Also, characteristically, the suicide was precipitated not by bullying, but by a friend's rejection, suggesting that Yana's psychopathology may have involved some borderline and avoidant-dependent traits. In both cases, the parents' neglectful and controlling parenting exemplified the affectionless control parenting style associated with suicide attempts.

Internet and Social Media

Among the opportunities and advancement that Internet and social media have brought to our lives, there are numerous risks and adverse effects of immersion in the digital age. The number of young people meeting the proposed diagnostic criteria for Internet addiction is on the rise, and aside from the ease of accessibility to all sorts of mentally distressing content, new phenomena like cyberbullying and communities of suicide affirmation have emerged (Niezen, 2013). Although the direction of causality remains unclear, recent cumulative evidence has established an independent association between heavy social media or Internet use and suicide attempts in young people under the age of 19 (Sedgwick et al., 2019).

On the other hand, the Internet, social media, and smartphone apps have made their way into mental health care, and the COVID-19 pandemic has catalyzed the widespread adoption of telehealth delivery in the United States and internationally. The rising use of new technologies in psychiatric care over the past decade has provided healthcare staff with the opportunity to reach a broader population of patients and to provide a variety of services remotely. An enormous number of different digital mental health interventions have been developed across various platforms, including through smartphone applications or through crisis texting lines. Many of these digital interventions have been tested empirically, and an emerging body of literature has identified promising online interventions for suicidality (Buscher et al., 2020; Robinson et al., 2016). Beyond the emerging interventions, the Internet and social media can be used to gain perspective into someone's mental health, as well as to identify potential expressions of suicide before they turn into behaviors, attempts, or completed suicides (Coppersmith et al., 2018; Pourmand et al., 2019). Overall, the Internet and social media are important features of contemporary psychiatry that require particular attention in suicide literature and assessment of patients.

Screen Time

According to a recent 10-year longitudinal study that followed over 500 youth, a high and increasing pattern of screen use throughout the course of adolescence was associated with heightened risk of suicide in early adulthood, particularly among girls (Coyne et al., 2021). Similarly, a recent systematic review investigating the relationship between social media use and self-harm found an association between increased time spent on social networking websites and SI in adolescents, based on five cross-sectional studies (Memon et al., 2018).

Meanwhile, the literature on the link between time spent on social networking and general mental well-being is mixed. A meta-analysis of 61 studies showed that the association between screen time and psychological well-being, self-esteem, life satisfaction, depression, and loneliness was negligible (Huang, 2017), a finding that was later replicated longitudinally (Coyne et al., 2020). On the other hand, another systematic review found a significant association between time spent on social media and depression and anxiety among adolescents. Nevertheless, the authors highlighted the complexity of the proposed relationship, the various mediating and moderating factors that have yet to be explored, and the methodological limitations of cross-sectional and meta-analytic studies (Keles et al., 2020). The inconclusive findings of the aforementioned studies emphasize the importance of assessing content and type of activity (Weinstein et al., 2021), adverse online experiences, and other potential reasons for increased screen time when attempting to understand the relationship between digital media usage, mental health, and suicide risk.

Internet Addiction

While Internet addiction is not an official diagnosis in the DSM, it has attracted the attention of many clinicians and researchers in the field (Hsu et al., 2015), as evidenced by the inclusion of Internet gaming disorder in the DSM-5 as a condition for further study. Although a number of variations in the classification of Internet addiction have been proposed (for a full review, see Mihajov & Vejmelka, 2017), the defining criteria of Internet addiction generally overlap with other formulations of behavioral addiction, including preoccupation with Internet usage, mood change as a result of attempting to stop or cut down Internet usage, staying online longer than intended, need to use the Internet in increased amounts to achieve desired effects, lying to others about the nature of one's Internet use, and unsuccessful efforts to stop using the Internet. A meta-analysis of 23 studies of more than 270,000 participants showed a strong association, after adjusting for demographics and depression, between Internet addiction and SI and suicide attempts (Cheng et al., 2018). Further research demonstrated that the effect of Internet addiction on SI is closely linked to sleep disturbances (Sami et al., 2018). Taken together, the extant literature supports a link between Internet addiction and suicide, although the directionally of the relationship has yet to be established.

Cyberbullying

Among the various digital phenomena linked to suicide, online bullying, also called cyberbullying, has the most substantial body of empirical support demonstrating its association with suicidal thoughts and behaviors. Among individuals under the age of 25, numerous studies have documented a strong link between cybervictimization and SI, suicidal behavior, and suicide attempts, independently (John et al., 2018). Moreover, cyberbullying was found to be the strongest predictor of SI, outperforming traditional (noncyber) bullying (van Geel et al., 2014). It has been proposed that perceived stress mediates the effect of cyberbullying on SI, and that this relationship is intensified by feelings of revenge and avoidance (Quintana-Orts et al., 2022). Furthermore, among youth who report having been a target of cyberbullying, adolescent girls consistently report higher levels of suicidal thinking and behavior than are reported by their male counterparts (Bauman et al., 2013; Reed et al., 2015). In a sample of over 10,000 adolescent students in Canada, one study found that having been a victim of cyberbullying was associated with increased odds of psychological distress and SI in both girls and boys; however, more frequent exposure to cyberbullying victimization increased the odds of SI only in adolescent girls (Kim et al., 2019). Taken together, these findings highlight the association between cyberbullying victimization and suicide in all adolescents, with particular vulnerability among teenage girls.

COVID-19 Pandemic

The COVID-19 pandemic is unlike any other public health crisis we have encountered in our lifetime. With respect to the number of deaths and economic consequences, the last comparable pandemic was the Spanish Flu of 1918–1919, a crisis that coincided with a significant increase in suicide rates (Wasserman, 1992). Since the outbreak of COVID-19, clinicians and researchers have voiced concern over the mental effects of the pandemic, speculating that the COVID-19 crisis and its enormous consequences will exacerbate known factors associated with suicide, such as financial crisis or death of a loved one. While the majority of large-scale studies examining suicide rates during the COVID-19 era have yet to reach publication, preliminary CDC data suggest that suicide rates decreased in 2020 (Curtin et al., 2021). Nevertheless, there are emerging lines of evidence that reveal a complex picture of suicide amid the global pandemic (Wu et al., 2021).

Most of the stressful events discussed in this chapter can potentially be either caused or exponentiated by a pandemic like COVID-19. Some examples of stressful events triggered by the COVID-19 pandemic include job loss, economic hardship during lockdowns, relationship stressors, or worsening of preexisting medical illnesses as healthcare staff, resources, and attention are overwhelmed by COVID-19 cases (Rogers et al., 2020). Increased drug and alcohol use during the COVID-19 pandemic has also been recorded; more than one in ten adults have reported starting or increasing the use of alcohol or drugs to cope with the pandemic (Czeisler et al., 2020). Additionally, fear of being infected by the virus and social isolation related to quarantine measures have been linked to suicide deaths (Leaune et al., 2020). Like other stressful life events, COVID-19-related stressors have a hypothesized role in the development of suicidal thoughts and behaviors that can be conceptualized through various models of suicide, including the interpersonal model, stress-diathesis model, cognitive vulnerability model (Raj et al., 2021), and the NCM.

Recent evidence points to distinct trends in rates of suicidal thoughts and behaviors across demographic subgroups during the COVID-19 pandemic. One large-scale cross-sectional study across 10 countries found that SI was significantly associated with male gender, younger age, being single, and differences in health beliefs (Cheung et al., 2021), which appear to be somewhat similar to the factors associated with suicide outside the pandemic. Another meta-analytic study partially replicated these findings, suggesting that younger people, women, and individuals from democratic countries were more susceptible to SI during the COVID-19 pandemic (Dubé et al., 2021). Gender differences in suicide rates are especially notable in Japan: although the population observed a 14% decrease in suicide mortality rates in the first few months of the pandemic, this decline was followed by a 16% increase later in the pandemic's course, with the largest spikes observed in Japanese women (37%) and children and adolescents (49%; Tanaka & Okamoto 2021). Given the likelihood that the COVID-19 pandemic may have exacerbated gender-linked mental health challenges, especially among pregnant women (Lopez-Morales et al., 2021) and victims of domestic violence (Sediri et al., 2020), understanding the acute effects of the pandemic on women and youth is critical for assessing suicide risk during the pandemic.

Like Japan in the early months of the pandemic, the United States experienced a decrease in suicide deaths during the first year of the COVID-19 pandemic, as evidenced by preliminary CDC reports on 2020 suicide mortality rates (Curtin et al., 2021). One proposed explanation for the decrease in suicide deaths is that it reflects a "pulling together phenomenon" that can emerge during times of national crises. Characterized by increased social cohesion and community connectedness in the immediate aftermath of a crisis, the pulling together phenomenon is theorized to coincide with a sudden drop in suicide rates, as was observed in the midst of events like Hurricane Katrina in 2005 or the 9/11 terrorist attacks in 2001 (Kõlves et al., 2013). In each of these instances, however, sudden drops were ultimately followed by steady increases in suicide rates, possibly suggesting a lagged effect of the psychological consequences of a global health crisis. Thus, mental health professionals must be vigilant about the long-term effects of the COVID-19 pandemic on the development and expression of suicidal crises.

References

Afifi, T. O., Enns, M. W., Cox, B. J., Asmundson, G. J., Stein, M. B., & Sareen, J. (2008). Population attributable fractions of psychiatric disorders and suicide ideation and attempts associated with adverse childhood experiences. *American Journal of Public Health*, 98(5), 946–952. https://doi.org/10.2105/ajph.2007.120253

Ahlm, K., Lindqvist, P., Saveman, B. I., & Björnstig, U. (2015). Suicidal drowning deaths in northern Sweden 1992–2009: The role of mental disorder and intoxication. *Journal of Forensic and Legal Medicine, 34,* 168–172. https://doi.org/10.1016/j.jflm.2015.06.002

Akiskal, H. S., & Benazzi, F. (2005). Psychopathologic correlates of suicidal ideation in major depressive outpatients: Is it all due to unrecognized (bipolar) depressive mixed states? *Psychopathology, 38*(5), 273–280.

Akiskal, H. S., & Benazzi, F. (2006). The DSM-IV and ICD-10 categories of recurrent [major] depressive and bipolar II disorders: Evidence that they lie on a dimensional spectrum. *Journal of Affective Disorders, 92*(1), 45–54.

American Foundation for Suicide Prevention. (2022). *Suicide statistics.* https://afsp.org/suicide-statistics

American Psychiatric Association. (2013). *Diagnostic and statistical manual of mental disorders* (5th ed.). American Psychiatric Association Publishing.

American Psychological Association. (2020, November 17). *Psychologists report large increase in demand for anxiety, depression treatment* [Press release]. https://www.apa.org/news/press/releases/2020/11/anxiety-depression-treatment

Amiri, S., & Behnezhad, S. (2020). Alcohol use and risk of suicide: A systematic review and meta-analysis. *Journal of Addictive Diseases, 38*(2), 200–213. https://doi.org/10.1080/10550887.2020.1736757

Ammerman, B. A., Burke, T. A., Jacobucci, R., & McClure, K. (2021). Preliminary investigation of the association between COVID-19 and suicidal thoughts and behaviors in the U.S. *Journal of Psychiatric Research, 134,* 32–38. https://doi.org/10.1016/j.jpsychires.2020.12.037

Baldwin, D. S., Montgomery, S. A., Nil, R., & Lader, M. (2007). Discontinuation symptoms in depression and anxiety disorders. *International Journal of Neuropsychopharmacology, 10*(01), 73–84.

Bagge, C. L., Lee, H. J., Schumacher, J. A., Gratz, K. L., Krull, J. L., & Holloman, G. (2013). Alcohol as an acute risk factor for recent suicide attempts: A case-crossover analysis. *Journal of Studies on Alcohol and Drugs, 74*(4), 552–558. https://doi.org/10.15288/jsad.2013.74.552

Bagge, C. L., & Sher, K. J. (2008). Adolescent alcohol involvement and suicide attempts: Toward the development of a conceptual framework. *Clinical Psychology Review, 28*(8), 1283–1296.

Bagley, C., Bolitho, F., & Bertrand, L. (1995). Mental health profiles, suicidal behavior, and community sexual assault in 2112 Canadian adolescents. *Journal of Crisis Intervention and Suicide Prevention, 16*(3), 126–131. https://doi.org/10.1027/0227-5910.16.3.126

Bauman S., Toomey, R. B., & Walker, J. L. (2013) Associations among bullying, cyberbullying, and suicide in high school students. *Journal of Adolescence, 36,* 341–350. http://dx.doi.org/10.1016/j.adolescence.2012.12.001

Beautrais, A. L., Joyce, P. R., & Mulder, R. T. (1997). Precipitating factors and live events in serious suicide attempts among youths aged 13 through 24 years. *Journal of the American Academy of Child & Adolescent Psychiatry, 36*(11), 1543–1551. https://doi.org/10.1016/S0890-8567(09)66563-1

Benazzi, F. (2007). Bipolar disorder—Focus on bipolar II disorder and mixed depression. *Lancet, 369*(9565), 935–945.

Benazzi, F., & Akiskal, H. S. (2001). Delineating bipolar II mixed states in the Ravenna–San Diego collaborative study: The relative prevalence and diagnostic significance of hypomanic features during major depressive episodes. *Journal of Affective Disorders*, 6, 115–122.

Bielefeldt, A. Ø., Danborg, P. B., & Gøtzsche, P. C. (2016). Precursors to suicidality and violence on antidepressants: systematic review of trials in adult healthy volunteers. *Journal of the Royal Society of Medicine*, 109(10), 381–392. https://doi.org/10.1177/0141076816666805

Bloch-Elkouby, S., Barzilay, S., Gorman, B., Lawrence, O., Rogers, M. L., Richards, J., Cohen, L., Johnson, B. N., & Galynker, I. (2021). The revised Suicide Crisis Inventory (SCI-2): Validation and assessment of near-term suicidal ideation and attempts. *Journal of Affective Disorders*, 295, 1280–1291. https://doi.org/10.1016/j.jad.2021.08.048

Bloch-Elcouby, S., Zilcha-Maro, S., Rogers, M., Park, J-Y., Krumerman, M., Manlogat, K., & Galynker, I. (2022). Who are the patients who deny suicidal intent? Exploring patients' characteristics associated with self-disclosure and denial of suicidal intent. *Acta Psychiatrica Scandinavica*, https://doi.org/10.1111/acps.13511

Borges, G., & Loera, C. R. (2010). Alcohol and drug use in suicidal behaviour. *Current Opinion in Psychiatry*, 23(3), 195–204. https://doi.org/10.1097/YCO.0b013e3283386322

Borges, G., & Rosovsky, H. (1996). Suicide attempts and alcohol consumption in an emergency room sample. *Journal of Studies on Alcohol*, 57(5), 543–548.

Brent, D. A., & Mann, J. J. (2006). Familial pathways to suicidal behavior—Understanding and preventing suicide among adolescents. *New England Journal of Medicine*, 355, 2719–2721.

Brent, D. A., Perper, J. A., Moritz, G., Allman, C., Friend, A., Roth, C., Schweers, J., Balach, L., & Baugher, M. (1993). Psychiatric risk factors for adolescent suicide: A case-control study. *Journal of the American Academy of Child & Adolescent Psychiatry*, 32(3), 521–529. https://doi.org/10.1097/00004583-199305000-00006

Bridge, J. A., Greenhouse, J. B., Weldon, A. H., Campo, J. V., & Kelleher, K. J. (2008). Suicide Trends Among Youths Aged 10 to 19 Years in the United States, 1996–2005. *JAMA*, 300(9), 1025–1026. doi:10.1001/jama.300.9.1025

Bridge, J. A., Asti, L., Horowitz, L. M., Greenhouse, J. B., Fontanella, C. A., Sheftall, A. H., Kelleher, K. J., & Campo, J. V. (2015). Suicide trends among elementary school-aged children in the United States from 1993–2012. *JAMA Pediatrics*, 169(7), 673–677. https://doi.org/10.1001/jamapediatrics.2015.0465

Brooks, D. (2015, June 12). How adulthood happens. *The New York Times*. http://www.nytimes.com/2015/06/12/opinion/david-brooks-how-adulthood-happens.html?_r=0

Brown, J., Cohen, P., Johnson, J. G., & Smailes, E. M. (1999). Childhood abuse and neglect: Specificity of effects on adolescent and young adult depression and suicide. *Journal of the American Academy of Child & Adolescent Psychiatry*, 38(2), 1490–1496. https://doi.org/10.1097/00004583-199912000-00009

Büscher, R., Torok, M., Terhorst, Y., & Sander, L. (2020). Internet-based cognitive behavioral therapy to reduce suicidal ideation: A systematic review and meta-analysis. *JAMA Network Open*, 3(4), e203933. https://doi.org/10.1001/jamanetworkopen.2020.3933

Caetano, R., Kaplan, M. S., Huguet, N., McFarland, B. H., Conner, K., Giesbrecht, N., & Nolte, K. B. (2013). Acute alcohol intoxication and suicide among United States ethnic/racial groups: Findings from the National Violent Death Reporting System. *Alcoholism: Clinical and Experimental Research*, 37(5), 839–846.

Campbell, G., Darke, S., Degenhardt, L., Townsend, H., Carter, G., Draper, B., Farrell, M., Duflou, J., & Lappin, J. (2020). Prevalence and characteristics associated with chronic noncancer pain in suicide decedents: A national study. *Suicide and Life-Threatening Behavior, 50*(4), 778–791. https://doi.org/10.1111/sltb.12627

Cantor, C. H., & Slater, P. J. (1995). Marital breakdown, parenthood and suicide. *Journal of Family Studies, 1*(2), 91–102. https://doi.org/10.5172/jfs.1.2.91

Cash, S. J., & Bridge, J. A. (2009). Epidemiology of youth suicide and suicidal behavior. *Current Opinion in Pediatrics, 21*(5), 613–619. https://doi.org/10.1097/mop.0b013e328 33063e1

Centers for Disease Control and Prevention. (2015a). *Suicide facts at a glance*. https://www.cdc.gov/violenceprevention/pdf/suicide-datasheet-a.PDF

Centers for Disease Control and Prevention. (2015b). *Suicide prevention*. http://www.cdc.gov/violenceprevention/suicide/youth_suicide.html

Centers for Disease Control and Prevention. (2016). *Drug overdose*. https://www.cdc.gov/drugoverdose

Chang, B., Gitlin, D., & Patel, R. (2011). The depressed patient and suicidal patient in the emergency department: Evidence-based management and treatment strategies. *Emergency Medicine Practice, 13*(9), 1–23.

Chang, S. S., Stuckler, D., Yip, P., & Gunnell, D. (2013). Impact of 2008 global economic crisis on suicide: Time trend study in 54 countries. *BMJ, 347*, f5239. https://doi.org/10.1136/bmj.f5239

Cheatle, M. D. (2011). Depression, chronic pain, and suicide by overdose: On the edge. *Pain Medicine, 12*(Suppl. 2), S43–S48. https://doi.org/10.1111/j.1526-4637.2011.01131.xs

Chen, Y. Y., Wu, K. C., Yousuf, S., & Yip, P. S. (2012). Suicide in Asia: Opportunities and challenges. *Epidemiological Reviews, 34*(1), 129–144. https://doi.org/10.1093/epirev/mxr025

Cheng, A. T. A., Chen, T. H. H., Chen, C. C., & Jenkins, R. (2000). Psychosocial and psychiatric risk factors for suicide: Case–control psychological autopsy study. *British Journal of Psychiatry, 177*(4), 360–365.

Cheng, Y. S., Tseng, P. T., Lin, P. Y., Chen, T. Y., Stubbs, B., Carvalho, A. F., Wu, C. K., Chen, Y. W., & Wu, M. K. (2018). Internet addiction and its relationship with suicidal behaviors: A meta-analysis of multinational observational studies. *The Journal of Clinical Psychiatry, 79*(4), 17r11761. https://doi.org/10.4088/JCP.17r11761

Cherpitel, C. J., Borges, G. L., & Wilcox, H. C. (2004). Acute alcohol use and suicidal behavior: A review of the literature. *Alcoholism: Clinical and Experimental Research, 28*(Suppl. 1), 18S–28S.

Cheung, G., Merry, S., & Sundram, F. (2015a). Late-life suicide: Insight on motives and contributors derived from suicide notes. *Journal of Affective Disorders, 185*, 17–23. https://doi.org/10.1016/j.jad.2015.06.035

Cheung, G., Merry, S., & Sundram, F. (2015b). Medical examiner and coroner reports: Uses and limitations in the epidemiology and prevention of late-life suicide. *International Journal of Geriatric Psychiatry, 30*(8), 781–792. https://doi.org/10.1002/gps.4294

Cheung, T., Lam, S. C., Lee, P. H., Xiang, Y. T., Yip, P., & International Research Collaboration on COVID-19 (2021). Global imperative of suicidal ideation in 10 countries amid the COVID-19 pandemic. *Frontiers in Psychiatry, 11*, 588781. https://doi.org/10.3389/fpsyt.2020.588781

Cohen, L. J. (1994). Psychiatric hospitalization as an experience of trauma. *Archives of Psychiatric Nursing, 8*(2), 78–81. https://doi.org/10.1016/0883-9417(94)90037-x

Čoklo, M., Stemberga, V., Cuculić, D., Šoša, I., Jerković, R., & Bosnar, A. (2008). The methods of committing and alcohol intoxication of suicides in southwestern Croatia from 1996 to 2005. *Collegium Antropologicum, 32*(2), 123–125.

Conner, K. R., Beautrais, A. L., & Conwell, Y. (2003). Risk factors for suicide and medically serious suicide attempts among alcoholics: Analyses of Canterbury Suicide Project data. *Journal of Studies on Alcohol, 64*(4), 551–554.

Conner, K. R., Huguet, N., Caetano, R., Giesbrecht, N., McFarland, B. H., Nolte, K. B., & Kaplan, M. S. (2014). Acute use of alcohol and methods of suicide in a US national sample. *American Journal of Public Health, 104*(1), 171–178.

Consoli, A., Payre, H., Speranza, M., Hassler, C., Falissard, B., Touchette, E., Cohen, D., Moro, M., & Revah-Levy, A. (2013). Suicidal behaviors in depressed adolescents: Role of perceived relationships in the family. *Child and Adolescent Psychiatry and Mental Health, 7*(1), 1. https://doi.org/10.1186/1753-2000-7-8

Cook, C. R., Williams, K. R., Guerra, N. G., Kim, T. E., & Sadek, S. (2010). Predictors of bullying and victimization in childhood and adolescence: A meta-analytic investigation. *School Psychology Quarterly, 25*(2), 65–83. https://doi.org/10.1037/a0020149

Coope, C., Donovan J., Wilson, C., Barnes, M., Metcalfe, C., Hollingworth, W., Kapur, N., Hawton, K., & Gunnell, D. (2015). Characteristics of people dying by suicide after job loss, financial difficulties and other economic stressors during a period of recession (2010–2011): A review of coroners' records. *Journal of Affective Disorders, 183*(1), 98–105. https://doi.org/10.1016/j.jad.2015.04.045

Coppersmith, G., Leary, R., Crutchley, P., & Fine, A. (2018). Natural language processing of social media as screening for suicide risk. *Biomedical Informatics Insights, 10*, 1178222618792860. https://doi.org/10.1177/1178222618792860

Coyne, S. M., Hurst, J. L., Dyer, W. J., Hunt, Q., Schvanaveldt, E., Brown, S., & Jones, G. (2021). Suicide risk in emerging adulthood: Associations with screen time over 10 years. *Journal of Youth and Adolescence, 50*(12), 2324–2338. https://doi.org/10.1007/s10964-020-01389-6

Coyne, S. M., Rogers, A. A., Zurcher, J. D., Stockdale, L., & McCall, B. (2020). Does time spent using social media impact mental health? An eight year longitudinal study. *Computers in Human Behavior, 104*, 106160. https://doi.org/10.1016/j.chb.2019.106160

Culpepper, L., Davidson, J. R., Dietrich, A. J., Goodman, W. K., & Schwenk, T. L. (2004). Suicidality as a possible side effect of antidepressant treatment. *Journal of Clinical Psychiatry, 65*(6), 742–749.

Curtin, S. C., Hedegaard, H., & Ahmad, F. B. (2021). *Provisional numbers and rates of suicide by month and demographic characteristics: United States, 2020.* National Center for Health Statistics. https://www.cdc.gov/nchs/data/vsrr/VSRR016.pdf

Curtin, S., Warner, M., & Hedegaard, H. (2016). *Increase in suicide in the United States, 1999–2014* (NCHS data brief No. 241). National Center for Health Statistics. https://www.cdc.gov/nchs/products/databriefs/db241.htm

Czeisler, M. É., Lane, R. I., Petrosky, E., Wiley, J. F., Christensen, A., Njai, R., Weaver, M. D., Robbins, R., Facer-Childs, E. R., Barger, L. K., Czeisler, C. A., Howard, M. E., & Rajaratnam, S. M. W. (2020). Mental health, substance use, and suicidal ideation during the COVID-19 pandemic—United States, June 24–30, 2020. *Morbidity and Mortality Weekly Report, 69*, 1049–1057. http://dx.doi.org/10.15585/mmwr.mm693 2a1external icon

Donath, C., Graessel, E., Baier, D., Bleich, S., & Hillemacher, T. (2014). Is parenting style a predictor of suicide attempts in a representative sample of adolescents? *BMC Pediatrics, 14*(1), 1–13. https://doi.org/10.1186/1471-2431-14-113

Dougall, N., Lambert, P., Maxwell, M., Dawson, A., Sinnott, R., McCafferty, S., Morris, C., Clark, D., & Springbett, A. (2014). Deaths by suicide and their relationship with general and psychiatric hospital discharge: 30-year record linkage study. *British Journal of Psychiatry, 204*(4), 267–273. https://doi.org/10.1192/bjp.bp.112.122374

Dilillo, D., Mauri, S., Mantegazza, C., Fabiano, V., Mameli, C., & Zuccotti, G. V. (2015). Suicide in pediatrics: Epidemiology, risk factors, warning signs and the role of the pediatrician in detecting them. *Italian Journal of Pediatrics, 41*(1), 49. https://doi.org/10.1186/s13052-015-0153-3

Duan, S., Duan, Z., Li, R., Wilson, A., Wang, Y., Jia, Q., Yang, Y., Xia, M., Wang, G., Jin, T., Wang, S., & Chen, R. (2020). Bullying victimization, bullying witnessing, bullying perpetration and suicide risk among adolescents: A serial mediation analysis. *Journal of Affective Disorders, 273,* 274–279. https://doi.org/10.1016/j.jad.2020.03.143

Dubé, J. P., Smith, M. M., Sherry, S. B., Hewitt, P. L., & Stewart, S. H. (2021). Suicide behaviors during the COVID-19 pandemic: A meta-analysis of 54 studies. *Psychiatry Research, 301,* 113998. https://doi.org/10.1016/j.psychres.2021.113998

Dufort, M., Stenbacka, M., & Gumpert, C. H. (2015). Physical domestic violence exposure is highly associated with suicidal attempts in both women and men. Results from the National Public Health Survey in Sweden. *European Journal of Public Health, 25*(3), 413–418. https://doi.org/10.1093/eurpub/cku198

Dufrasne, S., Roy, M., Galvez, M., & Rosenblatt, D. S. (2011). Experience over fifteen years with a protocol for predictive testing for Huntington disease. *Molecular Genetics and Metabolism, 102*(4), 494–504. https://doi.org/10.1016/j.ymgme.2010.12.001

Edwards, A. C., Ohlsson, H., Sundquist, J., Sundquist, K., & Kendler, K. S. (2020). Alcohol use disorder and risk of suicide in a Swedish population-based cohort. *American Journal of Psychiatry, 177*(7), 627–634. https://doi.org/10.1176/appi.ajp.2019.19070673

Elbogen, E. B., Lanier, M., Montgomery, A. E., Strickland, S., Wagner, H. R., & Tsai, J. (2020). Financial strain and suicide attempts in a nationally representative sample of US adults. *American Journal of Epidemiology, 189*(11), 1266–1274. https://doi.org/10.1093/aje/kwaa146

Elman, I., Borsook, D., & Volkow, N. D. (2013). Pain and suicidality: Insights from reward and addiction neuroscience. *Progress in Neurobiology, 109,* 1–27.

Erlangsen, A., Stenager, E., & Conwell, Y. (2015). Physical diseases as predictors of suicide in older adults: A nationwide, register-based cohort study. *Social Psychiatry and Psychiatric Epidemiology, 50*(9), 1427–1439. https://doi.org/10.1007/s00127-015-1051-0

Esposito, C. L., & Clum, G. A. (2002a). Psychiatric symptoms and their relationship to suicidal ideation in a high-risk adolescent community sample. *Journal of the American Academy of Child & Adolescent Psychiatry, 41*(1), 44–51. https://doi.org/10.1097/00004583-200201000-00010

Esposito, C. L., & Clum, G. A. (2002b). Social support and problem-solving as moderators of the relationship between childhood abuse and suicidality: Applications to a delinquent population. *Journal of Traumatic Stress, 15*(2), 137–146. https://doi.org/10.1023/a:1014860024980

Fang, F., Fall, K., Mittleman, M. A., Sparén, P., Ye, W., Adami, H., & Valdimarsdóttir, U. (2012). Suicide and cardiovascular death after a cancer diagnosis. *New England Journal of Medicine, 367*(3), 276–277. https://doi.org/10.1056/nejmc1205927

Fergusson, D. M., Horwood, L. J., & Lynskey, M. T. (1996). Childhood sexual abuse and psychiatric disorder in young adulthood: II. Psychiatric outcomes of childhood sexual abuse. *Journal of the American Academy of Child & Adolescent Psychiatry, 35*(10), 1365–1374. https://doi.org/10.1097/00004583-199610000-00024

Fergusson, D. M., Woodward, L. J., & Horwood, L. J. (2000). Risk factors and life processes associated with the onset of suicidal behavior during adolescence and early adulthood. *Psychological Medicine, 30*(1), 23–39.

Fergusson, D. M., Beautrais, A. L., & Horwood, L. J. (2003). Vulnerability and resiliency to suicidal behaviours in young people. *Psychological Medicine, 33*(1), 61–73. https://doi.org/10.1017/S0033291702006748

Fiedorowicz, J. G., Leon, A. C., Keller, M. B., Solomon, D. A., Rice, J. P., & Coryell, W. H. (2009). Do risk factors for suicidal behavior differ by affective disorder polarity? *Psychological Medicine, 39*(05), 763–771.

Foster, T. (2011). Adverse life events proximal to adult suicide: A synthesis of findings from psychological autopsy studies. *Archives of Suicide Research, 15*(1), 1–15. https://doi.org/10.1080/13811118.2011.5402213

Fowler, K. A., Gladden, M., Vagi, K. J., Barnes, J., & Frazier, L. (2015). Increase in suicides associated with home eviction and foreclosure during the US housing crisis: From 16 national violent death reporting system states, 2005–2010. *Research and Practice, 105*(312), 311–316. https://doi.org/10.2105/AJPH.2014.301945

Freuchen, A., Kjelsberg, E., Lundervold, A. J., & Groholt, B. (2012). Differences between children and adolescents who commit suicide and their peers: A psychological autopsy of suicide victims compared to accident victims and a community sample. *Child and Adolescent Psychiatry and Mental Health, 6*(1), 1–12. https://doi.org/10.1186/1753-2000-6-1

Friedman, R. A., & Leon, A. C. (2007). Expanding the black box—Depression, antidepressants, and the risk of suicide. *New England Journal of Medicine, 356*(23), 2343–2346.

Fudalej, S., Ilgen, M., Fudalej, M., Wojnar, M., Matsumoto, H., Barry, K. L., Ploski, R., & Blow, F. C. (2009). Clinical and genetic risk factors for suicide under the influence of alcohol in a Polish sample. *Alcohol and Alcoholism, 44*(5), 437–442.

Galdas, P. M., Cheater, F., & Marshall, P. (2005). Men and health help-seeking behaviour: Literature review. *Journal of Advanced Nursing, 49*(6), 616–623. https://doi.org/10.1111/j.1365-2648.2004.03331.x

Galynker, I., Yaseen, Z. S., Cohen, A., Benhamou, O., Hawes, M., & Briggs, J. (2016). Prediction of suicidal behavior in high risk psychiatric patients using an assessment of acute suicidal state: The suicide crisis inventory. *Depression and Anxiety, 34*(2), 147–158. https://doi.org/10.1002/da.22559

Glowinski, A. L., Bucholz, K. K., Nelson, E. C., Fu, Q., Madden, P. A., Reich, W., & Heath, A. C. (2001). Suicide attempts in an adolescent female twin sample. *Journal of the American Academy of Child & Adolescent Psychiatry, 40*(11), 1300–1307. https://doi.org/10.1097/00004583-200111000-00010

Gold, M. S., Pottash, A. L. C., Sweeney, D. R., & Kleber, H. D. (1980). Efficacy of clonidine in opiate withdrawal: A study of thirty patients. *Drug and Alcohol Dependence, 6*(4), 201–208.

Goldsmith, S. K., Pellmar, T. C., Kleinman, A. M., & Bunney, W. E. (2002). *Reducing suicide: A national imperative*. National Academies Press.

Goschin, S., Briggs, J., Blanco-Luten, S., Cohen, L. J., & Galynker, I. (2013). Parental affectionless control and suicidality. *Journal of Affective Disorders, 151*(1), 1–6. https://doi.org/10.1016/j.jad.2013.05.096

Gould, M. S. (1996). Psychosocial risk factors of child and adolescent completed suicide. *Archives of General Psychiatry, 53*(12), 1155. https://doi.org/10.1001/archpsyc.1996.01830120095016

Groholt, B., Ekeberg, O., Wichstrom, L., & Haldorsen, T. (1998). Suicide among children and younger and older adolescents in Norway: A comparative study. *Journal of the American Academy of Child & Adolescent Psychiatry, 37*(5), 473–481. https://doi.org/10.1097/00004583-199805000-00008

Gunnell, D., Brooks, J., & Peters, T. J. (1996). Epidemiology and patterns of hospital use after parasuicide in the south west of England. *Journal of Epidemiology and Community Health, 50*(1), 24–29. 10.1136/jech.50.1.24

Gunnell, D., Appleby, L., Arensman, E., Hawton, K., John, A., Kapur, N., Khan, M., O'Connor, R. C., Pirkis, J., & The COVID-19 Suicide Prevention Research Collaboration (2020). Suicide risk and prevention during the COVID-19 pandemic. *The Lancet Psychiatry, 7*(6), 468–471. https://doi.org/10.1016/S2215-0366(20)30171-1

Gunnell, D., Eddleston, M., Phillips, M. R., & Konradsen, F. (2007). The global distribution of fatal pesticide self-poisoning: Systematic review. *BMC Public Health, 7*(1), 357. https://doi.org/10.1186/1471-2458-7-357

Harper, S., Charters, T. J., Strumpf, E. C., Galea, S., & Nandi, A. (2015). Economic downturns and suicide mortality in the USA, 1980–2010: Observational study. *International Journal of Epidemiology, 44*(3), 956–966. https://doi.org/10.1093/ije/dyv009

Hasin, D. S., Keyes, K. M., Alderson, D., Wang, S., Aharonovich, E., & Grant, B. F. (2008). Cannabis withdrawal in the United States: A general population study. *Journal of Clinical Psychiatry, 69*(9), 1354.

Hawton, K., Fagg, J., & McKeown, S. P. (1989). Alcoholism, alcohol and attempted suicide. *Alcohol and Alcoholism, 24*(1), 3–9. https://doi.org/10.1093/oxfordjournals.alcalc.a044864

Hawton, K., & Gunnell, D. (2015). Characteristics of people dying by suicide after job loss, financial difficulties and other economic stressors during a period of recession (2010–2011): A review of coroners records'. *Journal of Affective Disorders, 183*, 98–105. https://doi.org/10.1016/j.jad.2015.04.045

Hawton, K., & Van Heeringen, K. (2009). Suicide. *Lancet, 373*(9672), 1372–1381. https://doi.org/10.1016/S0140-6736(09)60372-x

Heikkinen, M., Aro, H., & Lönnqvist, J. (1992). The partners' views on precipitant stressors in suicide. *Acta Psychiatrica Scandinavica, 85*(5), 380–384. https://doi.org/10.1111/j.16000447.1992.tb10323.x

Heikkinen, M., Aro, H., & Lönnqvist, J. (1994). Recent life events, social support and suicide. *Acta Psychiatrica Scandinavica, 89*(s377), 65–72.

Hengartner, M. P., Amendola, S., Kaminski, J. A., Kindler, S., Bschor, T., & Plöderl, M. (2021). Suicide risk with selective serotonin reuptake inhibitors and other new-generation antidepressants in adults: A systematic review and meta-analysis of observational studies. *Journal of Epidemiology and Community Health, 7*(6). https://doi.org/10.1136/jech-2020-214611

Hinze, V., Crane, C., Ford, T., Buivydaite, R., Qiu, L., & Gjelsvik, B. (2019). The relationship between pain and suicidal vulnerability in adolescence: A systematic review. *The Lancet Child & Adolescent Health, 3*(12), 899–916. https://doi.org/10.1016/S2352-4642(19)30267-6

Houle, J. N., & Light, M. T. (2014). The home foreclosure crisis and rising suicide rates, 2005 to 2010. *American Journal of Public Health, 104*(6), 1073–1079. https://doi.org/10.2105/ajph.2013.301774

Howarth, E. J., O'Connor, D. B., Panagioti, M., Hodkinson, A., Wilding, S., & Johnson, J. (2020). Are stressful life events prospectively associated with increased suicidal ideation and behaviour? A systematic review and meta-analysis. *Journal of Affective Disorders, 266,* 731–742. https://doi.org/10.1016/j.jad.2020.01.171

Howland, R. H. (2010). Potential adverse effects of discontinuing psychotropic drugs—Part 3: Antipsychotic, dopaminergic, and mood-stabilizing drugs. *Journal of Psychosocial Nursing and Mental Health Services, 48*(8), 11–14.

Høyen, K. S., Solem, S., Cohen, L. J., Prestmo, A., Hjemdal, O., Vaaler, A. E., Galynker, I., & Torgersen, T. (2021). Non-disclosure of suicidal ideation in psychiatric inpatients: Rates and correlates. *Death Studies, 46*(8), 1823–1831. https://doi.org/10.1080/07481187.2021.1879317

Hsu, W. Y., Lin, S. S., Chang, S. M., Tseng, Y. H., & Chiu, N. Y. (2015). Examining the diagnostic criteria for Internet addiction: Expert validation. *Journal of the Formosan Medical Association, 114*(6), 504–508. https://doi.org/10.1016/j.jfma.2014.03.010

Huang, C. (2017). Time spent on social network sites and psychological well-being: A meta-analysis. *Cyberpsychology, Behavior, and Social Networking, 20*(6), 346–354. https://doi.org/10.1089/cyber.2016.0758

Hufford, M. R. (2001). Alcohol and suicidal behavior. *Clinical Psychology Review, 21*(5), 797–811.

Isometsä, E. (2014). Suicidal behaviour in mood disorders—Who, when, and why? *Canadian Journal of Psychiatry, 59*(3), 120–130.

Jacobson, C., Batejan, K., Kleinman, M., & Gould, M. (2013). Reasons for attempting suicide among a community sample of adolescents. *Suicide and Life-Threatening Behavior, 43*(6), 646–662. https://doi.org/10.1111/sltb.12047

Jia, C., Wang, L., Xu, A., Dai, A., & Qin, P. (2014). Physical illness and suicide risk in rural residents of contemporary China. *Crisis, 35*(5), 330–337. https://doi.org/10.1027/0227-5910/a000271

John, A., Glendenning, A. C., Marchant, A., Montgomery, P., Stewart, A., Wood, S., Lloyd, K., & Hawton, K. (2018). Self-harm, suicidal behaviours, and cyberbullying in children and young people: Systematic review. *Journal of Medical Internet Research, 20*(4), e129. https://doi.org/10.2196/jmir.9044

Johnson, J. G., Cohen, P., Gould, M. S., Kasen, S., Brown, J., & Brook, J. S. (2002). Childhood adversities, interpersonal difficulties, and risk for suicide attempts during late adolescence and early adulthood. *Archives of General Psychiatry, 59*(8), 741. https://doi.org/10.1001/archpsyc.59.8.741

Kapfhammer, H., & Lange, P. (2012). Suicidal and infanticidal risks in puerperal psychosis of an early onset. *Neuropsychiatrie, 26*(3), 129–138. https://doi.org/10.1007/s40211-012-0023-9

Katz, C., Yaseen, Z. S., Mojtabai, R., Cohen, L. J., & Galynker, I. I. (2011). Panic as an independent risk factor for suicide attempt in depressive illness. *Journal of Clinical Psychiatry, 72*(12), 1628–1635. https://doi.org/10.4088/jcp.10m06186blus

Kazan, D., Calear, A. L., & Batterham, P. J. (2016). The impact of intimate partner relationships on suicidal thoughts and behaviours: A systematic review. *Journal of Affective Disorders, 190,* 585–598. https://doi.org/10.1016/j.jad.2015.11.003

Keles, B., McCrae, N., & Grealish, A. (2020) A systematic review: The influence of social media on depression, anxiety and psychological distress in adolescents. *International Journal of Adolescence and Youth, 25*(1), 79–93. https://doi.org/10.1080/02673843.2019.1590851

Kessler, R. C., Chiu, W. T., Demler, O., & Walters, E. E. (2005). Prevalence, severity, and comorbidity of 12-month DSM-IV disorders in the National Comorbidity Survey replication. *Archives of General Psychiatry, 62*(6), 617. https://doi.org/10.1001/archpsyc.62.6.617

Kim, S., Kimber, M., Boyle, M. H., & Georgiades, K. (2019). Sex differences in the association between cyberbullying victimization and mental health, substance use, and suicidal ideation in adolescents. *Canadian Journal of Psychiatry/Revue Canadienne de Psychiatrie, 64*(2), 126–135. https://doi.org/10.1177/0706743718777397

Kirtley, O. J., Rodham, K., & Crane, C. (2020). Understanding suicidal ideation and behaviour in individuals with chronic pain: A review of the role of novel transdiagnostic psychological factors. *The Lancet Psychiatry, 7*(3), 282–290. https://doi.org/10.1016/S2215-0366(19)30288-3

Kisiel, C. L., & Lyons, J. S. (2001). Dissociation as a mediator of psychopathology among sexually abused children and adolescents. *American Journal of Psychiatry, 158*(7), 1034–1039. https://doi.org/10.1176/appi.ajp.158.7.1034

Kitagawa, Y., Shimodera, S., Togo, F., Okazaki, Y., Nishida, A., & Sasaki, T. (2014). Suicidal feelings interfere with help-seeking in bullied adolescents. *PLOS One, 9*(9), e106031. https://doi.org/10.1371/journal.pone.0106031

Kleber, H., & Gawin, F. (1986). Psychopharmacological trials in cocaine abuse treatment. *American Journal of Drug and Alcohol Abuse, 12*(3), 235–246.

Kõlves, K., Kõlves, K. E., & De Leo, D. (2013). Natural disasters and suicidal behaviors: A systematic literature review. *Journal of Affective Disorders, 146*, 1–14. http://dx.doi.org/10.1016/j.jad.2012.07.037

Kõlves, K., Värnik, A., Schneider, B., Fritze, J., & Allik, J. (2006). Recent life events and suicide: A case–control study in Tallinn and Frankfurt. *Social Science & Medicine, 62*(11), 2887–2896. https://doi.org/10.1016/j.socscimed.2005.11.048

Krug, E. G., Dahlberg, L. L., Mercy, J. A., Zwi, A. B., & Lozano, R. (2002). *World report on violence and health.* World Health Organization.

Large, M., Sharma, S., Cannon, E., Ryan, C., & Nielssen, O. (2011). Risk factors for suicide within a year of discharge from psychiatric hospital: A systematic meta-analysis. *Australian and New Zealand Journal of Psychiatry, 45*(8), 619–628. https://doi.org/10.3109/00048674.2011.590465

Lawrence, D. M., Holman, C. D. J., Jablensky, A. V., & Fuller, S. A. (1999). Suicide rates in psychiatric in-patients: An application of record linkage to mental health research. *Australian and New Zealand Journal of Public Health, 23*(5), 468–470. https://doi.org/10.1111/j.1467-842x.1999.tb01300.x

Leaune, E., Samuel, M., Oh, H., Poulet, E., & Brunelin, J. (2020). Suicidal behaviors and ideation during emerging viral disease outbreaks before the COVID-19 pandemic: A systematic rapid review. *Preventive Medicine, 141*, 106264. https://doi.org/10.1016/j.ypmed.2020.106264

Lester, D. (1997). The role of shame in suicide. *Suicide and Life-Threatening Behavior, 27*(4), 352–361. https://doi.org/10.1111/j.1943-278X.1997.tb00514.xs

Libby, A. M., Orton, H. D., & Valuck, R. J. (2009). Persisting decline in depression treatment after FDA warnings. *Archives of General Psychiatry, 66*(6), 633. https://doi.org/10.1001/archgenpsychiatry.2009.46

Lim, M., Kim, S. W., Nam, Y. Y., Moon, E., Yu, J., Lee, S., Chang, J. S., Jhoo, J. H., Cha, B., Choi, J. S., Ahn, Y. M., Ha, K., Kim, J., Jeon, H. J., & Park, J. I. (2014). Reasons for desiring death: Examining causative factors of suicide attempters treated in emergency rooms in Korea. *Journal of Affective Disorders, 168,* 349–356. https://doi.org/10.1016/j.jad.2014.07.026

Liu, B. P., Zhang, J., Chu, J., Qiu, H. M., Jia, C. X., & Hennessy, D. A. (2019). Negative life events as triggers on suicide attempt in rural China: A case-crossover study. *Psychiatry Research, 276,* 100–106. https://doi.org/10.1016/j.psychres.2019.04.008

Locke, T. F., & Newcomb, M. D. (2005). Psychosocial predictors and correlates of suicidality in teenage Latino males. *Hispanic Journal of Behavioral Sciences, 27*(3), 319–336. https://doi.org/10.1177/0739986305276745

López-Morales, H., Del Valle, M. V., Canet-Juric, L., Andrés, M. L., Galli, J. I., Poó, F., & Urquijo, S. (2021). Mental health of pregnant women during the COVID-19 pandemic: A longitudinal study. *Psychiatry Research, 295,* 113567.

Lundholm, L., Thiblin, I., Runeson, B., Leifman, A., & Fugelstad, A. (2014). Acute influence of alcohol, THC or central stimulants on violent suicide: A Swedish population study. *Journal of Forensic Sciences, 59*(2), 436–440.

Luo, F., Florence, C. S., Quispe-Agnoli, M., Ouyang, L., & Crosby, A. E. (2011). Impact of business cycles on US suicide rates, 1928–2007. *American Journal of Public Health, 101*(6), 1139–1146. https://doi.org/10.2105/AJPH.2010.300010

Luxton, D. D., June, J. D., & Comtois, K. A. (2013). Can postdischarge follow-up contacts prevent suicide and suicidal behavior? *Crisis, 34*(1), 32–41. https://doi.org/10.1027/0227-5910/a000158

Machado, D. B., Rasella, D., & Santos, D. N. (2015). Impact of income inequality and other social determinants on suicide rate in Brazil. *PLOS One, 10*(4), e0124934. https://doi.org/10.1371/journal.pone.0124934

Martin, G., Bergen, H. A., Richardson, A. S., Roeger, L., & Allison, S. (2004). Sexual abuse and suicidality: Gender differences in a large community sample of adolescents. *Child Abuse & Neglect, 28*(5), 491–503. https://doi.org/10.1016/j.chiabu.2003.08.006

Martin, J. A. (2005). Annual summary of vital statistics—2003. *Pediatrics, 115*(3), 619–634. https://doi.org/10.1542/peds.2004-2695

Marttunen, M. J., Aro, H. M., & Lonnqvist, J. K. (1993). Adolescence and suicide: A review of psychological autopsy studies. *European Child & Adolescent Psychiatry, 2*(1), 10–18. https://doi.org/10.1007/BF02098826

Memon, A. M., Sharma, S. G., Mohite, S. S., & Jain, S. (2018). The role of online social networking on deliberate self-harm and suicidality in adolescents: A systematized review of literature. *Indian Journal of Psychiatry, 60*(4), 384–392. https://doi.org/10.4103/psychiatry.IndianJPsychiatry_414_17

Merrall, E. L. C., Kariminia, A., Binswanger, I. A., Hobbs, M. S., Farrell, M., Marsden, J., Hutchinson, J. S., & Bird, S. M. (2010). Meta-analysis of drug-related deaths soon after release from prison. *Addiction, 105*(9), 1545–1554. https://doi.org/10.1111/j.1360-0443.2010.02990.x

Mihajlov, M., & Vejmelka, L. (2017) Internet addiction: A review of the first twenty years. *Psychiatria Danubina, 29*(3), 260–272. https://doi.org/10.24869/psyd.2017.260

Miller, A. B., Esposito-Smythers, C., Weismoore, J. T., & Renshaw, K. D. (2013). The relation between child maltreatment and adolescent suicidal behavior: A systematic review and critical examination of the literature. *Clinical Child and Family Psychology Review, 16*(2), 146–172. https://doi.org/10.1007/s10567-013-0131-5

Miller, M., Azrael, D., & Barber, C. (2012). Suicide mortality in the United States: The importance of attending to method in understanding population-level disparities in the burden of suicide. *Annual Review of Public Health, 33*(1), 393–408. https://doi.org/10.1146/annurev-publhealth-031811-124636

Mills, J. A., & Strawn, J. R. (2020). Antidepressant tolerability in pediatric anxiety and obsessive-compulsive disorders: A Bayesian hierarchical modeling meta-analysis. *Journal of the American Academy of Child & Adolescent Psychiatry, 59*(11), 1240–1251. https://doi.org/10.1016/j.jaac.2019.10.013

Montgomery, S. A. (2008). Tolerability of serotonin norepinephrine reuptake inhibitor antidepressants. *CNS Spectrums, 13*(Suppl. 11), 27–33. https://doi.org/10.1017/s10928 52900028297

Mortensen, P. B., & Juel, K. (1993). Mortality and causes of death in first admitted schizophrenic patients. *British Journal of Psychiatry, 163*(2), 183–189. https://doi.org/10.1192/bjp.163.2.183

Mościcki, E. K. (2001). Epidemiology of completed and attempted suicide: Toward a framework for prevention. *Clinical Neuroscience Research, 1*(5), 310–323. https://doi.org/10.1016/s1566-2772(01)00032-9

Murphy, S. M., & Tyrer, P. (1991). A double-blind comparison of the effects of gradual withdrawal of lorazepam, diazepam and bromazepam in benzodiazepine dependence. *British Journal of Psychiatry, 158*(4), 511–516.

Niezen, R. (2013). Internet suicide: Communities of affirmation and the lethality of communication. *Transcultural Psychiatry, 50*(2), 303–322. https://doi.org/10.1177/13634 61512473733

Nordentoft, M., Mortensen, P. B., & Pedersen C. B. (2011). Absolute risk of suicide after first hospital contact in mental disorder. *JAMA Psychiatry, 68*(10), 1058–1064. doi:10.1001/archgenpsychiatry.2011.113

Nordentoft, M., Pedersen, C. B., & Mortensen, P. B. (2012). Absolute risk of suicide following first hospital contact with mental disorder. *Schizophrenia Research, 136*, S73–S74. https://doi.org/10.1016/s0920-9964(12)70268-2

Novick, D. M., Swartz, H. A., & Frank, E. (2010). Suicide attempts in bipolar I and bipolar II disorder: A review and meta-analysis of the evidence. *Bipolar Disorders, 12*(1), 1–9.

Olfson, M., & Marcus, S. C. (2008). A case–control study of antidepressants and attempted suicide during early phase treatment of major depressive episodes. *Journal of Clinical Psychiatry, 69*(3), 425–432. https://doi.org/10.4088/jcp.v69n0313

Oquendo, M. A., Perez-Rodriguez, M. M., Poh, E., Sullivan, G., Burke, A. K., Sublette, M. E., Mann, J. J., & Galfalvy, H. (2014). Life events: A complex role in the timing of suicidal behavior among depressed patients. *Molecular Psychiatry, 19*(8), 902–909. https://doi.org/10.1038/mp.2013.128

Orri, M., Séguin, J. R., Castellanos-Ryan, N., Tremblay, R. E., Côté, S. M., Turecki, G., & Geoffroy, M. C. (2020). A genetically informed study on the association of cannabis, alcohol, and tobacco smoking with suicide attempt. *Molecular Psychiatry, 26*, 5061–5060. https://doi.org/10.1038/s41380-020-0785-6

Ortega, L. A., & Karch, D. (2010). Precipitating circumstances of suicide among women of reproductive age in 16 U.S. states, 2003–2007. *Journal of Women's Health, 19*(1), 5–7. https://doi.org/10.1089/jwh.2009.1788

Orth, M., Handley, O. J., Schwenke, C., Dunnett, S. B., Craufurd, D., Ho, A. K., Wild, E., Tabrizi, S. J., Landwehrmeyer, G. B., & Investigators of the European Huntington's Disease Network. (2010). Observing Huntington's disease: The European Huntington's Disease Network's registry. *PLOS Currents, 2*, RRN1184. https://doi.org/10.1371/curre nts.RRN1184

Owens, D., Horrocks, J., & House, A. (2002). Fatal and non-fatal repetition of self-harm: Systematic review. *British Journal of Psychiatry, 181*, 193–199.

Pan, Y., Stewart, R., & Chang, C. (2013). Socioeconomic disadvantage, mental disorders and risk of 12-month suicide ideation and attempt in the National Comorbidity Survey Replication (NCS-R) in US. *Social Psychiatry and Psychiatric Epidemiology*, *48*(1), 71–79. https://doi.org/10.1007/s00127-012-0591-9

Pavarin, R. M., Sanchini, S., Tadonio, L., Domenicali, M., Caputo, F., & Pacetti, M. (2021). Suicide mortality risk in a cohort of individuals treated for alcohol, heroin or cocaine abuse: Results of a follow-up study. *Psychiatry Research*, *296*, 113639. https://doi.org/10.1016/j.psychres.2020.113639

Penttinen, J. (1995). Back pain and risk of suicide among Finnish farmers. *American Journal of Public Health*, *85*(10), 1452–1453. 10.2105/ajph.85.10.1452-a

Philipsen, A., Schmahl, C., & Lieb, K. (2004). Naloxone in the treatment of acute dissociative states in female patients with borderline personality disorder. *Pharmacopsychiatry*, *37*(5), 196–199.

Phillips, M. R., Yang, G., Zhang, Y., Wang, L., Ji, H., & Zhou, M. (2002). Risk factors for suicide in China: A national case-control psychological autopsy study. *Lancet*, *360*(9347), 1728–1736. https://doi.org/10.1016/s0140-6736(02)11681-3

Plunkett, A., O'Toole, B., Swanston, H., Oates, R. K., Shrimpton, S., & Parkinson, P. (2001). Suicide risk following child sexual abuse. *Ambulatory Pediatrics*, *1*(5), 262–266.

Pompili, M., Innamorati, M., Szanto, K., Di Vittorio, C., Conwell, Y., Lester, D., Tatarelli, R., Girardi, P., & Amore, M. (2011). Life events as precipitants of suicide attempts among first-time suicide attempters, repeaters, and non-attempters. *Psychiatry Research*, *186*(2-3), 300–305. https://doi.org/10.1016/j.psychres.2010.09.003

Pompili, M., Serafini, G., Innamorati, M., Möller-Leimkühler, A. M., Giupponi, G., Girardi, P., Tatarelli, R., & Lester, D. (2010). The hypothalamic-pituitary-adrenal axis and serotonin abnormalities: A selective overview for the implications of suicide prevention. *European Archives of Psychiatry and Clinical Neuroscience*, *260*(8), 583–600. https://doi.org/10.1007/s00406-010-0108-z

Pourmand, A., Roberson, J., Caggiula, A., Monsalve, N., Rahimi, M., & Torres-Llenza, V. (2019). Social media and suicide: A review of technology-based epidemiology and risk assessment. *Telemedicine Journal and E-Health*, *25*(10), 880–888. https://doi.org/10.1089/tmj.2018.0203

Prigerson, H. G., Maciejewski, P. K., & Rosenheck, R. A. (1999). The effects of marital dissolution and marital quality on health and health service use among women. *Medical Care*, *37*(9), 858–873. https://doi.org/10.1097/00005650-199909000-00003

Qin, P., Hawton, K., Mortensen, P., & Webb, R. (2014). Combined effects of physical illness and comorbid psychiatric disorder on risk of suicide in a national population study. *British Journal of Psychiatry*, *204*(6), 430–435. https://doi.org/10.1192/bjp.bp.113.128785

Qin, P., Mortensen, P. B., & Pedersen, C. B. (2009). Frequent change of residence and risk of attempted and completed suicide among children and adolescents. *Archives of General Psychiatry*, *66*(6), 628. https://doi.org/10.1001/archgenpsychiatry.2009.20

Qin, P., & Nordentoft, M. (2005). Suicide risk in relation to psychiatric hospitalization: Evidence based on longitudinal registers. *Archives of General Psychiatry*, *62*(4), 427–432. https://doi.org/10.1001/archpsyc.62.4.427

Quan, H., Arboleda-Flórez, J., Fick, G. H., Stuart, H. L., & Love, E. J. (2002). Association between physical illness and suicide among the elderly. *Social Psychiatry and Psychiatric Epidemiology*, *37*(4), 190–197. https://doi.org/10.1007/s001270200014

Quintana-Orts, C., Rey, L., & Neto, F. (2022). Beyond cyberbullying: Investigating when and how cybervictimization predicts suicidal ideation. *Journal of Interpersonal Violence, 37*(1-2), 935–957. https://doi.org/10.1177/0886260520913640

Raj, S., Ghosh, D., Singh, T., Verma, S. K., & Arya, Y. K. (2021). Theoretical mapping of suicidal risk factors during the COVID-19 pandemic: A mini-review. *Frontiers in Psychiatry, 11*, 589614. https://doi.org/10.3389/fpsyt.2020.589614

Randall, J. R., Walld, R., Chateau, D., Finlayson, G., Sareen, J., & Bolton, J. M. (2014). Risk of suicide and suicide attempts associated with physical disorders: A population-based, balancing score-matched analysis. *Psychological Medicine, 45*(3), 495–504. https://doi.org/10.1017/s0033291714001639

Reed, K. P., Nugent, W. R., & Cooper, L. (2015) Testing a path model of relationships between gender, age, and bullying victimization and violent behavior, substance abuse, depression, suicidal ideation, and suicide attempts in adolescents. *Children and Youth Services Review, 55*, 128–137. https://doi.org/10.1016/j.childyouth.2015.05.016

Reeves, A., McKee, M., & Stuckler, D. (2014). Economic suicides in the great recession in Europe and North America. *British Journal of Psychiatry, 205*(3), 246–247. https://doi.org/10.1192/bjp.bp.114.144766

Reger, M. A., Gahm, G. A., Kinn, J. T., Luxton, D. D., Skopp, N. A., & Bush, N. E. (2011). *Department of Defense Suicide Event Report (DoDSER) calendar year 2010 annual report*. National Center for Telehealth and Technology.

Rehkopf, D. H., & Buka, S. L. (2006). The association between suicide and the socio-economic characteristics of geographical areas: A systematic review. *Psychological Medicine, 36*(2), 145. https://doi.org/10.1017/s003329170500588x

Rew, L., Thomas, N., Horner, S. D., Resnick, M. D., & Beuhring, T. (2001). Correlates of recent suicide attempts in a triethnic group of adolescents. *Journal of Nursing Scholarship, 33*(4), 361–367. https://doi.org/10.1111/j.1547-5069.2001.00361.x

Rihmer, Z., & Akiskal, H. (2006). Do antidepressants t(h)reat(en) depressives? Toward a clinically judicious formulation of the antidepressant–suicidality FDA advisory in light of declining national suicide statistics from many countries. *Journal of Affective Disorders, 94*(1), 3–13.

Robinson, J., Cox, G., Bailey, E., Hetrick, S., Rodrigues, M., Fisher, S., & Herrman, H. (2016). Social media and suicide prevention: A systematic review. *Early Intervention in Psychiatry, 10*(2), 103–121. https://doi.org/10.1111/eip.12229

Rogers, J. P., Chesney, E., Oliver, D., Pollak, T. A., McGuire, P., Fusar-Poli, P., Zandi, M. S., Lewis, G., & David, A. S. (2020). Psychiatric and neuropsychiatric presentations associated with severe coronavirus infections: A systematic review and meta-analysis with comparison to the COVID-19 pandemic. *The Lancet Psychiatry, 7*(7), 611–627. https://doi.org/10.1016/S2215-0366(20)30203-0

Rogers, M. L., Bloch-Elkouby, S., & Galynker, I. (2022). Differential disclosure of suicidal intent to clinicians versus researchers: Associations with concurrent suicide crisis syndrome and prospective suicidal ideation and attempts. *Psychiatry Research, 314*, 114522. https://doi.org/10.1016/j.psychres.2022.114522

Rogers, M. L., Cao, E., Richards, J., Mitelman, S., Barzilay, S., Blum, Y., Chistopolskaya, K., Çinka, E., Dudeck, M., Husain, I., Kantas Yilmaz, E., Kuśmirek, O., Menon, V., Nikolaev, E., Pilecka, B., Titze, L., Valvassori, S., Luiz, T., You, S., & Galynker, I. (under review). Associations between long-term and near-term stressful life events, suicide crisis syndrome, and suicidal ideation. *7*.

Rogers, M. L., Vespa, A., Bloch-Elkouby, S., & Galynker, I. (2021). Validity of the Modular Assessment of Risk for Imminent Suicide in predicting short-term suicidality. *Acta Psychiatrica Scandinavica, 144*(6), 563–577. https://doi.org/10.1111/acps.13354

Rosenberg, H. J., Jankowski, M. K., Sengupta, A., Wolfe, R. S., Wolford, G. L., & Rosenberg, S. D. (2005). Single and multiple suicide attempts and associated health risk factors in New Hampshire adolescents. *Suicide and Life-Threatening Behavior, 35*(5), 547–557. https://doi.org/10.1521/suli.2005.35.5.547

Routley, V. H., & Ozanne-Smith, J. E. (2012). Work-related suicide in Victoria, Australia: A broad perspective. *International Journal of Injury Control and Safety Promotion, 19*(2), 131–134. https://doi.org/10.1080/17457300.2011.635209

Runeson, B., Tidemalm, D., Dahlin, M., Lichtenstein, P., & Langstrom, N. (2010). Method of attempted suicide as predictor of subsequent successful suicide: National long term cohort study. *BMJ, 341*, c3222. https://doi.org/10.1136/bmj.c3222

Saad, A. M., Gad, M. M., Al-Husseini, M. J., AlKhayat, M. A., Rachid, A., Alfaar, A. S., & Hamoda, H. M. (2019). Suicidal death within a year of a cancer diagnosis: A population-based study. *Cancer, 125*(6), 972–979. https://doi.org/10.1002/cncr.31876

Sami, H., Danielle, L., Lihi, D., & Elena, S. (2018). The effect of sleep disturbances and Internet addiction on suicidal ideation among adolescents in the presence of depressive symptoms. *Psychiatry Research, 267*, 327–332.

Santos, J., Martins, S., Azevedo, L. F., & Fernandes, L. (2020). Pain as a risk factor for suicidal behavior in older adults: A systematic review. *Archives of Gerontology and Geriatrics, 87*, 104000. https://doi.org/10.1016/j.archger.2019.104000

Schilling, E. A., Aseltine, R. H., Glanovsky, J. L., James, A., & Jacobs, D. (2009). Adolescent alcohol use, suicidal ideation, and suicide attempts. *Journal of Adolescent Health, 44*(4), 335–341. https://doi.org/10.1016/j.jadohealth.2008.08.006

Smith, S. M., Edwards, R., & Duong, H. C. (2021). Unemployment rises in 2020, as the country battles the COVID-19 pandemic. Monthly Labor Review, U.S. Bureau of Labor Statistics, June 2021, https://doi.org/10.21916/mlr.2021.12

Sedgwick, R., Epstein, S., Dutta, R., & Ougrin, D. (2019). Social media, Internet use and suicide attempts in adolescents. *Current Opinion in Psychiatry, 32*(6), 534–541. https://doi.org/10.1097/YCO.0000000000000547

Sediri, S., Zgueb, Y., Ouanes, S., Ouali, U., Bourgou, S., Jomli, R., & Nacef, F. (2020). Women's mental health: Acute impact of COVID-19 pandemic on domestic violence. *Archives of Women's Mental Health, 23*(6), 749–756. https://doi.org/10.1007/s00737-020-01082-4

Serby, M. J., Brody, D., Amin, S., & Yanowitch, P. (2006). Eviction as a risk factor for suicide. *Psychiatric Services, 57*(2), 273–274. https://doi.org/10.1176/appi.ps.57.2.273-b

Shaffer, D., Gould, M., & Hicks, R. C. (1994). Worsening suicide rate in Black teenagers. *American Journal of Psychiatry, 151*(12), 1810–1812. https://doi.org/10.1176/ajp.151.12.1810

Shiratori, Y., Tachikawa, H., Nemoto, K., Endo, G., Aiba, M., Matsui, Y., & Asada, T. (2014). Network analysis for motives in suicide cases: A cross-sectional study. *Psychiatry and Clinical Neurosciences, 68*(4), 299–307. https://doi.org/10.1111/pcn.12132

Simon, T. R., Swann, A. C., Powell, K. E., Potter, L. B., Kresnow, M. J., & O'Carroll, P. W. (2002). Characteristics of impulsive suicide attempts and attempters. *Suicide and Life-Threatening Behavior, 32*(Suppl. 1), 49–59.

Singhal, A., Ross, J., Seminog, O., Hawton, K., & Goldacre, M. J. (2014). Risk of self-harm and suicide in people with specific psychiatric and physical disorders: Comparisons between disorders using English national record linkage. *Journal of the Royal Society of Medicine, 107*(5), 194–204. https://doi.org/10.1177/0141076814522033

Smith, J. C., Mercy, J. A., & Conn, J. M. (1988). Marital status and the risk of suicide. *American Journal of Public Health, 78*(1), 78–80. https://doi.org/10.2105/ajph.78.1.78

Smith, S. G., Zhang, X., Basile, K. C., Merrick, M. T., Wang, J., Kresnow, M., & Chen, J. (2018). *The national intimate partner and sexual violence survey (NISVS): 2015 data brief—Updated release.* Centers for Disease Control and Prevention. 1–32. https://www.cdc.gov/violenceprevention/pdf/2015data-brief508.pdf

Spiegel, B., Schoenfeld, P., & Naliboff, B. (2007). Systematic review: The prevalence of suicidal behaviour in patients with chronic abdominal pain and irritable bowel syndrome. *Alimentary Pharmacology & Therapeutics, 26*(2), 183–193. https://doi.org/10.1111/j.1365-2036.2007.03357.x

Stack, S., & Wasserman, I. (1993). Marital status, alcohol consumption, and suicide: An analysis of national data. *Journal of Marriage and the Family, 55*(4), 1018–1024. https://doi.org/10.2307/352781

Sublette, M. E., Carballo, J. J., Moreno, C., Galfalvy, H. C., Brent, D. A., Birmaher, B., Mann, J. J., & Oquendo, M. A. (2009). Substance use disorders and suicide attempts in bipolar subtypes. *Journal of Psychiatric Research, 43*(3), 230–238.

Sue, D., Sue, D., Sue, S., & Sue, D. (2013). *Cengage advantage books: Essentials of understanding abnormal behavior.* Wadsworth.

Takeshima, M., & Oka, T. (2013). A comprehensive analysis of features that suggest bipolarity in patients with a major depressive episode: Which is the best combination to predict soft bipolarity diagnosis? *Journal of Affective Disorders, 147*, 150–155.

Tanaka, E., Sakamoto, S., Ono, Y., Fujihara, S., & Kitamura, T. (1998). Hopelessness in a community population: Factorial structure and psychosocial correlates. *Journal of Social Psychology, 138*(5), 581–590. https://doi.org/10.1080/00224549809600413

Tanaka, T., & Okamoto, S. (2021). Increase in suicide following an initial decline during the COVID-19 pandemic in Japan. *Nature Human Behaviour, 5*(2), 229–238. https://doi.org/10.1038/s41562-020-01042-z

Tang, N. K., & Crane, C. (2006). Suicidality in chronic pain: A review of the prevalence, risk factors and psychological links. *Psychological Medicine, 36*(5), 575. https://doi.org/10.1017/s0033291705006859

Tanriverdi, D., Cuhadar, D., & Ciftci, S. (2014). Does the impairment of functional life increase the probability of suicide in cancer patients? *Asian Pacific Journal of Cancer Prevention, 15*(21), 9549–9553. https://doi.org/10.7314/apjcp.2014.15.21.9549

Terra, M. B., Figueira, I., & Barros, H. M. T. (2004). Impact of alcohol intoxication and withdrawal syndrome on social phobia and panic disorder in alcoholic inpatients. *Revista do Hospital das Clínicas, 59*(4), 187–192.

Thompson, A. H., Dewa, C. S., & Phare, S. (2012). The suicidal process: Age of onset and severity of suicidal behavior. *Social Psychiatry and Psychiatry Epidemiology, 47*(8), 1263–1269. https://doi.org/10.1007/s00127-011-0434-0

U.S. Food and Drug Administration. (2007). *FDA proposes new warnings about suicidal thinking, behavior in young adults who take antidepressant medications* [Press release]. http://www.fda.gov/NewsEvents/Newsroom/PressAnnouncements/2007/ucm108905.htm

Valtonen, H. M., Suominen, J., Sokero, P., Mantere, O., Arvilommi, P., Leppämäki, S., & Isomesta, E. T. (2009). How suicidal bipolar patients are depends on how suicidal ideation is defined. *Journal of Affective Disorders, 118*(1-3), 48–54. https://doi.org/10.1016/j.jad.2009.02.008

Van Geel, M., Vedder, P., & Tanilon, J. (2014). Relationship between peer victimization, cyberbullying, and suicide in children and adolescents. *JAMA Pediatrics, 168*(5), 435. https://doi.org/10.1001/jamapediatrics.2013.4143

Viguera, A. C., Baldessarini, R. J., Hegarty, J. D., van Kammen, D. P., & Tohen, M. (1997). Clinical risk following abrupt and gradual withdrawal of maintenance neuroleptic treatment. *Archives of General Psychiatry, 54*(1), 49–55.

Voshaar, R. C. O., Couvée, J. E., Van Balkom, A. J., Mulder, P. G., & Zitman, F. G. (2006). Strategies for discontinuing long-term benzodiazepine use. *British Journal of Psychiatry, 189*(3), 213–220.

Waldrop, A. E., Hanson, R. F., Resnick, H. S., Kilpatrick, D. G., Naugle, A. E., & Saunders, B. E. (2007). Risk factors for suicidal behaviors among a national sample of adolescents: Implications for prevention. *Journal of Traumatic Stress, 20*(5), 869–879. https://doi.org/10.1002/jts.20291

Walsh, S. L., Stoops, W. W., Moody, D. E., Lin, S. N., & Bigelow, G. E. (2009). Repeated dosing with oral cocaine in humans: Assessment of direct effects, withdrawal, and pharmacokinetics. *Experimental and Clinical Psychopharmacology, 17*(4), 205–216. https://doi.org/10.1037/a0016469

Warner, C. H., Bobo, W., Warner, C., Reid, S., & Rachal, J. (2006). Antidepressant discontinuation syndrome. *American Family Physician, 74*(3), 449–456.

Wasserman, M. (1992). The impact of epidemic, war, prohibition, and media on suicide: United States, 1910-1920. *Suicide and Life-Threatening Behavior, 22*(2), 240–254.

Weinstein, E., Kleiman, E. M., Franz, P. J., Joyce, V. W., Nash, C. C., Buonopane, R. J., & Nock M. K. (2021). Positive and negative uses of social media among adolescents hospitalized for suicidal behavior. *Journal of Adolescence, 87*, 63–73. https://doi.org/10.1016/j.adolescence.2020.12.003

Wojnar, M., Ilgen, M. A., Jakubczyk, A., Wnorowska, A., Klimkiewicz, A., & Brower, K. J. (2008). Impulsive suicide attempts predict post-treatment relapse in alcohol-dependent patients. *Drug and Alcohol Dependence, 97*(3), 268–275.

Wu, T., Jia, X., Shi, H., Niu, J., Yin, X., Xie, J., & Wang, X. (2021). Prevalence of mental health problems during the COVID-19 pandemic: A systematic review and meta-analysis. *Journal of Affective Disorders, 281*, 91–98. https://doi.org/10.1016/j.jad.2020.11.117

Wyder, M., Ward, P., & De Leo, D. (2009). Separation as a suicide risk factor. *Journal of Affective Disorders, 116*(3), 208–213. https://doi.org/10.1016/j.jad.2008.11.007

Yamaguchi, T., Fujii, C., Nemoto, T., Tsujino, N., Takeshi, K., & Mizuno, M. (2015). Differences between subjective experiences and observed behaviors in near-fatal suicide attempters with untreated schizophrenia: A qualitative pilot study. *Annals of General Psychiatry, 14*(17), 1–8. https://doi.org/10.1186/s12991-015-0055-1x

Yaseen, Z. S., Chartrand, H., Mojtabai, R., Bolton, J., & Galynker, I. I. (2013). Fear of dying in panic attacks predicts suicide attempt in comorbid depressive illness: Prospective evidence from the National Epidemiological Survey on Alcohol and Related Conditions. *Depression and Anxiety, 30*(10), 930–939. https://doi.org/10.1002/da.22039

Yaseen, Z. S., Kopeykina, I., Gutkovich, Z., Bassirnia, A., Cohen, L. J., & Galynker, I. I. (2014). Predictive validity of the Suicide Trigger Scale (STS-3) for post-discharge suicide attempt in high-risk psychiatric inpatients. *PLOS One, 9*(1), e86768. https://doi.org/10.1371/journal.pone.0086768

Zayas, L. H., Bright, C. L., Álvarez-Sánchez, T., & Cabassa, L. J. (2009). Acculturation, familism and mother–daughter relations among suicidal and non-suicidal adolescent Latinas. *Journal of Primary Prevention, 30*(3-4), 351–369. https://doi.org/10.1007/s10935-009-0181-0

Zhang, J., & Ma, Z. (2012). Patterns of life events preceding the suicide in rural young Chinese: A case-control study. *Journal of Affective Disorders, 140*(2), 161–167. https://doi.org/10.1016/j.jad.2012.01.010

Zisook, S., Trivedi, M. H., Warden, D., Lebowitz, B., Thase, M. E., Stewart, J. W., Moutier, C, Fava, M., Wisniewski, S. S., Luther, J., & Rush, A. J. (2009). Clinical correlates of the worsening or emergence of suicidal ideation during SSRI treatment of depression: An examination of citalopram in the STAR*D study. *Journal of Affective Disorders, 117*(1), 63–73.

6

Suicidal Narrative

The Seven Stages of the Suicidal Narrative

Suicide may be conceptualized as the ultimate state of alienation from the world when all connections to everything a person loves in it—people, achievements, aspirations, or possessions—become irreversibly lost in one final action. This level of alienation is perceived by a suicidal person as a literal "end" from which there is no way out. Patients describe it variously as running out of options, having no good solutions, being in a tunnel with no light ahead, being backed into a corner, or being stuck in a dark department store after hours.

According to the narrative-crisis model (NCM) proposed in this book, people with long-term risk factors for suicidal behavior develop a fatalistic perception of their future. When stressors accumulate, these individuals increasingly see their lives as moving toward "a dead end" with no possibility of an acceptable or livable outcome. This perception of having no future and no power to affect change is unbearable and gives rise to the suicide crisis syndrome (SCS). Establishing the extent to which the suicidal person's state of mind corresponds to this process is critical to the assessment of imminent suicide risk, as well as to the development of corresponding interventions. To underscore the storylike process that characterizes the mind's progression toward the SCS as well as the narrative quality of a person's perception of their life, we've termed it the *suicidal narrative* (SN).

As mentioned in Chapter 3, as a theoretical construct, the SN echoes the concept of life narrative from a psychological theory of narrative identity (McAdams et al., 2001). Currently, the similarities between the SN and the narrative identity are semantic and conceptual. Because both are new, this hypothetical relationship has not been tested experimentally and warrants future studies.

According to McAdams et al. (2001), narrative identity is a person's internalized and evolving life story, integrating the reconstructed past, the present, and the imagined future to provide life with some degree of unity and purpose. Research into the relationship between life narratives and psychological adaptation shows that narrators who find redemptive meanings in suffering and adversity, and who construct life stories that feature themes of personal agency and exploration, tend to enjoy higher levels of mental health, well-being, and maturity (McLean et al., 2007; Pals, 2006). Conversely, those who cannot find positive meaning in adverse experiences and for whom the future becomes unimaginable may find themselves entrapped with no alternate solutions, placing them at increased suicide risk. This is a testable hypothesis, and future research will need to examine the relationship between narrative identity, the construct of SN, and suicidal ideation and behavior.

The content and structure of the SN are based on information gleaned from research studies on static risk factors underlying the second-generation *suicide risk models*, which have revealed pervasive themes in how acutely suicidal individuals perceive the evolution of their suicidality in response to stressful life events. Very common among these themes are perfectionism (O'Connor, 2007), setting up unrealistic life goals (O'Connor et al., 2015), failure to meet these unattainable life goals (Zhang & Lester, 2008), failure to redirect to more realistic goals (O'Connor, 2007), humiliating personal or social defeats (Siddaway et al., 2015), perception of being a burden to others (Joiner et al., 2002), and alienation (Joiner et al., 2005).

As introduced in Chapter 3, the SN component of the NCM organizes these themes into seven stages that follow a coherent life story of progressive failure and alienation, leading to a dead end when the future becomes impossible:

- Stage 1: Unrealistic life goals
- Stage 2: Entitlement to happiness
- Stage 3: Failure to redirect to more realistic goals
- Stage 4: Humiliating personal or social defeat
- Stage 5: Perceived burdensomeness
- Stage 6: Thwarted belongingness
- Stage 7: Perception of no future

Although the body of experimental evidence linking the individual themes of the SN to suicide is substantial (Cohen et al., 2019; Chistopolskaya et al., 2020; Menon et al., 2022) to date there are few data on how their exact sequences overlap and evolve over time to interact and form causal pathways, making suicide possible. Moreover, the available data are conflicting. Some reports suggest that defeat and entrapment are distinct constructs, each associated with increased risk for suicidal ideation and behavior, whereas one study suggests that defeat and entrapment are closely related and form a single construct (Taylor et al., 2009). In addition, there are no data to explain whether someone who has a tendency to set unrealistic life goals and has also suffered a humiliating career setback is at higher risk for suicide than someone who has had a similar career setback but does not have such tendencies.

The individual stressors that induce these themes and contribute to the formation of the SN may differ between individuals. As discussed later, some of these stressors, such as not being invited to a party, receiving a B on a college exam, or being scolded by a parent, may appear insignificant or even trivial to an outsider. Other stressors, such as overwhelming financial loss, death of a spouse, or divorce, are significant and tragic by any standard. Still, the vast majority of people eventually overcome even catastrophic losses, viewing them as an inevitable part of life. Although one can hypothesize that people with trait vulnerability for suicide are more likely than others to become suicidal when facing relatively trivial life stressors, little is known about what exactly in the interaction of stressful life events and trait vulnerabilities leads to suicide.

In contrast to the dearth of research addressing the hypothetical relationship between the SN and narrative identity, several recent reports examined whether a perception of one's life as a sequence of the suicide narrative stages increases one's risk of developing the suicidal crisis syndrome and of dying by suicide in the near future. One of the aims of these studies was to design a clinical scale to evaluate the intensity of the SN and its relationship to suicide risk.

In the first of these studies, Cohen et al. (2019) first investigated, the previously hypothetical construct of the SN, and its relationship with near-term suicidal risk and SCS, through the newly developed instrument, the Suicide Narrative Inventory (SNI), which combined the previously documented risk factors of thwarted belongingness, perceived burdensomeness, humiliation, social defeat, goal disengagement, and goal reengagement. In this cross-sectional study, factor analysis of the SNI yielded two factors, termed interpersonal (comprising perceived burdensomeness, social defeat, humiliation, and thwarted belongingness) and goal orientation (comprising goal disengagement and goal reengagement, and to a lesser extent, humiliation). While the interpersonal factor correlated with both SCS severity and suicidal phenomena, the goal orientation factor correlated with no other variable. Thus, their findings supported the SN as a viable construct, distinct from SCS and related to suicidal behaviors, while suggesting that the Interpersonal factor would have a stringed association with SCS compared to the goal-orientation factor.

In the subsequent prospective study, Bloch-Elkouby et al. (2020) investigated the SN within the NCM framework as a whole. The researchers used structural equation modeling to examine the main underlying hypothesis of the NCM, that individuals with long-term risk factors for suicide may develop distorted perceptions of themselves and society, which culminate in a sense of no future and make them more likely to experience SCS. Since the data was collected at three time points, that is, at admission to the inpatient unit, at discharge, and at post-discharge follow-up, it was possible to illustrate the temporal sequence of the NCM. The results of the study supported the model as a whole, including its temporal progression from long-term risk factors to SN, to SCS, to SA. The researchers found that each temporal stage of the model was significantly predicted by the precedent stage and there is progression from trait vulnerabilities to suicidal outcomes, as proposed by the NCM, with a strong effect size for the model of this complexity.

Similar to Cohen et al. (2019), this study also found a significant correlation between the interpersonal factor (and not goal orientation) of NCM and the SCS.

In contrast, however, recent data from Pia et al. (2020) suggest that goal orientation may connect to SCS and subsequent suicidal outcomes through mediation of ruminative flooding. Figure 6.1 further illustrates these associations.

Underscoring the importance of the SN in suicide risk assessment, recently, in 2021, Ying et al. found that only the SNI scores and perceived burdensomeness subscale scores were significantly associated with clinician therapist response scores, and that a higher SNI score was significantly related to higher distress and lower affiliation scores among clinicians. They therefore concluded that clinicians appear to respond emotionally to their patients' SN and future investigations of such narratives and potential to improve imminent suicide risk is therefore warranted.

Several further studies have investigated the SNI in international samples. In the Russian sample, confirmatory factor analysis (CFA) was used to test the fit of the hypothesized seven-factor structure of the SNI in the population, including thwarted belongingness, perceived burdensomeness, fear of humiliation, defeat, goal reengagement, goal disengagement, entrapment

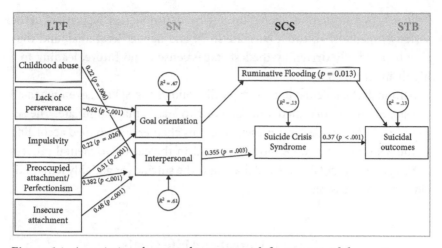

Figure 6.1 Associations between long-term risk factors, suicidal narrative, suicide crisis syndrome, and suicidal outcomes.

(Chistopolskaya et al., 2020; Menon et al., 2022). These analyses also included the long-term risk factor of perfectionism, which separated into an eighth factor. In the Russian sample, CFA indicated good model fit, though construct validity indicated further work was needed for Goal Redirection (Stage 3), potentially due to the personal style and strategies of the suicidal person. Additionally, the more established subscales of Thwarted Belongingness, Perceived Burdensomeness, Defeat, and Fear of Humiliation were found useful for SN studies, while the new domains of goal adjustment and perception of no future may require more elaborate questionnaires. Similar to the Russian sample, the study conducted in India, also indicated good model fit for the seven-factor SNI structure with the majority of factors correlated with one-another. In this study, perceived burdensomeness, fear of humiliation, defeat, and entrapment were positively correlated with stressful life events, perceived stress, suicidal ideation and lifetime suicide attempt. Both these studies have supported the SN.

Although all SNs share a common last stage, the perception of no future, the relative importance of the other stages varies among people. Many SNs are dominated by unrealistic expectations of success, either in work or in personal life, and they are driven by unfulfilled narcissism. Many college student suicides, failed business-related suicides, and some suicides related to romantic rejection fall into this category. Life goals of those who killed themselves due to relentless bullying may be quite realistic, and their SN is driven primarily by humiliation, alienation, and burdensomeness. Narratives of the seriously mentally ill could be quite short and appear irrational, and they may be primarily driven by the last stage's sense of no future, leading to a highly intense SCS.

Although the suicidal process typically follows the SN arc, even when all the stages can be identified, only one or two stages may dominate. The series of real-life suicide cases presented in this chapter are grouped according to the SN stages that were most dominant in the causative mental process leading to the suicidal crisis and that made the suicide (or a highly lethal suicide attempt) possible.

Stage 1: Unrealistic Life Goals

Life is a pursuit of happiness, but happiness is often achieved by pursuing goals. Some life goals are unique and individualistic, but many are shared by a vast majority of people in most cultures. Most of us set life goals to be employed and independent, to create and maintain a happy home, to have a family, or to acquire material possessions ranging from smartphones to automobiles and homes. Very few of us, however, fulfill all our hopes, and those who do so, quickly expand their horizons to goals that were previously unimaginable. The most common goals are tangible and related to achievements and relationships; other less quantifiable goals pertain to emotions such as happiness, contentment, curiosity, or agency.

The first stage of the SN, setting up unrealistic life goals, originates in trait perfectionism. Individuals with trait perfectionism tend to set lofty life goals, particularly if they carry a belief that others hold unrealistically high expectations of their behaviors and will only be satisfied if these expectations are met (socially prescribed perfectionism or social perfectionism). As mentioned in Chapter 4 on trait vulnerability to suicidal behaviors, cross-sectional and population studies in the past have supported the association of social perfectionism with both suicidal ideation and behavior (O'Connor & Forgan, 2007; Smith et al., 2017). Additionally, perfectionism has also been strongly correlated with suicidal behavior in qualitative studies within clinical and community samples (Katzenmajer-Pump & Balázs, 2021). Such associations tend to have a less significant effect on suicidal thoughts than the interpersonal factors of the SN. Recently, Pia et al. (2020) found that although the direct effect of trait perfectionism (see Chapter 4) on suicidal thoughts and behavior was not significant, the indirect effect, through mediation of fear of humiliation (Stage 4) and the SCS, was significant.

Perfectionism is a powerful motivating trait that can be easily assessed during an interview, often by the direct question, "Do you think or do others think that you are a perfectionist?" with a proper follow-up. Setting up life goals appropriate to one's strengths, weaknesses, and available resources is an exceedingly complicated task. Assessing the suicidal patient's life goals in relation to his or her talents, flaws, personality features, and social aspects of the person's background will give an astute clinician invaluable clinical material for understanding the first stage of the SN and its assembly. Life goals taken for granted by an individual can be perceived as realistic by someone else and completely unachievable for others. As a simple example, the goals of having a family, owning a home, and having an income at the level of national average would be taken for granted by a young person from a middle-class background with traits of social perfectionism, and they would be a realistic goal for the child of a first-generation immigrant, while they would be unreachable for a high-school dropout with a drug problem and an impoverished family.

Although unrealistic life goals often relate to money and status, they are invariably symbolic of larger social expectations of behavior, such as the social roles of providers, parents, children, leaders, or community members. For example, over 250,000 Indian farmers killed themselves over 16 years after droughts because they failed to deliver on the microloans they had received (Bhise & Behere, 2016; Kannuri & Jadhav, 2021).

The following two cases exemplify how unrealistic life goals contributed to the SN of failure, leading to the dead end of the acute suicidal crisis.

Case 24

Kimiko was a 21-year-old Japanese woman who was brought up in Japan as the only daughter in a wealthy family who owned a financial business. She was a bright girl, and her parents had shown off her talents to their friends since her early childhood. Kimiko was raised with the expectation that she would attend a prestigious university and succeed her father as head of the family business. She was privately tutored and had little free time, and thus she had very few friends. As a teenager, she attended a private school in Massachusetts where she was the only Asian student. She did not get along with her classmates but was by far the best student in her grade and quickly became her teachers' favorite.

Kimiko was a hard worker and was meticulous in her assignments. She had developed very close relationships with her teachers, who all told her, as did her parents, that she had unlimited potential and a spectacular future. This made Kimiko feel proud and special. However, she continued to have very few friends and spent most of her time reading and dreaming about joining her father's company at age 21 as a highly paid executive. In the last year of high school, she started having panic attacks, which were treated with a selective serotonin reuptake inhibitor (SSRI) and an "as needed" benzodiazepine.

Kimiko graduated first in her class and was accepted at Princeton University. There, she had very few friends and again tried to distinguish herself with professors. Princeton was a large school, however, and her professors were busy. Kimiko felt lost and insignificant. Her grades were good but so were those of other students, and people no longer lauded her "unlimited potential." She got B pluses and A minuses on her midterms, which made her feel embarrassed. She could not bring herself to reveal her grades to her parents. She felt trapped and, not knowing how to face her parents, took all the prescription medications prescribed for her panic disorder. After the overdose, she got scared and went to the emergency department, where she was treated; she survived.

Kimiko's SN arc is a story of unrealistic expectations set for her by her parents, her single-minded pursuit of goals at the expense of age-appropriate social and emotional development, and her abrupt and catastrophic humiliating personal defeat after getting Bs in college, all of which led to her perception that her life narrative was heading for a dead end. In her case, the dead end was "I will not be the CEO of my father's company."

Her narrative was dominated by an unrealistic life goal set up for her by her parents. Becoming a company CEO by merit is a setup for failure, even if one's father is the owner.

Kimiko's parents fueled her single-minded drive for a success so narrow that her failure was inevitable. Kimiko's Millon Clinical Multiaxial Inventory personality testing scores were high on narcissistic, dependent, avoidant, and schizotypal traits, as well as on anxiety and depression. At the time of her suicide attempt, she was convinced that she had failed her family, that she was unworthy of her parents, and that she was not smart enough to ever achieve what was rightly expected of her. After Kimiko was released from the hospital, she was treated with an SSRI for her depression and anxiety, as well as with an intensive crisis intervention in individual and family psychotherapy, which helped Kimiko accept alternative measures of success.

Case 25

Stella was a 33-year-old woman who overdosed on Tylenol the day before her planned move into an independent living facility after 10 years in a psychiatric residence. Stella grew up in a middle-class family as a shy and reclusive girl with very few friends, but she studied hard and was a B student. She had one brother with attention deficit hyperactivity disorder and a sister with a drug abuse problem who had dropped out of high school. Her father killed himself when Stella was 10 years old, and since his death, her mother relied heavily on Stella for emotional support and for housework help, to the extent that Stella assumed a parent role with her mother (paternalized child). Her mother was unaware of the parental burden she was placing on Stella; Stella was always simply "the good kid."

However, in the last year of high school, Stella's grades started dropping. She could not concentrate and started having fears that classmates were laughing at her behind her back for being awkward and overweight. She stopped going to school, stopped eating, her hygiene worsened, and finally she locked herself in her bedroom and refused to leave because she said the TV started sending her coded threatening messages. Stella was hospitalized in an inpatient psychiatric unit and was diagnosed with schizophrenia. She was treated with neuroleptics and had several more hospitalizations before she was stabilized on clozaril and placed in a psychiatric residence, where she lived until her eventual suicide.

The residence staff members liked Stella and, just like her mother, called her "a good kid." Over time, she became a "star patient" who attended all the group meetings and activities, knew the residence rules better than some of the staff, and even helped the staff members with taking care of sicker patients, assuming the same role she had in her own family. Her treatment goals included job training and eventual transition to independent living. However, several times throughout the years as she approached transition, she required hospitalization for acute psychosis.

After a staff change, Stella's new psychiatrist decided that she was too high functioning for the residence, and as Stella was being prepared for discharge and a transition to independent living, the psychiatrist added a first-generation antipsychotic. To everybody's surprise and relief, Stella did not become psychotic, and Stella's discharge was scheduled for a Monday. On Friday, the residence held a goodbye party for Stella. At the party, she seemed upbeat and cheerful, and she thanked everybody for all they had done for her.

Stella overdosed on two bottles of Tylenol on Friday evening. She wrote a suicide note explaining that she was killing herself because she knew she would get sick again and would let everybody down. After taking the Tylenol, she got scared of what staff would think when they found her dead and told a health aide about her overdose. She was taken to a local hospital and was placed in the intensive care unit. She told the visiting residence staff that she was happy not to have died so that she could have another chance at transitioning to a residence. However, the next day she died of liver failure.

The first stage of Stella's SN was written when she assumed the role of caretaker for her mother. Stella had a family history of serious mental illness and also suffered childhood trauma from her father's suicide, which increased her trait risk for suicide and for developing a major Axis I disorder. After her father's death, when Stella assumed a caretaker role for her mother, she also internalized her mother's unrealistic expectations of her as a perfect caretaker. The stress of these expectations most likely contributed to her developing schizoaffective disorder. During her 10 years in residence, Stella stepped into the role of perfect caretaker and was fulfilled by it. Graduation to independent living was a setup for certain failure; she would have nobody to take care of, she was destined to lose her sense of belongingness to the residence, and she felt like a burden to the new doctor. Even her opportunity of escape into psychosis was taken from her by the addition of the second antipsychotic.

Consequently, Stella's life fell into the SN of an unfulfillable expectation of being a perfect caretaker, followed by a 10-year experience of acting like one in a psychiatric setting, and ending in suicide due to fear of humiliation and the expected defeat of letting down her substitute family, in addition to losing her connection with them. This fear was the dead end that led to the suicide crisis and suicide.

Two additional points in Stella's case are worth noting. First, unlike Kimiko's life goals, which had a concrete performance aspect and could be measured in grades, Stella's goals were entirely emotional. Concrete performance-oriented SNs like Kimiko's are easier to detect and monitor clinically. Purely emotional life aims are much more difficult to identify, track, and monitor.

Second, although losing a supportive structure could be catastrophic for seriously mentally ill and psychotic patients like Stella, patients may lack the cognitive skills to communicate their distress and fears appropriately. Such cases are further complicated by alexithymia, which prevents patients like Stella from recognizing their own emotional distress. As a result, the danger of such transitions may be underestimated by staff, who have limited resources and are typically under pressure to discharge patients who are doing well. Many suicides of seriously mentally ill patients at the time of a reduction in level of care fall into this category.

Stage 2: Entitlement to Happiness

Suicide is an irreversible act that ends a person's life and, with it, puts an end to all expectations that a person may have had for the future. Everyone has expectations for the future that start developing early in childhood. As a person grows older, expectations are encouraged and often actively cultivated by parents and other parental figures—grandparents, teachers, college professors, and mentors. Life partners, friends, and acquaintances also actively support our expectations. Finally, society, industry, and the media bombard us with messages of success and happiness, creating the expectation that once we succeed in our goals, happiness and fulfillment will follow. Often, however, our expectations are not met, and we are left to come to terms with reality. This is particularly true for individuals who are brought up with unrealistic expectations of success that are not commensurate with their talents and who lack the resilience and the psychological tools needed to cope with life's disappointments.

Psychological entitlement is a personality trait characterized by pervasive feelings of deservingness, specialness, and exaggerated expectations, characteristics that contribute to having unrealistic life goals and subject the individual to a continual vulnerability to unmet expectations. Moreover, entitled individuals are likely to interpret unmet expectations in ways that foster disappointment, ego threat, and a sense of perceived injustice, all of which may lead to indicators of psychological distress, such as dissatisfaction across multiple life domains, anger, and generally volatile emotional responses. Furthermore, in the wake of disappointment, ego threat, or perceived injustice, entitled individuals are likely to attempt to bolster their entitled self-concept, leading to a reinforcement of entitled beliefs and failure to redirect

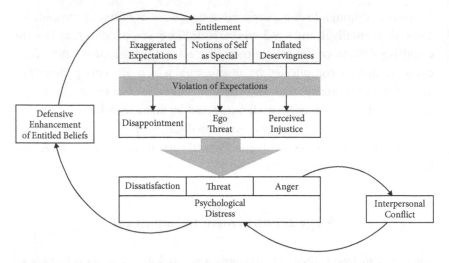

Figure 6.2 Proposed model illustrating the various pathways by which entitlement might lead to psychological distress (Grubbs & Exline, 2016).

to more realistic and less inflated life goals (Stage 3), thereby initiating the cycle again, with each cycle being more unrealistic than the preceding one. At each stage of this process, entitlement presents the individual with the possibility of experiencing distress, predisposes the person to further risk factors for distress (e.g., the subsequent steps in the model), and increases the risk of interpersonal conflict, again leading to distress, which may include fear of humiliation and crushing personal defeat (Stage 4). Figure 6.2, from Grubbs and Exline (2016), demonstrates these relationships.

Although psychological entitlement is a trait and thus constitutes a long-term risk factor for suicide, the recurrent and self-reinforcing cognitive constructs in the wake of inevitable disappointments to bolster entitled self-concept represent the "entitlement to happiness" stage of the SN. This stage is a cognitive and subacute state, which may wax and wane, often in concert with other individual stages of the SN, or SN as a whole, depending on how threatening the current perceived failures are to the individual's life narrative.

Recent research suggests that the origins of today's youths' sense of entitlement may lie in their inflated self-esteem as children. Moreover, some have argued that entitlement, along with other narcissistic attitudes, such as vanity, exploitativeness, and manipulativeness, have increased as a result of a recent emphasis on increasing adolescents' level of self-esteem (Twenge, 2006). Indeed, self-esteem has risen substantially over the last 40 years, and

Twenge and Campbell (2001) found that the average student in the mid-1990s had a higher self-esteem score than 73% of their late 1960s peers. The self-esteem "movement," an effort designed to protect adolescents' sense of self-worth from parents' and teachers' harsh criticism and negative appraisals, began in the 1970s and became more prevalent during the 1980s and 1990s. Twenge et al. (2008) and Twenge (2006) contended that this movement was largely responsible for the observed increases in self-esteem over time, but it has had the unanticipated side-effect of artificially inflating adolescents' feelings of self-worth, independent of their actual abilities and accomplishments (Crocker & Knight, 2005). The result, they argued, has led to an increase in attitudes like entitlement. By the late 1980s, for example, 80% of adolescents, compared to only 12% in the 1950s, agreed that they were an important person (Newsom et al., 2003), and in the early 2000s there was an increased expectation of success and higher-level goal attainment among adolescents (Reynolds et al., 2006; Twenge, 2006). Additionally, 63% of high school graduates were expected to be working in a professional job by age 30, compared to only 18% of 30-year-olds who actually held such positions (Reynolds et al., 2006). Twenge and Campbell (2001) found a modest association between the Psychological Entitlement Scale and the Rosenberg Self-Esteem Scale (RSE), in addition to a strong association between self-esteem and narcissism. In another study, adolescents agreed with 24% of the entitlement subscale items of the Narcissitic Personality Inventory (NPI) (Moeller et al., 2009). While both the clinical and research evidence is strong for the association between self-esteem and entitlement, there are some reports that indicate the contrary (Bogart et al., 2004; Strelan, 2007), so the connection between the two concepts needs to be tested further experimentally.

Hopelessness has been identified as one of the strongest predictors of suicide (Beck et al., 1975; Fawcett et al., 1990). However, hopelessness is only predictive of suicide in the long term, over a period of 10 to 20 years, and is not a predictor of imminent suicide (Simon, 2006), or even of a suicide within 12 months after the assessment. One possible reason is that although hopelessness is often experienced acutely in the present, and is thus viewed as a state condition, it is largely a temperament and a trait (Mann et al., 1999). Moreover, hopelessness and pessimism are also cultural phenomena and may carry adaptive advantages in some cultures (e.g., Russia) but be maladaptive in others (e.g., the United States; Kassinove & Sukhodolsky, 1995). Thus, hopelessness may not necessarily be related to short-term risk for suicide.

The ability or inability to think positively about the future is a state rather than a trait phenomenon, which may be more directly related to short-term suicide risk. Positive future thinking is defined as anticipation of positive experiences in the future, and it can be assessed experimentally via the future thinking task (MacLeod et al., 1997), during which participants are asked to generate as many future events or experiences as possible that they are looking forward to. Most of these questions can also be asked during a clinical interview. Future positive experiences are divided into the following categories (O'Connor et al., 2015):

- Social/interpersonal expectancies involve at least one other person (e.g., marriage).
- Financial and home expectations refer to any aspect of financial or material gain or home improvement (e.g., making money, saving, buying a car, and decorating the house).
- Achievement relates to the anticipation of an accomplishment (not including earning money), such as an accomplishment at work, a promotion, or fame.
- Leisure/pleasure refers to fun or pleasure (e.g., vacation).
- Health of others describes expectations of health for friends and family.
- Intrapersonal positive thinking involves the individual and nobody else.
- The last category, "other," is applied to expectations not classified elsewhere.

Although all of these categories are related to suicide risk and are often intercorrelated (e.g., those who expect to achieve in one category tend to also expect an achievement in others), the primary expectation most directly connected with the risk of suicidal ideation/suicide attempt in the next several months is intrapersonal thinking (i.e., expectation of happiness). Thus, short-term suicide risk seems to be intimately connected to a patient's failure to achieve their fulfilling inner state, such as a state of exhilaration or that of inner calm and peace.

The relationship between expectations of happiness and suicide risk is not straightforward. Some reports suggest that low levels of positive future thinking are associated with suicidality, and this association is independent of depression and some other possible confounds (O'Connor et al., 2000). In other words, high levels of intrapersonal positive future thinking appear to be protective from suicide. This finding is intuitive and could also be clinically important because creating positive future thinking would provide intuitive and easily understood treatment targets for clinicians. In a short-term suicide risk study, Morrison and O'Connor (2008) found that low levels of positive future thinking were better predictors of suicidal ideation (there were no data on attempts) than global hopelessness two or three months after a suicide attempt.

On the other hand, a 15-month study showed the opposite finding (O'Connor et al., 2015), and the likelihood of a repeat suicide attempt was elevated among those who reported more intrapersonal positive future thinking at baseline. These findings are crucial because they show that high levels of positive future thinking are not always protective. On the face of it, this may seem counterintuitive, given the generally accepted view that high levels of positive thinking buffer against distress in the face of life stressors (O'Connor et al., 2004). However, if a person's expectation of future happiness is so high that it is unrealistic, this positive future thinking becomes an unreachable life goal of the kind described in the previous section.

A good way to probe the entitlement to happiness is to ask if the patient expects to be happy in life and how much unhappiness is reasonable to expect and tolerate. If the answer to "How are you feeling today?" is "I have never felt this bad in my life," it should bring on a probing "Did you think that you should be feeling happier than you are now?" or "How did you expect to feel at this point in your life?" The answer "I thought if I do all that is asked of me, I would be happy" should serve as a red flag that the person being interviewed felt entitled to happiness that is now starting to slip out of reach.

Entitlement to happiness appears to be a prominent stage in SNs among young people, or "millennials," who have come of age in the first two decades of the third millennium. In the United States, Japan, and the countries of the European Union, many millennials continued their education and remained dependent on their parents well into their young adult years. This historically new social behavior created a whole generation of highly educated young people entering an oversaturated job market with few jobs available requiring a high level of education, thus frustrating their future expectancies of success and happiness (Knowlton & Hagopian, 2013) and creating fertile ground for SNs based on thwarted entitlement to happiness.

A new life stage, emergent adulthood, was defined to describe young people 18 to 25 years old who, although adult in biological age, continue to live lives of adolescents. The term *moratorium* was coined to describe the decade between ages 20 and 30 years when millennials typically postpone making both career and personal commitments, taking time to enjoy themselves and to find occupations that will bring them future happiness (Knowlton & Hagopian, 2013). At the end of the moratorium, some the 30-year-olds do not have the emotional maturity needed to make age-appropriate decisions necessary for full financial independence. This often requires accepting jobs they believe they are overqualified for with salaries well below those they believe they are entitled to, given their level of education. Many millennials believe that they have been cheated out of the bright future promised to them by society and by their parents. This generational conflict is a frequent stressor, which often precipitates the suicidal crisis.

Following are case examples of the early stages of the SN anchored in unrealistic positive future expectancies and in the entitlement to happiness.

Case 26

Angelia, a 27-year-old woman with a history of heroin and cocaine use disorder and an externalizing personality disorder, nearly died of a heroin overdose after her mother told her she was cutting off her financial support. Angelia's mother was a writer and an untreated alcoholic who drank daily and had frequent blackouts. When she was pregnant with Angelia, she divorced Angelia's father to marry a well-known artist 30 years her senior, who was also an alcoholic. Angelia's mother and stepfather fought frequently, and they split occasionally for short periods of time. Her mother's parenting style was unpredictable, alternating between hands-off and smothering and overbearing. Angelia dealt with her mother's erratic parenting and lack of boundaries primarily by trying to avoid her and by lying when necessary.

Having only episodic parental oversight, Angelia started using drugs in ninth grade but was able to hide it from her mother until her mid-20s, when she started using her mother's credit cards to support her heroin habit. Despite her drug use, Angelia was a good student, showed some promise as a writer, and was accepted into a good private university, where she was an English major. Her college grades, however, were mediocre. When her parents suggested during her junior year that she should consider an alternative career, Angelia flatly said that only writing could make her happy and that if her mother would not help her pursue her passion, she would never speak to her again. Angelia's mother continued her financial support.

Because of Angelia's heroin and cocaine addiction, it took her six years to complete college. During this time, she was supported primarily by her parents, but she also made some money by tutoring and occasional freelance writing. During these years, she became dependent on prescription opiates and Adderall. Her drugs were prescribed by several doctors, but because none was illegal, she was able to keep her parents in the dark about the extent of her drug misuse for several years. However, after she developed a stimulant-induced psychotic episode and was hospitalized, her parents finally appreciated the severity of the problem. Angelia's addiction treatment was not successful. She skillfully used confidentiality and HIPAA laws to manipulate her parents into continuing to support her drug habit and her so-called writing career. She was hospitalized three times for low-lethality suicide attempts. After her mother canceled all her credit cards, Angelia made a high-lethality attempt with the intent to die.

Angelia was not a perfectionist. Her modest life goals consisted of becoming an intellectual like her parents and stepfather. She grew up expecting a bright and happy future. However, like some millennials, she felt entitled and expected her good fortune to arrive without much effort. Her SN was anchored in her entitlement to happiness. Her family supported her entitlement because they set high goals for Angelia; in a way, the first stage of her narrative was written by proxy (as is often the case with helicopter parenting).

With substance abuse history on her mother's side of the family, Angelia discovered early on that using drugs was the easiest way to relieve her dysphoria and maintain the illusion of a happy future. The later stages of her SN were related to her drug use, but it was the entitlement to happiness that laid the foundation of her future setbacks, alienation, and eventual suicide attempt.

Case 27

David was a 29-year-old man who died by hanging after his parents refused to fund his cannabis-growing enterprise following the legalization of marijuana in Colorado. David grew up in New Jersey, one of two children in a middle-class family. His family had no significant psychiatric history, his parents were happily married, and he had a happy childhood. On the surface, he was a well-adjusted student who was able to get As and Bs effortlessly.

He was a recreational marijuana user, smoking weed weekly with his many friends.

David went to college without an idea for a major. He expected that he would get As and Bs without studying, but the courses were difficult, and he flunked his midterms. He was embarrassed to tell his parents the truth, so he told them that everything was fine. In reality, he stopped going to classes and spent all day in his dorm smoking weed and binge-watching TV. When his parents found out, they suggested that David take a semester off. David searched for a job but could not find anything he liked. Instead of working, he stayed at home and tried to become a professional poker player. He was initially successful but soon quit, saying that the game involved luck and no skill.

It took David six years to graduate from college. He changed majors several times and ended up majoring in English. His parents paid his tuition and living expenses. David had several short-lived part-time jobs, which he lost due to his inability to handle feedback. After graduation, he got a job as an assistant at a start-up company but was let go after three months. He moved back in with his parents and lived there for several years rent-free. He worked occasionally, but he used his income as spending money. His parents eventually retired, sold their house, and rented a small apartment. They began living on a fixed income. For David's 30th birthday, they gave him $30,000 and told him that from that point on he would have to be independent.

David moved to Florida, where he rented an inexpensive apartment and invested most of his money in a friend's Facebook-based dating app. Eventually, the start-up folded. David's parents bailed him out "for the last time," telling him to get a job. He did so, only to be fired. When David's parents told him they could not afford to support him anymore, David threatened to kill himself. His parents gave him more money, taken from their individual retirement accounts.

David ran out of money and asked for his parents' support several more times. They would initially refuse but would cave to his threats of suicide. They consulted a psychiatrist on how to give their son financial independence and whether his suicide threats were real.

Just like Angelia, David grew up expecting a happy future but had neither the talent nor the work ethic to back his expectancies of success and happiness. The SN of his life trajectory was rooted in his entitlement to happiness. His goals were quite achievable when he was in college, but they became increasingly unrealistic as he aged. With time, his lack of age-appropriate life experiences made it increasingly difficult for him to keep up with his peers. His parents repeatedly let him know that he was burdensome to them. A quick business success remained the only viable option until, in his mind, that door was shut by his parents' refusal to support his cannabis business. In summary, David's SN had all the usual stages, but it was driven by his entitlement to happiness.

Stage 3: Failure to Redirect to More Realistic Goals

Striving for goals is a universal human experience. People work to attain goals with expectations of self-fulfillment, happiness, and other positive emotions. When goals cannot be attained, humiliation, anxiety, depression, and other negative emotions result. People's goals change throughout their life cycle. As people mature, inevitably some unattainable goals need to be discarded (Carver & Scheier, 1998). With age, the number of unattainable goals that need to be re-evaluated grows. Goal losses accumulating with age can be disheartening, but older adults have the highest life satisfaction (Stone et al., 2010), as a result of the many realistic goals they have accomplished after discarding unattainable ones (Morrison & O'Connor, 2008). If Kimiko and David had been able to appreciate that their life goals were unattainable, their life stories may not have become SNs.

When goal accomplishment is thwarted, the brain activates psychological processes of goal regulation, which differ for each individual. These processes result in response patterns used to abandon commitment to a goal that has become unachievable (Wrosch et al., 2003). From an evolutionary perspective, continuing the quest for an unachievable goal could result in exhaustion of cognitive, behavioral, or emotional resources (Gilbert, 2001; Wrosch et al., 2003). When goal attainment is unlikely, disengagement helps avoid feelings of failure (associated with suicide risk; Nesse, 2000) and allows redirection of efforts toward more realistic goals in a process called goal re-engagement (Heckhausen et al., 2010). The latter adaptive process is associated with lower suicide risk and involves the process of reducing efforts toward unachievable goals or unsuccessful activities, or it serves as a means to deal with loss or threatened attachment relationships (Wetherall et al., 2019).

Disengaging from unattainable goals is adaptive only when there are alternative meaningful goals available (O'Connor & Kirtley, 2018; Wrosch et al.,

2003). O'Connor et al. (2009) studied the relationship between goal disengagement, goal re-engagement, and suicidal ideation in a general hospital population and found that those who reported high levels of goal disengagement, but low levels of re-engagement, exhibited significantly more suicidal ideation at follow-up compared with those who reported high levels of goal re-engagement and disengagement. Availability of goals varies by age (Wrosch et al., 2003). Older populations who possess limited options (Heckhausen et al., 2010) may be forced to abandon difficult-to-attain goals without re-engagement with new goals. Disengagement without re-engagement in older populations is associated with emptiness, thoughts of meaninglessness, and feeling irrelevant (Wrosch et al., 2003). Consequently, depression, hopelessness, and increased suicide risk may result (Carver & Scheier, 1998). Interestingly, a recent national Scottish study among adolescents found that neither goal disengagement nor re-engagement was significantly associated with either suicidal ideation or attempt, when adjusted for in a multivariate model (Wetherall et al., 2018).

In industrialized societies, redirection after retirement is essential for well-being. Failure to disengage from decades-old career goals to new goals may bring tragic consequences, particularly for men (Andreassen et al., 2016). With the slow disappearance of the glass ceiling and emerging equal opportunities in the workplace, women approaching retirement are increasingly experiencing the same problem. It is not surprising that recent data from the Centers for Disease Control and Prevention show that some the highest increases in suicide rates are among women in their 50s and 60s, followed by men of the same age group (Kemp Cooney, 2019).

Recent increases in suicide rates for professionals of both genders in the later years of their careers suggest that without new worthwhile goals to engage in, goal redirection may not be adaptive. In these cases, retiring without having a groundwork for new meaningful activities may be more harmful than continuing work, even when work goals become unrealistic. The most adaptive pre-retirement strategy may be trying to identify goals and to redirect one's engagement in them (Leinonen et al., 2013).

In contrast to older populations, young people have numerous choices for goal redirection. For them, low levels of goal re-engagement are strongly associated with higher levels of depressive psychopathology and suicide (Wrosch et al., 2003). Those who continue to pursue unachievable goals may do so because of "painful engagement"—a dysphoric state defined by the perception of being painfully trapped in thwarted goal pursuit (MacLeod

& Conway, 2007). Some instances of painful engagement are invaluable in teaching young people to recognize attainable goals.

Extended pursuit, against the odds, of a high-risk career path that promises stardom, such as acting, music, or professional sports, is a common example of painful engagement. Most aspirants, realizing that their chances are low, disengage from unachievable goals of stardom and re-engage in pursuit of a lower-risk, more realistic goal with higher chances for success. Those who do not disengage may become entrapped in increasingly painful experiences of repeated failure, which bring on depression and increased suicide risk.

Another common setting for painful engagement, both literally and figuratively, is a once-promising romantic relationship gone wrong. The pain the couple experiences may feel unbearable. Often, the more intense the initial attraction that brought the couple together, the more difficult it is to accept that the goal of mutual happiness has become unattainable. The following case examples illustrate situations in which individuals were aware that their goals had become unattainable but were unable to quit and to find alternatives.

Case 28

Irena was a 32-year-old divorced woman of Polish descent who worked as a social worker. She had one 7-year-old son. She had recently divorced her husband of seven years. Nothing was particularly wrong with her marriage, but Irena wanted something more. She met another social worker, Mark, at a meeting and fell in love. For her, it was love at first sight, but being Catholic, she considered infidelity a sin. Mark was the director of a department at a large hospital and had recently separated from his wife. He was Armenian, which Irena found exciting and exotic. Irena knew Mark was attracted to her, too.

Once she made it known she was available, Irena and Mark started an affair. They were both madly in love and could not get enough of each other. Mark was everything Irena wanted—smart, ambitious, attractive, and sensitive. Their tastes were the same, their conversations were great, and their sex was fantastic. Irena thought she found a perfect man with whom to spend the rest of her life.

After approximately 10 weeks of bliss, Mark suddenly changed. Without warning, he told Irena that he needed space. Irena tried to give him space, but because she was afraid that he might leave her, she kept a close watch on him and kept finding different reasons to call or text him. That irritated Mark, who kept telling her he loved her, that he had no intention of leaving her, and that he just needed breathing room. Irena tried to give him space, but she could not.

Their fights were upsetting to Irena but also to Mark, who started pulling away. Irena resented him for ruining their perfect relationship. They had many talks and attempted to bring back the blissful first weeks of their relationship but could not. Mark wanted to break up. Irena told him that she could not live without him and if they just tried harder—if he tried to appreciate her love for him—they would be happy again. But the clock could not be reversed.

This continued for months. All Irena's girlfriends were telling her that she needed to stop seeing Mark and to look for somebody else. They were telling her that she was young, beautiful, had a wonderful personality, and that Mark just did not appreciate her. They found him shallow and selfish. Irena agreed that this may have been the case, but she could not stop seeing him.

There were many breakups and reconciliations initiated by Irena. Mark thought Irena was "unstable" and could not see himself living with her long term. But he was also attracted to her and could not resist seeing her when she reached out. Passionate sex would ensue, followed by fighting and another breakup. Despite everything, Irena was not willing to let Mark go. One night after yet another breakup, Mark stopped answering her frantic text messages. Irena could not bear his silence. She left work and waited for him at his hospital. Mark appeared, laughing and flirting with another woman. Devastated, Irena went home and jumped to her death from her 21st-floor balcony. Her son was at home in his room.

Irena's case is a typical example of a romantic painful engagement. What makes it typical is the realization that the relationship is doomed and the inability to end it. This cognitive–emotional dissonance results in a rollercoaster of breakups and reconciliations, which are prompted by extremes of attraction and despair and are rationalized by cognitive schemes of "working on the relationship." In the end, Irena's inability to disengage from a doomed relationship was at the core of her SN.

Case 29

Andrew was a promising assistant professor of geology in one of the larger Midwestern universities. He joined the faculty when he was in his 30s, which was later than most of his colleagues. Once he joined, he published often, was popular among students, and was quickly promoted from instructor to associate professor. However, when he was an associate professor, he had an affair with a student that resulted in a sexual harassment complaint, followed by a meeting with a dean. The dean was discreet but firm. Because he liked Andrew, he would keep the allegations quiet on the condition that Andrew resign.

Andrew was devastated. His life was derailed, and his life goals were destroyed. He contacted two of his graduate school friends working in academic institutions, but no comparable positions were available.

Becoming desperate, Andrew called the student who had filed the complaint to demand she retract it. The graduate student instead went to the student newspaper, which published an article about Andrew's harassment. Later that day, the chairman called Andrew into his office and told him that his teaching and research careers were over and that he had himself to blame.

In the evening, Andrew tried to kill himself with sleeping pills. Andrew was usually prompt in answering phone calls, so one of his friends, worried by Andrew's unresponsiveness, went to his apartment. Andrew did not answer the door, and his friend called 911. When the police broke in, Andrew was lying on the floor unconscious. He was taken to a hospital and later was transferred to an inpatient psychiatric unit.

Upon discharge from the hospital, Andrew resigned. While job searching, he saw an ad for a naturalist–lecturer on a cruise ship and decided to apply for the job. The cruise ship company hired Andrew. Andrew liked teaching, and the passengers very much enjoyed him.

At the end of his first contract with the shipping company, Andrew was surprised at how good he felt about his job. He renewed his contract for another year and then for many years afterward. He still works as the cruise ship naturalist and is one of the major draws for customers.

Andrew's inability to change his career nearly cost him his life. Fortunately, he survived his suicide attempt, and his next job was a great fit for him, illustrating his ability to recover when a viable option presented itself.

Stage 4: Humiliating Personal or Social Defeat

Human social structure is highly organized. Attaining a particular social position can be a major aspiration. Negotiation of social hierarchies and determining when to yield to others in social situations are universal human experiences. Whether one is born into nobility, fame, fortune, or poverty, there is always room for advancement.

According to social rank theory (Price et al., 1994), the term *social defeat* applies to a failure or struggle to obtain a particular social status or to maintain it as a result of an external event or social circumstances. In both major and minor social conflicts, those who win the prize become victors and those who fail suffer a defeat. The ability to cope with social defeat is central to well-being, happiness, and, at times, survival.

From the evolutionary perspective, depression can be adaptive in circumstances of social defeat. When adjusting to the realities of social hierarchies, depression may help reduce the level of arousal, initiative, and activity generated by noradrenergic fight-or-flight responses. The latter are useful during a conflict over power because they help maximize intellectual, physical, and emotional resources, but they can be harmful afterward, when a yielding approach is essential.

Depressed affect after a social defeat signals resignation and acceptance that can also be adaptive because they may reassure the social conflict victor that the depressed competitor is no longer a threat. Consistent with this theory, research indicates that acute suicidal states involve anxiety, panic, mental anguish, and desperation rather than depression (Fawcett et al., 1990).

A person's perception of their social defeat is a cognitive understanding of the outcome of the particular social conflict. As such, it is distinct from negative mood, hopelessness, and depression. A person who understands and appreciates a defeat experienced in a social conflict may not necessarily be depressed or hopeless and, in fact, could be hopeful for a victory or revenge. Research indicates that the acknowledgment of social defeat carries a near-term suicide risk that is independent of depression and hopelessness (O'Connor et al., 2013; Pollak et al., 2021; Taylor et al., 2011).

The consequences of social defeat are as varied as the conflicts from which they arise. One aspect of social defeat is its objective magnitude. From an impartial perspective, the defeat of not getting on the debate team, not being invited to a birthday party, or being criticized at work would be considered relatively minor. On the more serious end of the spectrum are devastating losses, such as being evicted from one's home, being fired from a job for fraud, or being exposed as a pedophile priest.

Importantly, the magnitude of a social defeat involves not only the size of the "prize" but also the extent of the emotional toll the defeat imparts on the person who has suffered it. The latter could take the form of public embarrassment, shame, indignity, and dishonor. The social defeats of eviction, job loss, and conviction for sexual molestation are devastating not only because of the income or social status loss but also due to the disgrace and ostracism that accompany the defeat.

Consequently, of many possible social defeats, those associated with public disgrace and humiliation dramatically increase near-term risk of suicidal ideation (Höller et al., 2020; O'Connor & Kirtley, 2018) and attempt (Höller et al., 2020). The most common examples are suicides of tycoons who have lost their fortune and have been in the news (Herszenhorn, 2013); business owners who have lost, or are about to lose, their businesses and will have to face their friends or investors (Keneally et al., 2014); and men who have recently lost their homes (Serby et al., 2006). A recent study by Pollak et al. (2021) looked at a sample of community-based adolescents and found that defeat predicted future suicidal ideation, while controlling for history of ideation, and the link was strongest among adolescents with greater positive future thinking abilities, driven by the tendency to set less realistic and achievable goals (Stage 3).

Interestingly, suicides are often triggered by personal defeats that most people would consider trivial, such as getting a B+ on an organic chemistry exam as a college freshman. Strikingly, most people who have suffered life-altering defeats, such as being removed from a public office for sexual misconduct, do not die by suicide (Feuer, 2008). Thus, in determining imminent suicide risk, the individual's perception of the magnitude of the social defeat is more important than the objective magnitude.

Perception of failure and subsequent risk for imminent suicide can be dramatically influenced by the person's culture, history, and personality. Cultural aspects of suicide risk include acceptability of suicide.

Receiving Bs in college can have overwhelming negative meaning for students who equate good grades with success, whereas socially minded students may consider Bs to be good grades. For immigrant children who were raised to fulfill their authoritarian parents' expectations of success and higher social status, two Bs in science courses may spell the end to their parents' dreams. The students' anticipated humiliation and fear of their parents' reaction to their failure may be so strong as to result in panic attacks and anguished turmoil, characteristics of the acute suicidal state.

The following case examples illustrate situations in which humiliating defeat was the core stage of the SN.

Case 30

Dan was a 44-year-old, married, California wine distributor executive who was good at his job and rose quickly to the position of vice president of marketing. During the first Internet bubble in the late 1990s, he left the company to start his own online wine distributing company. He raised a large amount of money from his friends, added his own, and opened his business as sole owner, confident that he would succeed. However, his business was soon failing, and his friends' investments were lost. He tried to borrow more money but could not find new investors.

Dan's business failure was a terrible blow financially and psychologically. His savings were depleted, and he was in debt. His image of himself as an exceptional business visionary was shattered. More than anything, however, Dan was ashamed that he had let his friends down. Dan was a gregarious, athletic man, a team player, and a leader. His friends invested in his business because they trusted his business sense and knew that they could rely on him.

In a last-ditch attempt to raise funds, Dan flew to New York for a meeting with a new group of potential investors. On the eve of the meeting, an article about his failing business appeared in a local newspaper. Several of his friends read it and called him to ask about their investments. Feeling humiliated and unable to face his associates, Dan hanged himself in his hotel room. He left a suicide note apologizing for letting everybody down and asking for forgiveness for being unable to live with his shame.

The most prominent feature of Dan's SN was the feeling of humiliation after he lost his friends' investments. Dan was a man known for his drive but also for his kindness, ethics, and morals. Losing his friends' investments shattered Dan. To him, telling his friends about the loss was a fate worse than death, making a very compelling humiliating social defeat stage of the SN. If Dan had borrowed the money from venture capitalists, his life may have turned out differently.

Case 31

Adrianna was a 55-year-old woman who at the time of her death was unemployed and living in a psychiatric residence on disability income. She died of prescription opiate and benzodiazepine overdose after her son Luke called her residence administrators and demanded that they keep his mother away from him. Adrianna had previously reported that her son had died of heart failure years earlier.

Adrianna had a history of severe borderline personality disorder. She had many psychiatric hospitalizations for depression and suicidal behavior. She had three suicide attempts resulting in medical intensive care unit (MICU) admission. On one occasion, she was intubated and required ventilatory support for days. Adrianna was obese, weighing more than 350 pounds. She had been diagnosed with type 1 diabetes mellitus, and her blood glucose was poorly controlled. She had few friends and had poor relationships with the residence staff and her neighbors.

A former sales representative, Adrianna was divorced three times and had two adult children. Luke, who was 28 years old at the time of her death, had a congenital heart malformation that carried a life expectancy of 25 years. He had an office job, was married, and had two children. He lived in rural Pennsylvania 100 miles away from his mother. Adrianna's other son lived on the West Coast.

The last known encounter between Adrianna and Luke took place during her final psychiatric hospitalization and was humiliating. Luke attended the family meeting and instead of being empathetic, he told Adrianna that he was tired of her manipulating him with her illnesses and said that he would never visit her in the hospital again. "I have been dealing with this since I can remember," he told the treatment team. "Imagine what it was like to call 911 because your mother threatened to kill herself starting in middle school all through high school," he said. "I have had enough."

Several days later, Adrianna was discharged. According to the residence staff, she and Luke sometimes talked on the phone, but he never visited. There was a lot of screaming. After their phone calls, Adrianna would say how she regretted her difficult relationship with him and that she wanted to see her grandchildren—another one was on the way. One day, Adrianna got off the phone crying and said that Luke had died of a heart attack. She took a day off, ostensibly to go to his funeral. The reality was that Luke's wife had given birth, and Luke told his mother that she was not invited to the christening and, if she came, she would never see her grandchildren again.

As in Dan's case, Adrianna's suicide was driven by humiliation. In her case, the humiliating event was personal. Facing the other residents, knowing that they were aware of her lies about her son's death and of her failure as a mother, was a fate worse than death to her. Adrianna's connections to others were based on a lie. Once that lie was exposed, there was nothing left.

Stage 5: Perceived Burdensomeness

Joiner's interpersonal theory of suicidal behavior suggests that concurrent feelings of burdensomeness and thwarted belongingness increase an individual's desire for death. *Burdensomeness* is defined as the sense that one is a burden to their family or loved ones, whereas *thwarted belongingness* is akin to social alienation and isolation. This model has been implicated extensively in suicidal behavior, but the duration of these psychological states remains unclear. Further research is necessary to more precisely understand the role of burdensomeness and thwarted belongingness in the acute period.

In a 2009 study of patients referred to the hospital for "severe suicidal symptoms," "recent" suicide attempt (a specific time frame was not indicated), or serious suicidal ideation, burdensomeness and thwarted belongingness were significantly predictive of current suicide attempt, but only when combined with previous number of attempts. (Joiner et al., 2009). In a psychological autopsy study comparing the suicide notes of 20 people who attempted suicide and lived versus 20 people who died by suicide, the notes from those who died by suicide reflected greater levels of burdensomeness compared to the notes from those who survived. The decedents' suicide methods were more lethal than the methods used by those who survived their attempts (Joiner et al., 2002).

Failure to achieve unrealistic goals or failure to achieve financial gains anticipated either due to perfectionism or to expectations of others often involves financial hardship. The resulting financial difficulties may force a person to seek help from others. Asking friends or relatives for money or moving in with one's elderly parents can make many people feel like a burden. According to some suicide notes, suicidal individuals come to perceive themselves as a burden to the extent that they believe that their close others would be better off without them—that is, they are high on perceived burdensomeness (Joiner et al., 2002).

Perceived burdensomeness is the result of thinking that others would "be better off if I were gone," which manifests when the need for social competence that is posited by frameworks including self-determination theory (Ryan & Deci, 2000) is unmet. Furthermore, greater perception of burdensomeness in suicide notes is associated with more lethal means of suicide. A person's perception that they are a burden to others is an independent predictor of suicidal ideation in a range of samples, including older adults (Jahn & Cukrowicz, 2011), people with chronic pain (Kanzler et al., 2012), and people with a physical disability (Khazem, 2018). Perceived burdensomeness also has been shown to mediate the association between perfectionism and suicidal ideation (Rasmussen et al., 2012) and to remain predictive of ideation even after controlling for factors like depression and hopelessness. The sense that one is a burden to one's family or loved ones has been shown to be a predictor of suicidal ideation in a number of samples, independently of reports of depression or hopelessness (Joiner et al., 2006). Perceived burdensomeness is the fifth stage of the SN.

Case 32

Penny, a 28-year-old single woman, was diagnosed with bipolar disorder (BD) after an extensive prodromal state, which manifested as recurrent mood lability and impulsive behavior. Penny completed high school with good grades and was accepted into Emory University, but she took a leave of absence after her freshman year to pursue activist work. She was active in feminist organizations, and she often worked through the night, constantly moving from place to place. At age 26, she fell in love with a woman. When her love was not reciprocated, she left the country and had her first manic episode in Europe. Severe, treatment-resistant depression followed. Penny moved in with her mother and left the house only for doctors' appointments. She stopped talking to friends. She was treated as an inpatient for depression with suicidal ideation and with postdischarge follow-up in dialectical behavior therapy (DBT) programs and by esteemed therapists. Despite the expensive treatments, her condition did not improve. She did not find group therapy helpful and did not connect with the other patients, who did not share her passion for social causes. After the DBT program let her go and after she got the "maximum" benefit from participation, her mother let her know that she would no longer pay for ineffective, expensive treatment and that Penny should snap out of it and get a job. Feeling alienated from the world and knowing that she had become a burden to her mother, Penny attempted suicide by asphyxiation. She survived this attempt and was admitted to an inpatient psychiatric unit. She was later discharged to a long-term residential treatment facility.

Penny's SN was complicated and had several components. Her goals of saving the world were unattainable, her return home from Europe and her discharge from the day program were humiliating, and her withdrawal from her friends was a typical response to the shame of her current life situation. However, the most compelling stage prompting her suicide attempt was feeling like she was a financial and emotional burden to her mother as well as an emotional burden to her friends. The latter feeling led to her self-imposed isolation, which worsened her feeling of alienation. She had no source of income. Her depression was so severe that she lacked the concentration and initiative to work or study. Her stress tolerance was too low to negotiate the conflict with her mother. As a result, Penny believed that her life had reached a dead end, and she attempted suicide.

Case 33

Craig was a married 47-year-old unemployed lawyer who ended his life by jumping in front of an oncoming train after his wife told him she was tired of borrowing money from her parents for living expenses while he chased crazy projects.

Initially, Craig was an Ivy League law school graduate who had a very promising career, but he later suffered several setbacks, resulting in increasingly severe depressions. Three years before his suicide, he was diagnosed with BD II, and at the time of his death, he was being treated with lithium, aripiprazole, and bupropion. Craig's first job was a partner-track position at a large law firm. He was the hardest-working, brightest associate, who was nevertheless difficult to get along with because he had a big ego and responded poorly to feedback. Nevertheless, he did well until he antagonized the partner with whom he worked on an important case to the extent that Craig was let go just short of making partner himself.

Craig was depressed for months, but then he found a partner-track job in a smaller firm. He was initially happy with the firm, and the firm was happy with him until history repeated itself: Craig insulted a senior attorney and was fired. After a second depressive episode, Craig was able to find a short-lived job in the district attorney's office, but he was soon let go.

After this third setback, Craig could not find another job. His wife Jackie was a homemaker caring for their daughter, who had a learning disability. Craig's third depressive episode was more serious than the first two. He changed psychiatrists twice and was finally diagnosed with BD II. Craig's bipolar depression was treatment-resistant. The medications were not effective, and he refused electroconvulsive therapy. The longer he stayed unemployed, the more difficult it was for him to find another job. However, he was hopeful and resistant to taking just any job to survive.

Initially, Craig and his family lived off savings, but soon the money ran out and they had to borrow money from Jackie's parents. This was humiliating for Jackie, who was resentful of Craig's failure to provide for the family, and for Craig, who felt like a burden. Jackie told Craig that he was a failure who could not even support his only daughter and that his BD was just an excuse for laziness. She told him to "snap out of it" and to do what all normal men do and get a job, or they would have to take their daughter out of her school, which specialized in learning disabilities.

Although Craig was cocky when manic, during his depressions he was prone to guilty ruminations, blaming himself for his family's predicament. He felt especially guilty for not being able to pay his daughter's tuition. Pressed by Jackie, he searched for a lower-paying job but was unsuccessful because he was overqualified. The money they had borrowed from Jackie's parents was running out. They could either ask for another loan, take their daughter out of private school, or sell their apartment. The atmosphere at home was reaching a boiling point: Jackie told Craig she wanted out of the marriage. Craig killed himself the day he discovered Jackie had consulted a divorce lawyer. In his suicide note, he said that he was ending his life because he could not go on living feeling like a burden to his family.

Craig's SN was driven by failure to disengage, humiliation, and perceived burdensomeness. His BD probably had strongly contributed to his suicidal process. The goals he had set for himself during hypomanic stages were most likely unrealistic, and his grandiosity impaired his reality testing, making it rigid and inflexible. As a result, Craig had difficulty accepting feedback and could not redirect his efforts when necessary. Because he was fired during manic episodes, the humiliation of losing the job was buffered by his in-flated self-image. However, when he developed his most serious depressive episode, his failure as a provider was amplified by feelings of worthlessness and intense guilty ruminations (see Chapter 7), resulting in his feeling like a burden to his family.

Stage 6: Thwarted Belongingness

The other main component of the interpersonal theory of suicidal behavior (Joiner, 2005) is the unmet fundamental human need to be socially integrated or to "belong." Individuals are at greater risk for suicidal behavior when this need is not met, and those who attempt suicide often experience loneliness or thwarted belongingness that leads to their suicidal behavior (Van Orden et al., 2008).

Numerous studies have suggested that the sense of belonging associated with community involvement or participation in social events serves as a protective factor against suicidal ideation (Joiner et al., 2006; Van Orden et al., 2008; Kessler et al., 2006). Kleiman et al. (2013) examined variations in suicidal ideation by college semester, and they isolated belongingness as a mediating factor.

People who have failed in their life goals and have been forced into a position of real or perceived financial and/or emotional dependency are often ashamed of their predicament and embarrassed to disclose their failures to others. As a result, such people, even though they desperately want support and companionship, often isolate themselves and avoid social contact, and being isolated thwarts a their basic need to connect, to be accepted, and to belong.

In contrast to perceived burdensomeness, which originates in self-determination theory, the construct of thwarted belongingness has multiple origins and is an amalgam of theories of the human need to connect. Thwarted belongingness is a psychologically painful mental state that results when the fundamental need for connectedness or the "need to belong" is unmet (Baumeister & Leary, 1995; see also Cacioppo & Patrick, 2008).

A number of theories suggest that the various indices of social isolation—living alone (Heikkinen et al., 1994), loneliness (Koivumaa-Honkanen et al., 2001), and low social support (Qin & Nordentoft, 2005)—are associated with suicide across the life span because they are indicators that the need to belong has been thwarted. Retrospective studies showed that both men and women who were socially well integrated had substantially lower long-term risk for suicide (Tsai et al., 2015), regardless of burdensomeness, which was not examined. Thus, thwarted belongingness is a unique construct and plays a prominent role in Stage 6 of the SN.

Joiner's (2005) interpersonal theory of suicide posits that when a person feels both hopelessly alienated from others and a burden to them, he or she starts to develop suicidal ideation. According to Joiner, suicidal ideation is a necessary but not sufficient cause for suicide. Suicide takes place when a person with suicidal ideation loses fear of death, which prevents most people with suicidal ideation from taking their lives. Joiner's theory equates losing fear of death with acquiring the capability for suicide, attained through practicing increasingly lethal means of ending one's life and through habituation to death.

Joiner's two-step theory readily explains why most people with suicidal ideation do not attempt suicide and do not die by suicide. However, the interpersonal theory does not explain why the average time interval from the first thought of taking one's life to the suicide attempt is 15 minutes (Deisenhammer et al., 2009) and why some survivors of serious impulsive suicide attempts report having no prior suicidal ideation. Joiner's framework does not quite account for the state of desperation felt by many suicidal individuals, with suicide being an urge to escape the intolerable pain of the moment rather than a rational plan.

However, there is a substantial body of research indicating that the two central concepts of the interpersonal theory of suicide—the thwarted belongingness and perceived burdensomeness predisposing individuals to the development of suicidal thoughts and attempts (Shneidman, 1998)—are associated with long-term suicide risk. Subjective perception of lack of social connections and of thwarted belongingness specifically is associated with suicide attempts (Fässberg et al., 2012; Hatcher & Stubberfield, 2013). Similarly, a person's perception that he or she is a burden to others is a predictor of suicidal ideation in the elderly and people with chronic pain (Kanzler et al., 2012). Consistent with the interpersonal theory of suicide, the interaction of thwarted belongingness and perceived burdensomeness is predictive of suicidal ideation independent of depression (Joiner et al., 2009). A systematic review and meta-analysis of the literature on the interpersonal theory of suicide supported the interaction between thwarted belongingness and perceived burdensomeness and their association with suicidal ideation. The study also found that the two feelings and the capability for suicide was significantly related to a greater number of suicide attempts (Chu et al., 2017). Quite recently, a review of suicidal risk factors during the COVID-19 pandemic revealed that perceived burdensomeness and thwarted belongingness, along with stress sensitivity and cognitive factors, are probably the reasons behind elevated risk of suicide seen during the pandemic (Raj et al., 2021).

In addition to the interactions between feelings of perceived burdensomeness and thwarted belongingness, trait perfectionism, associated with the SN's first stage, unrealistic life goals, has been shown to moderate and augment the relationship between these interpersonal distress variables and suicide ideation in adolescents (Sommerfeld & Malek, 2019).

The following two cases illustrate SNs defined by alienation and thwarted belongingness.

Case 34

Adam was a 22-year-old college senior who wanted to kill himself by jumping off a bridge near his campus but was talked out of it by a passer-by who then called the police.

Adam was a typical American college senior with an average GPA and $50,000 in student loans. He was on a debate team, was a fraternity member, and had joined several other clubs because he liked the feeling of belonging to his class, college, and generation. Adam's parents were helping to pay for his education as an investment in his future, but they expected him to support himself after graduation. Adam imagined a bright future and felt justified to receive his parents' support, never believing that he was a burden to his parents.

Unexpectedly, after graduation, Adam, unlike his friends, was unable to find a job. His Facebook feed was full of entries from friends who were furnishing their new apartments and hanging out with coworkers and new friends. Adam, on the other hand, had to move back in with his parents. Time passed and still Adam could not find a suitable job. As Adam's friends seemed to move into the next stages of their lives, he seemed to move backward. The only jobs available were menial and did not even require a high school diploma. Taking such a job symbolized defeat, social and otherwise. To add insult to injury, his parents, who worked hard to put him through college, wanted him to start doing "something."

This turn of events led to a drastic change in Adam's state of mind. His feeling of belonging to a cohort of people marching forward to happy futures had been shattered. Reading his friends' Facebook entries was making him depressed, so he stopped using Facebook altogether, telling everybody that he was taking a break from it because it was taking too much time. Time, however, was all he had, and he spent it smoking weed and playing video games.

Some of Adam's high school classmates never went to college and were living at home. Adam tried to hang out with them several times, but he never really fit in. Eventually, he made his suicide attempt.

In Adam's case, getting a good job after college signified continued belonging in a group with his socioeconomic status. His failure to get a job thwarted his attempt at continued belongingness. Adam's sense of thwarted belongingness became even more acute after his ill-designed attempt to belong to the "bad crowd" from his high school. His parents never explicitly told him he had become a burden, but Adam imagined that they must be thinking it, adding perceived burdensomeness to thwarted belongingness.

Therefore, over time, Adam fell into both thwarted belongingness and, to a lesser degree, perceived burdensomeness. For somebody without other risk factors, this change in mental state alone would not increase the imminent suicide risk. However, Adam was led to believe that he was destined for success in life, and his entitlement to happiness further increased the intensity of his SN. Moreover, Adam was competitive, perfectionistic, and conscious of his family's social status. This led him view his failure as a personal social defeat, increasing his suicide risk dramatically.

Case 35

Shirley was a 59-year-old divorced woman who jumped to her death from the window of her apartment building several weeks after the death of her only friend, Susan, who was also a mother figure for Shirley.

Shirley had been diagnosed with borderline personality disorder and had a long history of depression, anxiety, and panic attacks. She graduated from a good college and obtained a law degree from a prestigious law school, but because she was never able to get along with her peers or supervisors, a career never manifested. After college, Shirley had several jobs at law firms, but the jobs never lasted long because she was soon fired or asked to leave.

Shirley's parents divorced when she was in elementary school, and she was estranged from her father, who remarried and had three more children. After her mother died when Shirley was in her forties, Shirley entered a legal battle for an inheritance that was left mostly to her sister, her mother's favorite. Shirley died before the endless lawsuit was settled.

Shirley's longest employment lasted seven years, when she worked for a nonprofit organization. After she was asked to resign, she filed a discrimination lawsuit, which dragged on for several years before it was settled.

Shirley was married for a year when she was in her thirties. Her husband left her because she was "impossible to be around." This was the consensus of most of the people who knew Shirley. Shirley had no friends except for Susan, who made a lifelong habit of helping people like Shirley survive. Shirley was chronically depressed and suicidal, and her wrists were covered with scars from self-inflicted razor wounds.

Shirley often talked to Susan about how she liked people and wanted to get along with them. When Shirley would meet a man on the Internet, or a potential girlfriend in a class she was taking, Susan coached her through relationship basics—be nice, ask questions, and give them space—but it never worked. Everyone Shirley met quickly became disturbed by her blend of aggression, possessiveness, and lack of boundaries. "If not for me," Susan would say, "she would be dead. She has nobody else."

That was not quite true. Throughout her life, Shirley saw many psychiatrists and therapists. After Susan died, Shirley's therapist wanted to hospitalize her, but Shirley refused, saying that she was not suicidal. Shirley's suicide followed a canceled dinner with Susan's daughter. Shirley left a note saying that she did not belong in this world.

It would be difficult to find a clearer illustration of SN dominated by thwarted belongingness than Shirley's case. Borderline personality disorder is characterized by difficulty regulating emotions, which leads to unstable mood, impulsivity, and poor self-image, along with constant fear of abandonment. Repeated and frantic attempts to avoid abandonment come across as hostile and needy, resulting in stormy relationships. Borderline personality disorder often manifests in self-harm or suicide attempts. While Susan was alive, she was the only person who Shirley could trust to be there for her. Given her borderline personality structure, Shirley experienced Susan's death as her final abandonment, which she did not survive.

Stage 7: Perception of No Future

Perception of no future is a new cognitive construct defined as the absence of positive thinking and the inability to imagine a viable and acceptable future. It can be conceptualized as the reverse of positive future thinking (Pollak et al., 2021). Some studies have shown positive future thinking to be a protective factor against suicide; however, other reports suggested that anticipation of future positive experiences was associated with increased risk of suicidal behavior due to more intense experiences of defeat (O'Connor et al., 2015; Pollak et al., 2021). Patients with the SN are unable to think about the future, even with an active effort. The perception of no future, which is the framework for describing this cognitive process, is hypothesized to have an unambiguous prospective association with suicidal behavior. Like entitlement to happiness, this concept needs to be refined and tested in future research with scales, which may be initially derived from future expectancy scales. Since no data on the perception of no future are yet available, the literature on suicide, positive future thinking, and future expectancies is reviewed here.

The integrated motivational-volitional (IMV) model of suicide posits that motivational moderators (MMs), such as future thoughts, influence the transition to suicidal ideation and intent. Thus, when present and protective, the MMs allow the individual to see alternatives and a positive future. Namely, positive future thinking is thought to serve as a buffer against the emergence of suicidal ideation and intent (O'Connor & Kirtley, 2018). Conversely, negative future thoughts, which occur prior to any suicidal ideation and behavior, can be conceptualized as the SN's perception of no future.

Only a few studies have assessed the relationship between positive future thinking (or lack thereof) and suicide risk, and its association with entrapment, defeat, and unrealistic life goals. However, the studies' conclusions have remained hypothesis-generating.

A study by Hunter and O'Connor (2003), for example, found that social perfectionism and positive future thinking discriminated between parasuicidal patients and controls, beyond the effects of hopelessness, depression, and anxiety. Similarly, MacLeod et al. (1997) and Conaghan and Davidson (2002) have supported the relationship between reduced positive thinking and parasuicidality, although no study has confirmed the role of negative future thinking.

Paradoxically, several reports by O'Connor's group found that positive future thinking may predict repeat suicide attempts, which the authors attributed to unrealistic goals and expectations about self, which when not realized may increase the risk of suicide by contributing to the individual's sense of entrapment (O'Connor et al., 2015).

O'Connor and Portzky (2018) suggested that entrapment (Chapter 7) could increase suicide risk via its association with positive future thinking. Moreover, Tucker et al. (2016) demonstrated that hope, a trait related to positive future thinking, significantly moderated the relationship between entrapment and suicidal ideation (Tucker et al., 2016). This finding is consistent with the proposal that perception of no future may give rise to the entrapment criterion of SCS (see Chapter 7).

The following cases illustrate the SN's essential last stage, perception of no future.

Case 36

Peter was a 58-year-old married engineer with three adult children who shot himself in the head in front of his wife Carrie during an argument.

Peter married Carrie when they were both 19 years old because she was pregnant with their first child, a boy. They had two more boys. At the time of Peter's death, his oldest son was married and lived in another state with his family; his middle son was single, lived at home, and worked at a local bank; and his youngest son, Dan, who had a severe congenital disorder, also lived at home, requiring 24-hour care. Peter's insurance was paying for most of Dan's care, but his income was essential for keeping his ill son out of an institution.

Peter knew his marriage was unhappy and so did everybody else. His wife was viewed as selfish, prickly, and manipulative. The two met as freshmen in college and dated for several months. The relationship was rocky even then. When Peter decided to break up because he did not love Carrie and wanted to meet somebody else, Carrie told him she was pregnant. They got married one month later because Peter decided to "do the right thing." After they had their third son and learned that he was ill, the marriage became truly difficult. The couple decided to care for Dan at home, regardless of cost, and his care had drained their savings. Peter's income was barely sufficient, and Carrie did not contribute financially because she was Dan's full-time caretaker.

Peter had to take a second job. That solved the financial problem, but he was never at home, so Carrie essentially raised their sons on her own. With time, she became increasingly bitter. She believed that life has passed her by and blamed Peter for it. As time went on, Carrie became hostile, and her treatment of Peter became harsh. She angrily berated him for being a poor provider, a miserable lover, and a failure in all aspects of life. There were shouting matches every evening. Their older son left the house for college and never came back. Their middle son moved to a friend's basement. Dan was nonverbal and did not react.

Unable to bear the thought of living like this five or 10 years into the future, Peter finally decided to file for divorce. However, the divorce lawyer told him that if he did divorce, Peter would lose the house and would have to continue to support his son while paying his wife a hefty maintenance. Peter did not file for divorce and vicious arguments at home continued. The atmosphere became so toxic that the two older sons would not come home for the holidays.

Being at home was so painful that Peter often stayed with friends, who urged him to leave Carrie. "Nobody would want me with a disabled son. I cannot leave Carrie to take care of him all alone. She is a good woman. I have not been there for her enough," Peter would respond. Carrie had gotten into his head.

When he finally went to a psychiatrist, he was diagnosed with major depression and was prescribed an antidepressant. Unable to either see his future with Carrie or to leave, Peter started having suicidal thoughts but no plans. However, he did have visions of himself crashing the car into a wall when driving. With Peter in his office, the psychiatrist called Carrie and alerted her to Peter's state of mind and high suicide risk. He asked her to remove all firearms from the house and to come in for a family session. Carrie became defensive and said that she would not take the blame for Peter's failures.

The psychiatrist advised Peter to stay with his friends. Peter did so for one week, but when he returned home to do his laundry, an argument quickly ensued, and Peter shot himself in the head. His life insurance was valid and had enough coverage to pay for Dan's care for 20 years.

Peter's case is an example of somebody reaching the stage of perception of no future while having few other stages of the SN. His life goals were realistic, he was not entitled, he did not perceive himself as a burden (just the opposite), and he was connected to many people. The only other significant stage in his SN was the failure to disengage, in his case from his commitment to keeping Dan at home and from his toxic marriage. And yet, his enmeshed relationship with his wife had evolved so far that looking into the future, he could not picture a life that was acceptable to him. When thinking about his options, he could not imagine himself staying married unless his wife stopped treating him like dirt, which seemed highly unlikely because, in his words, "people don't change." On the other hand, he could not imagine himself living alone or being with somebody else. His final argument with Carrie escalated the already present SN to the level of SCS, as defined by an unbearable state of entrapment and emotional pain.

Case 37

Marissa, a 40-year-old separated woman diagnosed with BD, was admitted to an inpatient psychiatric unit after she was found unconscious in a bathtub with cuts on her wrists. Marissa was recently removed from her position as CEO of a small start-up company after her main investor (with whose son she was having an affair) discovered that the bylaws of the company were in disarray and that she did not actually own the company product.

Although Marissa had been diagnosed with BD only recently, she always had mood swings. When she was down, she had difficulty getting out of bed and was unmotivated but was still very functional. During hypomania, she was incredibly charismatic, creative, and energetic. Since the beginning of her last hypomanic episode three years earlier, she had been able to start a company, raise millions in venture capital, hire a staff of 20 people, and create a prototype of her product. "This is what I always knew I was capable of," she told her friends, "and it is finally happening."

However, as she was building her company, Marissa made many mistakes, which led to her removal from her position. She failed to hire a legal team, used company funds for personal expenses, and had an affair with the principal investor's son, who was employed by the company as her assistant. When a competitor sued for the rights to the product, the investors discovered the improprieties, and she was removed from the company she had founded.

Her affair quickly ended. After learning about the affair, the young man's father swore that he would never work with Marissa again and would make sure that nobody else would either. He sought legal action to block Marissa's access to the company accounts and remove her from the company, which Marissa had thought would become her life's success. Looking into the future and thinking about her options, Marissa could not picture a future when she would be running the company with the young man's father, nor could she imagine the future doing anything else. Heavily in debt and depressed, Marissa attempted suicide.

Marissa's case is typical of a SN of a person with BD. Her life goal of making it "really big" could be seen as unachievable, her company collapse could be considered a public humiliating defeat, and the end of her affair could qualify as thwarted belongingness. Nevertheless, it was her inability to imagine a viable future either with or without her company that brought her to the brink of SCS and first-ever suicidal behavior. Inability to generate imagery of an acceptable future brings on very real emotional pain and the desperate state of entrapment, which is at the heart of the suicide crisis and forms the defining component of the SCS.

Constructing the Suicidal Narrative

The SN interview portion of the imminent risk assessment consists of two parts. The first part is a systematic assessment of each of the SN's stages, in which the patient is asked whether, and to what extent, the constructs previously described are applicable to the story of his or her life. After the clinician obtains enough information to construct a formulation of the patient's SN, the clinician cautiously discusses this formulation with the patient to establish if the SN accurately reflects the patient's perception of his or her life. The clinician then suggests a possible alternative life narrative, so as to not strengthen the SN with a new and more articulate formulation.

The seven stages of the SN discussed in this chapter—unrealistic life goals, entitlement to happiness, failure to redirect to more realistic goals, humiliating personal or social defeat, thwarted belongingness, perceived burdensomeness, and perception of no future options—read like a general outline of a life story gone wrong. Published research supports the relationships of each of the concepts outlined in these stages with suicidal behavior, and research efforts to test the narrative are ongoing.

The life events of suicidal patients are different, and so are the details of their SNs. However, some generalizations apply to all, or almost all, suicidal individuals. For example, setting up unrealistic life goals will frequently result in failure. Entitlement to happiness makes it difficult to accept current failure in chasing a life's dream or to imagine alternative paths to happiness and fulfillment. In turn, this makes it difficult to disengage from the now hopeless undertaking and re-engage in pursuit of a more realistic goal. The more one persists in a failed endeavor, the more likely the failure will be experienced as humiliating defeat. Such defeats often result in financial losses and unwanted dependence on others (often loved ones) for economic support, which could be perceived as burdensome and shameful. In addition, reluctance and embarrassment in admitting the failure may result in feelings of thwarted belongingness and a perceived sense of having no future.

These generalizations provide an outline of a typical SN. The goal of the narrative portion of the imminent suicide risk assessment is to establish to what extent the suicidal patient's perception of their life (or the patient's life narrative) fits this outline. In a comprehensive clinical assessment, all seven domains must be assessed. However, the "end" of the SN—the sense of having no future—carries the most weight, should be assessed most explicitly, and must be countered.

The assessment sequence does not need to follow the stages in order, but it should depend on the course of the conversational interview. For example, if a patient's presenting complaint is suicidal ideation because they have no good options, then one may start by exploring the patient's perception of entrapment, which is the end of the SN. Alternatively, if a patient has not spontaneously expressed suicidal ideation or intent, one may start the narrative section of the interview by exploring the life goals and expectations of happiness—that is, the beginning of the narrative.

When conducting the SN part of the imminent risk assessment, it is important to "translate" the terminology used in this chapter, including most stage titles, into accessible language. The terms *attainable or unattainable goals* and *failure to disengage or redirect* are neither intuitive nor familiar to the general public or, as a matter of fact, to many clinicians. Clinicians' use of psychiatric terminology (or "psychobabble") is often perceived as condescending, cold, and insensitive, and an effort should be made to use simple vocabulary accessible to all.

A good entry into a discussion of the realism of the patient's life goals and their ability or failure to achieve them is a simple question about the patient's life, such as "How are things working out in your life?" or "How has life treated your lately?" Any response is likely to mention either a work situation or a relationship and provide an opening for follow-up questions. For example, the answer "I have had trouble with my boss" could lead to follow-up questions about the patient's occupation and career goals and the realism thereof.

Occasionally, the patient may feel too tense or too distressed to answer the opening question or will give an evasive answer, such as "Everything is fine," making a life goals discussion slightly more difficult. One interviewing strategy in these cases is to use some factual knowledge of the person's life and offer the interviewer's best guess on what the problem might be, such as "I know you had some issues with (your boss, your boyfriend) lately." After the patient acknowledges the issue, the interviewer can start the discussion in earnest by saying, "Please tell me more about this." Usually, the following questions are sufficient to formulate a clinical opinion about the patient's life goals: "What are your life goals?" "What would you like to achieve in life?"

"How close are you to achieving them?" "Are they realistic?" "What would your life be like if you fail?"

After the life goals are identified, a good second question is "How important are these to you?" An answer to this question could be pivotal for understanding both the goals' importance and the degree of the patient's investment in them. For example, the answer "I have been working there for 30 years, and this job has been my life" is quite revealing of potential difficulty in disengaging from a lifelong ambition. Alternatively, the answer "I thought he was the one" reveals how difficult it may be for the patient to give up a romance and start searching for a new relationship. Once the aim is identified, the interview can explore how central and meaningful the issue is to the person's life, as well as possible alternatives.

Because most patients know what they feel, discussing their entitlement to happiness is often easier than talking about their life goals, which some people may have never defined consciously. Usually, the following questions are sufficient to formulate a clinical opinion about patients' expectations of happiness: "Are you happy now?" "How happy did you expect to feel at this point in your life?" "Did you expect to feel this bad?" "Do you deserve to feel the way you are feeling?"

Like unattainable goals, the notion of humiliating social defeat is an abstract concept foreign to most patients. Even patients who are aware that they have just lost a social battle may not consciously appreciate to what degree their defeat has been humiliating. Other patients may not even be aware that the stress and emotional turmoil they have been experiencing were brought on by a social defeat. Fortunately, whether patients did or did not suffer defeat can be deciphered from their recent histories.

Often, patients will spontaneously bring up their losses and embarrassments. Statements such as "I lost this lawsuit," "I got laid off," "I am getting Cs, it is so competitive," and "This is so embarrassing" are explicit acknowledgments of a defeat or humiliating situation, and they should be interpreted as such during an interview. In these instances, to formulate the opinion about the intensity of the defeat stage, the clinician needs to assess the extent of defeat or humiliation by asking, "How bad is it?" When the patient does not respond, one option is to wait for the patient to identify the conflict—for example, "I have been going through a bad divorce"—and then ask about its implications. For example, the question "Do you feel like you are losing this battle?" frames the divorce as a social struggle and sets up a discussion of possible losses and humiliations.

States of thwarted belongingness and perceived hopelessness are often very labile and can change rapidly depending on life circumstances. A rejection letter from one's dream college or failure to land a good job can be perceived as a thwarted attempt to belong to a group of successful people and generate an acute sense of thwarted belongingness. If a person in one of the previously mentioned situations is financially dependent on others, perceived burdensomeness may follow.

Although the terms *thwarted belongingness* and *perceived burdensomeness* are very cumbersome, the corresponding themes may be easier to talk about and empathize with during a psychiatric interview than the other concepts discussed in previous chapters. Most people can relate to feeling alienated or like a burden. Hence, simply asking if the patient feels alone and like a burden will often provide enough information to assess the severity of these two stages of the narrative. Several follow-up questions from the interview algorithm presented later or from the sample cases are most often sufficient to complete the assessment.

Finally, the assessment of either thwarted belongingness or perceived burdensomeness can be transitioned to the discussion of whether either or both could be seen by the patient as relenting in the future.

In addition to not being able to imagine a livable future, many patients at a higher risk of suicide will spontaneously report feelings of entrapment. In these cases, it is important not to miss that the patient has just reported one of the symptoms of SCS, and to pursue this inquiry (see Chapter 7). That is, the clinician should use such patient's cue as an opportunity to follow-up and assess whether the patient thinks the trap has an exit by simply asking "Are there any exits to your situation?" "Is there anything that can be done to open some doors for you?" and "What if X happens?" The more negative the answers to the "What if" questions are, the likelier it is that the patient will attempt suicide in the near future.

Probing the Suicidal Narrative: An Interview Algorithm

Patients' openness about their suicidal ideation or intent depends on the clinical setting and the individual. Many patients coming to the emergency department for help and protection from their suicidal thoughts and impulses are open about their suicidal intent. Patients who are either invested in hiding their intent or unaware of it may be less forthcoming. The algorithm outlined here should be used for guarded patients who do not disclose their suicidality in the first minutes of the interview. For patients who answer the first question by acknowledging their entrapment, such as by saying "I am suicidal and I am trapped in a horrible situation," the algorithm should be reversed and transitioned to the assessment of SCS. The interviewer should first explore the entrapment and suicidality and conclude by assessing perfectionism and entitlement to happiness.

All patients and clinical situations are unique. The guideline should be personalized for each patient according to his or her history and circumstances. The case examples that follow show how the algorithm can be adjusted depending on the course of the interview.

- Forming rapport
  - How are you feeling today?
  - What happened (or what has been happening)?
- Perfectionism
  - Do you believe that whatever you do, you should always give it 100%?
  - Are you a perfectionist?
- Unrealistic life goals
  - Please tell me about your life goals and plans
  - Do you think that these are realistic?
  - What makes you think that your goals are realistic?
- Entitlement to happiness
  - Do you work hard to achieve what you want in life?
  - You said you feel miserable. Is it fair that you feel this way, given how hard you have been working?
  - For all the hard work you have put in, do you deserve to be happy?
- Failure to redirect to more realistic goals
  - Can you tell me more about your (work situation or relationship)?
  - How important is this to you?
  - Can you find an alternative?
  - How hard would it be to live without it?
- Humiliating personal or social defeat
  - How bad was it?
  - Was it humiliating?
  - Did (do) you feel defeated?
  - Is it possible that it just seemed that way to you?
  - Do many people know about this?

- • How hard would it be for you to face them?
- • Perceived burdensomeness
  - ▪ Do you feel like you are a burden to others?
  - ▪ How bad a burden?
  - ▪ Would they be relieved if you were not there?
  - ▪ Will others miss you if you are gone?
- • Thwarted belongingness
  - ▪ Do you feel alone (in this)?
  - ▪ Even when you are with people?
  - ▪ Do you feel disconnected even from people who are closest to you?
- • Perception of no future
  - ▪ What are you looking forward to in the future?
  - ▪ Can you picture life five years from now? Ten years from now?
  - ▪ Please tell me about your future plans
  - ▪ Where do you think your life is going?
  - ▪ Do you think you could be happy in the future?
  - • Constructing a SN
  - ▪ It seems that . . . (Describe the SN created from answers to the previous questions).
  - ▪ Does this apply to you?
  - ▪ What does and what does not?

Case Examples

Case 38: High Risk for Imminent Suicide

Gary is a 30-year-old single Jewish man with a history of BD I and two previous psychiatric hospitalizations who is currently living in an apartment with his parents. He returned to the United States six months ago after teaching English in Croatia, and his parents referred him for a psychiatric assessment by a bipolar specialist "so he can get the best possible treatment because his is a difficult case." Gary has no previous suicide attempts, but his parents are concerned that he may kill himself because "there is just something scary about him that makes us very uncomfortable."

DR: How are you feeling today? (*Forming rapport*)
GARY: Not so great. Trying to adjust to living with my parents.

DR: What happened?

GARY: I had been living in Croatia for two years, tutoring college students in English, and it was going great but then they did not renew my contract, and I figured I needed to get back home to regroup. So, I moved back in with my parents, temporarily, until I find a job.

DR: Is this making you upset?

GARY: Very. I am 35 years old. I did not expect to be living with my parents at 35.

DR: Did you imagine something different? (*Perfectionism*)

GARY: Of course I did, because I always tried to do my best. Straight As and all that.

DR: Are you a perfectionist?

GARY: You could say so.

DR: Can you tell me a little more about your life plans and your life goals? (*Unrealistic life goals*)

GARY: I always wanted to be a writer and a professor. My father is a writer, my mother teaches at NYU. I was writing and publishing when I was in high school. I could not get an academic job after college, but I worked for a publishing house and wrote two novels. I also tutored, until I got a university job in Croatia. It worked great for two years and then I got into a fight with the stupid administrator, and they did not renew my contract. I thought I had a good CV, but I applied to several teaching jobs and nothing.

DR: Do you think you could still be a professor?

GARY: Why shouldn't I? I am working hard for it.

DR: Did you think you would be happier at 35? (*Entitlement to happiness*)

GARY: Of course. Who expects to be miserable? Ten years ago, I thought I would be on top of the world by now.

DR: Are you saying that from where you were 10 years ago, you should be feeling a lot happier than you are now?

GARY: Exactly. I graduated from Cornell, did all the right things, even after I was diagnosed with bipolar.

DR: I am sorry, it must have been rough for you. Do you think from everything that you've done, you deserve to be happy?

GARY: I have put in more than enough effort, a lot more than other people I know. This is just so unfair.

DR: Are you saying that life has not been fair to you?

GARY: Isn't this what I just said? Do you think I planned on having a manic break in the first year of college?

DR: How important is this career to you? (*Failure to redirect to more realistic goals*)

GARY: I cannot see myself doing anything else. I am a great teacher—all my students say so. I am also a good writer, and I have been published. I should be in academics.

DR: Can you see yourself doing other things?

GARY: Like what? Driving a cab?

DR: Well, some people would do that, but maybe for you something more intellectual. Would you consider becoming a schoolteacher, or perhaps changing careers and going to social work school?

GARY: After all that I have been through? All my college classmates have academic jobs or are doctors and lawyers. There is a job opening at Stony Brook I am a perfect fit for. I should hear from them this week.

DR: What if you are not able to get the right job? How hard would it be to live without it?

GARY: I must get it. There is nothing else out there and I cannot continue living off my parents, it is just too embarrassing.

DR: What part was embarrassing? Everybody goes through difficult times. (*Humiliating defeat*)

GARY: It would be a disaster. I have no money, my parents are sick of supporting me. They keep saying that I must get a job. My sister is a lawyer, and she is not as smart as I am. And here I am. I was not able to get an academic job in the States, I lost one in Croatia, and here I am again, living off my parents.

DR: You sound defeated. Is this how you feel?

GARY: Exactly.

DR: Is it humiliating?

GARY: It is beyond humiliating. I cannot take a girl out on a date—I have to ask my parents for money. And what will I tell her? That I am an unemployed writer at 35 living with my parents?

DR: Do many people know about this?

GARY: When my contract didn't get renewed in Croatia, it was pretty public. All my friends knew. My girlfriend dumped me—good riddance:She did not love me, and she just wanted a green card. This is one of the reasons I came back to the US. And here—I am sure my parents are talking to their friends, unless they are ashamed to. I tried to call a couple of my old friends. Can't talk to any of them; I feel so small by comparison.

DR: Do you think you may be exaggerating?

GARY: I am not exaggerating. I went to a club last Friday. I had to go alone, and no girl would even dance with me.

DR: Do you feel alone? (*Thwarted belongingness*)

GARY: Terribly.

DR: Even when you are with people?

GARY: What people? I told you I have lost all my friends; I have nothing in common with them. And girls wouldn't even look at me.

DR: This sounds worse than alone; this sounds like you feel alienated. Is there anybody or anything that you feel connected to? Maybe professionally?

GARY: Well, I should feel connected to other writers, or academics—but everybody is so self-centered. And successful. And I am not.

DR: How about people closest to you, your parents and your sister? (*Perceived burdensomeness*)

GARY: I cannot talk to my parents. My sister is too busy with her children and her Wall Street shark husband.

DR: Do you feel like you are a burden to them?

GARY: I know. My parents said they cannot support me forever, and that if I cannot find a job, I should go on disability. I can't ask my sister for money, it is too humiliating, and she needs it for her own family.

DR: How bad a burden do you think you are?

GARY: They are certainly acting like I am a burden. I am not asking them to support me "forever," just until I get a good teaching job. I will pay them back. . . . I think they can afford it—look at their lifestyle!

DR: Would they be relieved if you were not there?

GARY: Probably. . . . I don't think that they look forward to facing me every day.

DR: Do you think they would miss you if you weren't around?

GARY: Not sure.

DR: How do you see your future? (*Perception of no future*)

GARY: I can't. I need a teaching job, which looks more and more like a miracle. There are no jobs out there.

DR: Do you see other alternatives for yourself? Five years from now?

GARY: Like what? I can try to look for an editor job, but I have not done any editing for years. And they do not pay well. I can try to finish my novel, but that is not a job.

DR: Other choices? Maybe tutoring, some tutors make a lot of money, much more than college professors.

GARY: I can't stand tutoring! And I am not good at it—I get too impatient with stupid students. . . . Tutor at 35? After being a professor? I would rather kill myself!

DR: Have you been thinking about killing yourself? (*Suicide intent and plan*)

GARY: Yes, but I would never do it. . . . I don't have the guts.

DR: I may come back to this a little later, if you do not mind, but now I have just a few questions about your life situation. Do you feel trapped in it?

GARY: Yes.

DR: Do you see any exits?

GARY: Not really.

DR: Is there anything that can be done to improve the situation?

GARY: Do you have a job for me?

DR: (*Constructing Suicidal Narrative*) Let me make sure I understand. From what you are telling me, it seems that you do not see a future for yourself because the only professional life goal you see—the academic career—is unreachable. You are a perfectionist and you have been working hard to make your dreams come true. It is just so unfair that despite that you are forced into living with your parents, who make you feel like a burden. I condensed it a little, but does this ring a bell?

GARY: Yeah, I can identify with this, and the humiliation is just unbearable.

DR: What do you mean by unbearable?

GARY: I am not sure if I can take it much longer.

Gary identifies with all seven aspects of the SN: The goal of the academic career he is chasing is unattainable, he feels defeated and alienated, he believes that he is a burden to his parents, and, finally, he understands that he does not have good options. His false hope for a miracle job opening and even more miraculous interview is likely to be dashed soon. Gary's SN suggests very high risk (Table 6.1).

Case 39: Moderate Risk for Imminent Suicide

Bernie is a 53-year-old single gay man with a history of generalized anxiety disorder who came for treatment of his depression with suicidal ideation after he discovered that his just deceased partner of 20 years had a family and children. Bernie had a plan to kill himself with a barbiturate and alcohol overdose. He has just retired from his teaching job. He has one brother and a large circle

Table 6.1 Suicide narrative risk assessment, Case 38

Component	Risk Level				
	Minimal	Low	Moderate	High	Severe
Unrealistic life goals				X	
Entitlement to happiness					X
Failure to redirect to more realistic goals					X
Humiliating personal or social defeat					X
Perceived burdensomeness					X
Thwarted belongingness					X
Perception of no future				X	
Total					X

of friends. He had seen a therapist twice in the past following relationship breakups, but he was never on medications and had no past suicide attempts.

DR: How are you feeling today? (*Forming rapport*)

BERNIE: I am still in shock from everything that happened.

DR: What exactly has been happening?

BERNIE: Well, he was the love of my life, he died in my arms, it was a fairy tale. . . . Twenty years together, he would come home, I would make dinner. Twenty years . . .

DR: And?

BERNIE: He got diagnosed with liver cancer last month, it was really quick, and I took him home, he wanted to die in our bed. And I took care of the funeral, and then this Korean woman shows up I have never met, with two teenagers, and tells me she is his wife! He had a wife!

DR: Are you angry?

BERNIE: I am not angry, I love him.

DR: You said your relationship was perfect. . . . Let me ask you maybe a strange question, but trust me, it is not strange: Are you a perfectionist? (*Perfectionism*)

BERNIE: Strange question, you're right. No, I am not, I am actually pretty easy-going. I do my job, but I don't go crazy about it, I am not too hard on my students.

DR: What about your relationship? You said it was perfect. . . . Were you a perfectionist about that?

BERNIE: I am not sure, it just happened. He was on a tour with this dance company, and we met in a bar. It was love at first sight, and then he defected, and we stayed together, and it was perfect.

DR: Still, do you think that somewhere out there may be somebody like John . . . but truthful?

BERNIE: What do you mean?

DR: Well, it sounds he was not truthful with you for many years. . . . Some people would say that he betrayed your trust.

BERNIE: I am not sure what you mean. . . . We loved each other. I had coffee with his wife. I talked to her about how I could help her with the kids.

DR: But what if it does not work?

BERNIE: I should make it work, it is his family, and I do not need anybody else.

DR: Did you ever expect to be this happy?

BERNIE: Never. But after John and I got together, among all my friends, I was the happiest.

DR: Do you deserve to be happy? (*Entitlement to happiness*)

BERNIE: Everybody deserves to be happy, and I am not sure if I will ever be happy again.

DR: It sounds like the life was hard on you lately. . . . Now, after all that happened, would it be possible for you to be with somebody else? (*Failure to redirect to achievable goals*)

BERNIE: Never. I am trying to get to know his wife and his children. . . . I don't even know what he told them about me. Probably that I was a roommate and that he was saving money that way. I don't remember much from the funeral, all this feels like nightmare . . . a horror movie, and everything is in a fog.

DR: How about the fact that John was not truthful to you for 20 years? Don't you deserve somebody who would?

BERNIE: I don't know, I feel no anger. . . . I only feel love and sadness. Nothing will ever match it. And I don't need anything. Or anybody (crying).

DR: When you discovered that John was married . . . was, or is, this embarrassing for you? (*Social defeat*)

BERNIE: I understand why you would think so, but it was not. I have many friends, and they are all very supportive and sympathetic. Everybody is concerned; that's why I am here.

DR: What is everybody concerned about? Did you tell them about John's wife?

BERNIE: No, I didn't . . . I could not . . . I did not want them to think badly about him.

DR: What did you tell them?

BERNIE: That he died in my arms.

DR: Are you saying that telling them the truth would have been too humiliating for him? For his memory I mean.

BERNIE: Yes. . . . He was a saint.

DR: Do you feel alone (in this)? (*Thwarted belongingness*)

BERNIE: Not at all, as I said, I have a lot of support.

DR: I heard what you said. I meant do you know anybody else who ended up in your situation—having lived with somebody for 20 years, who was leading a . . . double life?

BERNIE: How dare you call it a "double life"?! John was incapable of lying.

DR: But he got married and had two children while you were together, and he did not tell you about it.

BERNIE: He must have had his reasons. . . . I can't think about it, I cannot talk about it.

DR: And you don't feel like you are a burden to them? (*Perceived burdensomeness*)

BERNIE: I try not to be a burden. I have enough friends and I am very considerate. Nobody complained. So far, that is.

DR: What are your plans in life? (*Perception of no future*)

BERNIE: I don't have any. I just retired and we planned to spend the rest of our lives together, and now it is impossible. That's why I think that my life is pointless. I would rather kill myself.

DR: I will have to ask you more about that later, but now I need to talk about something else. It may sound like an insensitive question to ask, but when one comes in suicidal, we must do everything to protect them. Do you think you can ever get over John's death, and maybe have another relationship?

BERNIE: You can't find another fairy tale. You are rationed just one in your lifetime, if any. I cannot have another fairy tale.

DR: But . . .

BERNIE: How can you go on living when your fairy tale has ended? There was no happy ending. . . . There cannot be—he is no longer with me. There is nothing I can do to bring him back. I see no future for myself. What is the point?

DR: Is there anything that can be done to improve the situation?

DR: (*Constructing Suicidal Narrative*) Let me make sure I understand the situation correctly. It seems that you wanted a perfect relationship and were incredibly lucky to have one for 20 years. It ended tragically and you learned some shocking things about John that put you in a bind:If your relationship was what you thought it was, a fairy tale, then nothing can ever match it, there is no point in living, and you want to kill yourself. Admitting that John was lying to you would ruin the fairy tale—and then what?

BERNIE: Nothing can ruin my fairy tale. . . . I loved him so much.

DR: Fortunately, you have friends to support you and as a considerate person you try not to burden them too much. Does this sound right?

BERNIE: Most of it. Except he wasn't lying.

DR: How is this possible?

BERNIE: I don't know; he just wasn't. . . . I will never meet anybody like him, even if I try.

DR: Will you try?

BERNIE: I don't know.

In contrast to Gary, who does not volunteer suicidal thoughts or plans, Bernie's presenting complaint is active suicidal ideation and intent. Yet, at this moment, Bernie's narrative is less alarming than Gary's. Bernie's drive for a perfect relationship is as strong as Gary's aspiration for an academic career, and he has seemingly achieved it in his 20-year fairy tale relationship with John, except, of course, it was based on a lie. Bernie's image of his life is as elusive as Gary's hope for an academic job, if not more. For Bernie, acknowledging the truth to himself and to others appears to signify destruction of the only thing that made his life meaningful—his love for John. Bernie is also very conscious that he is trapped between a rock and a hard place with very few options: He will try to date, but he is not emotionally available, and his dating is likely to lead nowhere. However, his social support is fairly strong, and he feels neither defeated, alienated, nor like a burden. Hence, at this moment, he should be considered a moderate risk for imminent suicide (Table 6.2). This risk will increase drastically if he is unable to come to terms with his past and move on to another relationship.

Case 40: Low Risk for Imminent Suicide

Kate is a 28-year-old woman who was admitted to a psychiatric unit for a suicide attempt. Kate repeatedly cut her left arm and left thigh with a razor blade

Table 6.2 Suicide narrative risk assessment, Case 39

Component	Minimal	Low	Moderate	High	Severe
			Risk Level		
Unrealistic life goals			X		
Entitlement to happiness			X		
Failure to redirect to more realistic goals				X	
Humiliating personal or social defeat				X	
Perceived burdensomeness			X		
Thwarted belongingness		X			
Perception of no future				X	
Total		X			

after she was let go from a nonprofit after a falling out with her supervisor. The cuts were deep enough for her thigh wounds to require sutures. Kate had a long psychiatric history and was diagnosed with attention deficit disorder as a child and with major depressive disorder, generalized anxiety disorder, panic disorder, and borderline personality disorder in high school. She was accepted to, but never completed, college, despite several attempts to do so. She worked only sporadically, mainly for environmental causes, and was supported by her father. During the interview, Kate was confrontational and provocative.

DR: How are you feeling today? (*Forming rapport*)
KATE: I am feeling awful.
DR: What is making you feel awful?
KATE: I was in Europe traveling, working for a cause, and then I met somebody who was nice at first, but then horrible to me, and I was in so much pain that I cut myself. I was bleeding and went to the ER, and they sutured me but then put me onto the psych unit. I don't know why.
DR: I will ask you about your suicide attempt a little later if you do not mind; Please tell me what cause were you working on?
KATE: The environment. We are sucking the life out of the environment. If we continue like this, soon there will be no resources left. We used up most of the oil already and so many species are endangered. We need to organize and stop this. I have been canvassing and organizing people.
DR: And what was so special about this person to you that you attempted suicide when things did not work out?

KATE: He also cared about environment and was working for this non-profit ... or pretended to care. ... In either case, I volunteered for him and then he turned out to be a jerk—I always meet jerks. That hurts.

DR: Do you always meet jerks, as you say, or are you a perfectionist? (*Perfectionism*)

KATE: Certainly not. I am very accepting of people's faults, except they must be liberal. I always try to give it my best, but it does not always work ... and my room is a mess.

DR: Can you tell me more about your causes? (*Unrealistic life goals*)

KATE: I only have one:the environment. Nobody understands how serious the damage is we are causing our planet. Do you want me to elaborate?

DR: Please do; that's why I asked.

KATE: Global warming is the biggest immediate problem. The climate has already changed, yearly temperature just keeps setting records. Hurricane Sandy was the worst ever, and then ... there are the natural resources:We are running out of oil, and there's deforestation in the Amazon. People just don't understand how bad it is going to get. ... Nobody listens ... they just don't get it.

DR: Does fighting for the environment make you happy?
(*Entitlement to happiness*)

KATE: Hah, I wish I were happy. I am either unhappy or depressed.

DR: Do you think this will change?

KATE: It better—one can't live like this. I hope it does, but I have been on this depression rollercoaster for so long that it's hard to keep the hope.

DR: This question may feel strange to you, but bear with me:Do think that you deserve to be happy?

KATE: Everybody does ...

DR: But at the moment I am not concerned with everybody, I'm asking about you:Are you entitled to happiness?

KATE: In a fair world I would be: I am a fair person, I care for others, I fight for causes ... I always do my best.

DR: How important is this cause to you?
(*Failure to redirect to more realistic life goals*)

KATE: It is my whole life!

DR: If for some reason you can't champion this cause—will you champion another?

KATE: What can be more important than the environment? And I don't see why I would need to.

DR: You attempted suicide after a conflict with your supervisor.

KATE: There are other supervisors. . . . I live for the environment.

DR: You said that people don't listen. Does this make you feel defeated? (*Social defeat*)

KATE: It can be frustrating, but I don't give up.

DR: You cut yourself after you were let go. Why? Was it humiliating?

KATE: It wasn't humiliating; it was infuriating. I felt so betrayed, and so angry, and did not know how to live at that moment, and so I cut myself.

DR: Did the meeting with your supervisor make you feel defeated?

KATE: I am not defeated. I am a fighter. I will find another organization.

DR: Do many people know about this?

KATE: My family and friends; everybody knows!

DR: How hard was it for you to face them?

KATE: Well, it was not fun, but I did, didn't I? That's why I am here . . .

DR: What do your friends think? I mean your close friends? (*Thwarted belongingness*)

KATE: I only have two close friends, and they think I should not be cutting myself and that I should get some help.

DR: So, do you feel disconnected even from people who are closest to you?

KATE: Sometimes. They get tired of me . . .

DR: Do you feel like you are a burden to them? (*Perceived burdensomeness*)

KATE: Not really . . . maybe emotionally . . .

DR: Not financially? I thought your job was a volunteer job.

KATE: They only pay my rent. I have inherited some money from my grandmother. It should last another year.

DR: And after that?

KATE: After that I will have to get a job.

DR: Have you ever had a paying job?

KATE: No, but my volunteer job was very important, and I am very responsible.

DR: Did your supervisor feel that way?

KATE: He turned out to be a jerk.

DR: So, what does the future hold for you? (*Perception of no future*)

KATE: I will take some time off and maybe go on a yoga retreat.

DR: And then?

KATE: And then I will look for a job.

DR: What kind?

KATE: For the cause, of course. . . . Something to do with environment.

DR: What are your options?

KATE: I will find something.

DR: Do you have people you can ask for a reference letter? I suspect your supervisor is not one of them.

KATE: No, and I would not ask him if you would pay me. I will find somebody.

DR: (*Constructing Suicidal Narrative*) It seems that you met somebody who you thought had the same goals that you did and really understood you, but then he turned on you—unexpectedly—and that was so painful that you wanted to die. But then you didn't, and it sounds like you have a pretty good support system and that you still have options for how to volunteer for the cause . . . as long as you still have your inheritance. Does this sound right?

KATE: Sounds about right . . . . You are very smart.

DR: Thank you. Does all this apply to you?

KATE: Even worse: I really started caring for the guy. . . . I thought we were going to be a couple.

DR: Twice disappointed!

KATE: I have got to go back out there and start looking . . .

Although Kate attempted suicide and may do so again in the future, her current suicide risk is relatively low (Table 6.3), primarily because she does not feel trapped and thinks she has options for the future. However, Kate only has options because her inheritance shelters her from the need to support herself. She has few friends, her goal of converting everybody into an

Table 6.3   Suicide narrative risk assessment, Case 40

Component	Minimal	Low	Moderate	High	Severe
Unrealistic life goals		X			
Entitlement to happiness			X		
Failure to redirect to more realistic goals					X
Humiliating personal or social defeat			X		
Perceived burdensomeness	X				
Thwarted belongingness		X			
Perception of no future	X				
Total		X			

environmentalist is unattainable, and her approach to life lacks maturity. There is a good chance that once she runs out of funds, she will become a burden on her parents, with very few options. At that point, her life may take the shape of the SN, and her risk for imminent suicide will increase.

Test Case 2

Zhang is a 20-year-old Chinese student at Queens College who was admitted to a local hospital after being admitted to the emergency department for a suicide attempt by methanol poisoning. He was dialyzed in the MICU and was transferred to an inpatient psychiatric unit. Zhang was treated with medications, and the following interview was conducted on the eve of his discharge:

DR: How are you feeling today?

ZHANG: Much better, I feel much better, I am ready to go home.

DR: You were admitted after a suicide attempt; what has changed? What is different now, after two weeks in the hospital?

ZHANG: My thoughts are better, and I don't think the same thing all the time. I am not depressed anymore.

DR: What was making you depressed when you came in?

ZHANG: I had these bad thoughts I could not stop.

DR: What were you thinking?

ZHANG: I cannot talk about them, it is private.

DR: Were these thoughts getting in the way of what you were trying to achieve in life?

ZHANG: I could not study, the thoughts were just too upsetting . . . and they just keep coming, over and over . . . like in a loop. My grades dropped.

DR: Did your parents get upset?

ZHANG: Yes, I am pre-med, and they sacrificed everything for me when they came from China. They want me to be a doctor and they always ask about grades. I had good grades in high school.

DR: Are you a perfectionist?

ZHANG: I have to be, I don't have a choice.

DR: If you are a perfectionist, you must be working very hard. Are you a hard worker?

ZHANG: I am a hard worker, but I should work harder.

DR: In a fair world, for the effort you put in, do you deserve to be happy?

ZHANG: Not now, but if get into medical school, I do.

DR: How important is a medical career for you?

ZHANG: Very important. It is everything for me. I always wanted to be a doctor for as long as I can remember.

DR: Why?

ZHANG: I don't know. It is something I always wanted to do.

DR: Do your parents want you to be a doctor?

ZHANG: Yes, they are very supportive.

DR: Can you find an alternative?

ZHANG: I never thought of that. Like what?

DR: Like other medical professions. Like a PA, a nurse, or even a social worker. Social workers help people.

ZHANG: I don't know. Maybe. Not sure (*silence, staring into space*).

DR: You seem hesitant, why?

ZHANG: I don't think my parents would like it. They will be disappointed . . .

DR: After you saw your grades and thought that you may not get into med school, you almost killed yourself. Can you go on living without med school?

ZHANG: Now I can, I feel much better than before.

DR: What is the worst thing about possibly dropping out of the pre-med program?

ZHANG: I just would not know how to tell my parents; I would let them down. I would let the whole family down. I would die of embarrassment.

DR: You almost did. Would it be humiliating?

ZHANG: Very humiliating.

DR: Is it possible that these are just your fears, but they would actually understand?

ZHANG: No, they would be very upset. They are very proud of me. They always talk about me being a doctor to the rest of the family. They say, they immigrated for me, so I could be happy. If I don't get in, they would tell me they immigrated for nothing . . .

DR: Your parents come to visit you in the hospital every day. Do they know about your grades?

ZHANG: No, I didn't tell them. They always compare me to Xu—he always gets straight As and he is at Cornell, and I am in Queens College, I didn't get in.

DR: You sound like this is a race, and you have been losing even before you got any grades.

ZHANG: I did, but I thought if I get straight As I could make up for not getting into an Ivy League.

DR: Are your parents supporting you?

ZHANG: Yes, they pay my tuition, and they give me money for books and lunch. I also live at home, and they pay for my food.

DR: Do you feel like you are a burden to them?

ZHANG: I know I am—they always talk about money, and they are in their grocery store 16 hours a day.

DR: Are you close to your parents?

ZHANG: I guess so.

DR: I mean, do you do things together? Do you tell them about what is happening in your life? Do they tell you what is happening in theirs?

ZHANG: Aah. This is, like, American. We do things together—like sharing work around the house, but we don't talk very much.

DR: What about your friends? Are you the type of person who always has many friends or one or two best friends?

ZHANG: One or two best friends.

DR: When is the last time you talked to one of them?

ZHANG: I don't know. Maybe a month. I am too busy at school and helping my parents around the house.

DR: Did you tell them you are here?

ZHANG: No, I can't. I am too ashamed.

DR: You must feel very alone. How about here, in the hospital?

ZHANG: Not here—there are always nurses and staff.

DR: You said earlier: I just would not know how to tell my parents; I would let them down.

ZHANG: I would let the whole family down. I would die of embarrassment.

DR: Does this mean you have not told them?

ZHANG: Yes.

DR: Are you planning to tell them?

ZHANG: I don't have a choice.

DR: Are there any good choices in your situation?

ZHANG: No.

DR: Have you thought about your possible options, when you are discharged? I mean if you were no longer a pre-med?

ZHANG: No. I don't want to think about it.

DR: But you will have to, right?

ZHANG: (*Silence, looks down*)

DR: (*Constructing Suicidal Narrative*) From what you are saying, it seems that your family planned for you to be a doctor and that you have been working toward this goal almost since you remember yourself. But not all goals are attainable, and it seems that you have not thought of any alternatives, Plan B, so to speak. So, if pre-med does not work out, there do not seem to be any good choices for you. Dropping out of the pre-med program may feel like a defeat in the battle for med school you have been fighting, and also very hard on your parents, who will feel like they have failed in the eyes of your community. You also said that you feel ashamed to be a burden to them, and it seems that you are kind of by yourself. Does this sound right?

ZHANG: Yeah . . . (*Silence*)

Zhang's whole life may be seen as one evolving SN (Table 6.4). Perfectionist since childhood, devoted to the goal of becoming a doctor to uphold the honor of his family, he does not have the mental aptitude to achieve his goal, nor does he have the flexibility to disengage from it. Abandoning a medical career will signify disgrace for his family and ostracism in his community. He is not even in a position to seek support from his family or friends, which leaves him isolated, internally humiliated and defeated, without any chance for support from others. His failure is about

Table 6.4 Suicide narrative risk assessment, Test Case 2

	Risk Level				
Component	Minimal	Low	Moderate	High	Severe
Unrealistic life goals					
Entitlement to happiness					
Failure to redirect to more realistic goals					
Humiliating personal or social defeat					
Perceived burdensomeness					
Thwarted belongingness					
Perception of no future					
Total					

to become public, and he is at a very high risk of ending his life, either to avoid the pain of admitting his failure to his parents or after facing their inevitable extreme disappointment.

References

Andreassen, C. S., Griffiths, M. D., Sinha, R., Hetland, J., & Pallesen, S. (2016). The relationships between workaholism and symptoms of psychiatric disorders: A large-scale cross-sectional study. *PLOS One, 11*(5), e0152978. https://doi.org/10.1371/jour nal.pone.0152978

Baumeister, R. F., & Leary, M. R. (1995). The need to belong: Desire for interpersonal attachments as a fundamental human motivation. *Psychological Bulletin, 117*(3), 497–529. https://doi.org/10.1037/0033-2909.117.3.497

Beck, A. T., Kovacs, M., & Weissman, A. (1975). Hopelessness and suicidal behavior: An overview. *JAMA, 234*(11), 1146–1149. https://doi.org/10.1001/jama.234.11.1146

Bhise, M. C., & Behere, P. B. (2016). Risk ractors for farmers' suicides in central rural India: Matched case-control psychological autopsy study. *Indian Journal of Psychological Medicine, 38*(6), 560–566. https://doi.org/10.4103/0253-7176.194905

Bloch-Elkouby, S., Gorman, B., Lloveras, L., Wilkerson, T., Schuck, A., Barzilay, S., Calati, R., Schnur, D., & Galynker, I. (2020). How do distal and proximal risk factors combine to predict suicidal ideation and behaviors? A prospective study of the narrative crisis model of suicide. *Journal of Affective Disorders, 277*, 914–926. https://doi.org/10.1016/j.jad.2020.08.08

Bogart, L. M., Benotsch, E. G., & Pavlovic, J. D. (2004). Feeling superior but threatened: The relation of narcissism to social comparison. *Basic and Applied Social Psychology, 26*(1), 35–44. https://doi.org/10.1207/s15324834basp2601_4

Cacioppo, J. T., & Patrick, W. (2008). *Loneliness: Human nature and the need for social connection.* W.W. Norton.

Carver, C. S., & Scheier, M. F. (1998). *On the self-regulation of behavior.* Cambridge University Press.

Chistopolskaya K. A., Rogers M. L., Cao, E., Galynker, I., Richards, J., Enikolopov, S. N., Nikolaev, E. L., Sadovnichaya, V. S., & Drovosekov, S. E. (2020). Adaptation of the suicidal narrative inventory in a Russian sample [in Russian]. *Suicidology, 11*(4), 76–90. https://doi.org/10.32878/suiciderus.20-11-04(41)-76-90

Chu, C., Buchman-Schmitt, J. M., Stanley, I. H., Hom, M. A., Tucker, R. P., Hagan, C. R., Rogers, M. L., Podlogar, M. C., Chiurliza, B., Ringer, F. B., Michaels, M. S., Patros, C., & Joiner, T. E. (2017). The interpersonal theory of suicide: A systematic review and meta-analysis of a decade of cross-national research. *Psychological Bulletin, 143*(12), 1313–1345. https://doi.org/10.1037/bul0000123

Cohen, L. J., Gorman, B., Briggs, J., Jeon, M. E., Ginsburg, T., & Galynker, I. (2019). The suicidal narrative and its relationship to the suicide crisis syndrome and recent suicidal behavior. *Suicide and Life-Threatening Behavior, 49*(2), 413–422.

Conaghan, S., & Davidson, K. M. (2002). Hopelessness and the anticipation of positive and negative future experiences in older parasuicidal adults. *The British Journal of Clinical Psychology, 41*(3), 233–242. https://doi.org/10.1348/014466502760379208

Crocker, J., & Knight, K. M. (2005). Contingencies of self-worth. *Current Directions in Psychological Science*, 14(4), 200–203. https://doi.org/10.1111/j.0963-7214.2005.00364.x

Deisenhammer, E. A., Ing, C. M., Strauss, R., Kemmler, G., Hinterhuber, H., & Weiss, E. M. (2009). The duration of the suicidal process: How much time is left for intervention between consideration and accomplishment of a suicide attempt? *The Journal of Clinical Psychiatry*, 70(1), 19–24.

Fässberg, M. M., van Orden, K. A., Duberstein, P., Erlangsen, A., Lapierre, S., Bodner, E., Canetto, S. S., De Leo, D., Szanto, K., & Waern, M. (2012). A systematic review of social factors and suicidal behavior in older adulthood. *International Journal of Environmental Research and Public Health*, 9(3), 722–745. https://doi.org/10.3390/ijerph9030722

Fawcett, J., Scheftner, W. A., Fogg, L., Clark, D. C., Young, M. A., Hedeker, D., & Gibbons, R. (1990). Time-related predictors of suicide in major affective disorder. *American Journal of Psychiatry*, 147(9), 1189–1994.

Feuer, A. (2008, March 7). Four charged with running online prostitution ring. *The New York Times*. http://www.nytimes.com/ 2008/03/07/nyregion/07prostitution.html?_r=0

Gilbert, P. (2001). Depression and stress: A biopsychosocial exploration of evolved functions and mechanisms. *Stress (Amsterdam, Netherlands)*, 4(2), 121–135. https://doi.org/10.3109/10253890109115726

Grubbs, J. B., & Exline, J. J. (2016). Trait entitlement: A cognitive-personality source of vulnerability to psychological distress. *Psychological Bulletin*, 142(11), 1204–1226. https://doi.org/10.1037/bul0000063

Hatcher, S., & Stubbersfield, O. (2013). Sense of belonging and suicide: A systematic review. *Canadian Journal of Psychiatry/Revue canadienne de psychiatrie*, 58(7), 432–436. https://doi.org/10.1177/070674371305800709

Heckhausen, J., Wrosch, C., & Schulz, R. (2010). A motivational theory of life-span development. *Psychological Review*, 117(1), 32–60. https://doi.org/10.1037/a0017668

Heikkinen, M., Aro, H., & Lönnqvist, J. (1994). Recent life events, social support and suicide. *Acta Psychiatrica Scandinavica Supplementum*, 377, 65–72. https://doi.org/10.1111/j.1600-0447.1994.tb05805.x

Herszenhorn, D. M. (2013, March 23). Russian oligarch and sharp critic of Putin dies in London. *The New York Times*. http:// www.nytimes.com/2013/03/24/world/europe/boris-a-berezovsky-a-putin- critic-dies-at-67.html

Höller, I., Teismann, T., Cwik, J. C., Glaesmer, H., Spangenberg, L., Hallensleben, N., Paashaus, L., Rath, D., Schönfelder, A., Juckel, G., & Forkmann, T. (2020). Short Defeat and Entrapment Scale: A psychometric investigation in three German samples. *Comprehensive Psychiatry*, 98, 152160. https://doi.org/10.1016/j.comppsych.2020.152160

Hunter, E. C., & O'Connor, R. C. (2003). Hopelessness and future thinking in parasuicide: The role of perfectionism. *The British Journal of Clinical Psychology*, 42(4), 355–365. https://doi.org/10.1348/014466503322528900

Jahn, D. R., & Cukrowicz, K. C. (2011). The impact of the nature of relationships on perceived burdensomeness and suicide ideation in a community sample of older adults. *Suicide and Life-Threatening Behavior*, 41(6), 635–649.

Joiner, T. E. (2005). *Why people die by suicide*. Harvard University Press.

Joiner, T. E., Jr., Brown, J. S., & Wingate, L. R. (2005). The psychology and neurobiology of suicidal behavior. *Annual Review of Psychology*, *56*, 287–314.

Joiner, T. E., Jr., Hollar, D., & Van Orden, K. (2006). On Buckeyes, Gators, Super Bowl Sunday, and the Miracle on Ice: "Pulling together" is associated with lower suicide rates. *Journal of Social and Clinical Psychology*, *25*(2), 179–195. https://doi.org/10.1521/ jscp.2006.25.2.179

Joiner, T. E., Jr., Pettit, J. W., Walker, R. L., Voelz, Z. R., Cruz, J., Rudd, M. D., & Lester, D. (2002). Perceived burdensomeness and suicidality: Two studies on the suicide notes of those attempting and those completing suicide. *Journal of Social and Clinical Psychology*, *21*(5), 531–545. https://doi.org/10.1521/jscp.21.5.531.22624

Joiner, T. E., Van Orden, K. A., Witte, T. K., Selby, E. A., Ribeiro, J. D., Lewis, R., & Rudd, M. D. (2009). Main predictions of the interpersonal-psychological theory of suicidal behavior: Empirical tests in two samples of young adults. *Journal of Abnormal Psychology*, *118*(3), 634–646. https://doi.org/10.1037/a0016500

Kannuri, N. K., & Jadhav, S. (2021). Cultivating distress: Cotton, caste and farmer suicides in India. *Anthropology & Medicine*, *28*(4), 558–575. https://doi.org/10.1080/13648 470.2021.1993630

Kanzler, K. E., Bryan, C. J., McGeary, D. D., & Morrow, C. E. (2012). Suicidal ideation and perceived burdensomeness in patients with chronic pain. *Pain Practice*, *12*(8), 602–609.

Kassinove, H., & Sukhodolsky, D. G. (1995). Optimism, pessimism and worry in Russian and American children and adolescents. *Journal of Social Behavior & Personality*, *10*(1), 157–168.

Katzenmajer-Pump, L., & Balázs, J. (2021). Perfectionism and suicide: A systematic review of qualitative studies. *Psychiatria Hungarica*, *36*(1), 4–11.

Kemp Cooney, J. (2019). Suicide rates have soared among middle-aged white women in the U.S. *Population Health Research Brief Series*, March 2019(2). https://surface.syr. edu/lerner/5

Keneally, M., Nathan, S., & Collins, L. (2014, March 18). Designer L'Wren Scott was "embarrassed and millions in debt" when she committed suicide in her Manhattan apartment while "devastated" lover Mick Jagger was on tour in Australia. *Daily Mail*. http:// www.dailymail.co.uk/news/article-2582815/Mick-Jaggers-girlfriend- designer-LWren-Scott-commits-suicide.html

Kessler, R. C., Galea, S., Jones, R. T., Parker, H. A., & Hurricane Katrina Community Advisory Group. (2006). Mental illness and suicidality after Hurricane Katrina. *Bulletin of the World Health Organization*, *84*(12), 930–939. https://doi.org/10.2471/ blt.06.033019

Khazem, L. R. (2018). Physical disability and suicide: Recent advancements in understanding and future directions for consideration. *Current Opinion in Psychology*, *22*, 18–22. https://doi.org/10.1016/j.copsyc.2017.07.018

Kleiman, E., Adams, L., & Kashdan, T., & Riskind, J. (2013). Gratitude and grit indirectly reduce risk of suicidal ideations by enhancing meaning in life: Evidence for a mediated moderation model. *Journal of Research in Personality*, *47*, 539–546. https://doi. org/10.1016/j.jrp.2013.04.007.

Knowlton, D. S., & Hagopian, K. J. (Eds.). (2013). *From entitlement to classroom: New directions for teaching and learning*. John Wiley & Sons.

Koivumaa-Honkanen, H., Honkanen, R., Viinamäki, H., Heikkilä, K., Kaprio, J., & Koskenvuo, M. (2001). Life satisfaction and suicide: A 20-year follow-up study. *The*

American Journal of Psychiatry, 158(3), 433–439. https://doi.org/10.1176/appi. ajp.158.3.433

Leinonen, T., Martikainen, P., Laaksonen, M., & Lahelma, E. (2013). Excess mortality after disability retirement due to mental disorders: Variations by socio-demographic factors and causes of death. *Social Psychiatry and Psychiatric Epidemiology, 49*(4), 639–649.

MacLeod, A. K., & Conway, C. (2007). Well-being and positive future thinking for the self versus others. *Cognition & Emotion, 21*(5), 1114–1124. https://doi.org/10.1080/026999 30601109507

MacLeod, A. K., Pankhania, B., Lee, M., & Mitchell, D. (1997). Brief communication: Parasuicide, depression and the anticipation of positive and negative future experiences. *Psychological Medicine, 27*(4), 973–977.

Mann, J. J., Waternaux, C., Haas, G. L., & Malone, K. M. (1999). Toward a clinical model of suicidal behavior in psychiatric patients. *American Journal of Psychiatry, 156*(2), 181–189.

McAdams, D. P., Josselson, R., & Lieblich, A. (2001). *Turns in the road: Narrative studies of lives in transition* (pp. xxi, 310). American Psychological Association. https://doi.org/ 10.1037/10410-000

McLean, K. C., Pasupathi, M., & Pals, J. L. (2007). Selves creating stories creating selves: A process model of self-development. *Personality and Social Psychology Review, 11*(3), 262–278. https://doi.org/10.1177/1088868307301034

Menon, V., Bafna, A. R., Rogers, M. L., Richards, J., & Galynker, I. (2022). Factor structure and validity of the Revised Suicide Crisis Inventory (SCI-2) among Indian adults. *Asian Journal of Psychiatry, 73*, 103119. https://doi.org/10.1016/j.ajp.2022.103119

Moeller, S. J., Crocker, J., & Bushman, B. J. (2009). Creating hostility and conflict: Effects of entitlement and self-image goals. *Journal of Experimental Social Psychology, 45*(2), 448–452. https://doi.org/10.1016/j.jesp.2008.11.005

Morrison, R., & O'Connor, R. C. (2008). A systematic review of the relationship between rumination and suicidality. *Suicide and Life-Threatening Behavior, 38*(5), 523–538. https://doi.org/10.1521/suli.2008.38.5.523

Nesse, R. (2000). Is depression an adaptation? *Archives of General Psychiatry, 1*, 14–20.

Newsom, C. R., Archer, R. P., Trumbetta, S., & Gottesman, I. I. (2003). Changes in adolescent response patterns on the MMPI/MMPI-A across four decades. *Journal of Personality Assessment, 81*(1), 74–84. https://doi.org/10.1207/S15327752JPA8101_07

O'Connor, E., Gaynes, B. N., Burda, B. U., Soh, C., & Whitlock, E. P. (2013). Screening for and treatment of suicide risk relevant to primary care: A systematic review for the U.S. Preventive Services Task Force. *Annals of Internal Medicine, 158*(10), 741–754. https:// doi.org/10.7326/0003-4819-158-10-201305210-00642

O'Connor R. C. (2007). The relations between perfectionism and suicidality: A systematic review. *Suicide and Life-Threatening Behavior, 37*(6), 698–714. https://doi.org/10.1521/ suli.2007.37.6.698

O'Connor, R. C., Connery, H., & Cheyne, W. M. (2000). Hopelessness: The role of depression, future directed thinking and cognitive vulnerability. *Psychology, Health & Medicine, 5*(2), 155–161. https://doi.org/10.1080/713690188

O'Connor, R. C., & Forgan, G. (2007). Suicidal thinking and perfectionism: The role of goal adjustment and behavioral inhibition/activation systems (BIS/BAS). *Journal of Rational-Emotive & Cognitive-Behavior Therapy, 25*(4), 321–341.

O'Connor, R. C., Fraser, L., Whyte, M. C., MacHale, S., & Masterton, G. (2009). Self-regulation of unattainable goals in suicide attempters: The relationship between goal disengagement, goal reengagement and suicidal ideation. *Behaviour Research and Therapy*, 47(2), 164–169. https://doi.org/10.1016/j.brat.2008.11.001. PMID:19103433.

O'Connor, R. C., & Kirtley, O. J. (2018). The integrated motivational-volitional model of suicidal behaviour. *Philosophical Transactions of the Royal Society of London*, 373(1754), 20170268. https://doi.org/10.1098/rstb.2017.0268. PMID:30012735. PMCID:PMC6053985.

O'Connor, R., O'Connor, D., O'Connor, S., Smallwood, J., & Miles, J. (2004). Hopelessness, stress, and perfectionism: The moderating effects of future thinking. *Cognition & Emotion*, 18(8),1099–1120. https://doi.org/10.1080/02699930441000067

O'Connor, R. C., & Portzky, G. (2018). The relationship between entrapment and suicidal behavior through the lens of the integrated motivational-volitional model of suicidal behavior. *Current Opinions in Psychology*, 22, 12–17. https://doi.org/10.1016/j.copsyc.2017.07.021. PMID:30122271.

O'Connor, R. C., Smyth, R., & Williams, J. M. G. (2015). Intrapersonal positive future thinking predicts repeat suicide attempts in hospital-treated suicide attempters. *Journal of Consulting and Clinical Psychology*, 83(1), 169–176. https://doi.org/10.1037/a0037846

Pals, J. L. (2006). Narrative identity processing of difficult life experiences: Pathways of personality development and positive self-transformation in adulthood. *Journal of Personality*, 74(4), 1079–1109. https://doi.org/10.1111/j.1467-6494.2006.00403.x

Pia, T., Galynker, I., Schuck, A., Sinclair, C., Ying, G., & Calati, R. (2020). Perfectionism and prospective near-term suicidal thoughts and behaviors: The mediation of fear of humiliation and suicide crisis syndrome. *International Journal of Environmental Research and Public Health*, 17(4), 1424. https://doi.org/10.3390/ijerph17041424

Pollak, O. H., Guzmán, E. M., Shin, K. E., & Cha, C. B. (2021). Defeat, entrapment, and positive future thinking: Examining key theoretical predictors of suicidal ideation among adolescents. *Frontiers in Psychology*, 12, 590388. https://doi.org/10.3389/fpsyg.2021.590388

Price, J. S., Sloman, L., Gardner, R., Jr., Gilbert, P., & Rohde, P. (1994). The social competition hypothesis of depression. *British Journal of Psychiatry*, 164, 309–315.

Qin, P., & Nordentoft, M. (2005). Suicide risk in relation to psychiatric hospitalization: Evidence based on longitudinal registers. *Archives of General Psychiatry*, 62(4), 427–432. https://doi.org/10.1001/archpsyc.62.4.427

Raj, S., Ghosh, D., Singh, T., Verma, S. K., & Arya, Y. K. (2021). Theoretical mapping of suicidal risk factors during the COVID-19 pandemic: A mini-review. *Frontiers in Psychiatry*, 11, 589614. https://doi.org/10.3389/fpsyt.2020.589614

Rasmussen, K. A., Slish, M. L., Wingate, L. R. R., Davidson, C. L., & Grant, D. M. M. (2012). Can perceived burdensomeness explain the relationship between suicide and perfectionism? *Suicide and Life-Threatening Behavior*, 42(2), 121–128.

Reynolds, J., Stewart, M., Macdonald, R., & Sischo, L. (2006). Have adolescents become too ambitious? High school seniors' educational and occupational plans, 1976 to 2000. *Social Problems*, 53(2), 186–206. https://doi.org/10.1525/sp.2006.53.2.186

Ryan, R. M., & Deci, E. L. (2000). Self-determination theory and the facilitation of intrinsic motivation, social development, and well-being. *American Psychologist*, 55(1), 68–78.

Serby, M. J., Brody, D., Amin, S., & Yanowitch, P. (2006). Eviction as a risk factor for suicide. *Psychiatric Services*, 57(2), 273–274.

Shneidman, E. S. (1998). *The suicidal mind*. Oxford University Press.

Siddaway, A. P., Taylor, P. J., Wood, A. M., & Schulz, J. (2015). A meta-analysis of perceptions of defeat and entrapment in depression, anxiety problems, posttraumatic stress disorder, and suicidality. *Journal of Affective Disorders, 184*, 149–159.

Simon, R. I. (2006). Imminent suicide: The illusion of short-term prediction. *Suicide and Life-Threatening Behavior, 36*(3), 296–301. https://doi.org/10.1521/suli.2006.36.3.296

Smith, M. M., Sherry, S. B., Chen, S., Saklofske, D. H., Mushquash, C., Flett, G. L., & Hewitt, P. L. (2017). The perniciousness of perfectionism: A meta-analytic review of the perfectionism-suicide relationship. *Journal of Personality, 86*(3), 522–542. https://doi.org/10.1111/jopy.12333

Sommerfeld, E., & Malek, S. (2019). Perfectionism moderates the relationship between thwarted belongingness and perceived burdensomeness and suicide ideation in adolescents. *The Psychiatric Quarterly, 90*(4), 671–681. https://doi.org/10.1007/s11126-019-09639-y

Stone, A. A., Schwartz, J. E., Broderick, J. E., & Deaton, A. (2010). A snapshot of the age distribution of psychological well-being in the United States. *Proceedings of the National Academy of Sciences, 107*(22), 9985–9990. https://doi.org/10.1073/pnas.1003744107

Strelan, P. (2007). The prosocial, adaptive qualities of just world beliefs: Implications for the relationship between justice and forgiveness. *Personality and Individual Differences, 43*(4), 881–890. https://doi.org/10.1016/j.paid.2007.02.015

Taylor, P. J., Gooding, P., Wood, A. M., & Tarrier, N. (2011). The role of defeat and entrapment in depression, anxiety and suicide. *Psychological Bulletin, 137*(3), 391–420.

Taylor, P. J., Wood, A. M., Gooding, P. A., Johnson, J., & Tarrier, N. (2009). Are defeat and entrapment best defined as a single construct? *Personality and Individual Differences, 47*, 795–797.

Tsai, A. C., Lucas, M., & Kawachi, I. (2015). Association between social integration and suicide among women in the United States. *JAMA Psychiatry, 72*(10), 987–993. https://doi.org/10.1001/jamapsychiatry.2015.1002

Tucker, R. P., O'Connor, R. C., & Wingate, L. R. (2016). An investigation of the relationship between rumination styles, hope, and suicide ideation through the lens of the integrated motivational-volitional model of suicidal behavior. *Archives of Suicide Research, 20*(4), 553–566. https://doi.org/10.1080/13811118.2016.1158682

Twenge, J. M. (2006). *Generation Me: Why today's young Americans are more confident, assertive, entitled—And more miserable than ever before.* Free Press.

Twenge, J. M., & Campbell, W. K. (2001). Age and birth cohort differences in self-esteem: A cross-temporal meta-analysis. *Personality and Social Psychology Review, 5*(4), 321–344. https://doi.org/10.1207/s15327957pspr0504_3

Twenge, J. M., Konrath, S., Foster, J. D., Campbell, W. K., & Bushman, B. J. (2008). Further evidence of an increase in narcissism among college students. *Journal of Personality, 76*(4), 919–928. https://doi.org/10.1111/j.1467-6494.2008.00509.x

Van Orden, K. A., Witte, T. K., James, L. M., Castro, Y., Gordon, K. H., Braithwaite, S. R., Holler, D. L., & Joiner, T. E. (2008). Suicidal ideation in college students varies across semesters: The mediating role of belongingness. *Suicide and Life-Threatening Behavior, 38*(4), 427–435.

Wetherall, K., Cleare, S., Eschle, S., Ferguson, E., O'Connor, D. B., O'Carroll, R. E., & O'Connor, R. C. (2018). From ideation to action: Differentiating between those who think about suicide and those who attempt suicide in a national study of young adults. *Journal of Affective Disorders, 241*, 475–483. https://doi.org/10.1016/j.jad.2018.07.074

Wetherall, K., Robb, K. A., & O'Connor, R. C. (2019). Social rank theory of depression: A systematic review of self-perceptions of social rank and their relationship with depressive symptoms and suicide risk. *Journal of Affective Disorders, 246*, 300–319. https://doi.org/10.1016/j.jad.2018.12.045

Wrosch, C., Scheier, M. F., Miller, G. E., Schulz, R., & Carver, C. S. (2003). Adaptive self-regulation of unattainable goals: Goal disengagement, goal reengagement, and subjective well-being. *Personality and Social Psychology Bulletin, 29*(12), 1494–1508. https://doi.org/10.1177/0146167203256921

Ying, G., Chennapragada, L., Musser, E. D., & Galynker, I. (2021). Behind therapists' emotional responses to suicidal patients: A study of the narrative crisis model of suicide and clinicians' emotions. *Suicide and Life-Threatening Behavior, 51*(4), 684–695. https://doi.org/10.1111/sltb.12730

Zhang, J., & Lester, D. (2008). Psychological tensions found in suicide notes: A test for the strain theory of suicide. *Archives of Suicide Research, 12*(1), 67–73.

7

Suicide Crisis Syndrome

Distinction between Chronic Long-Term and Acute
Short-Term Suicide Risk

In routine clinical work, mental health professionals are required to conduct daily assessments of imminent suicide risk. This routine task provides clinicians with a unique opportunity for suicide prevention. Of note, between 60% and 98% of all suicide decedents worldwide carry a psychiatric diagnosis (Bachmann, 2018; Chang et al., 2011), while 50% to 70% of decedents saw a clinician within the month preceding their death (Chang et al., 2011). Moreover, close to 80% had contact with their primary care clinician within one year of their death (Stene-Larsen & Reneflot, 2019). As discussed in previous chapters, serious mood and psychotic disorders carry a 4- to 50-fold increased risk for completed suicide (Appleby et al., 2012; Van Os & Kapur, 2009), with half of all completed suicides having been related to depressive and other mood disorders (Bachmann, 2018). Thus, clinicians are in an opportune position to identify those at imminent risk for suicide. However, given the 4% completion rate among those with mental illness, coupled with the absence of reliable methods for assessment of imminent risk, the task of detecting those who will go on to attempt suicide in the immediate future is very difficult.

Recognizing the constraints of relying on long-term risk factors to predict imminent suicide, Fawcett and colleagues (1990) were among the first researchers to investigate short-term suicide risk. In a sample of individuals with affective disorders, they discovered that the clinical features related to suicides within one year and those related to suicides over two to 10 years after the study intake were different: three well-known suicide risk factors—severe hopelessness, suicidal ideation (SI), and past suicide attempt—were predictive of suicide in two to 10 years of follow-up, but they were not predictive of suicide within one year. On the other hand, among the six clinical factors predictive of suicide within one year, only one factor—severe loss of interest or pleasure (anhedonia)—was directly related to the symptoms of major depression. The other short-term predictors the researchers discovered were largely related to anxiety, including panic attacks, psychic anxiety, diminished concentration, insomnia, and moderate alcohol abuse.

Fawcett et al.'s (1990) study provided empirical support for the existence of an acute, transdiagnostic suicidal state. While Fawcett did not conceptualize the symptoms associated with short-term risk as a psychiatric syndrome, his work and that of others laid the groundwork for the concept of "warning signs of suicide," described in the next section. At the same time, because of the complexity of suicidal behavior, as well as the logistical and ethical difficulties in conducting prospective research on suicidal patients, a well-validated and universally accepted tool for assessing imminent suicide risk has yet to be implemented.

Suicide Warning Signs

In tandem with the increasing empirical focus on short-term risk factors, the construct of warning signs has become a central area of study in the field of suicide research over the past few decades. Interestingly, warning signs, although popular in other medical fields, were not applied to suicide or other psychiatric crises until relatively recently. In 2006, Rudd and colleagues proposed that warning signs of imminent suicide are theoretically and practically distinct from risk factors, and that establishing and disseminating knowledge about warning signs would enable intervention to prevent imminent suicidal behavior. Through expert consensus, Rudd and others set out to identify warning signs among many suicide-specific risk factors, including emotional, cognitive, behavioral, social, and demographic characteristics, although suicide research often isolates these domains, studying them separately.

For example, a Medline search using the keywords *suicide* + [*negative affect*] revealed that the most studied clinical constructs were depression and anxiety, which are both very common in suicide attempters. Most depressed and anxious people are not acutely suicidal; thus, these emotions are of little use in assessing suicidal states and imminent suicide. On the other hand, the least-studied clinical factors in the literature were the arousal states and negative affects predictive of imminent suicide risk, including insomnia, hopelessness, despair, entrapment, and desperation. To date, this body of research has provided very limited data on which of the factors are considered warning signs and which clusters confer incremental and additive suicide risk.

For instance, although some of the factors have been linked to SI (Kessler et al., 1999), they do not differentiate people with SI who have or have not attempted suicide (Klonsky & May, 2014). Moreover, no direct correlation has been found between the number of possible risk factors or warning signs endorsed by a patient and his or her degree of short-term risk (Moscicki, 1997). At present, the website for the Substance Abuse and Mental Health Services Association (SAMHSA; https://www.samhsa.gov/find-help/suic ide-prevention) and the Suicide Prevention Lifeline (https://suicideprevent ionlifeline.org/help-someone-else/) list 11 suicide warning signs (Table 7.1), which differ somewhat from the original signs defined by the expert consensus of the American Association of Suicidology (Rudd et al., 2006). The first two warning signs are explicit SI and suicide intent, while the others include changes in affect and behavior (Table 7.1). Despite the intellectual appeal of such a framework, there is currently no clear experimental evidence of the construct validity and clinical usefulness of warning signs. Given these limitations, Fowler (2012) proposed that clinicians should not simply rely on risk factors or warning signs independently when assessing safety but should use the factors and signs together in a collaborative, patient-specific manner to facilitate the understanding of unique suicidal mental processes and the clinical syndrome.

Table 7.1 Suicide warning signs (SAMHSA, 2022)

Suicide Warning Signs*
Talking about wanting to die or to kill oneself
Looking for a way to kill oneself, such as searching online or buying a gun
Increasing the use of alcohol or drugs
Acting anxious or agitated; behaving recklessly
Sleeping too little or too much
Withdrawing or feeling isolated
Talking about feeling hopeless or having no reason to live
Talking about feeling trapped or in unbearable pain
Talking about being a burden to others
Showing rage or talking about seeking revenge
Displaying extreme mood swings

* Risk is greater if a behavior is new or has increased and if it seems related to a painful event, loss, or change.

Bolded warning signs coincide with SCS symptom criteria.

The evidence-based suicide crisis syndrome (SCS) criteria described in this book overlap somewhat with six of the 11 warning signs in the 2022 iteration, which are bolded in Table 7.1. Since the initial results of implementation of the SCS diagnostic assessment were encouraging (Karsen et al., under review), the use of the proposed DSM-5 SCS diagnosis may have better clinical utility and efficacy in reducing suicidal outcomes than the warning signs, although more research is needed to support this hypothesis.

Suicidal Ideation and Suicide Intent

It is a common notion that suicide cannot occur without a wish to die and a suicidal act. However, either could be either conscious or unconscious. A self-inflicted shooting death with a suicide note is an example of a conscious and planned suicide, whereas deaths by unintentional overdose or due to reckless driving while intoxicated could result from an unconscious wish to die. Yet, questions about SI and suicide intent have always been central to any suicide risk assessment.

Suicidal Ideation

The term *suicidal ideation* refers to thoughts about suicide and encompasses a wide range of cognitions, from fleeting and infrequent to persistent and unrelenting. *Suicide intent*, which refers to SI that includes the purposeful plan to act, implies a more serious suicide risk and is considered separately. SI can vary in severity, from vague ideas with no plan to a detailed plan with intent to act on it. SI also ranges greatly in intensity, varying in terms of frequency, duration, and controllability of thoughts. For example, while one person may have relatively infrequent thoughts that can be easily suppressed, another individual might experience constant and uncontrollable thoughts of suicide.

Although SI is seemingly essential for any suicidal act, self-reported SI (as elicited in the assessment) predicts near-term suicidal behavior modestly at best. In teenagers and young adults (15 to 24 years old), SI severity and intensity (i.e., frequency and controllability) are significant independent predictors of future suicide attempts over a period of nine months, above and beyond the predictive power of past suicide attempts. However, this increase in suicide risk is minor in comparison to the sixfold increase in suicide risk due to history of suicide attempt(s). Moreover, the duration of suicidal thoughts is associated with higher risk only in men (Horwitz et al., 2015).

Self-reported SI was even less useful in predicting imminent suicidal behavior in a sample of suicidal callers who phoned crisis hotlines. These results were surprising, given that self-reported SI and plans would appear to be very reliable in crisis hotline settings. However, disclosure of SI did not predict either SI or suicide attempt(s) in the following two to eight weeks (Witte et al., 2012). A recent study by Rogers et al. (2022) indicated that patients who reported suicidal intent to anyone had higher levels of SCS symptoms, compared to those who denied intent. Additionally, severity of SI and rates of suicide attempt at one-month follow-up were higher among those who disclosed suicidal intent. Another study by Rogers and colleagues examined differential patient disclosure of suicidal intent to clinicians versus researchers (Rogers, Bloch-Elkouby, & Galynker, 2022). In this study, adult psychiatric outpatients preferentially disclosed their suicidal intent to research assistants, rather than clinicians. The authors proposed that these results may be explained by the longer duration of patient interviews with the assistants, allowing for the development of good rapport and mitigating the patients' shame and fear of judgment. The study also found that preferential disclosure to research assistants instead of clinicians was also predicted by personality traits. Specifically, patients who disclosed to assistants had higher levels of neuroticism and trait anxiety than those who did not disclose at all. Likewise, patients with higher extraversion and higher anxiety were more likely to disclose to research assistants, rather than clinicians.

When SI is measured using structured psychometric scales rather than clinical interviews, its value as a predictive tool for future ideation or behavior is only marginally better. At present, the Columbia Suicide Severity Rating Scale (C-SSRS) is the most widely used instrument for the assessment of both SI and suicidal behavior. (A more detailed description of the advantages and disadvantages of the C-SSRS is provided in Chapter 9.)

Other methods of assessing SI include the Scale for Suicidal Ideation (SSI), Hamilton Depression Scale (HAM-D) item 3, Beck Depression Inventory item 9, and simple questioning of patients on whether they had seriously considered suicide. All these methods have varying and relatively low predictive value for SI and attempts during a six-month follow-up period. In structured interviews, an SSI score > 8 seems to be best at predicting future suicide attempt over a period of six months, with a predictive value of 32% (Valtonen et al., 2009). A recent machine learning analysis of the predictive validity of

SCS symptoms for near-term suicidal behavior showed that adding current SI increased the area under the curve (AUC) by just 1% (89% versus 88%; McMullen et al., 2021).

Despite these findings, SI is one of the most frequently assessed warning signs of suicide, and it must continue to be incorporated in assessment of suicide risk. However, it must be acknowledged that this cornerstone of suicide risk assessment is not as useful in predicting imminent suicidal behavior, and it should not be relied on in isolation when making clinical decisions. Instead, SI assessment should be used as a modifier of SCS diagnosis, as described in the Suicide-Specific Modifiers for SCS section of this Chapter under Suicidal Ideation as a Modifier eponymous section included in this chapter.

Suicide Intent and Plan

The term *suicide intent* refers to a conscious desire to end one's life and, importantly, a resolve to act. The most prominent instrument for the assessment of the intensity and seriousness of suicide intent is the Suicide Intent Scale (SIS; Beck et al., 1974). The SIS consists of an objective component based on history (isolation, precautions against discovery, suicide note, and final preparations before death) and a subjective component based on self-report. Because patients with the most severe suicide intent usually go on to complete suicide, the SIS was designed for retrospective use immediately after a suicide attempt.

Generally, patients who make highly lethal suicide attempts have higher total SIS scores. The objective component of the SIS is highly correlated with the lethality of the most recent suicide attempt, as well as with communication difficulties in recent suicide attempters. The subjective component is associated with various mental pain factors, and these components are related to the intensity of the SCS. Suicide attempters with intense mental pain and communication difficulties have higher scores on the objective component of the scale (Horesh et al., 2012).

The same strong relationship between the lethality of the attempt and the degree of suicide intent holds true in clinical assessments of intent and for many cultures with diverse suicide statistics. On the other hand, the association between the degree of suicide intent and the degree of lethality of the attempt is dependent on the accuracy of expectations about the likelihood of dying as a result of the attempt: Higher levels of suicide intent were associated with more lethal attempts, but only for individuals who had more accurate expectations about the likelihood of dying from their attempts (Brown et al., 2004).

However, although the association between the suicide intent and potential lethality of past suicide attempts appears strong, repetition of suicide attempts in the future is not related to the seriousness of the intent of the original episodes. Thus, the relationship of lethality and suicide intent to further suicidal behavior does not appear to be straightforward (Haw et al., 2003), and suicide intent, just like SI, is not a reliable predictor of suicidal behavior in the near future.

The following are case examples of patient interviews assessing SI and suicide intent.

Case 41

Alina is a 17-year-old female with schizoaffective disorder, incorrectly diagnosed with bipolar disorder during her first manic episode. Alina had substantial negative symptoms and interpersonal deficits, was socially isolated, lacked initiative, and also admitted to having hallucinations since the age of 11 years. In high school, she had several psychotic episodes requiring hospitalization, which prevented her from graduating from high school with her classmates and disrupted her social life.

As a result, as a high school senior, Alina was a year behind and was trying to get her GED through an individualized tutoring program. She always appeared unhappy but denied being depressed. When asked about her state of mind, she would say that she was always thinking painful thoughts about how she was lazy and not trying hard enough to be successful.

One day, after returning from an Easter visit with her cousins, she came to her therapist's office looking particularly unhappy. Alina's mother texted the therapist that Alina had told her that she did not want to live anymore.

Alina's office interview with her therapist assessed SI and suicide intent.

SI

DR: Alina, your mother texted me that you told her you did not want to live anymore. Was she telling the truth?

ALINA: Yes.

DR: What's going on?

ALINA: I am just in so much pain, it's not worth it.

DR: Are you thinking about suicide?

ALINA: I just want to be gone. I don't want to suffer.

DR: And how long have you been having these thoughts? Days, weeks?

ALINA: All week.

DR: Are you having these thoughts now?

ALINA: Not now.

DR: These thoughts about not wanting to live, are they with you all the time?

ALINA: Almost.

Suicide intent and plan

DR: Have you thought about how you would kill yourself?

ALINA: Yes. I would take my mother's pills. She has like 10 bottles in her medicine cabinet.

DR: And what would happen if you took them?

ALINA: I would die and won't feel anything anymore. Life just is too painful.

DR: What prevents you from taking these pills tonight?

ALINA: She is with me all the time. And it would upset her. A lot.

DR: Can you picture yourself actually taking the pills?

ALINA: I can, but I don't think I would do it. I am too scared.

DR: What would it take for you to actually take the pills?

ALINA: To know that nobody cares.

DR: Did you pick the pill bottle you will use?

ALINA: I will use her sleeping pills.

DR: Did you hold the bottle in your hands?

ALINA: Yes.

DR: Did you open it?

ALINA: No.

The therapist was able to elicit Alina's persistent SI. Moreover, Alina acknowledged having conditional suicide intent with a specific plan, preparatory actions for suicide, and even practicing. Alina's description of her intent and plan is indicative of a high short-term risk. She had specific intent to end her life and had decided on a method. The self-report of SI by itself is not predictive of short-term risk, but in Alina's case, it is very congruent with her intent and plan, and it makes her admission of suicidality more credible.

Case 42

Richard is a 73-year-old retired dentist with a history of bipolar disorder and agoraphobia. He was depressed for several months as a freshman in college and had difficulty leaving his room and attending classes. He had prolonged undiagnosed hypomania through dental school and residency, followed by a second episode of depression after several years in practice. He was hospitalized, was treated with electroconvulsive therapy (ECT), and after discharge worked in a city hospital. He married a nurse, and they had two children. The couple divorced when Richard was 60 years old, and he married his 35-year-old dental hygienist.

When Richard was 65 years old, he was caught drinking alcohol at work, and the ensuing investigation uncovered that he was abusing sedatives. He was hospitalized with psychotic depression and was treated with ECT. At the time of the suicide risk assessment, he was in individual treatment for residual depression and severe agoraphobia. He and his wife were also in couples therapy because his symptoms were interfering with their social life. At the time of the interview, he was taking two antidepressants, a stimulant, and a low-dose antipsychotic. Richard's daughter called his psychiatrist after Richard told her, in speaking about his wife, that he was tired of "all her crap." Richard's daughter also alerted the psychiatrist that Richard was very angry at his wife for flirting with younger men.

Richard's office interview with his psychiatrist follows.

SI

DR: Hello Richard, how are you feeling?

RICHARD: Annoyed.

DR: Annoyed at what?

RICHARD: My wife is driving me crazy. She just keeps coming on to men right in front of me.

DR: What are you going to do?

RICHARD: I don't know, kill myself!

DR: Have you been thinking about suicide?

RICHARD: Sometimes.

DR: How frequently?

RICHARD: Not once a day but not once in a blue moon either. Maybe once a week.

DR: And what exactly do you think?

RICHARD: That I want to kill this flirt—my wife, that is. And since I don't want to spend the rest of my life in jail, I would rather shoot myself.

DR: How persistent are these thoughts? Do they last seconds, minutes, days?

RICHARD: Not long. Minutes.

DR: Is it hard to suppress these thoughts? Does it require effort, or do they just go away?

RICHARD: They go away. Unless she is flirting right in front of me. Then it's pretty hard.

DR: Do you have a gun at home?

RICHARD: Somewhere. Not sure.

DR: Do you have bullets at home?

RICHARD: Somewhere, not sure. But, doc, don't worry, these are just thoughts.

DR: When was the last time that you held your gun?

RICHARD: I don't remember. Two years ago, maybe.

DR: And what did you do with it?

RICHARD: I took it out of the box and put it back in.

DR: Where was it?

RICHARD: In the attic.

DR: Were you looking for it?

RICHARD: No, I was just organizing stuff.

DR: Was the gun loaded?

RICHARD: No.

DR: Did you load it?

RICHARD: No.

DR: Did you look for the bullets?

RICHARD: No.

DR: Did you aim the gun at yourself?

RICHARD: No.

DR: Did you aim it at anything?

RICHARD: No, I just looked at it and put it back.

DR: Were you thinking of shooting yourself at the time?

RICHARD: No.

DR: Where you thinking of shooting your wife?

RICHARD: No.

Richard's SI is less severe and persistent than that of Alina, and by his description, holding the gun in his hand may not be considered preparatory suicidal behavior. However, although flippant and impulsive, his description of losing control and shooting himself if his wife flirts too much is a conditional suicide plan, which carries with it a homicide or double homicide potential. This interview warrants an immediate intervention and removal of the firearm from the house.

Suicide Crisis Syndrome

SCS Diagnostic Structure

As described in Chapter 2, the concept of the suicide crisis originated in Baumeister's (1990) notion of suicide as an acute mental process and also in Shneidman's (1993) construct of psychache as a specific state of mind leading to suicide. The term *suicide crisis* was first used by Hendin et al. (2007), who described the construct of a suicide crisis as an acute, high-intensity, negative affect that may serve as a trigger for a suicide attempt.

Building on the work of Hendin and others, we have proposed that the mental state of the suicide crisis constitutes a distinct syndrome, SCS (which we originally called the "suicide trigger state"). Our initial research showed that SCS had three components: frantic hopelessness, an affective state of entrapment, dread, and hopelessness; ruminative flooding, a cognitive state of incessant and overwhelming rumination and a sense of one's head bursting with uncontrollable thoughts; and panic–dissociation, a state of strange somatic experiences in the context of severe anxiety and panic (Yaseen et al., 2010, 2012, 2014). Several studies established the predictive validity of SCS for near-term suicidal behaviors and its usefulness in describing a clinically meaningful syndrome in a high-risk population (Barzilay et al., 2020; Yaseen et al., 2019).

Our subsequent research indicated that SCS includes several other affective, cognitive, and behavioral symptoms (Schuck et al., 2019) that improve the predictive validity of the SCS for suicidal behavior. One symptom is emotional pain, which is a mental state of persistent inner anguish similar to psychache (Orbach, 2003b). Another symptom is acute anhedonia, or the inability to experience pleasure or to imagine past or future activities as enjoyable (Yaseen et al., 2012). Other symptoms that improve the predictive validity of the SCS are disturbance of arousal and acute social withdrawal.

Accumulating research demonstrates the reliability and concurrent incremental and predictive validity of tools that measure the SCS in its evolution with regard to SI and suicidal behavior (Barzilay et al., 2020; Bloch-Elkouby et al., 2020, 2021; Galynker et al., 1996; Hawes et al., 2018; Katz et al., 2011; Li et al., 2017; Rappaport et al., 2014; Yaseen et al., 2013). In particular, the SCS tools have shown concurrent validity in relation to recent and lifetime suicidality (Barzilay et al., 2020; Calati et al., 2020; Cohen et al., 2019; Galynker et al., 2017), incremental validity over self-reported SI in predicting near-term suicide attempts (Barzilay et al., 2020), and predictive validity with regard to SI one month postdischarge (Bloch-Elkouby et al., 2020), suicidal thoughts and behaviors (Bloch-Elkouby et al., 2021; Rogers, Vespa, et al., 2021), and suicide attempts (Barzilay et al., 2020; Galynker et al., 2017; Yaseen et al., 2019; Ying et al., 2020). Thus, at present, the predictive validity of the SCS for imminent suicidal risk is well documented.

Based on these findings and other published work related to the acute suicidal state, we have formulated the proposed *Diagnostic and Statistical Manual of Mental Disorders* (DSM; American Psychiatric Association, 2013) criteria for SCS, which are listed in the next section and in Table 7.2. SCS consists of five components, one Criterion A and four Criteria B (see Table 7.2). Criterion A is a persistent and intense feeling of frantic hopelessness/entrapment, which can be defined as an urge to escape a perceived inescapable life situation (Galynker et al., 2017; Yaseen et al., 2014). The four Criteria B include affective disturbances (B1), loss of cognitive control (B2), hyperarousal (B3), and acute social withdrawal (B4; Calati et al., 2020; Rogers et al., 2017; Schuck et al., 2019). Criterion A mediates the relationship between Criteria B and near-term suicidal behavior (Li et al., 2017). Those who meet Criterion A and have at least one symptom from all four Criteria B are diagnosed with SCS, and therefore are at high risk for a near-term suicide attempt.

Barzilay and colleagues (2020) tested the five-factor model of SCS, including entrapment, panic dissociation, ruminative flooding, fear of dying, and emotional pain, and found that it demonstrated good fit and excellent internal consistency. Chistopolskaya et al. (2020), Menon et al. (2022), Wu et al. (2022), and Park et al. (in press) tested the validity of SCS in Russian, Indian, Taiwanese, and Korean adults, respectively, and found mostly that the five-factor model, including entrapment, affective disturbances, loss of cognitive control, hyperarousal, and social withdrawal, had better fit than the one-factor model, with total and subscale scores showing excellent internal consistency and good convergent validity. These findings support the use of the Suicide Crisis Inventory (SCI) and SCS structure in suicide prevention

Table 7.2 Proposed criteria for the suicide crisis syndrome

Criterion	Symptom description
A: Frantic hopelessness/ entrapment	A persistent or recurring overwhelming feeling of urgency to escape or avoid an unbearable life situation that is perceived to be impossible to escape, avoid, or endure.
B: Associated disturbances[a]	
B1: Affective disturbance	Emotional pain; rapid spikes of negative emotions or extreme mood swings; extreme anxiety that may be accompanied by dissociation or sensory disturbances; acute anhedonia (i.e., a new or increased inability to experience or anticipate interest or pleasure).
B2: Loss of cognitive control	Intense or persistent rumination about one's own distress and the life events that brought on distress; cognitive rigidity (i.e., inability to deviate from a repetitive negative thought pattern); ruminative flooding, characterized by an overwhelming profusion of negative thoughts, accompanied by head pressure or pain and impairing ability to process information or make a decision; repeated unsuccessful attempts to suppress negative or disturbing thoughts.
B3: Hyperarousal	Agitation; hypervigilance; irritability; insomnia.
B4: Acute social withdrawal	Reduction in frequency and scope of social activity; evasive communication with close others.

[a] Criterion B, Associated disturbances, is met if there is at least one of the described symptoms present in *each* of the B1, B2, B3, and B4 criteria.

strategies in cross-cultural settings. On the other hand, Otte et al. (2020) tested the SCI with the same five-factor structure in a German forensic sample and found that factor structure was not supported by the sample, although item characteristics and reliability were very good. The results suggest a potentially different factorial structure or potentially fewer factors in SCS in a German forensic sample. Overall, however, SCS appears to be both a transdiagnostic and transcultural syndrome.

The exact criteria structure of SCS was examined in two studies of predictive validity of the proxy SCS Checklist (SCS-C), composed using the items from well-known validated scales approximating SCS symptoms (Bafna et al., 2022; Yaseen et al., 2019). In the latter replication study, we examined which configuration of SCS criteria demonstrates the strongest predictive validity for near-term suicidal behavior and pilot-tested the SCS-C on a subgroup of the study participants. The results revealed that, of all possible configurations, one-factor and five-factor models of proxy SCS-C variables exhibited the strongest model fit, supporting both the syndrome's unidimensionality and the optimal five-criteria structure. In addition, the proxy SCS-C and actual SCS-C symptom configurations were significant and positive. Overall, these results lend support to the proposed five-symptom structure of the SCS diagnostic criteria and demonstrate that SCS is a clinically meaningful syndrome predictive of near-term suicidal behavior. Thus, SCS assessment may significantly improve clinical evaluation of imminent suicide risk. Future studies are needed to further test the syndrome's utility in clinical settings.

We also proposed three exclusion criteria related to mental states of suicides (where SCS may not be a factor) due to medical or social issues:

- Mental states of delirium or confusion
- Mental states preceding suicides as a political statement
- Mental states preceding physician-assisted suicides.

The subsequent sections of this chapter examine the clinical utility of SCS and its proposed use, along with SI, suicidal behavior disorder, and acute suicidal affective disturbance. These discussions are followed by detailed descriptions of individual SCS symptoms, illustrated by corresponding case reports.

Clinical Utility of the SCS

In order for SCS to be a viable candidate for inclusion in the DSM, establishing the utility of SCS diagnosis for clinicians' decision-making is critical. Accordingly, the clinical utility of the SCS has been assessed in several ways. It has been implemented in a variety of clinical settings across several nations, and the feasibility, appropriateness, and acceptability of SCS and its corresponding self-report questionnaire have been surveyed in large samples of mental health providers. Likewise, our research team has tested the SCS's impact on clinical decision-making in outpatient settings.

First, SCS is being implemented in numerous healthcare systems, including inpatient and outpatient hospital settings, in New York, New York, Evanston, Illinois (Karsen et al., under review), Petah Tikva, Israel (Barzilay et al., under review), Trondheim, Norway (Hoyen et al., 2021), and Moscow, Russia (Bannikov et al., under review), as well as in school-based settings in Marin County, California, and Moscow, Russia. Moreover, although it

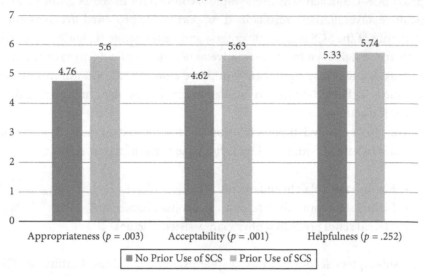

Average Survey Responses on a 1 (Strongly Disagree) to 7 (Strongly Agree) Scale

Figure 7.1 Perceived clinical utility of the suicide crisis syndrome (SCS) in three different settings.

is not yet an official diagnosis, SCS has been included in regional and national suicide risk assessments in the Central Norway Health Authority Helseplattformen (Health Platform) in Norway (Helseplattformen, 2021), Israel's national suicide prevention hotline (ERAN Suicide line, https://www.therapyroute.com/therapist/eranorgil-israel-il), and the Taiwan National Suicide Prevention Center (2022; https://sites.google.com/a/tsos.org.tw/english/). Of note, among the sites that have integrated SCS to various degrees, all agreed that SCS aids in clinical decision-making. Remarkably, when SCS diagnosis was implemented in emergency department (ED) electronic medical records alongside SI and suicidal behavior (SB), it played a dominant role in shaping clinicians' admissions/discharge decisions, while SI and SB were noncontributory (Figure 7.1). These results were especially pronounced in clinician decision-making about patients without psychosis. Studies assessing the impact of SCS assessments on suicidal outcomes are ongoing.

Second, a survey of the perceived clinical utility of SCS (feasibility, appropriateness, and acceptability of SCS diagnosis) was administered to mental health practitioners across three settings (Mount Sinai Beth Israel, Florida

International University, and Helseplattformen) to explore clinicians' attitudes toward the SCS. The survey asked clinicians to consider the feasibility, acceptability, and incremental helpfulness of SCS criteria relative to other traditional suicide risk assessments. Clinicians were also asked whether they had prior experience with using SCS directly with patients. The results of these analyses are presented below in Figure 7.1. Overall, clinicians found SCS diagnosis to be appropriate, acceptable, and incrementally more helpful than traditional forms of suicide risk assessment, and they viewed incorporating SCS into clinical practice as somewhat feasible. Moreover, clinicians who had used SCS in clinical practice had significantly higher ratings of its appropriateness and acceptability, as well as overall higher views of SCS, compared to clinicians with no prior use of the SCS. Furthermore, clinicians employed at NorthShore University Health System were polled using the same questionnaire after the SCS diagnosis was implemented in Epic EMR (electronic medical records), a healthcare software platform. The results were similar to those at the other three sites (see Figure 7.1). Together, these results support the clinical utility of the SCS and suggest that clinicians with prior training in, exposure to, and use of the SCS had even more favorable views.

Third, analyses were conducted in a large sample of psychiatric outpatients and their clinicians to determine whether the SCS criteria were incrementally informative in clinical decision-making regarding the intensity of treatment. Results indicated that, accounting for non-independence of clinician decision-making (i.e., patients were nested within clinicians), patients' self-reported SCS symptoms were more strongly associated with treatment intensification than patients' SI (Barzilay et al., 2021).

Finally, preliminary data suggest that the use of the SCS diagnostic assessment in the ED setting reduced psychiatric readmissions by 40% (Miller et al., in preparation). The detailed data analysis of the EMR data for the relationship between SCS diagnostic use and prospective suicidal outcomes, such as suicide deaths, suicide attempts, suicide attempt severity, SI, hospital readmission, and treatment utilization, is ongoing. Notably, however, over the two years since the SCS assessment was introduced, there has been no known suicide within the six-hospital NorthShore University Heath System.

Together, the use of the SCS across diverse settings, clinicians' reports on the feasibility, appropriateness, acceptability, and helpfulness of the SCS, as well as on its utility in clinical decision-making, provide substantial evidence that SCS has ample clinical utility.

Suicide-Specific Modifiers for SCS

As described in detail in this chapter and elsewhere, there is clear evidence that SCS is a unitary syndrome that can be diagnosed using five criteria, one criterion A and four criteria B (Bafna et al., 2022; Bloch-Elkouby et al., 2021; Calati et al., 2020; Rogers, Vespa, et al., 2021; Schuck et al., 2019; Yaseen et al., 2019). There is also evidence supporting the perceived and actual clinical utility of SCS (Karsen et al., under review; Mitelman et al., under review). The SCS clinical predictive validity for suicidal behavior is improved somewhat when it is used concurrently with SI (McMullen et al., 2021), and it may also improve when used along with two other clinical entities, suicidal behavior disorder (SBD; Oquendo & Baca-Garcia., 2014) and acute suicidal affective disturbance (ASAD; Stanley et al., 2016). SBD was temporarily listed in DSM-5 as a condition for further study and was recently finalized under the "Other conditions that may be a focus of clinical attention" modifier with its own diagnostic code. ASAD is hypothesized to be a pre-suicidal mental state characterized by rapid and exponential increase in suicidal intent over a period of days rather than weeks and months. In contrast to SCS, SI, SBD, and ASAD rely on self-reported SI or past SB as a centerpiece of their risk assessment, and yet both SI and past SB have been shown to be highly unreliable as predictors of imminent suicide (Berman, 2018). Still, while not imminent suicide predictors, all three constructs—SI, SBD, and ASAD—have been associated with past suicidal behavior and increase risk of suicide lifetime. Therefore, their clinical utility will be optimal if, like SBD, they are used as SCS modifiers, which when present, would further raise the SCS-associated suicide risk. The following three sections describe the suggested use of the three proposed modifiers for the SCS.

Suicidal Ideation as a Modifier

Evidence suggests that utilizing SCS along with SI is incrementally informative in predicting future suicidal behavior. As mentioned elsewhere in this book, SCS predicts suicide attempts within one month, above and beyond SI (Barzilay et al., 2020; Bloch-Elkouby et al., 2021; Galynker et al., 2017; Rogers, Vespa, et al., 2021; Yaseen et al., 2019). Other emerging evidence indicates that the combination of SCS and SI may be particularly pernicious with regard to imminent suicide risk. When clinical cutoff scores were used for the SCS, the combination of both SCS and SI was superior in predicting suicide attempts at one-month follow-up than either SCS or SI as an isolated predictor (Rogers et al., 2022). Finally, beyond simple prediction of suicide-related outcomes, clinicians perceive SCS as incrementally more helpful than existing suicide risk assessment protocols, and SCS is more strongly associated with clinical decision-making than patients' SI alone (Barzilay et al., 2021).

Although the predictive validity of SCS and SI for near-term suicidal behaviors was supported by machine learning analysis, the addition of SI increases SCS predictive validity only minimally (McMullen et al., 2021). Nonetheless, individuals who have both SCS and SI are at higher risk for imminent suicidal behavior than those with SCS alone. Altogether, these findings highlight the utility of SCS alone, but they also suggest a framework for the use of SI in combination with the SCS. Specifically, the inclusion of "with SI self-report" (regardless of its intensity of duration) or "without SI" as a modifier to the SCS DSM-5 diagnosis could serve as an additional indicator of potential severity of SCS and subsequent suicide risk, highlighting the need for management and evidence-based safety planning and intervention. Such a formulation would allow a diagnosis of SCS with or without SI, will integrate SCS and SI assessment, and will provide SI with a commensurate evidence-based place in suicide risk assessment protocols.

Suicidal Behavior Disorder as a Modifier
Suicidal behavior disorder SBD was originally included in DSM-5 as a "condition for further study." Recently, this status was changed to the modifier "Other conditions that may be a focus of clinical attention," which carries its own diagnostic code. The diagnostic criteria for SBD essentially equate to a suicide attempt within the past two years and specifically include:

- Within the last 24 months, the individual has made a suicide attempt.
- The act does not meet criteria for nonsuicidal self-injury.
- The diagnosis is not applied to SI or to preparatory acts.
- The act was not initiated during a state of delirium or confusion.
- The act was not undertaken solely for a political or religious objective.

As confirmed by the final decision of the steering committee, there are significant benefits to the inclusion of SBD in the DSM. Broadly, diagnoses are helpful in clarifying the essential features of a psychiatric condition, in communicating "clinical information to practitioners, patients and their families, and health care systems administrators" (First et al., 2004), in selecting an appropriate treatment, and in predicting the condition's future course (Obegi, 2019). SBD specifically may be useful in providing much-needed structure and training in obtaining suicidal behavior history during suicide risk assessment and management, in which many clinicians lack sufficient training (Schmitz et al., 2012). Additionally, some have argued for the utility of SBD in improving suicide risk assessment training, increasing the time spent assessing suicide in clinical intakes, and highlighting the potential for a future suicide attempt (Fehling & Selby, 2021), given associations between previous and future suicide attempts (Beautrais, 2004; Ribeiro et al., 2016).

However, SBD has several shortcomings as a diagnostic category of its own, as has been highlighted by multiple investigative teams (Fehling & Selby, 2021; Obegi, 2019; Schuck et al., 2019; Tucker et al., 2016). Most importantly, SBD does not include or describe a current phenomenon or presentation; rather, it describes behavior that has already occurred. Second, a previous suicide attempt is not necessarily indicative of a future suicide attempt, although it does reflect an increased risk period (Ribeiro et al., 2016). Thus, clinicians are unable to reliably identify or monitor current states with SBD, because SBD lacks specificity and acuity and therefore cannot improve the short-term prediction of future suicidal behavior (Glenn & Nock, 2014). Third, the reliance on past suicide attempts will miss a large proportion (approximately 50% or more) of individuals—especially those who use firearms in suicidal behavior (Anestis, 2016)—who die on their first suicide attempt (Bostwick et al., 2016).

Overall, given that SBD has utility in identifying a period of elevated suicide risk, and SCS has utility in understanding and predicting temporal fluctuations in suicide risk that precede short-term suicidal behavior, the combination of SCS and SBD as a modifier may be able to better identify those with SCS at the greatest risk for subsequent suicidal behavior.

Acute Suicidal Affective Disturbance as a Modifier

SCS is not the only proposed suicide-specific diagnosis. Independent efforts resulted in the development and validation of another proposed suicide-specific entity, acute suicidal affective disturbance (ASAD), which has some overlap with, and significant differences from, SCS (Rogers et al., under review; Galynker et al., 2017). The proposed criteria for ASAD include:

- An exponential increase in suicidal intent over the course of hours or days, as opposed to weeks or months.

- Marked social alienation (e.g., severe social withdrawal, disgust with others, perceived burdensomeness) and/or self-alienation (e.g., self-hatred, psychological turmoil/pain).
- Perceptions that one's suicidal intent and social/self-alienation are hopelessly intractable.
- Two or more manifestations of overarousal: agitation, marked irritability, insomnia, nightmares.

Much like SCS, ASAD has received research support for its factor structure and convergent, discriminant, and criterion validity in concurrent and retrospective studies. Specifically, several reports support a unidimensional factor structure for ASAD through the use of both proxy (Rogers et al., 2016; Rogers, Chiurliza, et al., 2017; Stanley et al., 2016) and standardized (Tucker et al., 2016) measures, as well as its convergent and discriminant validity with other psychiatric disorders and suicide-related risk factors and symptoms across samples of undergraduate students (Rogers & Joiner, 2019; Tucker et al., 2016), psychiatric outpatients (Rogers et al., 2016; Rogers, Chiurliza, et al., 2017), and psychiatric inpatients (Rogers, Chiurliza, et al., 2017; Stanley et al., 2016). Further, empirical evidence has provided support for ASAD as a proximal factor accounting for associations between more distal cognitive symptoms (Rogers et al., 2018), including suicide-specific rumination (Rogers & Joiner, 2018), and suicide attempts. However, to date, there has been no experimental evidence in support of the clinical utility of ASAD, the predictive validity of ASAD for near-term suicidal behavior, the impact of ASAD on clinical decision-making in real-life clinical settings, or the impact of ASAD on suicidal outcomes.

Both SCS and ASAD reflect acute, rapid-onset symptoms that are theorized to precede suicidal behavior, but there are substantial differences between the syndromes. Most importantly, ASAD is characterized by escalating, conscious suicidality, with its core symptom of drastically increasing suicidal intent; on the other hand, SCS does not require any conscious SI or suicide intent. Rather, loss of affective regulation and cognitive control in SCS represents a breakdown in emotional and executive functioning that leads to impaired problem-solving and increased susceptibility to selecting suicide as a solution (Galynker, 2017, Galynker et al., 2017). In other words, SCS describes interconnected affective, cognitive, and arousal symptoms that may escalate with a gradual, rapid, or fluctuating course. Finally, whereas SCS emphasizes affective, cognitive, and arousal symptoms as core components, ASAD places additional focus on extreme self-disgust and self-hatred.

Using data obtained from our ongoing COVID-19 and suicidality study, a recent network analysis showed that SCS and ASAD were two distinct syndromes. The only symptoms that ASAD and SCS have in common were related to disturbance of arousal and social withdrawal (Rogers et al., under review). In this analysis, disturbance of arousal symptoms—particularly irritability, insomnia, hypervigilance, and agitation—bridged SCS symptoms (i.e., frantic hopelessness/entrapment, affective disturbance, loss of cognitive control) and ASAD symptoms (i.e., acute self-hatred and exponential increases in suicidal intent). This evidence suggests that SCS and ASAD are two different syndromes, either representing two different pathways to suicide or, in combination, indicating higher risk for suicide.

Alternatively, given some overlap between the proposed SCS and ASAD criteria, it is possible that the two syndromes reflect different stages of the same process. For instance, ASAD may represent a later, even more transient, and more severe version of SCS, once suicidal intent has emerged and suicidal behavior is imminent. If this is indeed the case, it would highlight the clinical utility of jointly utilizing SCS and ASAD to better understand, predict, and prevent suicidal behavior. Accordingly, research is ongoing to empirically compare the similarities/differences across the two sets of criteria, as well as their reliability and incremental validity as a suicide-specific entity.

Regardless of the outcome of this research, two critical distinctions between SCS and ASAD remain that inform their potential utility in a real-world clinical setting. First, ASAD relies on the self-report of SI, yet the majority of suicide decedents do not disclose their ideation or intent to anyone (Berman, 2018; Busch et al., 2003; Stone et al., 2018). Second, in contrast to the SCS, which may last days (Galynker et al., 2017), the conscious SI and suicidal intent of ASAD may appear within minutes of suicidal behavior, when it may be too late to intervene (Deisenhammer et al., 2009). Both considerations make the SCS a potentially much broader and highly useful clinical category for a frontline clinician.

For all the above considerations, the primary possibility for inclusion of both syndromes would be the addition of a more acute but less readily identifiable ASAD as a modifier/specifier of SCS, such that SCS could be diagnosed both with and without accompanying ASAD, providing two degrees of acuity for the syndrome. Another prospect could be that SCS and ASAD could be two related, yet distinct, syndromes that could be included in DSM as separate diagnostic entities.

The Argument in Support of Three Modifiers

For conceptual simplicity and improved utility for the clinician, having SCS as one diagnostic entity that does not rely on self-report of SI, but in combination with three modifiers—SI, SBD, and ASAD—that do rely on it, is likely to result in the highest appropriateness and acceptability ratings by the frontline clinicians, which are critical for successful real-life implementation of SCS (Mitelman et al., in press). This is particularly true for clinicians in the high-risk inpatient and emergency settings, who are often pressed for time and would prefer few and clear categorical diagnoses to guide their decision-making (Barzilay et al., 2021). To this end, after one hospital unaffiliated with our research group implemented an abbreviated measure of SCS in their EDs, clinicians were dramatically more likely to rely on SCS over SI in admission and discharge decisions (Karsen et al., under review).

Clinical use of SCS is likely to identify a large group of those at risk who, for various reasons discussed previously, may not disclose their SI and suicidal intent. SI is a potent predictor of suicidal risk but with considerable limitations. Therefore, it is reasonable to add it as a modifier. Moreover, in our large-scale international online survey study, individuals who had SI in addition to SCS reported a greater number of recent stressful life events than those without SCS or SI, had larger changes in their cognitions and behaviors over time, and were more likely to seek suicide prevention resources than those with either SI or SCS alone (Rogers et al., under review –a, b, and c). It is possible that these individuals may be at higher risk than those with either SI or SCS alone. The same is likely to be true for SBD and ASAD modifiers. Although SBD is insufficient on its own as a basis for risk assessment, because so many suicides are completed on the first try, it remains a predictor of future attempts, and thus makes sense as a modifier of SCS. In the same vein, ASAD would be an appropriate modifier because although this syndrome may be a predictor of near-term suicidal behavior, its diagnosis would miss the 75% of suicide decedents who do not disclose their SI.

Finally, because SI, SBD, and ASAD are not mutually exclusive and may be used together, having the three modifiers would add additional dimension to suicide risk assessment. For example, a person may meet criteria for SCS, as well as for SI and SBD, or for SBD and ASAD. Hypothetically, a person meeting criteria for SCS and for all three modifiers will be a the highest risk for imminent suicide. This and related hypotheses will be tested in current and future studies.

Suicide Crisis Syndrome Criteria and Symptoms

Criterion A: Frantic Hopelessness/Entrapment

Criterion A of the proposed DSM criteria for SCS identifies frantic hopelessness/entrapment as the central feature of the acute suicidal state. The frantic hopelessness of SCS encompasses persistent and desperate feelings of entrapment, which is a frantic urgency to escape or avoid an unbearable life situation when escape is perceived as hopelessly impossible. Frantic hopelessness, as identified in our early studies of short-term suicide risk using the Suicide Trigger Scale (STS-3; Yaseen et al., 2010, 2012, 2014, 2016), is similar to entrapment (Tucker et al., 2016). Because the latter has been an accepted term used previously, in our subsequent studies in 2015 to 2019, we started using the term *entrapment* along with *frantic hopelessness* and sometimes interchangeably. However, subsequent network analysis (Bloch-Elkouby et al., 2020) showed that the most dominant SCS factor prominently includes both panic and hopelessness, underscoring the descriptive accuracy of the original term, *frantic hopelessness*. In order to minimize the confusion, this guide combines frantic hopelessness and entrapment into the term *frantic hopelessness/entrapment*, which is accurate, although somewhat cumbersome.

Entrapment has historically been implicated in social-rank theories of depression (Wetherall et al., 2019), the integrated motivational-volitional model of suicide, and the feedback loop hypothesis of the role of panic in the suicide trigger state (Katz et al., 2011; O'Connor & Portzky, 2018; Williams, 1997). The inability to escape from unbearable circumstances provides a setting for the emergence of SI (O'Connor, 2011; Williams, 1997), and the sense of entrapment distinguishes suicidal individuals from controls independently of depression, which predicts SI and attempts long-term (O'Connor, 2003; O'Connor et al., 2013). A relatively recent study assessed the relationship between feelings of frantic hopelessness/entrapment and the suicidal process and found that entrapment and emotional pain significantly and fully mediated the relationship of ruminative flooding, panic-dissociation, and fear of dying with SI, with no direct relationship between any of the variables and SI (Li et al., 2018). A similar study in a clinical cohort of high-risk adult psychiatric patients found that entrapment mediated the relationship between fearful attachment and suicidal behavior, suggesting that this stage could serve as a potential target to prevent suicidal behavior in these individuals (Li et al., 2017).

With regard to imminent suicide risk, the social aspect of entrapment has been found to play a minor role. It is often people's perception that the trap they find themselves in has no exit that may be one of the most critical factors in predicting whether they will attempt suicide in the immediate future. The word *entrapment* readily elicits visceral images of caged animals and captured people frantically trying to escape. Accordingly, it is the acute and almost physical sense of being locked up in a hopelessly bad situation that predicts imminent suicide.

As discussed in Chapter 2, entrapment has been proposed as a central psychological element of several models of suicidal behavior, notably the arrested flight/cry of pain model by Williams and Pollock, as well as O'Connor's integrated motivational-volitional model (O'Connor, 2011; Williams, 1997). The narrative-crisis model (NCM) separates the cognitive perception of no future from the emotional state of frantic hopelessness/entrapment. The cognitive perception of no future constitutes the last phase of the suicidal narrative (SN), whereas the affective state of entrapment is the key element of the suicidal crisis and therefore SCS.

Although a sense of entrapment may be associated with either objective or subjective stressful life events or circumstances (Brown et al., 1995), Gilbert and Allan (1998) suggested that entrapment could be divided into two subclasses: (1) external entrapment relating to external events or circumstances and (2) internal entrapment relating to internal thoughts, feelings, and perception. Thus, individual experiences of entrapment can emerge from a wide range of external hardships (Gilbert & Gilbert, 2003; Gilbert et al., 2004; Williams, 1997), and clinical assessment of entrapment should highlight how stressful life events are viewed (Lazarus & Folkman, 1984).

In agreement with these and other findings in cross-sectional and retrospective studies, our work has shown that, prospectively, among the SCS factors, frantic hopelessness/entrapment has the strongest association with short-term suicidal behavior, and the predictive validity of the entrapment subscale of the SCI for postdischarge suicidal behavior in high-risk psychiatric inpatients (odds ratio [OR] = 10) is just short of that of the full scale (OR = 13). Moreover, in acutely suicidal inpatients, entrapment fully mediates the relationship between the ruminative flooding, panic-dissociation, and SI, with no direct relationships between these variables and SI reaching statistical significance. Additionally, there were no reverse mediation relationships between the variables and SI, suggesting a unidirectional relationship. These findings suggest that frantic hopelessness/entrapment is related to suicide more intimately than the other SCS factors. In contrast, while entrapment mediated the relationship between emotional pain and SI, there was also a direct relationship between emotional pain and SI. Moreover, the reverse mediational analysis suggested that emotional pain was a partial mediator of the relationship between entrapment and SI (Li et al., 2018).

Desperation

Desperation is another symptom related to frantic hopelessness/entrapment that suicidal individuals often feel prior to attempting suicide. In a suicidal crisis, desperation may mediate the mental processes leading from frantic hopelessness/entrapment to suicide. Hendin et al. (2007) defined desperation as a state of anguish accompanied by the need for relief so urgent that any wait becomes unacceptable. The need for relief is so acute that the urge to relieve the pain becomes "the urge to end it all"—that is, the urge to end one's life by suicide. For a person in a state of desperation, the future possibility of relief from the current pain is so remote that it becomes irrelevant.

In the suicidal crisis, desperation, like frantic hopelessness/entrapment, is intertwined with the last phase of the SN: the perception of no future. The cognitive realization of being in a life situation with no good options does not automatically lead to desperation. However, such a perception is likely to worsen the emotional pain, with concomitant extreme anxiety and depressive turmoil—that is, to bring on the suicidal crisis and the dreadful urge to use suicide as the only perceived means to escape the dead end.

At present, desperation is not an SCS symptoms or criterion, and whether entrapment and desperation belong to the same syndrome remains an open question for future research. Currently, evidence suggesting that desperation is a central component of the mental state preceding imminent suicide derives primarily from interviews of clinicians with patients who died by suicide while in psychiatric treatment. For example, the following is an illustrative case of a 53-year-old clergyman with bipolar disorder (Hendin et al., 2007):

This patient's erratic behavior had caused him to be removed from his parish, which humiliated and enraged him. Despite his receiving treatment, which included hospitalization, his bipolar illness was not well controlled. His temper tantrums aimed at his wife and child and his irresponsible handling of money threatened his marriage. Because he was feeling that his life was falling apart, his anguish became intense and intolerable. Emotionally out of control, the patient appeared to have killed himself impulsively when he encountered frustration in getting started in a day treatment program.

As is clear from the description, the case described a man, demographically in a cohort with the highest suicide risk, suffering public humiliation, which led to a traplike life situation with no good options. As a result, he fell into a state of emotional instability, experienced as emotional disintegration, characteristic of depressive turmoil (discussed later). His emotional instability was worsened by his bipolar disorder. The patient killed himself impulsively after reaching a state of desperation when his anguished turmoil became intolerable. The final blow was when, in his mind, his last option for improvement, the day treatment program, failed him.

Note that desperation is often present in the context of hopelessness. However, desperation is sometimes seen where hopelessness is not, and when they do coexist, hopelessness is long-standing, whereas desperation is more acute. The same is true about the relationship between desperation and almost any other symptom, except acute physical pain. For patients who feel intensely desperate, the issue is not whether and when they would feel better but, rather, that they can no longer tolerate their present state.

The intense and brief states of desperation and urge to escape leading to suicide may leave no opportunity to evaluate the suicidal person and to intervene. However, levels of desperation fluctuate, and of course not every bout of desperation leads to suicide. On the other hand, the mere fact that a person is desperate dramatically increases his or her risk of imminent suicide. Thus, every imminent suicide risk assessment must probe the degree of the patient's desperation.

Asking a person about their options or the solutions they may see to their current life situation is a good way to start an SCS assessment interview. Such questions are viewed as caring, nonthreatening, and nonjudgmental, while the answers to these questions are of critical importance to the assessment of SCS and suicide risk.

The following continuing case examples illustrate the comprehensive assessment of the frantic hopelessness/entrapment aspect of SCS.

Case 41—Continued

Frantic Hopelessness/Entrapment

DR: When you are having these thoughts that nobody cares or that you don't want to be here, do you feel trapped?

ALINA: Last weekend I did.

DR: Or putting it differently, do you feel trapped by the pain?

ALINA: Yes! Often . . .

DR: Was this when you were with your cousins? And now?

ALINA: With them, yes. Now, not as much.

DR: How bad is the feeling of being trapped? Do you see any good options in your situation?

ALINA: Not really . . .

DR: If you think really hard . . . maybe medications?

ALINA: I have been sick for so long. Nothing seems to be working.

DR: I see. . . . I want to know more about how you felt last weekend when you were visiting your cousins. Did you feel so overwhelmed that you were losing control of your feelings?

ALINA: Yes, I felt so bad. . . . I don't want to remember how bad I felt, because I do not want to feel like that again.

DR: Does this feeling make you restless?

ALINA: Yeah . . . moving around helps. Last weekend I put my headphones on and went for a walk.

DR: Does listening to music make you feel better?

ALINA: Yes. And TV.

DR: How long can you tolerate being this upset?

ALINA: I do not know. Last weekend I was having suicidal thoughts.

DR: And now?

ALINA: Now not as much as last weekend but still pretty bad.

DR: Tell me about the last weekend. How painful was it?

ALINA: As painful as it gets. Somehow I managed to go to sleep and woke up feeling better. We need to do something, because if I feel like that again, I am not sure I will make it.

DR: What would you do?

ALINA: I don't know. I told you, I thought of taking pills. There are a lot of pills in the house. I need to feel better. I can't have another weekend like that.

DR: Medications should help, if not now, in the future.

ALINA: I can't wait for the future.

Alina's answers show that she feels both trapped in her current life situation and desperate to escape it. She sees no good options or treatments for her illness, which makes her feel anguished, isolated, and hopeless for the future. She has already rehearsed her suicidal actions, and her short-term risk is high.

Case 42—Continued

Frantic Hopelessness/Entrapment

DR: When you think about your situation—your wife's flirting, her out-of-control spending, your limited funds, your fixed income—do you feel trapped?

RICHARD: I told you I do—I can't talk to her about the money, and she just keeps buying designer outfits. I can't talk to her about her flirting either.

DR: What if you just don't give her the money?

RICHARD: Then she will leave and spend and flirt to her heart's desire.... And how am I going to be alone at 72 with agoraphobia? I can't leave the house by myself.

DR: Can you think of any good solutions to the problem?

RICHARD: I wish I could work, but I have been retired for a while. I can't start over.

DR: What about working for somebody else? Less headache managing the office.

RICHARD: I was never good with the bosses.

DR: What about talking to her about the finances, and how she makes you feel when she flirts?

RICHARD: Do you think I have not tried? I only feel worse afterward.

DR: How long can you tolerate this mental state that you are in?

RICHARD: It has been three years, and I will soon be at the end of my rope.

DR: How soon?

RICHARD: I don't know . . . six months maybe.

DR: Six months is good. I will take six months. Good couples' therapists can accomplish a lot in that time.

RICHARD: I hope so.

DR: Do you have hope that the pain will soon get better?

RICHARD: It has to, because if it does not, somebody will get hurt.

DR: Like who?

RICHARD: I do not know . . .

DR: The two of you are in therapy now, it may still help. You may just need to wait a little bit.

RICHARD: I am trying. . . . I like Dr. K. She is good.

Although the causes of Richard's sense of entrapment are different from those of Alina (romantic relationship conflict versus mental illness), their feelings of entrapment are similar in intensity. Neither Alina nor Richard sees any good options in their respective life situations. In contrast to Alina, however, Richard is not desperate, and he can tolerate his pain a little longer before, in his estimate, he may lose control and act out dangerously using the gun he has at home. This lack of desperation may give the interviewing doctor a feeling of confidence that Richard's life and that of his wife are not in imminent danger and that he has several weeks to remove the weapon and initiate couples' therapy.

Criterion B1: Affective Disturbance

Individuals in a suicidal crisis frequently experience extreme affective disturbance, which is a complex state of fluctuating negative affect. When suicidal individuals develop this highly aversive negative affect, it amplifies their desperate need to escape what has become an unbearable life situation.

Criterion B1 divides affective disturbance into four categories, which include the previously discussed negative affects, and it combines all anxiety symptoms into one category:

- *Emotional pain*: A painful state of mind, a psychache distinct from anxiety and depression.
- *Rapid spikes of negative emotions:* Abrupt changes in emotions or extreme mood swings.
- *Extreme anxiety:* A paniclike state with possible dissociative symptoms and sensory disturbances, which may include unusual bodily sensations and dissociative symptoms.
- *Acute anhedonia*: An inability to experience or imagine experiencing things as enjoyable (in individuals who previously have had that ability).

In the following discussion, for conceptual clarity and completeness, emotional pain, rapid spikes of negative emotions, extreme anxiety, and acute anhedonia are discussed separately. The same structure is retained in the case interviews.

Emotional Pain

Emotional pain (also called "mental pain" and "psychological pain") is a mixture of poorly differentiated but intense negative emotions, such as guilt, shame, hopelessness, disgrace, and rage. It arises when the essential needs to love, to have control, to protect one's self-image, to avoid shame, guilt, and humiliation, and to feel secure are frustrated (Williams et al., 2005). Emotional pain is similar to entrapment and is strongly correlated with, but distinct from, anxiety and depression. It can be so intense that the individual seeks to escape by committing suicide (Orbach, 2003b; Shneidman, 1993). Compared to entrapment, emotional pain may lack the desperation caused by the perception that all escape routes are blocked. Accordingly, although emotional pain and entrapment have equally immediate relationships to SI, in a multivariate analysis, entrapment was a stronger predictor of short-term suicidal behavior than emotional pain (Galynker et al., 2017).

An evaluation of emotional pain is a good starting point for the SCS part of the suicide risk assessment. Alternatively, asking if somebody feels emotional pain while thinking about a difficult or unbearable situation they find themselves in is an excellent beginning of the inquiry into the affective disturbance part of the SCS assessment.

Rapid Spikes of Negative Emotions

Rapid spikes of negative emotions, often defined in the literature as "depressive turmoil," describes a state of affective instability with rapid changes in negative moods, primarily depression and anxiety. Fawcett (1988, p. 7) defined depressive turmoil as "rapid switching of mood from anxiety to depression to anger, accompanied by agitation and perturbation." As such, this symptom partly resembles the "extreme mood swings" warning sign of suicide listed by the National Institute of Mental Health (2021). It is a state of affective instability with rapid changes in negative moods distinguishable from anxiety and depression by psychomotor agitation and anger, which are reflective of entrapment. This affective instability is common in recently discharged, depressed psychiatric inpatients and has been shown to be associated with increased risk of suicide (Angst et al., 1999).

Importantly, individuals in acute suicidal crises may experience rapid, alternating spikes of positive and negative emotions. Because of its strong anxiety and agitation component, this symptom also resembles depressive mixed states (Benazzi & Akiskal, 2001; Dilsaver et al., 2007). A depressed mixed state is observed predominantly in patients with bipolar depression, particularly those with bipolar II disorder (Akiskal & Benazzi, 2005; Takeshima & Oka, 2013), and it may be one of the strongest risk factors for suicidality (Valtonen et al., 2008).

Finally, depressive turmoil has many common features with activation syndrome (AS), which at times emerges during antidepressant therapy. As described in Chapter 4, AS consists of anxiety, agitation, panic attack, insomnia, irritability, hostility, aggressiveness, impulsivity, akathisia (psychomotor restlessness), and hypomania/mania. AS is similar to bipolar mixed states, but the fluctuating AS symptoms of agitation, insomnia, and hostility overlap with the affective disturbance and the depressive turmoil in SCS.

Extreme Anxiety

Extreme anxiety is a particularly severe form of anxiety frequently elicited in interviews with acutely suicidal individuals. It is characterized by an intense state of anxiety and panic accompanied by dissociation or sensory disturbances. Unlike the head pressure experienced during ruminative flooding, extreme anxiety involves the somatic experience of unfamiliar sensations felt all over the body, especially involving the skin. Indeed, prospective studies of acute suicidal states show that increased anxiety predicts suicidal behavior in the two months following the assessment (Kanwar et al., 2013; Lim et al., 2015; Nam et al., 2016; Nock et al., 2014; Rappaport et al., 2014). Anecdotally, in the words of eminent suicide expert Jan Fawcett, "There is anxiety and then there is suicidal anxiety; if you measure anxiety level on a 1 to 5 scale, the intensity of the suicidal anxiety is at 11."

Depending on their culture, history, and SN, suicidal patients may label extreme anxiety differently. However, most will identify with the sense of feeling strange sensations on their skin, often characterized by patients as feeling as if they have no skin. The raw sensitivity of unusual physical sensations in the body or on the skin often differentiates suicidal anxiety from situational anxiety and generalized anxiety disorder (GAD). Suicidal anxiety can be so intense and frenzied that it may reach the disorganized and undifferentiated state, in which it fuses with other negative affects described in this section—anhedonia, emotional pain, and rapid spikes of negative emotions—and reaches the level of desperation, where the promise of imminent relief becomes irrelevant because the pain is too great to bear even for another second.

Panic attacks are a heterogeneous syndrome comprising affective symptoms—primarily fear, cognitive symptoms congruent to fear, and autonomic nervous system activation symptoms, such as sweating and changes in heart rate (Fowles, 2007). Comorbid panic attacks aggravate the course of any psychiatric disorder, from severe and debilitating schizophrenia to relatively mild conditions like a social phobia. Panic attacks are significantly more frequent in those who go on to die by suicide than in those who do not (Fawcett et al., 1990). This is particularly true for patients with major depressive disorder (MDD) and panic attacks, who are 50% more likely to have SI and two times more likely to have attempted suicide than patients with MDD without panic attacks (Katz et al., 2011). Moreover, depressed patients with SI and panic attacks are two times more likely to attempt suicide.

The inclusion of extreme anxiety in SCS is supported by previous reports linking symptoms of panic attacks with increased suicide risk (Katz et al., 2011; Ozturk & Sar, 2008; Yaseen et al., 2012, 2013). Of note, in a prospective study, some panic symptoms, most notably catastrophic cognitions (fear of dying and fear of "losing control" or "going insane"), were more strongly and specifically associated with a suicide attempt, whereas others were more related to SI (Yaseen et al., 2013). Another study, however, indicated that the somatic symptoms of tingling, hot flushes or chills, and nausea were associated with past suicidal behavior, whereas dissociation was linked to SI (Rappaport et al., 2014).

The SCI data reliably indicate that somatic, paniclike symptoms included in extreme anxiety predict future suicidal behavior. The most prominent panic-related symptoms characterizing a suicidal crisis are sweating, nausea, problems breathing, and rapid heartbeat. Other strong predictors are strange sensations in the body or on the skin and a perception that the body may be changing. Likewise, in depressed individuals, a dissociative symptom that the world feels different or unreal also increases the short-term risk for suicide (Yaseen et al., 2012, 2014). Remarkably, in a recent machine learning analysis, the SCI item "Did you feel unusual physical sensations that you have never felt before?" was the strongest predictor for near-term suicidal behavior, on a par with self-reported SI (McMullen et al., 2021).

Acute Anhedonia

Anhedonia, defined as the inability to experience joy from activities that are normally found pleasurable, has long been considered primarily as one of the symptoms of major depression. Only relatively recently has it been recognized as a transdiagnostic symtom that is present in many disorders and is subserved by dopaminergic reward circuitry involving the nucleus accumbens (Wise, 1980). The severity of anhedonia appears to be associated with a deficit of activity of the ventral striatum (which includes the nucleus accumbens) and an excess of activity of the ventral region of the prefrontal cortex (including the ventromedial prefrontal cortex and the orbitofrontal cortex), with dopamine playing a pivotal, but not exclusive, role. The imbalance in neuronal activity is present in all major psychiatric disorders: schizophrenia, bipolar disorder, MDD, and borderline personality disorder (BPD). All carry a high risk for suicide, estimated to be 4% to 15% (Van Os & Kapur, 2009).

In schizophrenia, until recently, anhedonia had been subsumed by the broader term *negative symptoms*, which pertain primarily to the lack of motivation to embark on potentially rewarding activity—that is, the anhedonia motivational component. The consummatory component of anhedonia in schizophrenia manifests as the inability both to experience joy and to remember joy experienced previously (Treadway & Zald, 2011). Anhedonia as emptiness is most often seen in BPD, in which "chronic feelings of emptiness" are one of the criteria for the BPD diagnosis and are listed as Criterion 7 in DSM-V.

Whereas anhedonia in MDD and schizophrenia has a strong motivational component that reduces activity level, anhedonia in BPD is mostly consummatory, with motivation remaining relatively intact. As a result of this consummatory motivational imbalance, patients with BPD engage in frantic activity to escape their inner emptiness, searching for intense experiences that may include self-injurious behavior. Patients with BPD often state that they cut themselves to feel "something" because they feel empty. Paradoxically, the emptiness of BPD can be a quite intense and painful undifferentiated negative emotion, very similar to the concept of emotional pain. This mental pain can be so intense that patients with BPD seek the physical pain of self-injury to escape and find relief from the intolerable pain of inner emptiness.

Both emotional pain and anhedonia are frequently experienced by drug- and alcohol-addicted individuals in the course of acute and, more importantly, protracted withdrawal. Drug addiction directly engages the reward circuitry and nucleus accumbens, and it results in what is called an allosteric shift in the neurobiology of the brain, which adjusts to the drug of abuse, so the addicted state is perceived as neutral or normal. The absence of the drug is experienced as intense dysphoria and decreased ability to experience any positive emotions, including pleasure. The drug-seeking behavior shifts from craving euphoria in a euthymic state to craving normalcy in a dysphoric, anhedonic state.

Regardless of the categorical diagnosis, anhedonia, as a dimensional transdiagnostic entity, has been extensively correlated to SI in adolescents and adults (Gabbay et al., 2012). As a state, intensifying anhedonia is a component of the suicidal crisis and needs to be examined when assessing the risk for imminent suicide (Hawes et al., 2018). The intensifying nature of acute anhedonia differentiates it from a chronic anhedonic state, which is not a risk factor for suicidal behavior (Hawes et al., 2018). Interestingly, although not entirely unexpectedly, in the network analysis of the SCS, acute anhedonia was closely associated with acute social withdrawal (Bloch-Elkouby et al., 2021).

The following continuing case examples illustrate the comprehensive assessment of the affective disturbance criteria of SCS. Please note that while fear of dying is no longer part of SCS as a factor, it is still part of the extreme anxiety component, and hence has been kept as part of the case discussions.

Case 41—Continued

Emotional pain

DR: Alina, how are you feeling right now? You look like you are in pain.
ALINA: Yeah, I feel really awful. . . . Everybody keeps asking me about school, and which schools I have applied to, and I have nothing to say.
DR: Is that depression that you are feeling?
ALINA: It's not that; I am always depressed. It's like everything hurts, like I have the flu. My legs hurt, my back hurts, and my brain hurts. When they ask me questions, I can't think. It's too much pain and my mind goes blank.
DR: Are you anxious?
ALINA: I am always anxious. It's not that. It's like I have a headache, but it's different. It's excruciating. Like all my feelings need Tylenol or something.
DR: Do you feel that this pain is too much to live with?
ALINA: Sometimes.
DR: Do you feel that for you to go on this pain must be stopped right now?
ALINA: Sometimes.

Rapid spikes of negative emotions

DR: You said that you feel better now. . . . Do these feeling of being trapped in your pain, and being raw, and having no skin, can they appear suddenly? Do they come in waves?

ALINA: I could be fine one moment and then it just hits me. Out of the blue. And I start drowning.

DR: Like when Dorothy smirked?

ALINA: Yes. I was pretty OK until then, and then it was like somebody hit me. I could not catch my breath. And I got so angry I could not even talk anymore. I had to walk away.

DR: So, is it like a wave or like a punch?

ALINA: It can be ether. It's more like a punch when there is a trigger. Like Dorothy with her smirk, or my mother telling me to be like somebody I could never be. When there are no triggers, it comes and goes in waves.

DR: How do you feel when the wave passes?

ALINA: Better usually.

DR: Do you feel happy?

ALINA: Not happy; hyper.

Extreme anxiety

DR: When you felt trapped, did you feel emotionally raw?

ALINA: Yes! (*Emphatically, as if recognizing something*)

DR: Did you feel like even the smallest things were bothering you, that normally would not?

ALINA: Yeah, after I told Dorothy that I will take a gap year before college, she kind of smirked, like I was so inferior to her, and I kept thinking about it all evening. And then I dreamt about it. . . . Can you believe it; I had a dream about Dorothy's smirk!

DR: Do these feelings make you feel restless and make you want to escape?

ALINA: Yes! Escape and never come back . . .

DR: Last weekend after Dorothy smirked at you and you felt like a wave of a bad feeling hit you, did you feel that something was wrong with you physically?

ALINA: My skin was crawling. I wanted to leave, but my mother didn't let me.

DR: How about later that evening, when you felt trapped in your pain?

ALINA: I felt nauseous, and also my whole body was aching. I could barely move.

DR: It may sound like a strange question, but did your body or your body parts feel different?

ALINA: Yeah. . . . Now that you asked, my stomach was squashed.

DR: Did the world around you feel any different?

ALINA: Yes, the sounds were muffled, like from behind a wall, and everything was tilted.

DR: What do you mean?

ALINA: Like I would walk and the ground felt tilted and rubbery.

DR: Were you scared?

ALINA: I thought I was going to die. I did not know how much of this I could take.

DR: (*Gently*) But you did not answer my question.

ALINA: I was scared I was going to have a heart attack. That's not how I want to die.

DR: How?

ALINA: I told you, I would take the pills.

DR: Are you scared now?

ALINA: I am OK now, just a little nauseous and my hands are tingling.

Acute anhedonia

DR: What makes you feel good, usually?

ALINA: Watching TV or reading.

DR: Have you been doing that?

ALINA: There is nothing on. I watched *Game of Thrones* twice and read it twice.

DR: What about doing something with Sara? She called you a couple weeks ago if I remember.

ALINA: It hurts me even to think about this. And I am boring. I have very little to say. She is still on vacation anyway.

DR: What about going for a run with your mom? You used to like that.

ALINA: I used to like running in middle school, with my friend. I don't like it anymore. And my mother runs faster than me, she is all about winning. Just thinking about this is giving me a headache.

DR: Are you able to feel anything positive?

ALINA: Like what? Ice cream tastes good. There is only so much ice cream I can eat.

Alina's mental state at the time of the interview shows all aspects of affective disturbance. She clearly feels mental/emotional pain and distinguishes her "awful" state of mind both from depression and from anxiety. Her emotional pain is not constant, but fluctuates in intensity, which represents rapid spikes of negative emotions. The pain intensity depends on Alina's contact with the real world, which makes her feel damaged and inadequate. The pain comes in characteristic waves, and at their peak Alina feels the emotional rawness of extreme anxiety. The fantasy worlds of TV and fiction, which do not talk back, are her nonsuicidal escapes that make her feel good.

Alina describes extreme anxiety, including several essential somatic experiences, such as nausea, skin crawling, and tingling. Her experiences of sounds being muffled and the world being tilted, as well as the ground feeling rubbery, are typical dissociative experiences. She spontaneously says that she thought she was going to die, which means that the "death by distress" notion was very much in her consciousness and was also very intense.

Alina's lack of interest in searching for new shows on TV or for new books, as well as her lack of desire to shop for clothes and makeup and to dress up (activities she used to enjoy), is an example of motivational anhedonia. Her lack of pleasure when going on a run is an example of consummatory anhedonia.

Case 42—Continued

Emotional pain

DR: Richard, how have you been feeling lately?
RICHARD: Not so good.
DR: Are you depressed?
RICHARD: No, not depressed. It's like I am anxious, which is more painful than the depression.
DR: Would you say, regardless of how you label it, you feel emotional pain?
RICHARD: Yes, you could say that.
DR: Is it too much to bear?
RICHARD: Sometimes.
DR: How about right now?
RICHARD: Right now also.
DR: Do you feel that for you to go on it must be stopped?
RICHARD: It better be.
Rapid spikes of negative emotions
DR: This fear you just mentioned, that she would leave and you will be all alone in the end, is it there all the time or does it come in waves?

RICHARD: In waves.

DR: Waves of what? What feeling?

RICHARD: I just get very angry. I gave her everything I had, she spent all my money, and then she is going to leave. She makes me so mad.

DR: Mad or scared also?

RICHARD: Mad and scared. Nobody wants to be alone at the end.

DR: Do these feelings come out of the blue?

RICHARD: Sometimes. But mostly, it is when she is around. It gets so bad, I am afraid that if I speak, I will just scream.

Extreme anxiety

DR: Do you feel like you've lost control over the situation?

RICHARD: I never had any control, I just had the money.

DR: It sounds like you feel helpless to change the situation.

RICHARD: You could say so.

DR: Do you feel emotionally raw?

RICHARD: What do you mean?

DR: I mean, like having a very thin skin or no skin, like whatever she says will drive you crazy.

RICHARD: It does but I cannot show it. She will pick a fight and it will cost me.

DR: Does she get under your skin so much that you're afraid you will lose it?

RICHARD: She does, and I do lose it. I don't know what to do anymore. She just won't listen.

DR: Are you scared that she will leave?

RICHARD: Terribly. I can't stop thinking about this, particularly at night.

DR: When you are in the middle of a wave of bad feeling, anger, or anxiety, do you feel like something is wrong with you physically?

RICHARD: My eyes are hurting, and my stomach.

DR: Any strange sensations in your skin?

RICHARD: My eyelids are burning.

DR: Do you feel like something strange is happening in your body?

RICHARD: I feel my stomach shake in the morning and that I am disconnected from the world.

DR: Does all this feel scary to you?

RICHARD: Very.

DR: Are you scared that you might die?

RICHARD: Yes.

DR: What do you mean?
RICHARD: I mean my body will just give in and something will happen.
Acute anhedonia
DR: Does this pain make it difficult for you do things that you like?
RICHARD: Yes, it's hard.
DR: What is your most favorite thing to do?
RICHARD: I like watching movies.
DR: Have you been able to lately?
RICHARD: Not for a while. I can't make myself do it and when I try it feels like
    a chore.

Like Alina, Richard has most of the symptoms of SCS affective disturbance, but he is not very skilled at examining his feelings or talking about them. Richard acknowledges having emotional pain, which is distinct from anxiety and depression. Thinking about his wife's spending gives Richard extreme anxiety, mixed with waves of anger (rapid spikes of negative emotions), and his state of mind is so painful that he cannot stand it much longer (extreme anxiety). His hurting eyes and burning eyelids are somatic symptoms of panic, and his feeling of being disconnected from the world is a dissociative symptom. He admits to fear of dying—so scary that he does not want to think or talk about it. Finally, his anhedonic symptoms are demonstrated by his lack of pleasure from his favorite activities.

Criterion B2: Loss of Cognitive Control

Cognitive dysfunction is arguably the most studied and the most understood aspect of suicidal behavior. Many studies have shown that the suicidal crisis is characterized by a ruminative and rigid thought process (Halari et al., 2009), difficulties in decision-making and judgment (Leykin et al., 2011), problems with recall bias (Patten, 2003), and unsuccessful attempts to suppress unwanted thoughts (Van der Does, 2005).

In the proposed DSM definition of SCS, loss of cognitive control is the second of the four Criteria B. In suicidal individuals who experience the loss of cognitive control, the thought patterns identified in Criterion B2 may amplify the perception of the impossibility of escape from the unbearable life situation. These thought patterns are ruminations, cognitive rigidity, failed thought suppression, and ruminative flooding. In the proposed criteria, they are defined in colloquial clinical terms as follows.

Loss of cognitive control as manifested by

- *Ruminations:* intense and persistent thoughts about one's own distress and the life events that brought it on.
- *Cognitive rigidity:* inability to deviate from a repetitive negative pattern of thought.
- *Failed thought suppression:* repeated unsuccessful attempts to suppress negative or disturbing thoughts.
- *Ruminative flooding:* an experience of an overwhelming profusion of negative thoughts, accompanied by head pressure or pain, and impairing the ability to process information or make a decision.

Of the four loss-of-cognitive-control symptoms, ruminative flooding stands out as the most severe. Ruminative flooding is characterized not only by uncontrollable perseverative thinking involving continual thoughts about the causes, meanings, and consequences of one's negative mood (Katz et al., 2011; Yaseen et al., 2010, 2012, 2013, 2014, 2016) but also by somatic symptoms, including headaches and head pressure. In some studies, ruminative flooding had a stronger association with near-term suicidal behavior than frantic hopelessness/entrapment (Yaseen et al., 2010, 2012).

Ruminations

Ruminations can be defined as repetitive thoughts focused on one's own distress. The distress can be symptomatic, such as anguish, suffering, or guilt, or it can be factual, relating to difficult life situations and stressors. The more recently developed term *repetitive negative thinking* (RNT) also describes the ruminations and worry present in anxiety and depression, and it was hypothesized to be a transdiagnostic symptom present in many other disorders, including posttraumatic stress disorder, social phobia, obsessive-compulsive disorder, insomnia, eating disorders, panic disorder, hypochondriasis, alcohol use disorder, psychosis, and bipolar disorder (for a review, see Ehring & Watkins, 2008).

Ruminations have repeatedly been associated with suicidal thoughts and attempts (Morrison & O'Connor, 2008). Ruminations about one's own symptoms, or brooding ruminations, are more strongly associated with suicide attempts than ruminations about the events of one's life, or reflective pondering (Morrison & O'Connor, 2008). Brooding ruminations are very similar to, and may be identical to, RNT, although this remains to be proven through rigorous research.

Patients at risk for imminent suicide believe they are trapped in an endless loop of repetitive thinking from which there is no escape. Not surprisingly, in acutely suicidal people, ruminations are often focused on the perceived dead-end life situation from which there is no exit. The more they ruminate about their own failures, the more convinced they become that there are no viable solutions to improve their lives. Often the failures are related to the un-achievable goals they had set for themselves and the goal-orientation factor of the SN (Rogers et al., 2021; Vespa et al., 2021; see Chapter 5).

In a sense, acutely suicidal patients find themselves trapped in their own circular thinking about their own entrapment. When they try to break out of the loop with a willful effort, they either fail or succeed for only a very short time. Some patients with particularly intense ruminations experience them as a vortex rather than a loop, and they liken their attempts to stop their ruminations to trying to escape the vortex. Alternatively, they may feel like they are falling into a rabbit hole from which they cannot climb out. This imagery indicates that the ruminations have escalated to the level of ruminative flooding, which is a sign of a suicidal crisis and a symptom of SCS.

Cognitive Rigidity
Anecdotal accounts, the clinical experience of numerous clinicians over many years, and recent research data indicate that the thought process in acutely suicidal individuals is often inflexible and rigid.

Clinical experience repeatedly shows that acutely suicidal patients have difficulty changing their thinking patterns, having become locked into inflexible, repetitive thought patterns affixed to various aspects of their SN: failure to meet their own expectations, real or imagined social defeat or defeats, alienation, perceived burdensomeness, and, finally, increasingly desperate perception of no future. These thoughts are ruminative; circular ruminative thinking about the same matter is inflexible by nature. Notably, rigidity in thinking may be present even in impulsive suicide attempters, who may not develop ruminations. Thus, clinicians may attempt preventive interventions to improve flexibility in thinking before these patients decide that suicide is their only option.

In research studies, cognitive rigidity in patients with SI or a history of suicide attempts has been shown many times through testing rigidity in set-shifting—that is, the ability to change thinking and behavior in response to a changing environment (Marzuk et al., 2005). In the assessment of imminent suicide risk, cognitive rigidity can be evaluated following the assessment of ruminations by testing whether the patient can change their mind when presented with a hypothetical alternative interpretation of the patient's current life situation. If the patient is unable to do so, the clinician can offer an alternative interpretation. The patient's ability or inability to accept the proposed and less pernicious interpretation of their life will then reveal the degree of cognitive rigidity.

In recent network analysis studies, however, cognitive rigidity did not show a strong association with the rest of the SCS symptoms (Menon et al., 2022; Park et al., in press). While this may be due to the measures used, the matter requires further study.

Failed Thought Suppression

Thought suppression is the deliberate attempt to not think of something. It is often used as a strategy of conscious cognitive control when unpleasant thoughts need to be diminished or eliminated (Wegner, 1989), and it often fails. Research shows that this natural and intuitive strategy is counterproductive and achieves the opposite result. Thought suppression works for only a very short period of time, and when the strategy fails, unwanted thoughts return with both higher frequency and increased intensity (see reviews by Abramowitz et al., 2001, and Wegner, 1989). Remarkably, individuals with a greater tendency to suppress unwanted thoughts react to emotional thoughts more strongly and have a more difficult time regulating their emotions (Wegner & Zanakos, 1994). Conversely, those with less thought suppression are much more adept at regulating their emotions.

Thought suppression is a common strategy utilized by suicidal patients to reduce the thought pressure from unwanted ruminations. However, like all thought suppression, these willful attempts paradoxically increase the frequency of intrusive thoughts and amplify the intensity of suicidal thinking (Wegner et al., 1987). Findings from several studies showed that a tendency to suppress unwanted thoughts was associated with past SI and suicide attempts (Pettit et al., 2009) and that thought suppression was a mediator of the relationship between emotional reactivity and the occurrence of self-injurious thoughts and behavior (Najmi et al., 2007).

Ruminative Flooding

As the intensity of the suicidal crisis increases, the specific negative feelings attached to individual endeavors and activities converge into a state of psychic pain. Some people experience psychic pain physically as "head pain." This generalized intense sense of dysphoria must be assessed in depth during the assessment for imminent suicide risk.

The ruminative flooding component of SCS encompasses the uncontrollable onslaught of repetitive, automatic, affectively charged, negative thoughts characterized by ruminations and rigidity. However, unlike simple ruminations, ruminative flooding includes negativistic cognitive distortions with a paranoid flavor, which amplify with failed attempts at thought suppression, resulting in somatic symptoms in the brain. Ruminative flooding is distinguishable from simple ruminations by the presence of headaches or head pressure—migrainelike somatic symptoms in the head that confer an increased risk of SI and suicide attempts (Law & Tucker, 2018; Wetherall et al., 2019; Yaseen et al., 2012, 2013, 2014, 2016).

Thus, in ruminative flooding, the thought process disturbances reach such power and intensity that only the thoughts about the unbearable life situation are possible. The rigidity and the obsessive single focus of the circular thought process amplify the intensity of ruminations. As ruminative intensity increases, the subject matter further narrows, stultifying the thought process even more. In ruminative flooding, the endless feedback loop of ruminations and rigidity reaches a point at which the thought process becomes unbearably painful. The pain of uncontrollable ruminative negative thinking experienced by suicidal patients is distinct from that of a normal headache and is often described as head pain or pressure in the head that can be directly linked to the vortex of unwelcome thoughts.

The nature of the relationship between the head pain of ruminative flooding and suicide is worth investigating as a possible treatment target. Cluster headaches are associated with significant psychopathology, including suicide, and the relationship is so obvious clinically that cluster and migraine headaches are called suicide headaches (Robbins, 2013; Schneck & Andrasik, 2019). Patients with suicide headaches exhibit behaviors similar to SCS, such as overarousal, self-hurting behaviors, and agitation. This suggests that known treatments for migraine headaches have a potential as antisuicide agents.

In their loss of control over their thought process, ruminating patients are similar to patients with tangential thinking, looseness of associations, and flight of ideas, which are essential components of thought disorder. Hence, suicidal ruminations can arguably be considered a variant of thought disorder or psychosis. Although not all ruminations reach delusional intensity, almost all could be categorized as overvalued ideas. Of possible relevance, overvalued ideas are very common in patients with BPD (Zanarini et al., 2013), and meta-analyses show that a low-dose neuroleptic is the only treatment that appears to be beneficial for patients with BPD (Vita et al., 2011). Low-dose antipsychotics could be considered in suicidal individuals with loss of cognitive control as well.

Patients with a loss of cognitive control are very conscious of losing control over their thoughts. For that reason, the best way to assess Criterion B2 is by asking if the patients feel like they control their thoughts or if they feel that the thoughts are controlling them. A Yes answer to the latter, regardless of everything else, indicates that Criterion B2 has been met.

The following continuing case examples illustrate comprehensive assessment of the loss of cognitive control in SCS.

Case 41—Continued

Ruminations

DR: I want to talk a little bit more about last weekend, when you felt your worst. Was it after you thought that Dorothy smirked at you?
ALINA: Yes, but then I fell asleep.
DR: Well, do you remember, while you were alone in your room, before you fell asleep, did you keep thinking the same thoughts again and again?
ALINA: Yes.
DR: Were thoughts running, or was your head quiet?
ALINA: Running.
DR: What were you thinking exactly?
ALINA: I was trying to think of what to say to her so I would sound smart.
DR: Were you able to come up with anything?
ALINA: No, and then I started thinking about how miserable I was.
Cognitive rigidity
DR: Why are you so sure that Dorothy is happy in college?
ALINA: She looks happy. And she must be, she got into a very good school, what is there to be unhappy about?

DR: There are all kinds of reasons:difficult courses, too much work, stiff competition, no friends. I can go on.

ALINA: Why does she look happy then?

DR: Just good social skills. Never compare your insides with other people's
outsides.

ALINA: You are just making things up. She said that college was great and she
loved it.

Failed thought suppression

DR: These are pretty upsetting thoughts. What happens when you try not to
think them?

ALINA: It does not work very well.

DR: What happens?

ALINA: They just keep coming back.

DR: Does it work even a little? I mean, when Dorothy with her smirk comes
back, is her smirk the same, better, or worse?

ALINA: Worse.

Ruminative flooding

DR: Was your thinking clear or foggy? Did it feel noisy in your head?

ALINA: Noisy. Sometimes.

DR: Is it hard to figure out sometimes what exactly you are thinking?

ALINA: Sometimes.

DR: At those times when you were thinking so hard that your head was noisy
and confusing, did you feel pressure in your head?

ALINA: Yes.

DR: Were these thoughts and images of Dorothy smirking giving you a
headache?

ALINA: My brain hurt.

DR: Did you feel that your head could explode from having too many bad
thoughts you could not suppress?

ALINA: Yes.

DR: Did you feel that these thoughts and images were like a vortex pulling
you in, and you try to climb out, but you can't?

ALINA: I wasn't even trying to climb out. I gave in.

Although at the time of the office interview, Alina was not acutely suicidal,
the therapist's assessment of her state of mind during the preceding weekend

revealed most of the loss-of-cognitive-control symptoms of SCS. Alina described negativistic ruminations about her being inferior to Dorothy; she could not even consider alternative, less toxic interpretations of Dorothy's behavior (rigidity); she described unsuccessful attempts at thought suppression (Dorothy's smirk coming back with a vengeance); and she acknowledged the ruminative flooding (vortex). Thus, although Alina did not attempt suicide over the weekend, she was in the midst of a suicidal crisis.

Case 42—Continued

Ruminations

DR: Richard, you seem distracted to me; is your thinking right now clear or foggy?
RICHARD: I have a lot on my mind. It is hard to focus.
DR: Are you thinking about your wife and her spending?
RICHARD: That is all I can think about.
DR: Do you keep thinking the same thoughts again and again, like in a loop?
RICHARD: Yes.
DR: Is it worse at night before you fall asleep?
RICHARD: I have a hard time falling asleep.

Cognitive rigidity

DR: You know, there may be other approaches you could use to deal with your financial situations.
RICHARD: I can't think of any, I have tried. I am on a fixed income.
DR: Maybe she does not fully understand the situation. Did you try talking to her? Will you ask her to come in for a session?
RICHARD: No, she will leave. She thought she had married a rich man. I can't tell her we have no money.

Failed thought suppression

DR: You look distracted, like you are back in your endless thinking loop. What happens if you try to suppress these thoughts and think about something else?

RICHARD: I can't stop thinking about this; there is no point in thinking about anything else until I find a solution.

DR: What happens if you do try?

RICHARD: Nothing, the thoughts just come back.

DR: Worse, the same, or better than before you tried?

RICHARD: Worse.

Ruminative flooding

DR: Does all this thinking, these endless thoughts you cannot suppress, make you feel pressure in your head?

RICHARD: Yes. And pain in my skull, actually.

DR: Some liken their ruminative thoughts to a vortex, which just keeps getting deeper and deeper, and is sucking them in. Is that how you feel?

RICHARD: Kind of.

DR: Does it feel that you are trying to climb out, but you can't, and it is just pulling you back in?

RICHARD: Yes, this is exactly how it feels.

DR: For how long can you bear this head pressure or pain?

RICHARD: I can't. I have just about had it.

In contrast to Alina, who has somewhat recovered from the previous weekend's suicidal crisis, Richard's crisis is present and could be worsening. An outside observer may notice that he is internally preoccupied. Ruminations dominate his thinking, he is powerless to control or suppress them, and he admits to ruminative flooding. Loss of cognitive control, combined with Richard's affective disturbance, revealed in the first part of the previous interview, indicates that Richard is at high short-term risk for suicide.

Criterion B3: Hyperarousal

Hyperarousal is the third category of Part B symptoms required for the proposed DSM diagnosis of SCS. It can manifest as agitation—a state of extreme arousal, physical restlessness—as hypervigilance, as heightened irritability (Ballard et al., 2016; Bryan et al., 2014), or as insomnia. Hyperarousal is the energy that may fuel suicidal behavior.

Agitation and Irritability

On the surface, agitation may appear to be an uncomplicated symptom. It can be conceptualized as at least two different abnormal states: a state of extreme arousal or a state of heightened irritability and anxiety. The first definition of agitation, as an unpleasant arousal, places it in the same domain as other disturbances of arousal, such as lethargy, insomnia, and hypersomnia. On the other hand, the second definition of agitation, as a state of anxious excitement or disinhibition, consigns agitation to the spectrum of moods, together with anxiety, anhedonia, and anguish.

In short-term suicide risk evaluation, agitation is usually assessed as an objectively observed psychomotor behavior—that is, an abnormal state of arousal rather than a self-reported mood state (we rarely, if ever, ask patients if they feel agitated). Regardless of which definition is used, agitation has been repeatedly linked with suicidal behavior (Fawcett et al., 1997). Agitation has been hypothesized to be one potential mechanism through which bipolar disorder, medical illness, and prescription of certain psychiatric medications might increase the risk of suicidal behavior (Henry & Demotes-Mainard, 2006). This hypothesis remains to be tested, but it appears to be consistent with clinical experience: by definition, bipolar manic and mixed states involve increased arousal. Agitated delirium, which is common in medical illness, also involves increased arousal and akathisia, which is a side effect of many antipsychotics and some antidepressants.

Hypervigilance

Hypervigilance can be defined as a heightened sensory awareness and sensitivity to potential threats (Rollman, 2009). Increased attention to perceived threats in one's environment has been shown to increase anxiety levels (Taylor at al., 2011), which has been associated with an increase in suicidal behavior (Nepon et al., 2010). Additionally, patients with MDD and a history of suicide attempts demonstrated higher hypervigilance scores than patients without a history of suicide attempts and a healthy control group (Ahmadpanah et al., 2017). Hypervigilance has been shown to contribute to the predictive validity of the SCS diagnosis (Yaseen et al., 2019).

Insomnia

Insomnia is another aspect of disturbed arousal reported in the literature as preceding suicidal behavior (Hochard et al., 2016). Before completed suicides and serious suicide attempts, acutely suicidal individuals may experience difficulty falling asleep, waking up at night after initial sleep, or sometimes waking up every hour. Dreams, nightmares, night terrors (which could be nocturnal panic attacks), and being exhausted in the morning even after sleeping several hours were all reported to doctors or noted by relatives (Hochard et al., 2016). These clinical reports are consistent with the research findings of disturbed arousal in suicidal patients (Hochard et al., 2016; Ribeiro et al., 2014).

Insomnia is a very prevalent condition and is not specific to the acute suicidal state, which is also true of anxiety, ruminations, and panic—all of which are very common symptoms experienced by those with or without mental illness. However, prior to the suicide attempt, insomnia may escalate sharply, particularly in adolescents, for whom it is the second leading acute symptom, after emotional pain, that precedes high-lethality suicide attempts (Wong et al., 2016).

Although agitation and insomnia are risk factors for suicide in their own right, other components of the SCS may have agitation or insomnia as a part of their clinical presentation. Agitation, defined as extreme anxious arousal, overlaps with extreme anxiety. The symptoms of emotional pain and the ups and downs of depressive turmoil, desperation, and entrapment all include some elements of agitation and are frequently concomitant with insomnia.

Reports of withdrawal and hypersomnia in relation to suicide are less consistent. Some parents of adolescents who went on to die by suicide described their children as staying in their rooms and in bed prior to their death. Veterans Administration clinicians who treat suicidal veterans have reported the gradual withdrawal from life by suicidal veterans, who would not answer phone calls or would skip their appointments prior to their fatal suicide attempts.

The following continuing case examples describe the assessment of the disturbance of arousal.

Case 41—Continued

DR: You said that you did not know if you would make it last weekend, but then you fell asleep. Was it hard to fall asleep?
ALINA: Yeah, I just kept thinking the same thoughts, just as you said.
DR: What where you doing as you were thinking? Were you lying in bed?
ALINA: I tried. I could not. I could not stay in bed.

DR: What did you do?

ALINA: I tried to watch TV, but I could not concentrate. I could not sit still. So, I walked around the room.

DR: How did you fall asleep?

ALINA: I had two beers.

DR: Did you sleep through the night?

ALINA: No. I woke up two hours later when my mother came.

DR: Then?

ALINA: She tucked me in. Then I slept on and off. It was nice to have my mother next to me.

In the preceding weekend, Alina had both agitation (pacing around) and early and late insomnia. This adds to the evidence that she was in the midst of a suicidal crisis.

Case 42—Continued

DR: You seem restless; did you notice your leg is jumping up and down?

RICHARD: Not until you said it. You notice everything, don't you?

DR: Am I irritating you? Why are you getting up?

RICHARD: You make me feel like I am under a microscope. And I just can't sit still. There is too much on my mind.

DR: Do you feel restless inside, like you need to move?

RICHARD: No, I just feel like standing.

DR: You also look tired. Did you sleep well last night?

RICHARD: I always wake up a couple of times to go to the bathroom.

DR: Last night after you went to the bathroom, did you fall asleep right away?

RICHARD: No. I walked around a bit, and then I watched TV.

DR: Did pacing around help calm down your thoughts?

RICHARD: Not really. I just did not know what else to do.

In this interview in his doctor's office, Richard shows signs of psychomotor agitation (leg restlessness and jumping up). He is also irritable, telling the doctor he feels like he is under a microscope. Furthermore, he has developed insomnia, not being able to fall asleep in the middle of the night and pacing. Richard's psychomotor activity further confirms that he has developed SCS.

Criterion B4: Acute Social Withdrawal

Acute social withdrawal is the final component of SCS; it tends to manifest as a reduction in the frequency and scope of social activity as well as in evasive communication with others. Rejection of others and withdrawal of interpersonal support have been shown to increase the future risk of suicidal behavior (Stellrecht et al., 2006). Zhu et al. (2021) investigated prolonged social withdrawal among university students and found that it was associated significantly with increased self-harm and suicidal behavior, although not after adjusting for psychological factors, suggesting psychological symptoms may have stronger links with suicidality than social involvements. Another study by Kelley et al. (2019) among combat-wounded veterans found that social connectedness moderated the relationship between moral injury and suicidality, with lower levels of suicidality among those with higher social connectedness. In our prospective studies, distancing oneself from one's friends combined with not disclosing one's distress to others was one of the factors predictive of near-term suicidal behavior (Bloch-Elkouby et al., 2021).

SCS Assessment Algorithm

The assessment of SCS is more straightforward than the assessment and construction of the SN because it involves direct questions about a patient's mental state, which is the kind of patient engagement that clinicians are very familiar with. Here, we present a suggested SCS assessment algorithm. It was used in Cases 15 and 16, in the case examples presented later in this chapter, and in the test case in this chapter It does not include rapport building, which usually has been accomplished earlier, in the course of the SN part of the assessment.

The algorithm used is structured according to the proposed SCS DSM criteria. As in real clinical situations, in order to minimize misleading self-reports by individuals who have made up their minds to die by suicide and would like to hide their intent from the interviewing clinician, direct explicit questioning about the patient's SI and intent should be reserved until the end of the interview and is not discussed here. This change in the order of the assessment is illustrated in the overall interview strategies discussed in detail in Chapter 9.

Although during the course of a conversational interview the question order can be flexible and determined by the patient's answers, it is suggested that the interviewer evaluating SCS severity follow roughly the same order as in the guide and that the interviewer start with assessment of the criterion that has the most predictive validity for suicidal behavior, Criterion A, frantic hopelessness/entrapment. Ideally, this should be followed in order by the assessments of affective disturbance, loss of cognitive control, hyperarousal, and social withdrawal (for a detailed discussion of complete interview strategies, see Chapter 9). This order is important because the first boldface question in each criterion creates a narrative for the One-minute Assessment, to be used in high volume, high-pressure ED settings that may be understaffed and when clinicians may be overwhelmed with EMR documentation.

The affective disturbance part of the SCS assessment contains questions about the emotional state that, when asked sensibly, reveal concern and care. They should be asked before the questions about loss of cognitive control and arousal because the latter questions are more clinical and, if asked first, may seem uncaring and create a misperception that the clinician is "just doing a job."

In real life, when asking about affective disturbance, it is suggested that the interviewer start with the most intuitive and easy-to-understand questions about emotional pain, followed by more intrusive and specific questions about different aspects of entrapment. Similarly, when assessing loss of cognitive control, it makes sense to start with questions about less severe pathology, such as ruminations, and then to elaborate on the more severe and distressing pathology, such as ruminative flooding.

The Full SCS Assessment

Criterion A: Frantic hopelessness/entrapment

When you think about your current life situation that brought you here, do you feel trapped?
... do you see possible exits from your condition?
... do you see possible good solutions or ways out of your problem?
... do you see ways of improving the situation?
... do you see ways of solving your problem?
When you think about the (unbearable) life situation,

... how long can you tolerate living like this?

... is there hope that your life (your pain, your illness, your condition) will improve?

... can you wait for it to improve?

... how long can you wait?

... for you to go on, do you need for the pain to stop now?

... do you feel the urge to escape your situation now?

... is suicide an escape?

Criterion B1: Affective disturbance

Emotional pain

When you think about your current life situation that brought you here, are you in pain? Emotional pain?

Is this pain too much to bear?

Do you feel it needs to be stopped?

Do you feel this pain can get better?

Will it only get worse?

Rapid spikes of negative emotions

Do you feel waves of bad feelings or that your mood is even?

Do you feel waves of anxiety, anger, fear?

During these waves, are you afraid you might die or lose your mind? Which one?

Do these feelings come in waves out of the blue?

Do they make you feel restless and agitated?

Extreme anxiety

Do you feel that you have no control?

Do you feel that you have lost control to change things?

Do you feel powerless?

Do you feel helpless?

Do you feel overwhelmed with negative emotions?

Do you feel emotionally raw?

Do you feel like you have no skin?

Do you feel like the smallest things are bothering you, as if your life lies
in the balance?

Do you feel so nervous that you are on the verge of losing control?

With the waves of bad feelings, do you feel something is wrong with
you physically?

Do you feel unusual physical sensations that you have never felt before?

Do you also have physical symptoms, such as sweating? (Nausea?
Problems breathing? Rapid heartbeat?)

Do you feel strange sensations in your body or skin?

Do you feel something happening to (in, on) your body?

Do you feel that the world around you is different?

Do you also worry about bad things that may happen to you?

Do you have nightmares about death? (Which ones?)

Do you wake up at night in a sweat, so scared you might die it is hard
to breathe?

Do you fear for your life?

Acute anhedonia

What makes you feel good usually?

Has this activity become a burden to you?

Has this activity become painful?

Does it feel like torture?

Are you able to feel anything positive?

Is it hard to try to feel positive? How hard?

Criterion B2: Loss of cognitive control

**When you think about being trapped in your current life situation
(the one that causes you so much emotional pain), do you feel that
you can control your thoughts, or do your thoughts control you?**

Ruminations

Is your thinking clear or foggy?

Are your thoughts racing, running fast, or is your head quiet?

Is it hard to figure out exactly what you are thinking?

Do you have unpleasant thoughts in your head that keep running again
and again?

Do these thoughts come mostly at night before you go to sleep?

Do you think these thoughts also during the day?

Are you having these thoughts right now?

Do you feel pressure in your head from having too many thoughts?

Are you having headaches from having too many thoughts?

Do you feel like your head could explode from having too many thoughts?

Cognitive rigidity

You know, these negative thoughts you have been having about your life—this is not the only way to look at things. For example, here is an alternative interpretation . . .

But really—many people are happy doing this; can you see your life from this point of view?

How hard is it to see your problem in a different light?

Do you succeed? How often?

How long can you think other thoughts before you come back to the ones that bother you?

Failed thought suppression

Do you try to forcefully suppress these thoughts?

Can you?

Is it working?

Is trying to suppress your thoughts only making them worse?

Ruminative flooding

Do the out-of-control bad thoughts make you feel pressure in your head?

Do the out-of-control bad thoughts make you feel a headache or head pain?

Does this make you feel like your head could explode?

For some people, this endless thinking feels like a vortex, which just keeps getting deeper and deeper. Is that how you feel?

Does it feel like you are trying to climb out, but you can't?

Criterion B3: Hyperarousal

Do the out-of-control bad thoughts about the life situation you find yourself in come mostly at night? Can you sleep?

Agitation

> You seem agitated to me. Is this how you feel?
> Do you feel agitated inside?
> Is it hard to stay calm?

Hypervigilance

> Have you been kind of on edge, hypersensitive to the outside world lately?
> Like noticing things out of the corner of your eye, things that other people may miss or do not see?
> Have you been paying more attention to people's facial expressions, reading into their possible thoughts?
> Are bright colors, sounds, and smells bothering you more than usual?

Irritability

> Have you been more irritable lately?
> Do people get under your skin more than usual?
> Have you been losing your temper more?

Insomnia

> Does all this agitation prevent you from sleeping?
> Have you had problems falling asleep? Waking up in the middle of the night? Too early?
> When you have problems sleeping, do these thoughts we talked about a minute ago bother you?
> Criterion B4: Acute social withdrawal

> Have you felt isolated from others lately?
> Did you evade communications with people who care about you?
> Did you push away people who care about you?

The One-Minute Assessment

The order in the SCS assessment above is important because the first bold-face question in each criterion creates a narrative for the One-minute Assessment, which is comprised of five questions targeting the core of SCS. It can be used as a backbone to the SCS assessment, with other questions added as guided by the patients' answers and dictated by the clinical situation. In principle, the One-minute Assessment could be used in high volume, high-pressure ED settings that may be understaffed and when clinicians may be overwhelmed with EMR documentation. However, one should have no illusions that the One-minute Assessment is as good at detecting SCS as the full interview.

The five questions of the One-minute Assessment are:

1. When you think about your current life situation that brought you here, do you feel trapped?
2. When you think about your current life situation, do you feel pain? I mean either emotional pain or head pain.
3. Do you feel that you can control your thoughts, or are your thoughts controlling you?
4. Does this happen primarily at night, and can you sleep?
5. Have you told anybody about these thoughts? (probe for social withdrawal and evasive communication)

These five questions target SCS, which can be boiled down to one sentence, one snapshot, or one image of unending, painful, uncontrollable thoughts about being trapped in an unbearable life situation from which there is no exit; thoughts that are so intense that a person cannot sleep and cannot share these thoughts with anyone. This book aims to make this image known and accessible to every practicing clinician and, eventually, to everyone.

Case Examples—Continued from Chapter 6

Case 38: High Risk for Imminent Suicide—Continued

Gary is a 30-year-old single Jewish man with a history of bipolar I disorder and two previous psychiatric hospitalizations who is currently living in a two-bedroom apartment with his parents. He returned to the United States six months earlier after teaching English for two years in Croatia, and his parents referred him to a bipolar specialist for a psychiatric assessment "so he can get the best possible treatment because he is a difficult case." Gary has no previous suicide attempts, but his parents are concerned that he may kill himself because "there is just something scary about him that makes us very uncomfortable."

During the SN part of the assessment, Gary revealed all five components of the SN: He could not give up on an unrealistic expectation of an academic career; his professional and personal failures made him feel defeated and alienated, as well as a burden to his parents; and with the next job application rejection, he would find himself at a dead end with no good options, which would make him a very high suicide risk.

The SCS Assessment
Criterion A: Frantic hopelessness/entrapment

DR: When you think about your life situation, living with your parents, being supported by them, looking for a job, everything you told me about choices, do you want to escape?
GARY: Yes, it's close to intolerable . . .
DR: Do you feel an escape is possible?
GARY: Not sure. I need a miracle. I need a teaching job.
DR: Other than that, do you see any other good options?
GARY: None. I feel trapped. I feel horrible and I feel trapped.
DR: How long can you tolerate the mental pain you are in?
GARY: I don't know—sometimes I think I can't.
DR: Do you have hope that the pain will soon get better?
GARY: Yes—when I get a job.
DR: Can it get better if you do not?
GARY: I doubt it.
DR: I know you are expecting to hear from "College A." What if they say no?
GARY: That is going to be pretty bad. I am not sure I will be able to take it.
DR: What do you mean by that?
GARY: Don't worry doc, I am not going to kill myself now. There is still hope.

Criteria B: Associated disturbances
Criterion B1: Affective disturbance

Emotional pain

DR: Gary, you came to see me because you were feeling bad. You told me earlier that you were in pain. Is it emotional pain that you are in?

GARY: Yes, although at times everything hurts, even my legs.

DR: How bad is it?

GARY: Sometimes it feels unbearable. It can get so bad, I do not know how long I can take it.

DR: How long can you take it?

GARY: I don't know. That's why I am here. Maybe you will be able to stop it. I can't go on like this.

DR: Do you feel it all the time or it comes and goes?

GARY: It comes and goes. But when I have it, it is relentless. It's torture.

DR: Does anything make it better?

GARY: Nothing of late.

Rapid spikes of negative emotions

DR: Do the bad feelings that you feel come and go or is your mood even?

GARY: They come and go.

DR: Could these be waves of anxiety? Or fear?

GARY: Maybe.

DR: When they do come, do they come in waves out of the blue, or there is usually a reason?

GARY: Sometimes there is a reason. . . . Well, there used to be a reason, now they just come.

DR: During these waves, are you afraid you might die or lose your mind?

GARY: I feel like I am going crazy.

DR: Do you also have physical symptoms, such as sweating? Nausea? Problems breathing? Rapid heartbeat?

GARY: All of these.

DR: Do you sometimes wake up at night—just like that, nauseated, heart beating, short of breath and in a sweat, so you get scared you might die?

GARY: That too.

Extreme anxiety

DR: Do you feel scared of what is happening in your mind?

GARY: Yes, I do, sometimes it is really scary.

DR: Do you feel emotionally raw?

GARY: I don't know what I feel. I just know it feels like hell. Like I am in hell, that is.

DR: Are you able to make yourself feel differently? Or talk yourself into feeling differently?

GARY: It does not work. Still feel like sh . . .

DR: Do you feel like the smallest things that should not be bothersome, really get to you?

GARY: Yes, and they make me jumpy.

DR: Making you anxious, like you have no skin?

GARY: Like I have no skin.

DR: Do you feel anxious and scared of losing control?

GARY: I do, and I do lose it with my parents. And when I do, they look really scared of me.

DR: Do you become frantic when that happens?

GARY: You can say that, and this is what scares them, I guess.

DR: When this happens, do you feel strange sensations in your body or on your skin?

GARY: Yes, how did you know?

DR: Experience. Tell me what they are, please.

GARY: It is hard to describe. I have not felt anything like that until recently.

DR: Please try.

GARY: It's crazy. I can feel blood going through my veins, and I can feel my nerves.

DR: How?

GARY: The blood is kind of buzzing, and the nerves are burning. I can also feel my stomach move inside.

DR: Really? Anything else you could add?

GARY: Yes. At those times everything feels different. The world looks different.

DR: When this happens to you, do you ever get scared that you might die?

GARY: Yes.

DR: Literally, like your life is going to end?

GARY: Yes.

DR: Please explain.

GARY: I feel so bad mentally and physically that I am afraid that something must be at a breaking point somewhere inside me. One moment it will just snap and kill me.

DR: How frightening.

GARY: You are telling me.

Acute anhedonia

DR: What is your favorite thing to do for fun that usually makes you feel good?

GARY: Reading. I read a lot. And writing short stories. I used to be good at that.

DR: Have you been reading lately?

GARY: Only newspapers. And they are full of crap.

DR: Does it help relieve the emotional pain you have been feeling?

GARY: Not reading newspapers.

DR: Is reading newspapers painful to you?

GARY: It's never been fun. I like reading good fiction. Classics. Newspaper writers are illiterate.

DR: Have you been reading classics?

GARY: No. I have read and re-read most of them. . . . I thought I could learn how to be a good writer that way.

DR: And now?

GARY: Just opening the book makes my head hurt.

Criterion B2: Loss of cognitive control
Ruminations

DR: Is your thinking clear or foggy?

GARY: Yeah, a little foggy. I never thought I would say something like this. I think well—usually that is.

DR: Are your thoughts racing, running fast, or is your head quiet?

GARY: It is not that they are racing, it's like they are fragmented. Frequently flying fragments (*smiles*).

DR: Are these fragments hard to read?

GARY: They can be confusing.

DR: These fragments, are they repetitive? Do they keep running again and again? In circles?

GARY: Again and again, but not in circles.

DR: Do these thoughts come mostly at night before you go to sleep?

GARY: That's why I cannot sleep, I just keep thinking.

DR: Do you think these thoughts also during the day?

GARY: During the day, too, and in the morning. I wake up thinking about this stuff.

DR: What stuff?

GARY: What is going to happen if I lose this job. I can't not think about that.

DR: Do you feel pressure in your head from having too many thoughts?

GARY: No, they give me headaches.

DR: Do you feel like your head could explode from having too many thoughts?

GARY: That's too dramatic . . .

DR: Do you worry mainly about what's happening in your head, or trying to find a solution?

GARY: A solution—what's the point of worrying about worrying?

Cognitive rigidity

DR: Your thoughts about your life are pretty negative. You blame yourself a lot. Things may not be as black as they seem to be and not all the blame in the world lies with you.

GARY: How so?

DR: Well, you are a really smart guy, you are good at teaching. The academic jobs you are looking for are highly competitive and political. Your talents may be better used elsewhere.

GARY: You're kidding, right? (*Smirks*)

DR: No, I am not. You have been traveling a lot, which gives you a different perspective on life. You could teach high school, you could teach college ESL courses, you could tutor. You have a lot to offer.

GARY: Teaching ESL as a career? That's a great career goal. My parents would be really proud.

DR: Let's forget about your parents for a minute. There are quite a few happy ESL teachers. You could really make a difference.

GARY: Nice try, doc. You can't call teaching English at night a success.

Failed thought suppression

DR: What happens when you try to shut down these negative thoughts?

GARY: I can't.

DR: Do you try?

GARY: Of course I try, it just does not work. They keep coming back.

DR: Does trying to suppress your thoughts make them worse?

GARY: I never thought of this. Maybe it does. It certainly does not make them any better.

Ruminative flooding

DR: For some people, this endless irrepressible thinking feels like a vortex, which just keeps sucking you in deeper and deeper. Is that how you feel?

GARY: Yes, actually, now you got it. A vortex.

DR: Does it feel that you are trying to climb out, but you can't?

GARY: Yes.

DR: Like you are drowning?

GARY: Yes

Criterion B3: Hyperarousal
Agitation

DR: You seem agitated to me, is this how you feel?

GARY: I don't know how you can feel agitated.

DR: I meant, not being able to sit still, needing to move, getting up and pacing, the way you have been doing as we were talking.

GARY: Yes, I have been feeling kind of restless, not sure about agitated.

DR: Do you feel agitated inside?

GARY: Do you mean like stirred up? Yeah . . .

DR: Is it hard to stay calm?

GARY: It is very hard to stay calm, particularly around my parents.

Hypervigilance

DR: You seem to be very attuned to your parents.

GARY: Wouldn't you be? They are supporting me; they want to cut me off.

DR: Do you know what's on their mind?

GARY: I can read them really well. I know what they are thinking.

Irritability

DR: Can you keep your calm when you are talking to them?

GARY: It's getting harder and harder. I am blowing up on them more than I should . . .

Insomnia

DR: Does all this agitation prevent you from sleeping?
GARY: I have a hard time falling asleep.
DR: Are you waking up in the middle of the night? Too early?
GARY: In the middle of the night. I have a hard time waking up in the morning.

Criterion B4: Acute social withdrawal

DR: Have your told anybody about any of this?
GARY: I can't. It's too painful and embarrassing.
DR: Have been in touch with your friends?
GARY: Less and less—they all have jobs and families. We have nothing in common

End of the SCS part of the interview.

As would be true in real life, this interview did not follow the algorithm exactly because Gary gave answers to some of the questions before the questions were asked. By the end of the SCS assessment, however, almost all the questions were answered. Gary has an intense sense of frantic hopelessness/entrapment and is just short of being desperate due to his hope of getting an unlikely job offer. Gary's psychic pain is nearly intolerable. His fear of losing his mind and his anxiety are so expansive, they scare his parents. His anhedonia is painful and paralyzing, and his mood is unstable.

Despite his subjective feeling of being mostly in control of his thinking process, Gary has lost most of his capacity for rational thinking, which is reduced to reflective pondering. Gary appears to be dead set on his goal, incessantly thinking about becoming an academic; his looping thoughts cannot be derailed or suppressed, and he identifies with the experience of being flooded with these thoughts. The only component of ruminative flooding still missing is brooding ruminations about his loss of cognitive and emotional control of himself. Gary also exhibits signs of motor agitation while feeling agitated mentally inside. Overall, Gary's SCS symptoms are severe, and his short-term risk for suicide is high (Table 7.3).

Table 7.3 Gary's suicide crisis syndrome intensity assessment

Symptom	Symptom Severity				
	Minimal	Low	Moderate	High	Severe
Criterion A					
Frantic hopelessness/entrapment				X	
Criteria B					
B1: Affective disturbance					
Emotional pain					X
Rapid spikes of negative emotions					X
Extreme anxiety					X
Acute anhedonia					X
Affective disturbance summary					X
B2: Loss of cognitive control					
Ruminations					X
Cognitive rigidity					X
Failed thought suppression		X			
Ruminative flooding					X
Loss of cognitive control summary				X	
B3: Hyperarousal					
Agitation				X	X
Hypervigilance					X
Irritability					
Insomnia				X	X
Hyperarousal summary				X	X
B4: Acute social withdrawal					X
Reduction in social activities					
Evasive communication with others					
Acute social withdrawal summary					
Criteria B summary					X
Overall summary					X

Case 39: Moderate Risk for Imminent Suicide—Continued

Bernie is a 53-year-old single gay man with a history of a GAD who came for treatment of his depression with SI after discovering that his recently deceased partner of 20 years had a family and children whom Bernie knew nothing about. Bernie had a plan to kill himself with a barbiturate and alcohol overdose. He had also just retired from his teaching job. He has one brother and a large circle of friends. He saw a therapist twice in the past following relationship breakups, was never on medications, and had no past suicide attempts.

The SCS Assessment
Criterion A: Frantic hopelessness/entrapment

DR: When you think about your situation, about what Peter's death has revealed—his other family, his double life—do you feel trapped?
BERNIE: I do not feel trapped, but I am in pain. I do not understand what happened. I cannot reconcile this reality, when he is gone, and he has a wife and children, and our life together, when we only had each other.
DR: How long can you tolerate the condition you are in?
BERNIE: Until you help me feel better. I don't have a choice, do I?
DR: Your pain should get better with time. Time heals, medication and psychotherapy help. Do you have the strength to wait?
BERNIE: I am a pretty strong person.
DR: You still did not answer my question: How long do you think you can wait?
BERNIE: I don't know. Several weeks . . . months . . .
DR: And then? If you don't feel better?
BERNIE: And then, I don't know. We'll cross that bridge when we get there. Hopefully never.

Criteria B: Associated disturbances
Criterion B1: Affective disturbance
Emotional pain

DR: You must be in a lot of pain.
BERNIE: I am not sure the word "pain" describes it.
DR: Please describe what you feel inside, if you can.
BERNIE: It feels like a piece of me was ripped out . . . all that's left is a bleeding wound.
DR: It is emotional though, isn't it?
BERNIE: Yes, it is my soul that is bleeding.
DR: Do you feel that for you to go on, this pain must be stopped?
BERNIE: That's why I am here . . .

Rapid spikes of negative emotions

DR: When you say you feel on edge sometimes, do your bad feelings come in waves?

BERNIE: Yes.

DR: What are the feelings, besides "having no skin"?

BERNIE: Fear. Fear of the future.

DR: Depression?

BERNIE: Yes, depression.

DR: What about anger?

BERNIE: No anger. I am not an angry person. I can't feel angry at him. He was my life.

DR: Do these waves come out of the blue, or do you have some control over them?

BERNIE: These are two different things. The waves come without warning, but when they do, I can bear down and ride them out until I start feeling better.

Extreme anxiety

DR: Does thinking about the two irreconcilable realities make you feel unhinged?

BERNIE: Yes, it makes me feel on edge.

DR: When you feel on edge, do you feel like the smallest things are bothering you? As if you have no skin?

BERNIE: Sometimes.

DR: When you feel at your worst, do you feel like you may lose control?

BERNIE: Not really. I am pretty level-headed, always have been.

DR: I understand. Let's come back to the waves for a moment. When a wave of anxiety comes, do you feel any strange sensation in your body or skin?

BERNIE: I feel like my face is burning.

DR: The skin on your face?

BERNIE: Yes.

DR: How about inside your body?

BERNIE: Sometimes I feel like I am just one walking burning wound. It feels like all my insides are burning.

DR: Does it ever feel so bad that you fear for your life?

BERNIE: No, not that bad.

DR: Do you have nightmares about dying?

BERNIE: No, I have nightmares, but they are not about dying.

DR: What are they about?

BERNIE: Trains. Going into tunnels which never end.

Acute anhedonia

DR: What are the things you enjoy that usually make you feel good?

BERNIE: I like listening to jazz.

DR: Have you been doing that lately?

BERNIE: I tried, but I had to force myself.

DR: And how does it feel when you do?

BERNIE: It feels just OK. Even Miles is just OK.

DR: Are you able to feel anything positive at all?

BERNIE: Only the memories of our life together. We had a fairy tale life you know.

Criterion B2: Loss of cognitive control
Ruminations

DR: When you think about your situation, are your thoughts racing or is your head quiet?

BERNIE: Neither. The thoughts are orderly but just very persistent.

DR: Are your thoughts repetitive? Do they run in circles?

BERNIE: It is hard to think about anything else, but him, and how perfect it was.

DR: Do these thoughts come mostly at night before you go to sleep?

BERNIE: All the time, but worse at night.

DR: Are you having these thoughts right now?

BERNIE: Yes, although talking to you is distracting me.

Cognitive rigidity

DR: You know, these ruminations about the perfect fairy tale life you had . . . do you literally believe your life was perfect? Is it possible to have a perfect life? Most of us would gladly settle for "very good."

BERNIE: Well—you don't believe me, but ours was perfect.

DR: Really? Flawless?

BERNIE: Flawless. I loved him. He loved me. I loved his flaws. He had perfect flaws.

DR: "Perfect" is hard to match. Is it possible that he was not perfect? That maybe there were things about him you did not know?

BERNIE: When I think about this, my head feels like it would explode. He was perfect. And then this:his wife, his children . . . let's talk about something else.

Failed thought suppression

DR: What happens when you try to forcefully suppress these thoughts, or try not to think them?

BERNIE: It only works for a short while. Peter is all I can think about.

DR: Is trying to suppress your thoughts only making them worse?

BERNIE: Not sure. Trying to suppress thoughts about Peter does not make them better. It's not a very good strategy.

Ruminative flooding

DR: Do you feel that you can't really control your thoughts about Peter, that they come and go as they please?

BERNIE: If you put it this way, then yes.

DR: Do these out-of-control thoughts about Peter and about how to make sense of what happened make you feel pressure in your head?

BERNIE: Sometimes, mostly at night when I can't fall asleep.

DR: Does this make you feel like your head could explode?

BERNIE: It's not that dramatic.

DR: At those times, do these thoughts feel like a vortex pulling you in?

BERNIE: Yes, they do.

DR: And when they do, do you try to climb out? Can you?

BERNIE: Sometimes I can, and sometimes I can't.

Criterion B3: Hyperarousal
Agitation

DR: Have you been more tense than usual?

BERNIE: You may say that.

DR: Agitated? Hard to be still?

BERNIE: I do pace sometimes, but not frequently.

Hypervigilance

DR: Do you find yourself keyed up? Registering things you normally would not out of the corner of your eye?

BERNIE: Maybe. I have been oversensitive lately, trying to read people's faces . . . what people know and when then learned it

Irritability

DR: Do people irritate you?

BERNIE: Their matter-of-factness irritates me. They have no idea what it's like to be in my shoes.

Insomnia

DR: Have you had problems falling asleep?

BERNIE: Yes. Scotch helps.

DR: Are you waking up in the middle of the night?

BERNIE: Yes.

DR: And what happens?

BERNIE: I lie in bed thinking. Then I have another scotch.

DR: Do you wake up earlier than usual?

BERNIE: Yes, but that's OK. I try to exercise.

Criterion B4: Acute social withdrawal

DR: When you tell me your story you seem remarkably calm. Do you actually feel calm, or are you a good actor and in reality you feel agitated inside?

BERNIE: I am far from calm, but I do not believe in burdening others with my feelings.

DR: Including doctors?

BERNIE: Including doctors.

DR: Does this mean that you are staying away from your friends or just not being forthcoming when you are with them?

BERNIE: Both.

End of the SCS part of the interview.

Bernie's short-term suicide risk (Table 7.4) is lower than that of Gary, but it may increase if he is unable to reconcile his idyllic past with Peter with the reality of his partner's long deception. His emotional pain is severe, but his extreme anxiety and rapid spikes of negative emotions are not very significant. He has substantial symptoms of panic and dissociation, and his fear of dying is revealed symbolically in his dreams. With regard to loss of cognitive control, he is very high on ruminations and rigidity, but he does not have

Table 7.4 Bernie's suicide crisis syndrome intensity assessment

Symptom	Symptom Severity				
	Minimal	Low	Moderate	High	Severe
Criterion A					
Frantic hopelessness/entrapment		X			
Criteria B					
B1: Affective disturbance					
Emotional pain					X
Rapid spikes of negative emotions			X		
Extreme anxiety	X				
Acute anhedonia			X		
Affective disturbance summary			X		
B2: Loss of cognitive control					
Ruminations					X
Cognitive rigidity				X	
Failed thought suppression			X		
Ruminative flooding				X	
Loss of cognitive control summary				X	
B3: Hyperarousal					
Agitation	X	X	X		
Hypervigilance					
Irritability					
Insomnia		X	X		
Hyperarousal summary			X		
B4: Acute social withdrawal			X		
Reduction in social activity					
Evasive communication with others					
Acute social withdrawal summary					
Criteria B summary			X		
Overall summary			X		

ruminative flooding. He is also able to contain his state of inner agitation so that it is not visible to the outsider. He did, however, reduce his social activities and is not open with others. Overall, at the time of the interview, Bernie manifested an SCS of moderate intensity.

Case 40: Low Risk for Imminent Suicide—Continued

Kate is a 28-year-old woman who was admitted to a psychiatric unit for a suicide attempt. Kate repeatedly cut her left arm and left thigh with a razor blade after she was let go from a nonprofit after a falling out with her supervisor. The cuts were deep enough for her thigh wounds to require sutures. Kate had a long psychiatric history and was diagnosed with attention deficit disorder as a child and with MDD, GAD, panic disorder, and BPD in high school. She was accepted to, but never completed, college, despite several attempts to do so. She worked only sporadically, mainly for environmental causes, and was supported by her father. During the interview, Kate was confrontational and provocative.

The SCS Assessment
Criterion A: Frantic hopelessness/entrapment

DR: Do you feel sometimes that you've hit a dead end?
KATE: It felt like that at the time.
DR: When you think about your fight for the cause and all the frustrations involved, do you feel trapped?
KATE: I did before I came in. It is very frustrating, but I think once I feel better, I can still volunteer and be useful.
DR: How impatient are you for your emotional pain to get better?
KATE: I would like to feel better, of course, but I could be patient.
DR: How long can you tolerate the condition you are in?
KATE: Until I feel better, I guess. I hope not too long.
DR: It seems that before you came in, the pain was so strong you wanted it to stop then. Do you feel the urge for it to stop now?
KATE: I feel an urgent need, but I am not going to cut myself.
DR: Do you have an urge to escape it now?
KATE: Not anymore. The pills have helped.

Criteria B: Associated disturbances
Criterion B1: Affective disturbance
Emotional pain

DR: You just told me a lot about how you came to cut yourself so deeply that it required stitches and about what brought you to the hospital. Your cut seems to have healed. Do you still feel like you are in a state of emotional pain?

KATE: I do because I still believe in my cause.

DR: Do you feel that this inner pain is too much to bear?

KATE: No, after this admission, I can handle it. It makes me angry. It makes me work harder.

DR: What if the pain becomes worse?

KATE: I hope it does not. But if it does, I hope you will help me.

Rapid spikes of negative emotions

DR: OK. The way you are right now, is your mood even or could you have waves of anxiety or other bad feelings?

KATE: It's mainly anxiety. It was pretty bad earlier today before I took the pills.

DR: What about anger? You came in pretty angry at the world.

KATE: I am still angry.

DR: Were you angrier in the morning before you took the pills?

KATE: I guess . . . definitely, now that you say so.

DR: It sounds like you are still in a bit of turmoil. Do these feelings make you feel restless and agitated inside?

KATE: Yes.

Extreme anxiety

DR: You still sound pretty frustrated and anxious. Is this how you feel inside?

KATE: Yeah, I am pretty anxious but it's OK.

DR: How anxious do you feel, exactly? Do you feel emotionally raw?

KATE: Not as much as I did when I was admitted—that was really bad. Now I am almost my usual self.

DR: With you being so sensitive, does it sometimes feel like the smallest things bother you, like you have no skin?

KATE: Most of the time.

DR: Even now?

KATE: Even now. I am always like that.

DR: Like the smallest things make you feel off balance?

KATE: Kind of . . . but not as bad as before.

DR: Did you feel like you were losing control?

KATE: Then, but not now. I am pretty good now.

DR: Coming back to the waves . . . when the wave of bad feelings is at its peak, do you feel something is wrong with you physically?

KATE: I feel tightness in my chest; it's hard to breathe.

DR: Do you also feel strange sensations in your body or skin?

KATE: My fingers get numb.

DR: Do you feel something happening to your body?

KATE: I feel my nerves ring under my skin. . . . It sounds crazy, but I do. I just know where they are.

DR: And when you can sense your nerves, or at any other time, do you feel that the world around you is different?

KATE: No, it's always the same. Good old bad world that needs to change.

DR: When you can't breathe, do you get scared that it may get so bad that you die?

KATE: No, I know this is anxiety.

DR: Regardless of shortness of breath, can your waves of anxiety and anger feel so bad that you fear for your life?

KATE: Not really. It's not life threatening.

Acute anhedonia

DR: What do you do for fun that usually makes you feel good?

KATE: I like food. I have a sweet tooth. I know it's not good for you, but that's the truth. The food here is awful.

DR: What about the food that your family brings?

KATE: They brought Dunkin' Donuts. It made my day.

Criterion B2: Loss of cognitive control
Ruminations

DR: When you think about your fight for the cause and all the frustrations that led to your suicidal behavior, is your thinking clear or foggy?

KATE: Pretty clear.

DR: Though clear, are your thoughts racing, running fast, or is your head quiet?

KATE: My head is never quiet, and my thoughts are always fast. I'm not sure about racing.

DR: Are the thoughts still persistent, running in your head again and again?

KATE: Yes, I still think about my causes all the time.

DR: Are these thoughts worse at night when you try to go to sleep?

KATE: Yes, sometimes it is hard to fall asleep.

DR: And you are having these thoughts right now, as we speak?

KATE: Yes, I confirm!

Cognitive rigidity

DR: You know, with all due respect, many people would disagree with your point of view on the environment. The mineral depletion may not be as catastrophic as you say.

KATE: What do you mean? You can't be serious.

DR: I am not saying that this is my point of view, but one can argue that mankind has an inventive mind and will find other materials to create from and other sources of energy. Do you think this is possible, at least in theory?

KATE: I can't believe my ears. So you too are saying we can continue destroying our planet?

DR: I never said that. I just asked if you thought an alternative was possible.

KATE: I guess it is possible but very unlikely. It is very clear that mining and carbon emissions are the two main causes of global warming.

Failed thought suppression

DR: Do you ever try to forcefully suppress these thoughts?

KATE: Not particularly, why?

DR: They are not very comfortable thoughts to have.

KATE: It's OK, I have been living with these ideas for years.

Ruminative flooding

DR: Do you ever feel pressure in your head from having too many thoughts like these?

KATE: Not right now. When I was admitted, I did.

DR: Were you also having headaches from having too many thoughts?

KATE: No headaches. Well, maybe slightly, but not for a while.

DR: For some people this kind of endless thinking may feel like a vortex, which just keeps getting deeper and deeper. Have you ever felt like that?

KATE: Not quite . . . maybe a little, when I was admitted.

Criterion B3: Hyperarousal
Agitation

DR: You seem a little restless. Is this how you feel?

KATE: I am always restless—this is just me.

Hypervigilance

DR: Is your mind also restless? Does it jump to reading other people's facial expressions and imagining their thoughts?

KATE: Only when I need to, like at meetings.

DR: How about seeing things out of the corner of your eye that others may miss?

KATE: (*irritated*) I am not sure what you mean.

Irritability

DR: You seem irritated.

KATE: You are kind of irritating with your questions.

DR: Just me or others also?

KATE: Just you. Can I leave now?

Insomnia

DR: Yes, almost done. How are you sleeping?

KATE: Pretty well now, with the new pills. It takes me a while to fall asleep, but once I am asleep I sleep through the night.

DR: So, you are back to your usual self?

KATE: Pretty much. I want to be discharged.

Criterion B4: Acute social withdrawal
Reduction in social activities

DR: Are you planning to see your friends?
KATE: Yes, one of them will come to pick me up.

Evasive communications with others

DR: Will you tell them about your situation and experiences here?
KATE: They know my situation and I will definitely tell them about this place
   in great detail.

End of the SCS part of the interview.

   Kate is not in a suicide crisis, and her short-term suicide risk is low
(Table 7.5). From the interview, it can be gleaned that Kate's SCS severity at
admission was moderate. She has both anxiety and mood disorders, and at
the time of the interview she reports emotional pain, waves of panic, depressive turmoil, and ruminations. However, she has virtually no entrapment or
thought suppression, and her other SCS symptoms, including disturbance
in arousal, are minimal. Thus, overall, her SCS symptoms are mild, and her
short-term risk is low.

Test Case 3

Jackie is a 19-year-old woman who was referred for an evaluation after she
told her parents she would kill herself if they would not allow her to see
her friends (who her parents believed were a bad influence on her). Jackie
was recently discharged from an inpatient psychiatric unit, where she had
been admitted two months earlier with confusion following an overdose
with her stepmother's Klonopin. She was diagnosed with attention deficit
hyperactivity disorder (ADHD) and a learning disability as a child, with
depression and bulimia as an adolescent, and with borderline and narcissistic personality disorder during her recent psychiatric hospitalization.
Of relevance, Jackie's mother died of suicide by hanging when Jackie was
12 years old.

Table 7.5 Kate's suicide crisis syndrome intensity assessment

Symptom	Minimal	Low	Moderate	High	Severe
			Symptom Intensity		
Criterion A					
<u>Frantic hopelessness/entrapment</u>	X				
Criteria B					
<u>B1: Affective disturbance</u>					
Emotional pain			X		
Rapid spikes of negative emotions			X		
Extreme anxiety			X		
Acute anhedonia	X				
Affective disturbance summary		X			
<u>B2: Loss of cognitive control</u>					
Ruminations			X		
Cognitive rigidity		X			
Failed thought suppression	X				
Ruminative flooding		X			
Loss of cognitive control summary		X			
<u>B3: Hyperarousal</u>					
Agitation	X	X	X		
Hypervigilance					
Irritability					
Insomnia	X	X			
Hyperarousal summary					
<u>B4: Acute social withdrawal</u>					
Reduction in social activity	X	X			
Evasive communication with others					
Acute social withdrawal summary	X				
Criteria B summary		X			
Overall summary		X			

The SCS Assessment
Criterion A: Frantic hopelessness/entrapment

DR: Nice to meet you, Jackie. What brings you here?
JACKIE: My parents, you know they won't let me see my friends!
DR: That must be tough. . . . One needs one's friends. Do you see a solution to your situation?

JACKIE: Yes:My parents should allow me to see my friends. I am 19, I can make my own decisions about who I want to be friends with.

DR: Your parents seem to think that your friends are a bad influence on you. They drink and they do drugs and . . .

JACKIE: You don't know my friends, and neither do my parents. They are the only ones who don't put me down. They are the only ones who make me feel good.

DR: It's a problem, though, that your parents feel otherwise. Do you see any possible solutions to this problem?

JACKIE: Not with my parents. They never listen to me, and they always only see bad in me. Nothing I do is good enough.

DR: Do you have other friends?

JACKIE: What? I am not going to betray my friends to please my parents!

DR: How do you feel right now?

JACKIE: Miserable, angry, and frustrated.

DR: How long can you take feeling like this?

JACKIE: I don't know.

DR: To help your situation, we may need to do some family therapy with you, your father, and your stepmother. It may take some time. Can you live with your pain and frustration during this time?

JACKIE: As long as I can continue to be with my friends.

DR: And if not?

JACKIE: I will kill myself.

Criteria B: Associated disturbances
Criterion B1: Affective disturbance
Emotional pain

DR: Can your state of mind be described as emotional pain? Does this ring a bell?

JACKIE: Yes. I am in pain.

DR: Do you feel that this emotional pain is too much to bear?

JACKIE: Sometimes.

DR: How about right now?

JACKIE: I am bearing it right now.

DR: Do you feel this pain can get better?

JACKIE: Yes—I told you already. I am fine when I am with my friends.

Rapid spikes of negative emotions

DR: Does your emotional pain come in waves or is your mood even?
JACKIE: Neither. I am not sure what you mean.
DR: Do you feel waves of anxiety?
JACKIE: Yes.
DR: Do these feelings come in waves out of the blue?
JACKIE: Yes, they are not predictable.
DR: Do you feel bouts of anger?
JACKIE: Yes. I am trying to regulate that, though.
DR: Do you feel waves of fear?
JACKIE: No.
DR: Do the waves of anxiety and anger make you feel restless and agitated?
JACKIE: Sometimes.

Extreme anxiety

DR: Do you feel that you have lost control?
JACKIE: I am in control.
DR: I mean: Do you feel that you have lost control to change things?
JACKIE: I hope not.
DR: Do you feel overwhelmed with negative emotions?
JACKIE: Not now.
DR: Do you sometimes feel emotionally raw, like you have no skin?
JACKIE: What do you mean?
DR: Like the smallest things are bothering you, as if your life lies in the balance?
JACKIE: No, that's too dramatic.
DR: When you have waves of anxiety coming over you, do you feel something is wrong with you physically?
JACKIE: No.
DR: When you have waves of anxiety, do you also have physical symptoms, such as sweating? Nausea? Problems breathing? Rapid heartbeat?
JACKIE: Do you mean panic attacks? I have panic attacks.
DR: When you have panic attacks, do you feel strange sensations in your body or skin?
JACKIE: No.

DR: Do you feel something happening to (in) your body?
JACKIE: Other than nausea, no.
DR: When you panic, do you feel that the world around you is different?
JACKIE: I feel disconnected sometimes, like I am in a movie.
DR: Do you worry a lot about bad things that may happen to you?
JACKIE: Not usually.
DR: Do you have nightmares about death?
JACKIE: I have nightmares about my mother.
DR: Tell me about them.
JACKIE: I would rather not. Thinking about it makes me feel bad.
DR: Do you wake up at night in a sweat, so scared you might die that it is hard
    to breath?
JACKIE: Once or twice.
DR: Were you scared you may suddenly die?
JACKIE: Yes.

Acute anhedonia

DR: What makes you feel good usually?
JACKIE: Being with my friends.
DR: What else?
JACKIE: I like Chipotle, it's the best.
DR: Does it taste good?
JACKIE: Great! And they serve only "happy meat."

Criterion B2: Loss of cognitive control
Ruminations

DR: When you think about this impasse with your parents and your friends,
    is your thinking clear or foggy?
JACKIE: My thinking is always clear.
DR: Even when you took the overdose?
JACKIE: Yes.
DR: Right now, are your thoughts racing, running fast, or is your head quiet?
JACKIE: Quiet. My thoughts can be fast, though. I have ADHD. Sometimes it
    is hard to concentrate.
DR: In the last couple of days, did you have unpleasant thoughts in your head
    that kept running again and again?

JACKIE: Yes—like what to do about my parents.
DR: Do these thoughts come mostly at night before you go to sleep?
JACKIE: No.
DR: Do you think these thoughts also during the day?
JACKIE: Yes.
DR: Are you having these thoughts right now?
JACKIE: Yes, you are asking me all these questions.
DR: Do you feel pressure in your head from having too many thoughts?
JACKIE: No.
DR: Are you having headaches from having too many thoughts?
JACKIE: No.
DR: Do you feel like your head could explode from having too many thoughts?
JACKIE: No. That's crazy.

Cognitive rigidity

DR: You know, you are saying that your friends are the only people in the world that have ever liked you and will ever like you. It can't be this black and white.
JACKIE: That's how it is, though.
DR: Well, for example, did you make friends with other patients in the hospital?
JACKIE: There was one girl I liked.
DR: And? Did she like you?
JACKIE: Yeah, we talked. She cut herself.
DR: Well, that's another thing altogether. She liked you. People care about you more than you think, Jackie.
JACKIE: Hmm . . .

Failed thought suppression

DR: When you have the thoughts about taking pills, do you try to suppress them?
JACKIE: Not sure what you mean.
DR: People often try to suppress the disturbing thoughts that make them feel bad. Do you?
JACKIE: Not consciously.

Ruminative flooding

DR: It sounds like you feel the worst when your parents don't let you see your friends, in fact you feel so bad you think about suicide. Do these bad thoughts make you feel pressure in your head?

JACKIE: No.

DR: Do these thoughts make you feel like your head could explode?

JACKIE: No.

DR: For some people, thinking about suicide is like a vortex, which just keeps getting deeper and deeper and can suck you in.

JACKIE: Not really.

Criterion B3: Hyperarousal
Agitation

DR: A while back you said you felt miserable and angry to me. Is this how you still feel?

JACKIE: Yes, pretty much.

DR: Do you feel agitated inside?

JACKIE: Kind of.

DR: Is it hard to stay calm?

JACKIE: It's OK. I can stay in control.

Hypervigilance

DR: In the state you are in, do you find yourself keyed up?

JACKIE: What do you mean?

DR: Reading into people's facial expressions, imagining their thoughts, noticing little things out of the corner of your eye?

JACKIE: Not really.

DR: How about smells, noises, or colors bothering you?

JACKIE: Yeah . . . this place smells of horrible soap and these blue walls are ugly.

Irritability

DR: Do I irritate you with my questions?
JACKIE: Not particularly. People are generally irritating, especially my parents.

Insomnia

DR: Have you had problems falling asleep? Waking up in the middle of the night? Too early?
JACKIE: I am online a lot at night, talking to my friends.
DR: When you have problems sleeping, do these thoughts we talked about a minute ago bother you?
JACKIE: I sleep OK.

Criterion B4: Acute social withdrawal
Reduction in social activity

DR: So, coming back to the main issue, it is safe to say that you have not been withdrawing from your friends?
JACKIE: Yeah, I need my friends.

Evasive communication with others

DR: And you tell your friends about your problems?
JACKIE: That's what friends are for. We tell each other everything.

End of the SCS part of the suicide risk assessment.

Jackie's mother's death by suicide increases her suicide risk long term, whereas her recent overdose increases her suicide risk both long term and short term. Her Criterion A SCS assessment shows clear entrapment, which, however, is conditional on external circumstances. In contrast, her Criteria B assessment shows only minimal and low-intensity symptoms of affective disturbance, loss of cognitive control, hyperarousal, and acute social withdrawal. Thus, Jackie's overall short-term risk is moderate (Table 7.6). The divergent Criteria A and B symptom levels illustrate the usefulness of the full SCS assessment for short-term risk determination.

Table 7.6 Jackie's suicide crisis syndrome intensity assessment

| | Symptom Intensity | | | | |
Symptom	Minimal	Low	Moderate	High	Severe
Criterion A					
Frantic hopelessness/entrapment					
Criteria B					
B1: Affective disturbance					
Emotional pain					
Rapid spikes of negative emotions					
Extreme anxiety					
Acute anhedonia					
Affective disturbance summary					
B2: Loss of cognitive control					
Ruminations					
Cognitive rigidity					
Failed thought suppression					
Ruminative flooding					
Loss of cognitive control summary					
B3: Hyperarousal					
Agitation					
Hypervigilance					
Irritability					
Insomnia					
Hyperarousal summary					
B4: Acute social withdrawal					
Reduction in social activity					
Evasive communication with others					
Acute social withdrawal summary					
Criteria B summary					
Overall summary					

References

Abramowitz, J. S., Tolin, D. F., & Street, G. P. (2001). Paradoxical effects of thought suppression: A meta-analysis of controlled studies. *Clinical Psychology Review*, *21*(5), 683–703.

Ahmadpanah, M., Astinsadaf, S., Akhondi, A., Haghighi, M., Sadeghi Bahmani, D., Nazaribadie, M., Jahangard, L., Holsboer-Trachsler, E., & Brand, S. (2017). Early maladaptive schemas of emotional deprivation, social isolation, shame and abandonment are related to a history of suicide attempts among patients with major depressive disorders. *Comprehensive Psychiatry, 77*, 71–79. https://doi.org/10.1016/j.comppsych.2017.05.008

Akiskal, H. S., & Benazzi, F. (2005). Psychopathologic correlates of suicidal ideation in major depressive outpatients: Is it all due to unrecognized (bipolar) depressive mixed states? *Psychopathology, 38*(5), 273–280.

American Psychiatric Association. (2013). *Diagnostic and statistical manual of mental disorders* (5th ed.). American Psychiatric Association.

Anestis, M. D. (2016). Prior suicide attempts are less common in suicide decedents who died by firearms relative to those who died by other means. *Journal of Affective Disorders, 189*, 106–109. https://doi.org/10.1016/j.jad.2015.09.007

Angst, J., Angst, F., & Stassen, H. H. (1999). Suicide risk in patients with major depressive disorder. *Journal of Clinical Psychiatry, 60*, 57–62; discussion 75–76, 113–116.

Appleby, L., Kapur, N., Shaw, J., Hunt, I. M., Flynn, S., & Rahman, M. S.; University of Manchester Centre for Mental Health and Risk. (2012). *The national confidential inquiry into suicide and homicide by people with mental illness: Annual report.* http://research.bmh.manchester.ac.uk/cmhs/research/centreforsuicideprevention/nci

Bachmann, S. (2018). Epidemiology of suicide and the psychiatric perspective. *International Journal of Environmental Research and Public Health, 15*(7), 1425. https://doi.org/10.3390/ijerph15071425

Bafna, A., Rogers, M. L., & Galynker, II. (2022). Predictive validity and symptom configuration of proposed diagnostic criteria for the Suicide Crisis Syndrome: A replication study. *Journal of Psychiatric Research, 156*, 228–235. doi:10.1016/j.jpsychires.2022.10.027. Epub ahead of print. PMID: 36270061.

Ballard, E. D., Vande Voort, J. L., Luckenbaugh, D. A., Machado-Vieira, R., Tohen, M., & Zarate, C. A. (2016). Acute risk factors for suicide attempts and death: Prospective findings from the STEP-BD study. *Bipolar Disorders, 18*(4), 363–372.

Bannikov, G. S., Letova, A. V., Anisimova, Y. V., & Yakh"yayeva, P. K. (under review). *Cuitsidal'nyye intentsii studentov v period pandemii Kovid–19* [Suicidal intentions of students during the Covid-19 pandemic] [Unpublished manuscript]. *Irkutsk Suicidology Conference.*

Barzilay S, Apter A, & Levy-Betz, Y. (2021, September). *Assessment of suicide crisis syndrome in youth* [Paper presentation]. International Association for Suicide Prevention meeting.

Barzilay, S., Assounga, K., Veras, J., Beaubian, C., Bloch-Elkouby, S., & Galynker, I. (2020). Assessment of near-term risk for suicide attempts using the Suicide Crisis Inventory. *Journal of Affective Disorders, 276*, 183–190. https://doi.org/10.1016/j.jad.2020.06.053

Barzilay, S., Gagnon, A., Yaseen, Z. S., Chennapragada, L., Lloveras, L., Bloch-Elkouby, S., & Galynker, I. (2021). Associations between clinicians' emotion regulation, treatment recommendations, and patient suicidal ideation. *Suicide and Life-Threatening Behavior, 52*(22), 329–340. https://doi.org/10.1111/sltb.12824

Baumeister, R. F. (1990). Suicide as escape from self. *Psychological Review, 97*(1), 90–113. https://doi.org/10.1037/0033-295x.97.1.90

Beautrais, A. L. (2004). Further suicidal behavior among medically serious suicide attempters. *Suicide and Life-Threatening Behavior, 34*(1), 1–11. https://doi.org/10.1521/suli.34.1.1.27772

Beck, A. T., Schuyler, D., & Herman, J. (1974). Development of suicidal intent scales. In A. Beck, H. Resnik, & D. J. Lettieri (Eds.), *The prediction of suicide* (pp. 45–56). Charles Press.

Benazzi, F., & Akiskal, H. S. (2001). Delineating bipolar II mixed states in the Ravenna–San Diego collaborative study: The relative prevalence and diagnostic significance of hypomanic features during major depressive episodes. *Journal of Affective Disorders, 6*, 115–122.

Berman, A. L. (2018). Risk factors proximate to suicide and suicide risk assessment in the context of denied suicide ideation. *Suicide and Life-Threatening Behavior, 48*(3), 340–352. https://doi.org/10.1111/sltb.12351

Bloch-Elkouby, S., Barzilay, S., Gorman, B. S., Lawrence, O. C., Rogers, M. L., Richards, J., Cohen, L. J., Johnson, B. N., & Galynker I. (2021). The revised Suicide Crisis Inventory (SCI-2): Validation and assessment of prospective suicidal outcomes at one month follow-up. *Journal of Affective Disorders, 295*, 1280–1291. https://doi.org/10.1016/j.jad.2021.08.048

Bloch-Elkouby, S., Gorman, B., Lloveras, L., Wilkerson, T., Schuck, A., Barzilay, S., Calati, R., Schnur, D., & Galynker, I. (2020). How do distal and proximal risk factors combine to predict suicidal ideation and behaviors? A prospective study of the narrative crisis model of suicide. *Journal of Affective Disorders, 277*, 914–926. https://doi.org/10.1016/j.jad.2020.08.088

Bloch-Elkouby, S., Gorman, B., Schuck, A., Barzilay, S., Calati, R., Cohen, L. J., Begum, F., & Galynker, I. (2020). The suicide crisis syndrome: A network analysis. *Journal of Counseling Psychology, 67*(5), 595–607. https://doi.org/10.1037/cou0000423

Bloch-Elkouby, S., Zilcha-Mano, S., Roger, M. L., Park, J. Y., Manlongat, K., Krumerman, M., & Galynker, I. (2022). Who are the patients who deny suicidal intent? Exploring patients' characteristics associated with self-disclosure and denial of suicidal intent. *Acta Psychiatrica Scandinavica.* doi:10.1111/acps.13511. Epub ahead of print. PMID: 36263445.

Bostwick, J. M., Pabbati, C., Geske, J. R., & McKean, A. J. (2016). Suicide attempt as a risk factor for completed suicide: Even more lethal than we knew. *The American Journal of Psychiatry, 173*(11), 1094–1100. https://doi.org/10.1176/appi.ajp.2016.15070854

Brown, G. W., Harris, T. O., & Hepworth, C. (1995). Loss, humiliation and entrapment among women developing depression: A patient and non-patient comparison. *Psychological Medicine, 25*(1), 7–21.

Brown, G. K., Henriques, G. R., Sosdjan, D., & Beck, A. T. (2004). Suicide intent and accurate expectations of lethality: Predictors of medical lethality of suicide attempts. *Journal of Consulting and Clinical Psychology, 72*(6), 1170–1174. https://doi.org/10.1037/0022-006X.72.6.1170

Bryan, C. J., Hitschfeld, M. J., Palmer, B. A., Schak, K. M., Roberge, E. M., & Lineberry, T. W. (2014). Gender differences in the association of agitation and suicide attempts among psychiatric inpatients. *General Hospital Psychiatry, 36*(6), 726–731.

Busch, K. A., Fawcett, J., & Jacobs, D. G. (2003). Clinical correlates of inpatient suicide. *The Journal of Clinical Psychiatry, 64*(1), 14–19. https://doi.org/10.4088/jcp.v64n0105

Calati, R., Nemeroff, C. B., Lopez-Castroman, J., Cohen, L. J., & Galynker, I. (2020). Candidate biomarkers of suicide crisis syndrome: What to test next? A concept paper. *International Journal of Neuropsychopharmacology, 23*(3), 192–205. https://doi.org/10.1093/ijnp/pyz063

Chang, B., Gitlin, D., & Patel, R. (2011). The depressed patient and suicidal patient in the emergency department: Evidence-based management and treatment strategies. *Emergency Medicine Practice, 13*(9), 1–23.

Chistopolskaya, K. A., Rogers, M. L., Cao, E., Galynker, I., Richards, J., Enikolopov, S. N., Nikolaev, E. L., Sadovnichaya, V. S., & Drovosekov, S. E. (2020). Adaptation of the Suicidal Narrative Inventory in a Russian sample. *Suicidology, 11*(4), 76–90. https://doi.org/10.32878/suiciderus.20-11-04(41)-76-90

Cohen, L. J., Gorman, B., Briggs, J., Jeon, M. E., Ginsburg, T., & Galynker, I. (2019). The suicidal narrative and its relationship to the suicide crisis syndrome and recent suicidal behavior. *Suicide and Life-Threatening Behavior, 49*(2), 413–422. https://doi.org/10.1111/sltb.12439

Deisenhammer, E. A., Ing, C. M., Strauss, R., Kemmler, G., Hinterhuber, H., & Weiss, E. M. (2009). The duration of the suicidal process: How much time is left for intervention between consideration and accomplishment of a suicide attempt?. *The Journal of Clinical Psychiatry, 70*(1), 19–24.

Dilsaver, S. C., Benazzi, F., Akiskal, H., & Akiskal, K. (2007). Post-traumatic stress disorder among adolescents with bipolar disorder and its relationship to suicidality. *Bipolar Disorders, 9*, 649–655.

Ehring, T., & Watkins, E. R. (2008). Repetitive negative thinking as a transdiagnostic process. *International Journal of Cognitive Therapy, 1*(3), 192–205. https://doi.org/10.1680/ijct.2008.1.3.192

ERAN Association. (2022). *Suicide line.* https://en.eran.org.il

Fawcett, J. (1988). Predictors of early suicide: Identification and appropriate intervention. *Journal of Clinical Psychiatry, 49*, 7–8.

Fawcett, J., Busch, K. A., Jacobs, D., Kravitz, H. M., & Fogg, L. (1997). Suicide: A four-pathway clinical–biochemical model. *Annals of the New York Academy of Science, 836*, 288–301.

Fawcett, J., Scheftner, W. A., Fogg, L., Clark, D. C., Young, M. A., Hedeker, D., & Gibbons, R. (1990). Time-related predictors of suicide in major affective disorder. *American Journal of Psychiatry, 147*(9), 1189–1194.

Fehling, K. B., & Selby, E. A. (2021). Suicide in DSM-5: Current evidence for the proposed suicide behavior disorder and other possible improvements. *Frontiers in Psychiatry, 11*, 499980. https://doi.org/10.3389/fpsyt.2020.499980

First, M. B., Pincus, H. A., Levine, J. B., Williams, J. B. W., Ustun, B., & Peele, R. (2004). Clinical utility as a criterion for revising psychiatric diagnoses. *American Journal of Psychiatry, 161*, 946–954. https://doi.org/10.1176/appi.ajp.161.6.946

Fowler, J. C. (2012). Suicide risk assessment in clinical practice: Pragmatic guidelines for imperfect assessments. *Psychotherapy, 49*(1), 81–90. https://doi.org/10.1037/a0026148

Fowles, D. C. (2007). The three arousal model: Implications of Gray's two-factor learning theory for heart rate, electrodermal activity, and psychopathy. *Psychophysiology, 17*(2), 87–104.

Gabbay, V., Ely, B. A., Babb, J., & Liebes, L. (2012). The possible role of the kynurenine pathway in anhedonia in adolescents. *Journal of Neural Transmission, 119*(2), 253–260.

Galynker, I. (2017). *The suicidal crisis: Clinical guide to the assessment of imminent suicide risk.* Oxford University Press. https://doi.org/10.1093/med/9780190260859.001.0001

Galynker, I., Ieronimo, C., Perez-Acquino, A. Lee, Y., & Winston, A. (1996). Panic attacks with psychotic features. *Journal of Clinical Psychiatry, 57*(9), 402–406.

Galynker, I., Yaseen, Z. S., Cohen, A., Benhamou, O., Hawes, M., & Briggs, J. (2017). Prediction of suicidal behavior in high risk psychiatric patients using an assessment of acute suicidal state: The Suicide Crisis Inventory. *Depression and Anxiety*, 34(2), 147–158. https://doi.org/10.1002/da.22559

Gilbert, P., & Allan, S. (1998). The role of defeat and entrapment (arrested flight) in depression: An exploration of an evolutionary view. *Psychological Medicine*, 28(3), 585–598. https://doi.org/10.1017/s0033291798006710

Gilbert, P., & Gilbert, J. (2003). Entrapment and arrested fight and flight in depression: An exploration using focus groups. *Psychology and Psychotherapy*, 76(2), 173–188. https://doi.org/10.1348/147608303765951203

Gilbert, P., Gilbert, J., & Irons, C. (2004). Life events, entrapments, and arrested anger in depression. *Journal of Affective Disorders*, 79(1-3), 149–160.

Glenn, C. R., & Nock, M. K. (2014). Improving the short-term prediction of suicidal behavior. *American Journal of Preventive Medicine*, 47(3 Suppl. 2), S176–S180. https://doi.org/10.1016/j.amepre.2014.06.004

Halari, R., Premkumar, P., Farguharson, L., Fannon, D., Kuipers, E., & Kumari, V. (2009). Rumination and negative symptoms in schizophrenia. *Journal of Nervous and Mental Disease*, 197(9), 703–706.

Haw, C., Hawton, K., Houston, K., & Townsend, E. (2003). Correlates of relative lethality and suicidal intent among deliberate self-harm patients. *Suicide and Life-Threatening Behavior*, 33(4), 353–364. https://doi.org/10.1521/suli.33.4.353.25232

Hawes, M., Galynker, I., Barzilay, S., & Yaseen, Z. S. (2018). Anhedonia and suicidal thoughts and behaviors in psychiatric outpatients: The role of acuity. *Depression and Anxiety*, 35(12), 1218–1227. https://doi.org/10.1002/da.22814

Helseplattformen. (2021, September 19). *Helseplattformen: One common regional health record*. https://helseplattformen.no/om-oss/helseplattformen-one-common-regional-health-record

Hendin, H., Maltsberger, J. T., & Szanto, K. (2007). The role of intense affective states in signaling a suicide crisis. *Journal of Nervous and Mental Disease*, 195(5), 363–369.

Henry, C., & Demotes-Mainard, J. (2006). SSRIs, suicide and violent behavior: Is there a need for better definition of the depressive state? *Current Drug Safety*, 1, 59–62.

Hochard, K. D., Heym, N., & Townsend, E. (2016). Investigating the interaction between sleep symptoms of arousal and acquired capability in predicting Suicidality. *Suicide and Life-Threatening Behavior*, 47(3), 370–381. https://doi.org/10.1111/sltb.12285

Horesh, N., Levi, Y., & Apter, A. (2012). Medically serious versus non-serious suicide attempts: Relationships of lethality and intent to clinical and interpersonal characteristics. *Journal of Affective Disorders*, 136(2), 283–293. https://doi.org/10.1016/j.jad.2011.11.035

Horwitz, A. G., Czyz, E. K., & King, C. A. (2015). Predicting future suicide attempts among adolescent and emerging adult psychiatric emergency patients. *Journal of Clinical Child and Adolescent Psychology*, 44(5), 751–761. https://doi.org/10.1080/15374416.2014.910789

Høyen, K. S., Solem, S., Cohen, L. J., Prestmo, A., Hjemdal, O., Vaaler, A. E., Galynker, I., & Torgersen, T. (2021). Non-disclosure of suicidal ideation in psychiatric inpatients: Rates and correlates. *Death Studies*, 46(8), 1823–1831. https://doi.org/10.1080/07481187.2021.1879317

Kanwar, A., Malik, S., Prokop, L. J., Sim, L. A., Feldstein, D., Wang, Z., & Murad, M. H. (2013). The association between anxiety disorders and suicidal behaviors: A systematic review and meta-analysis. *Depression and Anxiety*, 30(10), 917–929.

Karsen, E., Cohen, L., Miller, F., De Luca, G., & White, B. (under review). Impact of the abbreviated Suicide Crisis Syndrome assessment on clinical decision making in the emergency department. *Acta Psychiatrica Scandinavica.*

Katz, C., Yaseen, Z. S., Mojtabai, R., Cohen, L. J., & Galynker, I. I. (2011). Panic as an independent risk factor for suicide attempt in depressive illness. *Journal of Clinical Psychiatry, 72*(12), 1628–1635. https://doi.org/10.4088/jcp.10m06186blu

Kelley, M. L., Bravo, A. J., Davies, R. L., Hamrick, H. C., Vinci, C., & Redman, J. C. (2019). Moral injury and suicidality among combat-wounded veterans: The moderating effects of social connectedness and self-compassion. *Psychological Trauma, 11*(6), 621–629. https://doi.org/10.1037/tra0000447

Kessler, R. C., Borges, G., & Walters, E. E. (1999). Prevalence of and risk factors for lifetime suicide attempts in the National Comorbidity Survey. *Archives of General Psychiatry, 56*(7), 617–626.

Klonsky, E. D., & May, A. M. (2014). Differentiating suicide attempters form suicide ideators: A critical frontier for suicidology research. *Suicide and Life-Threatening Behavior, 44*(1), 1–5. https://doi.org/10.1111/sltb.12068

Law, K. C., & Tucker, R. P. (2018). Repetitive negative thinking and suicide: A burgeoning literature with need for further exploration. *Current Opinion in Psychology, 22*, 68–72. https://doi.org/10.1016/j.copsyc.2017.08.027

Lazarus, R. S., & Folkman, S. (1984). *Stress, appraisal, and coping.* Springer.

Leykin, Y., Roberts, C. S., & DeRubeis, R. J. (2011). Decision-making and depressive symptomatology. *Cognitive Therapy and Research, 35*(4), 333–341.

Li, S, Galynker, I. I., Briggs, J., Duffy, M., Frechette-Hagan, A., Kim, H. J., Cohen, L. J., & Yaseen, Z. S. (2017). Attachment style and suicide behaviors in high risk psychiatric inpatients following hospital discharge: The mediating role of entrapment. *Psychiatry Research, 257*, 309–314. PMID:28797954. https://doi.org/10.1016/j.psych res.2017.07.072

Li, S., Yaseen, Z. S., Kim, H. J., Briggs, J., Duffy, M., Frechette-Hagan, A., Cohen, L. J., & Galynker, I. I. (2018). Entrapment as a mediator of suicide crises. *BMC Psychiatry, 18*(1), 4. https://doi.org/10.1186/s12888-018-1587-0

Lim, S. W., Ko, E. M., Shin, D. W., Shin, Y. C., & Oh, K. S. (2015). Clinical symptoms associated with suicidality in patients with panic disorder. *Psychopathology, 48*(3), 137–144.

Marzuk, P. M., Hartwell, N., Leon, A. C., & Portera, L. (2005). Executive functioning in depressed patients with suicidal ideation. *Acta Psychiatrica Scandinavica, 112*(4), 294–301.

McMullen, L., Parghi, N., Rogers, M. L., Yao, H., Bloch-Elkouby, S., & Galynker, I. (2021). The role of suicide ideation in assessing near-term suicide risk: A machine learning approach. *Psychiatry Research, 304*, 114–118. https://doi.org/10.1016/j.psych res.2021.114118

Menon, V., Bafna, A. R., Rogers, M. L., Richards, J., & Galynker, I. (2022). Factor structure and validity of the Revised Suicide Crisis Inventory (SCI-2) among Indian adults. *Asian Journal of Psychiatry, 73*, 103119. https://doi.org/10.1016/j.ajp.2022.103119

Mitelman, A., Bafna, A., Rogers, M. L., White, B., Karsen, E. F., Vaaler, A., & Galynker, I. (in press). Perceived clinical utility of Suicide Crisis Syndrome assessment: A multisite pilot study. *Psychological Services.*

Morrison, R., & O'Connor, R. C. (2008). A systematic review of the relationship between rumination and suicidality. *Suicide and Life-Threatening Behavior, 38*(5), 523–538. https://doi.org/10.1521/suli.2008.38.5.523

Mościcki, E. K. (1997). Identification of suicide risk factors using epidemiologic studies. *The Psychiatric Clinics of North America, 20*(3), 499–517. https://doi.org/10.1016/s0193-953x(05)70327-0

Najmi, S., Wegner, D. M., & Nock, M. K. (2007). Thought suppression and self-injurious thoughts and behaviors. *Behavior Research and Therapy, 45*(8), 1957–1965.

Nam, Y. Y., Kim, C. H., & Roh, D. (2016). Comorbid panic disorder as an independent risk factor for suicide attempts in depressed outpatients. *Comprehensive Psychiatry, 67*, 13–18.

National Institute of Mental Health. (August 2021). *Suicide prevention.* https://www.nimh.nih.gov/health/topics/suicide-prevention

Nepon, J., Belik, S. L., Bolton, J., & Sareen, J. (2010). The relationship between anxiety disorders and suicide attempts: Findings from the National Epidemiologic Survey on Alcohol and Related Conditions. *Depression and Anxiety, 27*(9), 791–798. https://doi.org/10.1002/da.20674

Nock, M. K., Stein, M. B., Heeringa, S. G., Ursano, R. J., Colpe, L. J., Fullerton, C. S., Hwang, I., Naifeh, J. A., Sampson, N. A., Schoenbaum, M., Zaslavsky, A. M., & Kessler, R. C. (2014). Prevalence and correlates of suicidal behavior among soldiers: Results from the Army Study to Assess Risk and Resilience in Service Members (Army STARRS). *Journal of the American Medical Association Psychiatry, 71*(5), 514–522.

Obegi, J. H. (2019). Rethinking suicidal behavior disorder. *Crisis, 40*(3), 209–219. https://doi.org/10.1027/0227-5910/a000543

O'Connor, R. C. (2003). Suicidal behavior as a cry of pain: Test of a psychological model. *Archives of Suicide Research, 7*(4), 297–308. https://doi.org/10.1080/713848941

O'Connor, R. C. (2011). The integrated motivational-volitional model of suicidal behavior [Editorial]. *Crisis, 32*(6), 295–298. https://doi.org/10.1027/0227-5910/a000120

O'Connor, R. C., & Portzky, G. (2018). The relationship between entrapment and suicidal behavior through the lens of the integrated motivational-volitional model of suicidal behavior. *Current Opinion in Psychology, 22*, 12–17. https://doi.org/10.1016/j.copsyc.2017.07.021

O'Connor, R. C., Smyth, R., Ferguson, E., Ryan, C., & Williams, J. M. (2013). Psychological processes and repeat suicidal behavior: A four-year prospective study. *Journal of Consulting and Clinical Psychology, 81*(6), 1137–1143. https://doi.org/10.1037/a0033751

Oquendo, M. A., & Baca-Garcia, E. (2014). Suicidal behavior disorder as a diagnostic entity in the DSM-5 classification system: Advantages outweigh limitations. *World Psychiatry, 13*(2), 128–130. https://doi.org/10.1002/wps.20116

Orbach, I. (2003b). Mental pain and suicide. *Israeli Journal of Psychiatry and Related Science, 40*(3), 191–201.

Otte, S., Lutz, M., Streb, J., Cohen, L. J., Galynker, I., Dudeck, M., & Büsselmann, M. (2020). Analyzing suicidality in German forensic patients by means of the German version of the Suicide Crisis Inventory (SCI-G). *Journal of Forensic Psychiatry & Psychology, 31*(5), 731–746. https://doi.org/10.1080/14789949.2020.1787487

Ozturk, E., & Sar, V. (2008). Somatization as a predictor of suicidal ideation in dissociative disorders. *Psychiatry and Clinical Neuroscience, 62*(6), 662–668. https://doi.org/10.1111/j.1440-1819.2008.01865.x.

Park, J. Y., Rogers, M. L., Bloch-Elkouby, S., Richards, J. A., Lee, S., Galynker, I., & You, S. (in press). Factor structure and validation of the revised Suicide Crisis Inventory (SCI-2) in a Korean population. *Asian Journal of Psychiatry.*

Patten, S. B. (2003). Recall bias and major depression lifetime prevalence. *Social Psychiatry and Psychiatric Epidemiology*, 38(6), 290–296.

Pettit, J. W., Temple, S. R., Norton, P. J., Yaroslavsky, I., Grover, K. E., Morgan, S. T., & Schatte, D. J. (2009). Thought suppression and suicidal ideation: Preliminary evidence in support of a robust association. *Depression and Anxiety*, 26(8), 758–763.

Rappaport, L. M., Moskowitz, D. S., Galynker, I., & Yaseen, Z. S. (2014). Panic symptom clusters differentially predict suicide ideation and attempt. *Comprehensive Psychiatry*, 55(4), 762–769.

Ribeiro, J. D., Franklin, J. C., Fox, K. R., Bentley, K. H., Kleiman, E. M., Chang, B. P., & Nock, M. K. (2016). Self-injurious thoughts and behaviors as risk factors for future suicide ideation, attempts, and death: a meta-analysis of longitudinal studies. *Psychological Medicine*, 46(2), 225–236. https://doi.org/10.1017/S0033291715001804

Ribeiro, J. D., Silva, C., & Joiner, T. E. (2014). Over arousal interacts with a sense of fearlessness about death to predict suicide risk in a sample of clinical outpatients. *Psychiatry Research*, 218(1-2), 106–112. https://doi.org/10.1016/j.psychres.2014.03.036

Robbins, M. S. (2013). The psychiatric comorbidities of cluster headache. *Current Pain and Headache Reports*, 17(2), 313. https://doi.org/10.1007/s11916-012-0313-8

Rogers, M. L., Bloch-Elkouby, S., & Galynker, I. (2022). Differential disclosure of suicidal intent to clinicians versus researchers: Association with concurrent Suicide Crisis Syndrome and prospective suicidal ideation and attempts. *Psychiatry Research, 312*, 114522. 10.1016/j.psychres.2022.114522

Rogers, M. L., Cao, E., Richards, J. A., Mitelman, A., Barzilay, S., Blum, Y., Chistopolskaya, K., Çinka, E., Dudeck, M., Husain, M. I., Kantas Yilmaz, F., Kuśmirek, O., Luiz, J. M., Menon, V., Nikolaev, E. L., Pilecka, B., Titze, L., Valvassori, S. S., You, S., & Galynker, I. (under review - a). Changes in daily cognitions and behaviors during the COVID-19 pandemic: Associations with Suicide Crisis Syndrome and suicidal ideation [Unpublished manuscript]. *Clinical Psychological Science*.

Rogers, M. L., Cao, E., Sinclair, C., & Galynker, I. (2021). Associations between goal orientation and suicidal thoughts and behaviors at one-month follow-up: Indirect effects through ruminative flooding. *Behaviour Research and Therapy, 145*, 103945. https://doi.org/10.1016/j.brat.2021.103945

Rogers, M. L., Chiurliza, B., Hagan, C. R., Tzoneva, M., Hames, J. L., Michaels, M. S., Hitschfeld, M. J., Palmer, B. A., Lineberry, T. W., Jobes, D. A., & Joiner, T. E. (2017). Acute suicidal affective disturbance: Factorial structure and initial validation across psychiatric outpatient and inpatient samples. *Journal of Affective Disorders, 211*, 1–11. https://doi.org/10.1016/j.jad.2016.12.057

Rogers, M. L., Galynker, I., Yaseen, Z., DeFazio, K., & Joiner, T. E. (2017). An overview and comparison of two proposed suicide-specific diagnoses: Acute suicidal affective disturbance and suicide crisis syndrome. *Psychiatric Annals*, 47(8), 416–420. https://doi.org/10.3928/00485713-20170630-01

Rogers, M. L., Jeon, M. E., Richards, J. A., Zheng, S., Joiner, T. E., & Galynker, I. (in prep). Two sides of the same coin? Empirical examination of two proposed characterizations of acute suicidal crises: Suicide Crisis Syndrome and Acute Suicidal Affective Disturbance.

Rogers, M. L., & Joiner, T. E. (2018). Lifetime acute suicidal affective disturbance symptoms account for the link between suicide-specific rumination and lifetime past suicide attempts. *Journal of Affective Disorders, 235*, 428–433. https://doi.org/10.1016/j.jad.2018.04.023

Rogers, M. L., & Joiner, T. E. (2019). Interactive effects of acute suicidal affective distur-bance and pain persistence on suicide attempt frequency and lethality. *Crisis*, *40*(6), 413–421. https://doi.org/10.1027/0227-5910/a000588

Rogers, M. L., Richards, J. A., Cao, E., Krumerman, M., Barzilay, S., Blum, Y., Chistopolskaya, K., Çinka, E., Dudeck, M., Husain, M. I., Kantas Yilmaz, F., Kravtsova, N. A., Kuśmirek, O., Menon, V., Peper-Nascimento, J., Pilecka, B., Titze, L., Valvassori, S. S., You, S., & Galynker, I. (under review - b). Associations between long-term and near-term stressful life events, Suicide Crisis Syndrome, and suicidal ideation. *International Journal of Stress Management*.

Rogers, M. L., Richards, J. A., Peterkin, D., Park, J., Astudillo-Garcia, C. I., Barzilay, S., Blum, Y., Chistopolskaya, K., Dudeck, M., Enikolopov, S., Husain, M. I., Jiménez, A., Kantas Yilmaz, F., Kuśmirek, O., Lee, M-B., Menon, V., Peper-Nascimento, J., Pilecka, B., Streb, J., . . . Galynker, I. (under review - c). Mental health and suicide prevention resource utilization among individuals with symptoms of Suicide Crisis Syndrome and/or suicidal ideation [Unpublished manuscript]. *International Journal of Stress Management*.

Rogers, M. L., Stanley, I. H., Hom, M. A., Chiurliza, B., Podlogar, M. C., & Joiner, T. E. (2018). Conceptual and empirical scrutiny of covarying depression out of suicidal ide-ation. *Assessment*, *25*(2), 159–172. https://doi.org/10.1177/1073191116645907

Rogers, M. L., Tucker, R. P., Law, K. C., Michaels, M. S., Anestis, M. D., & Joiner, T. E. (2016). Manifestations of overarousal account for the association between cognitive anxiety sensitivity and suicidal ideation. *Journal of Affective Disorders*, *192*, 116–124. https://doi.org/10.1016/j.jad.2015.12.014

Rogers, M. L., Vespa, A., Bloch-Elkouby, S., & Galynker, I. (2021). Validity of the mod-ular assessment of risk for imminent suicide in predicting short-term suicidality. *Acta Psychiatrica Scandinavica*, *144*(6), 563–577. https://doi.org/10.1111/acps.13354

Rogers, M. L., Bloch-Elkouby, S., & Galynker, I. (2022). Differential disclosure of sui-cidal intent to clinicians versus researchers: Associations with concurrent suicide crisis syndrome and prospective suicidal ideation and attempts. *Psychiatry Research*, *312*, 114522. doi:10.1016/j.psychres.2022.114522. Epub 2022 Mar 21. PMID: 35378454.

Rogers, M. L., Bafna, A., & Galynker, I. (2022). Comparative clinical utility of screening for Suicide Crisis Syndrome versus suicidal ideation in relation to suicidal ideation and attempts at one-month follow-up. *Suicide & Life-Threatening Behavior*, *52*(5), 866–875. https://doi.org/10.1111/sltb.12870

Rollman, G. B. (2009). Perspectives on hypervigilance. *Pain*, *141*(3), 183–184. https://doi.org/10.1016/j.pain.2008.12.030

Rudd, M. D., Berman, A. L., Joiner, T. E., Jr., Nock., M. K., Silverman, M. M., Mandrusiak, M., Van Orden, K., & Witte, T. (2006). Warning signs for suicide: Theory, research, and clinical application. *Suicide and Life-Threatening Behavior*, *36*(3), 255–262.

Substance Abuse and Mental Health Services Administration (SAMHSA). (2022). *Preventing suicide*. https://www.samhsa.gov/suicide

Schenck, L. A., & Andrasik, F. (2019). Behavioral and psychological aspects of cluster headache: An overview. *Neurological Sciences*, *40*(Suppl. 1), 3–7. https://doi.org/10.1007/s10072-019-03831-5

Schmitz, W. M., Jr., Allen, M. H., Feldman, B. N., Gutin, N. J., Jahn, D. R., Kleespies, P. M., Quinnett, P., & Simpson, S. (2012). Preventing suicide through improved training in suicide risk assessment and care: An American Association of

Suicidology Task Force report addressing serious gaps in U.S. mental health training. *Suicide and Life-Threatening Behavior, 42*(3), 292–304. https://doi.org/10.1111/j.1943-278X.2012.00090.x

Schuck, A., Calati, R., Barzilay, S., Bloch-Elkouby, S., & Galynker, I. (2019). Suicide Crisis Syndrome: A review of supporting evidence for a new suicide-specific diagnosis. *Behavioral Sciences & The Law, 37*(3), 223–239. https://doi.org/10.1002/bsl.2397

Shneidman, E. (1993). Suicide as psychache. *Journal of Nervous and Mental Disease, 181,* 147–149.

Stanley, I. H., Rufino, K. A., Rogers, M. L., Ellis, T. E., & Joiner, T. E. (2016). Acute suicidal affective disturbance (ASAD): A confirmatory factor analysis with 1442 psychiatric inpatients. *Journal of Psychiatric Research, 80,* 97–104.

Stellrecht, N. E., Joiner, T. E., Jr., & Rudd, M. D. (2006). Responding to and treating negative interpersonal processes in suicidal depression. *Journal of Clinical Psychology, 62*(9), 1129–1140. https://doi.org/10.1002/jclp.20298

Stene-Larsen, K., & Reneflot, A. (2019). Contact with primary and mental health care prior to suicide: A systematic review of the literature from 2000 to 2017. *Scandinavian Journal of Public Health, 47*(1), 9–17. https://doi.org/10.1177/1403494817746274

Stone, D. M., Simon, T. R., Fowler, K. A., Kegler, S. R., Yuan, K., Holland, K. M., Ivey-Stephenson, A. Z., & Crosby, A. E. (2018). Vital signs: Trends in state suicide rates—United States, 1999–2016 and circumstances contributing to suicide—27 states, 2015. *Morbidity and Mortality Weekly Report, 67*(22), 617–624. https://doi.org/10.15585/mmwr.mm6722a1

Taiwan National Suicide Prevention Center. (2022). https://sites.google.com/a/tsos.org.tw/english/

Takeshima, M., & Oka, T. (2013). A comprehensive analysis of features that suggest bipolarity in patients with a major depressive episode: Which is the best combination to predict soft bipolarity diagnosis? *Journal of Affective Disorders, 147,* 150–155.

Taylor, P. J., Gooding, P., Wood, A. M., & Tarrier, N. (2011). The role of defeat and entrapment in depression, anxiety, and suicide. *Psychological Bulletin, 137*(3), 391–420. https://doi.org/10.1037/a0022935

Treadway, M. T., & Zald, D. H. (2011). Reconsidering anhedonia in depression: Lessons from translational neuroscience. *Neuroscience and Biobehavioral Reviews, 35*(3), 537–555.

Tucker, R. P., Michaels, M. S., Rogers, M. L., Wingate, L. R., & Joiner, T. E. (2016). Construct validity of a proposed new diagnostic entity: Acute suicidal affective disturbance (ASAD). *Journal of Affective Disorders, 189,* 365–378. https://doi.org/10.1016/j.jad.2015.07.049

Tucker, R. P., O'Connor, R. C., & Wingate, L. R. (2016). An investigation of the relationship between rumination styles, hope, and suicide ideation through the lens of the integrated motivational–volitional model of suicidal behavior. *Archives in Suicide Research, 20*(4), 553–566. https://doi.org/10.1080/13811118.2016.1158682

Valtonen, H. M., Suominen, K., & Haukka, J. (2008). Differences in incidence of suicide attempts during phases of bipolar I and II disorders. *Bipolar Disorders, 10,* 588–596.

Valtonen, H. M., Suominen, K., Sokero, P., Mantere, O., Arvilommi, P., Leppämäki, S., & Isometsä, E. T. (2009). How suicidal bipolar patients are depends on how suicidal ideation is defined. *Journal of Affective Disorders, 118*(1-3), 48–54. https://doi.org/10.1016/j.jad.2009.02.008

Van der Does, W. (2005). Thought suppression and cognitive vulnerability to depression. *British Journal of Clinical Psychology, 44*(1), 1–14.

Van Os, J., & Kapur, S. (2009). Schizophrenia. *Lancet, 374*(9690), 635–645.

Vita, A., De Peri, L., & Sacchetti, E. (2011). Antipsychotics, antidepressants, anticonvulsants, and placebo on the symptom dimensions of borderline personality disorder: A meta-analysis of randomized controlled and open-label trials. *Journal of Clinical Psychopharmacology, 31*(5), 613–624.

Wegner, D. M. (1989). *White bears and other unwanted thoughts: Suppression, obsession, and the psychology of mental control.* Viking/Penguin.

Wegner, D. M., Schneider, D. J., Carter, S. R., & White, T. L. (1987). Paradoxical effects of thought suppression. *Journal of Personality and Social Psychology, 53*(1), 5–13.

Wegner, D. M., & Zanakos, S. (1994). Chronic thought suppression. *Journal of Personality, 62*(4), 616–640.

Wetherall, K., Robb, K. A., & O'Connor, R. C. (2019). Social rank theory of depression: A systematic review of self-perceptions of social rank and their relationship with depressive symptoms and suicide risk. *Journal of Affective Disorders, 246*, 300–319. https://doi.org/10.1016/j.jad.2018.12.045

Wetherall, K., Robb, K. A., & O'Connor, R. C. (2019). An examination of social comparison and suicide ideation through the lens of the integrated motivational–volitional model of suicidal behavior. *Suicide and Life-Threatening Behavior, 49*(1), 167–182.

Williams, J. M. G. (1997). *Cry of pain: Understanding suicide and self-harm.* Penguin.

Williams, J. M. G., Barnhofer, T., Crane, C., & Beck, A. T. (2005). Problem solving deteriorates following mood challenge in formerly depressed patients with a history of suicidal ideation. *Journal of Abnormal Psychology, 114*, 421–431.

Wise, R. A. (1980). The dopamine synapse and the notion of "pleasure centers" in the brain. *Trends in Neurosciences, 3*(4), 91–95. https://doi.org/10.1016/0166-2236(80)90035-1

Witte, T. K., Gordon, K. H., Smith, P. N., & Van Orden, K. A. (2012). Stoicism and sensation seeking: Male vulnerabilities for the acquired capability for suicide. *Journal of Research in Personality, 46*(4), 384–392. https://doi.org/10.1016/j.jrp.2012.03.004

Wong, M. M., Brower, K. J., & Craun, E. A. (2016). Insomnia symptoms and suicidality in the National Comorbidity Survey—Adolescent supplement. *Journal of Psychiatric Research, 81*, 1–8. https://doi.org/10.1016/j.jpsychires.2016.06.004

Wu, C. Y., Lee, M. B., Galynker, I., Rogers, M. L., Chen, C. Y., & Chan, C. T. (2022). The association between suicide crisis syndrome and psychosocial correlates under COVID-19 pandemic: An online survey in Taiwan. *Journal of Suicidology, 17*(3), 238–247. https://doi.org/10.30126/JoS.202209_17(3).0004

Yaseen, Z. S., Chartrand, H., Mojtabai, R., Bolton, J., & Galynker, I. I. (2013). Fear of dying in panic attacks predicts suicide attempt in comorbid depressive illness: Prospective evidence from the National Epidemiological Survey on Alcohol and Related Conditions. *Depression and Anxiety, 30*(10), 930–939. https://doi.org/10.1002/da.22039

Yaseen, Z. S., Galynker, I. I., Briggs, J., Freed, R. D., & Gabbay, V. (2016). Functional domains as correlates of suicidality among psychiatric inpatients. *Journal of Affective Disorders, 203*, 7–83. https://doi.org/10.1016/j.jad.2016.05.066

Yaseen, Z. S., Gilmer, E., Modi, J., Cohen, L. J., & Galynker, I. I. (2012). Emergency room validation of the revised Suicide Trigger Scale (STS-3): A measure of a hypothesized suicide trigger state. *PLOS One, 7*(9), e45157. https://doi.org/10.1371/journal.pone.0045157

Yaseen, Z. S., Hawes, M., Barzilay, S., & Galynker, I. (2019). Predictive validity of proposed diagnostic criteria for the suicide crisis syndrome: An acute presuicidal state. *Suicide and Life-Threatening Behavior, 49*(4), 1124–1135. https://doi.org/10.1111/sltb.12495

Yaseen, Z., Katz, C., Johnson, M. S., Eisenberg, D., Cohen, L. J., & Galynker, I. I. (2010). Construct development: The Suicide Trigger Scale (STS-2), a measure of a hypothesized suicide trigger state. *BMC Psychiatry, 10*(1), 110. https://doi.org/10.1186/1471-244x-10-110

Yaseen, Z. S., Kopeykina, I., Gutkovich, Z., Bassirnia, A., Cohen, L. J., & Galynker, I. I. (2014). Predictive validity of the Suicide Trigger Scale (STS-3) for post-discharge suicide attempt in high-risk psychiatric inpatients. *PLOS One, 9*(1), e86768. https://doi.org/10.1371/journal.pone.0086768

Ying, G., Cohen, L. J., Lloveras, L., Barzilay, S., & Galynker, I. (2020). Multi-informant prediction of near-term suicidal behavior independent of suicidal ideation. *Psychiatry Research, 291*, 113169. https://doi.org/10.1016/j.psychres.2020.113169

Zanarini, M. C., Frankenburg, M. D., Wedig, M. M., & Fitzmaurice, G. M. (2013). Cognitive experiences reported by patients with borderline personality disorder and Axis II comparison subjects: A 16-year prospective follow-up study. *American Journal of Psychiatry, 170*(6), 671–679.

Zhu, S., Lee, P. H., & Wong, P. (2021). Investigating prolonged social withdrawal behaviour as a risk factor for self-harm and suicidal behaviours. *British Journal of Psychiatry Open, 7*(3), e90. https://doi.org/10.1192/bjo.2021.47

8

Emotional Response to Suicidal Patients in the Assessment of Imminent Suicide Risk

With Benedetta Imbastaro, Olivia C. Lawrence, Inna Goncearenco, and Kimia Ziafat

Introduction

The Need for New Approaches in Risk Assessment

The global suicide epidemic has inspired tremendous efforts by clinicians and researchers to explore and understand the various factors that give rise to suicidal behavior. As discussed in the early chapters of this guide, acute suicide prediction has focused largely on long-term and proximal patient risk factors, such as stressful life events (Cohen et al., 2022; Rogers et al., 2022) and, more recently, on intense pre-suicidal affective and cognitive states (Rogers et al. 2017; Schuck et al., 2019). While such patient risk factors may be effectively identified retrospectively, a growing body of literature has revealed the various challenges and limitations of current clinical assessment of near-term suicide risk. To reiterate, the clinical utility of distal or long-term risk factors in predicting near-term suicidal behavior is limited (Glenn & Nock, 2014; Ribeiro et al., 2015; Tucker et al., 2015), and, furthermore, while standard assessment places significant value on patient disclosure of suicidal ideation (SI) and plans, studies have shown that up to 75% of individuals who died by suicide between 2000 and 2016 did not report SI or suicidal intent to anyone (Berman, 2018; Stone et al., 2018). Likewise, emerging evidence has highlighted the fluctuating nature of SI, suggesting that the onset of suicidal thoughts can develop rather abruptly in the moments preceding suicidal behavior (Bagge et al., 2022; Deisenhammer et al., 2009).

A conceptually new approach to improving our ability to assess imminent suicide risk focuses on clinicians' emotions that arise during therapeutic relationships with a suicidal patient. The nature of such relationships may span brief risk assessments in emergency department (ED) settings, time-limited intensive treatment on inpatient units, frequent or infrequent psycho-pharmacology appointments, short-term and long-term psychotherapies, or others. The therapeutic relationship has been shown to play a critical role in shaping treatment outcomes among suicidal patients (Barzilay et al., 2020), and clinicians' emotional responses to suicidal patients were related to their clinical decision-making and to prospective suicidal outcomes (Barzilay et al., 2022).

Yet, until recent decades, clinicians' emotional responses to suicidal patients have been largely overlooked in risk assessment theory, research, and practice (Galynker et al., 2017; Yaseen et al., 2013). While research investigating emotional responses to suicidal patients is limited, the existing literature generally suggests that clinicians experience negative emotional responses to suicidal patients, including anxiety, irritation, avoidance (Birtchnell, 1983; Varghese & Kelly, 1999), distress, hopelessness (Michaud et al., 2020), and aversion (Maltsberger & Buie, 1974). Although researchers have only recently attempted to study the clinical value of emotions in suicide risk assessment, quantifying clinicians' subjective emotional experiences when interacting with suicidal patients may serve as a meaningful component of suicide risk assessments.

Clinician's Emotional Responses to Suicidal Patients and Their Underlying Mechanisms

Experimental Evidence for Clinician's Emotional Responses

The phenomenon of a clinician's emotional reaction to a patient is conceptualized by the term *countertransference* in psychodynamic literature. From the time the term was coined by Freud in a letter to Jung in the early 1900s (Stefana, 2017), the meaning of the term has changed significantly over the years. Initially defined psychodynamically as the therapist's unconscious and conflict-based response to patient's transference, contemporary usage of the term often encompasses a transtheoretical description of the clinician's emotional response to a patient (Prasko et al., 2010). To underscore the psychodynamic nature of clinicians' responses, in this guide, the terms *countertransference* and *emotional response* are used interchangeably.

Healthcare professionals form clinical judgments based on logical considerations, such as patient clinical history and current symptomatology, as well as through unconscious emotional responses, such as "gut feelings" (Ægisdóttir et al., 2006). These emotions are difficult for clinicians to recognize and accept explicitly, regardless of the clinicians' experience (Nummenmaa et al., 2008). A systematic assessment of these responses, however, has the potential to ameliorate the inherent distortions of the clinician's judgment.

Maltsberger and Buie's (1974) seminal theoretical paper elaborated on an array of emotions and behaviors rooted in different defenses in response to negative countertransference toward the suicidal patient, which they combined under the construct *countertransference hate*. Later research confirmed their theories and found that negative countertransference and feelings of anxiety and hostility were prominently elicited by suicidal patients (Varghesse & Kelly, 1999). Of note, largely negative emotional responses to suicidal patients in clinicians were present even in situations of physician-assisted suicide: when confronted with patients' desire for death, clinicians' feelings were mostly anxiety, helplessness, and being overwhelmed (Groenewould et al., 1997).

Suicidal thoughts (as well as personality disorders) elicit strong emotional responses in clinicians, even after a single encounter, a phenomenon termed *instant countertransference* (iCT). The responses usually emerge in initial assessments in EDs and in outpatient clinics. Interestingly, there appears to be some overlap between clinicians' adverse emotional responses to SI and their responses to personality disorders. Both elicit feelings of low self-confidence, being tied, and feeling tense. On the other hand, personality disorders elicit, specifically, feelings of frustration, disaffiliation, and guilt, suggesting difficulties in establishing a connection, while suicidal thoughts are more associated with distress, lack of hope, confusion, and a sense that the patient's life has little worth, which may reflect the clinician's unconscious identification with the suicidal patient (Michaud et al., 2020).

Our research showed that clinicians treating imminently suicidal patients recalled somewhat positive feelings toward these patients, such as maintaining high hopefulness for treatment, while simultaneously finding themselves overwhelmed by, distressed by, and avoidant of them (Yaseen et al., 2013). Galynker et al. (2017) identified two distinct categories of countertransference phenomena that uniquely characterize the mixed emotional responses clinicians may experience while interacting with suicidal patients. The first type of conflicting countertransference response is referred to as rejection-avoidance, which is characterized by clinicians' manifestations of hostility and hopelessness toward the suicidal patient and may cause premature termination of treatment. The second classification of mixed clinician countertransference toward suicidal patients is termed anxious-overinvolvement, which is characterized by feelings of anxiety, unrealistic expectations for patient outcomes, and excessive efforts to help the suicidal patient. In support of mixed countertransference phenomena, research conducted by Yaseen et al. (2017) found that a pattern of clinicians' conflicting emotional responses—in particular, the combination of distress, avoidance, and optimism—was significantly associated with patients' future suicidal behavior. In addition, despite feeling slightly more positive in their responses preceding low-lethality suicide attempts, clinicians may also experience more sadness before either successful or highly lethal attempts (Yaseen et al., 2017).

The underlying mechanisms of negative emotional responses to patients with high suicide risk were recently investigated by Ying and colleagues (2021). Using the narrative-crisis model of suicide (NCM)—a framework that incorporates traditional long-term risk factors, suicidal narratives, and acute cognitive and affective markers of near-term suicide embodied in suicide crisis syndrome (SCS) criteria—the study revealed many notable findings.

First, the authors found that patients' suicidal narratives, as measured by the Suicidal Narrative Inventory (SNI; Cohen et al., 2019), exclusively elicited emotional responses from clinicians, while the other components of the NCM (long-term risk factors for suicidal behavior and SCS symptoms) did not (Ying et al., 2021). To explain the lack of clinicians' emotional response to patients' acute clinical symptoms, the authors suggested that the relatively minimal length of clinical experience reported by clinician participants in their sample may have accounted for underappreciation of the full range of possible symptoms associated with near-term suicidal behavior, therefore diminishing the strong clinician emotional response typically elicited by high-risk patients. On the other hand, because evidence has shown that experienced clinicians have developed the ability to compartmentalize emotional responses to patients' symptoms (Werner & Korsch, 1976), clinicians with more years of experience may engage this defense mechanism in dealing with the negative emotions that can emerge when working with suicidal patients.

Second, within the defining components of the suicidal narrative, the study found that patients' perceived burdensomeness was particularly significant in eliciting strong emotional responses from clinicians. These findings suggest that clinicians are more likely to respond emotionally to patients' life narratives and inner experiences rather than their presenting symptomology. As research has shown that clinicians generally connect with suicidal patients based on their life stories (Michel et al., 2002), these results highlight the foundational role of suicidal narratives in shaping the nature of the therapeutic relationship (Ying et al., 2021). Additionally, further results from the study showed that patients' suicidal narratives were significantly related to clinicians' negative emotional responses to them, specifically the responses of reduced affiliation and increased distress (Ying et al., 2021).

Last, Ying et al.'s study found an association between clinicians' therapeutic orientation and the valence of their emotional response to the patient: clinicians who identified as dynamically/analytically oriented experienced more negative responses to suicidal patients, while an integrative/eclectic orientation was associated with more positive emotional responses (Ying et al., 2021). While further research is needed to investigate the nature of these findings, such results cast light on the possible role of different theoretical backgrounds and training in dictating clinicians' interpretation of patients' suicidal presentations.

Clinicians' Defense Mechanisms in Psychotherapy with Suicidal Patients

In psychoanalytic theory, defense mechanisms are unconsciously used to make the "forbidden emotions," for example, hatred or attraction, more palatable (Schein, 2016). Clinicians are likely to use defense mechanisms, such as denial or repression, rather than acknowledge feelings of hate and/or sexual attraction toward a patient. Instead of feeling hatred toward patient A, a clinician may acknowledge and recognize a less threatening emotion, such as dislike. Similarly, instead of feeling lust toward patient B, a clinician may acknowledge a more acceptable emotion, such as feeling concerned. Maltsberger and Buie (1974) gave examples of five frequently encountered psychological defenses: reaction formation, denial, turning against self, projection, and repression. As mentioned before, psychological defenses interact with clinician and patient factors (e.g., personality traits, attachment styles, experiences) and shape the nature of the therapeutic relationship (Brewe et al., 2021; Cramer et al., 2015; Laconi et al., 2014.,). The next sections discuss the most common clinician-employed defense mechanisms that emerge while interacting with suicidal patients.

Reaction Formation

Reaction formation is a defense that turns an unacceptable emotion into its exact opposite. This defense is most characteristically used in situations in which a person is trapped, with no possibility of escape, and experiencing the unacceptable emotion is life-threatening. The most famous example of reaction formation is "Stockholm syndrome," in which a hostage or kidnap victim "falls in love" with his or her captor.

In suicide assessment work, a reaction formation would be attraction to, or even love for, a high-risk patient, who might otherwise provoke extreme anxiety. The clinician may experience a "rescue fantasy" of miraculously curing the patient, therefore projecting eagerness and urgency. Reaction formation often leads to overinvolvement with the patient, which is time-consuming, stressful, and ultimately unsustainable, resulting in physical withdrawal (referring the patient out) or emotional abandonment and disengagement.

Case 43

In July of his postgraduate year 3 (PGY-3), Dr. C is given a sign-out by the outgoing resident, who warns him about this most difficult case: Sarah, a 38-year-old bipolar woman, has made several previous suicide attempts. Sarah is known as one of the most challenging patients in the clinic; she has chronic SI, no social support, poor boundaries, and poor treatment adherence. Upon meeting the patient, Dr. C is surprised that Sarah is an attractive woman who seems eager to receive help and who is open to trying new medications. Sarah agrees to take a new selective serotonin reuptake inhibitor (SSRI), and as she is leaving, she gives Dr. C a bright smile. "She can't be so bad," thinks Dr. C, "and I am good at convincing people to take their meds. I will turn her around."

Repression

Repression is an unconscious defense mechanism that prevents disturbing emotions from becoming conscious. In psychiatry and in medicine overall, repression removes from consciousness intense negative feelings directed toward the patient, which are considered shameful and unprofessional. In clinicians working with suicidal patients, repression results in the desire to escape from the stress-laden engagement. When brought to consciousness, it is experienced as a thought like "I don't want this patient in my office." When doctors repress unacceptable feelings, patients see them as aloof and disconnected, and they feel rejected.

Case 44

Arthur is a 50-year-old obese, malodorous male with opiate use disorder, substance-induced mood disorder, and a history of near-lethal heroin overdose. Dr. D does not look forward to his sessions with Arthur, which often start late and run short and are limited to the assessment of Arthur's adherence to treatment, recent stressful life events, and SI. Arthur's answers are predictable, which gives Dr. D time during the session to check his e-mail and Facebook postings. In this example of repression of revulsion, Dr. D perceives himself as being professional, whereas Arthur views him as arrogant and indifferent.

Turning against the Self

Turning against the self is a defense mechanism in which a person becomes the target of his or her own unacceptable emotions. Turning against the self is a form of the displacement defense mechanism, in which unacceptable emotions are redirected to a substitute target. Typical examples of displacement are kicking the dog out of frustration with superiors at work or hating all members of the opposite sex when having romantic relationship difficulties.

Turning against the self is normally used in reference to hatred, anger, and aggression, and it is the Freudian explanation for feelings of inferiority, guilt, and depression. The idea that "depression is anger turned inward" has entered mainstream and pop psychology and is accepted by many laypeople.

When faced with a difficult suicidal patient, a clinician may feel incompetent and worthless and think that he or she should refer the patient to somebody else more competent. The danger of "turning against the self" is that doctor's actions reflect their inner hopelessness, and the patient may feel abandoned and rejected. The sense that their psychiatrist is giving up on them only adds to the patient's suicidal narrative elements of burdensomeness and alienation, as in the following case.

Case 45

Amy, a 55-year-old woman with treatment-resistant bipolar depression and several past suicide attempts, was admitted to an inpatient unit after she was taken off a bridge by the police. The patient's major fear was that she was a burden to her husband and to her doctors, and she feared they would collude to send her to a state hospital. Her psychiatrist of many years was feeling like he had run out of options. Seeing the patient was making him depressed, and he felt trapped by his commitment to her. "I have failed her," he thought, "I need to refer her out to more competent clinicians." When he told Amy that he would like to transfer her to the National Institute of Mental Health (NIMH) for a clinical trial of a new antidepressant, Amy said, "This is the end. You are shipping me off."

Projection

Projection is a defense in which a person attributes their own undesired emotions to another person. Projection often results from poor insight into one's motivations and feelings.

In working with suicidal patients, the unacceptable thoughts are hatred of the patients and even violent fantasies ("murder" as per Maltzberger). These thoughts are projected onto the patient, and the clinician believes that it is the patient who hates him or her. The clinician's conscious emotion is fear, which could result in unwarranted aggressiveness and poor judgment, as in the following case.

Case 46

Phoebe, an 18-year-old African American female, was admitted to an inpatient unit after a suicide attempt by drinking methanol. During the interview, she refused to get up and answer most questions, turning her back on the interviewer. The harried interviewing attending became frustrated. He touched the patient's shoulder. The girl looked at him and then turned her back again without saying a word. "She hates me," thought the attending, and said, "If you do not talk to us, we'll have security discharge you."

Denial

Denial is the refusal to accept reality, acting as if a painful event, thought, or feeling does not exist. It is considered the most primitive of the defenses because it is the first one to develop in small children, who escape into fantasy to avoid unpleasant reality. People often use denial to avoid dealing with problems in their lives that they do not wish to admit. For instance, alcoholics often deny they have a drinking problem, pointing to how well they function in their jobs. People often use denial when facing humiliating and potentially catastrophic problems, such as infidelity of spouses, deception by business partners, or emerging serious mental illness in children.

In suicide work, denial usually means that the clinician "does not notice" obvious features of the suicidal narrative or signs of a suicidal crisis. Both countertransference love and countertransference hate may underlie clinicians' denial. A clinician who likes a patient who is at high suicide risk may easily believe the patient's assurances that he or she has no suicidal intent. Strong dislike of a patient may result in the same outcome. In both scenarios, the suicidal patient may perceive the clinician's acceptance of his or her (false) assurances of safety as rejection.

Case 47

Linda, a 28-year-old disheveled woman with bipolar depression, was being evaluated in a clinic for patients with affective disorders. Linda told the evaluating clinician that she had tried all possible treatments, even electroconvulsive therapy, and nothing seemed to help. She told the doctor that she was suicidal and had even thought of the method: suffocation with a plastic bag. "I can help you," said the doctor, while thinking about how to avoid such a high-risk case: "You need psychotherapy. Let's make an appointment for next week with our therapist. Can you promise me that you will not harm yourself?" The patient committed to safety, but the following morning her parents found her, barely breathing, with a plastic bag over her head.

Rationalization

Rationalization is a defense mechanism in which unacceptable behavior, motives, or feelings are logically justified or made tolerable by plausible means (also known as making excuses). In the medical field, rationalization is sometimes seen in the covering up of mistakes (Banja, 2004).

Some common excuses are:

- "Why disclose the error? The patient was going to die anyway."
- "Telling the family about the error will only make them feel worse."
- "Well, we did our best. These things happen."
- "If we're not too certain the error caused the harm, we don't have to tell."

In suicide risk assessment, rationalization is used primarily to cover countertransference hate and disgust, which manifest as a lack of effort to properly assess risk. For example:

- "I am doing my job, aren't I? I can't go 'above and beyond' for every patient I see."
- "Given my workload, I am doing the best I can."
- "People determined to kill themselves will always manage to."
- "We can't predict suicide anyway."
- "This patient's life is miserable; they have nothing to live for."

Case 58

Edward, a 75-year-old-man with a history of Parkinson's disease, was admitted to an inpatient psychiatric unit for SI after a massive heart attack. He told the team that his life was over: He was sick, he was alone, and he could no longer do things he used to enjoy. The team was so affected by his despair that it left without doing a thorough evaluation of his suicidal risk. "If I were this sick, I would want to kill myself," one of the doctors said.

Clinicians' Pattern of Emotional Response

While transference and countertransference are global features of patient–clinician interactions, the nature of clinicians' emotional responses, as well as the defense mechanisms unconsciously employed to cope with these emotions, can manifest in particular patterns that are uniquely associated with working with high-risk suicidal patients. The clinician's ability to differentiate similar emotional states is critical to the use of emotions as diagnostic tools for assessing near-term suicide risk. The clinician's negative emotions, such as anxiety and dread, are closer to those targeted by mindfulness-based cognitive therapy (MBCT) and dialectical behavior therapy (DBT; Linehan, 1993a, 1993b; Segal et al., 2002), whereas positive responses, such as unreasonable optimism, have not been targeted. Regardless of their responses' emotional valence, clinicians face additional difficulties admitting to either due to ethical pressures, which result in disapproval of certain emotional responses to patients.

A recent study conducted by Soulié and colleagues (2018) investigated the nature of clinicians' countertransference to patients at risk for suicide on various dimensions of countertransference: entrapped/rejecting, fulfilled/engaging, aroused/reacting, informal/boundary-crossing, protective/overinvolvement, ambivalent/inconsistent, and mistreated/controlling. Factor analysis results showed that the entrapped/rejecting and fulfilled/engaging factors represented the greatest amount of variance in the sample of clinicians, highlighting the presence of a combination of ambivalent countertransference phenomena in their response to suicidal patients (Soulie et al., 2018). The authors suggest that the observed co-occurrence of entrapped/rejecting and fulfilled/engaging clinician responses may represent a manifestation of ambivalent countertransference that is unique to working with patients at risk for suicide. This interpretation aligns with findings that clinicians' conflicting emotional responses of distress and hopefulness effectively discriminated attempters from nonattempters and emerged as a strong predictor of short-term suicidal behavior (Yaseen et al., 2017).

Furthermore, Soulie et al. (2018) observed that not only did clinicians report low levels of endorsement on all negative countertransference factors, but also they reported the highest average level of endorsement for the fulfillment/engagement responses to patients at risk for suicide. Because female clinicians reported significantly more fulfilled/engaging responses than male clinicians in their sample, the authors suggested that social desirability response biases may explain these results. The researchers also discovered that psychodynamically oriented clinicians reported stronger negative countertransference than did eclectic and CBT-oriented clinicians (Soulie et al., 2018).

In interpreting the findings of the study collectively, the authors considered that the low levels of endorsement of all negative countertransference factors may be explained by the operation of defense mechanisms among clinicians. Drawing from Maltsberger and Buie's (1974) concept of countertransference hate, entrapped/rejecting responses from clinicians could represent countertransference hatred turned against the self (embodied by unwanted feelings of malice being redirected from the suicidal patient to self), repression of countertransference hatred, and/or reaction formation, or turning countertransference hatred into its opposite (for detailed description of these mechanisms, see Maltsberger & Buie, 1974, pp. 628–629). Furthermore, to explain the antagonistic combination of entrapped/rejection and fulfilled/engaging responses present among clinicians, Soulié and colleagues (2018) considered this countertransference pattern in the context of a specific coping strategy. Specifically, the authors noted important similarities between the clinicians' entrapment/rejecting countertransference and the feelings of entrapment often characteristic of the suicidal state. Indeed, the entrapped/rejecting dimension operationalized in this study outlines feelings of hopelessness and an urge to escape from a situation perceived as unavoidable. In what is referred to as a *countertransference montage*, clinicians empathize with their patients in a manner that involves the replication of the patient's inner state. As clinicians absorb their patients' feelings of entrapment, the affective discomfort of this experience may unconsciously lead clinicians to employ coping mechanisms aimed at manifesting positive feelings to offset feelings of entrapment (Soulié et al., 2018).

The patterns and types of clinician countertransference toward suicidal patients are ultimately shaped by a myriad of factors, such as defense mechanisms, clinicians' attachment styles, theoretical orientations, and patient narratives. Because treatment decisions are partly guided by clinicians' emotional experiences, assisting clinicians in developing skills in awareness and management of countertransference phenomena can serve as a meaningful step toward ethical and effective mental health practices informed by a healthy balance between unconscious emotions and rational judgments. Common clinicians' emotional responses, along with related clinical examples, are illustrated in the next sections.

From Rescue Fantasy to Helplessness and Anger

Although all patient–clinician encounters are unique, generally in psychotherapy, therapists are likely to respond positively to positive emotions and negatively to negative emotions. This emotional alignment may have many mechanisms, including emotional contagion, which makes one feel depressed around depressed people and happy around happy people (Bartel & Saavedra, 2000; Hatfield et al., 1993; Kramer et al., 2014; Sy et al., 2005). As psychotherapy or any other patient–clinician professional encounter progresses, patients' emotions evolve, as do those of their clinicians. An example of an emotional dynamic that may develop between a suicidal patient and a therapist is described next.

Case 49

When the suicidal patient Anne sees a new therapist, Dr. B, for the first time, she hopes that the therapist will be able to relieve her despair and to make her life at least tolerable. In Anne's mind, her new therapist will be able to put a healing balm, so to speak, on her psyche and cure her emotional pain.

In reality, Dr. B has certain clinical skills in which she has been trained. She will use her skills to the best of her ability, which is commensurate with her training and talent and is influenced by her personality and temperament, in addition to events taking place in her personal life. Although Dr. B's training allows her to minimize personal factors, they still influence her emotional response to Anne. Whether positive or negative, her emotions are never neutral, and they include some apprehension.

Initially, Anne likes Dr. B and finds her manner soothing, and Anne's emotional pain begins to ease. Anne starts thinking that she may have finally found a doctor who can help her in her long struggle with depression, as well as her recent sense that she is sinking into a deep hole of despair from which there is no escape. Feeling better, Anne begins to idealize Dr. B and tells her that she has finally met a doctor who understands her. Flattered, and seeing that Anne's affect is brightening, Dr. B feels relieved and hopeful for her new patient, whom she finds likable. "I may actually save this woman," she thinks, not quite realizing that she is experiencing a rescue fantasy.

Anne's improved mood is short-lived, and her repetitive, ruminating thoughts soon push her back toward the feeling of anguish from which there seems to be no exit. Her suicidal urges return, and the hope she felt after meeting Dr. B dissipates. "She does not care about me," thinks Anne, "She is listening to me because she is getting paid.... Does she really care?"

Anne is late for her session with Dr. B, and the first words out of her mouth are "I forgot my checkbook. Do you care, or are you only seeing me for the money?" Dr. B is well trained and understands that she is being tested. However, wanting to show Anne that she cares and to develop a therapeutic alliance, Dr. B says something she knows she should not: "It's OK, you will pay me later. . . . You need therapy." She also offers Anne her cell phone number, should Anne be particularly down. Anne agrees to continue, and Dr. B breathes a sigh of relief: "I dodged a bullet, I really understand her, and I can prevent her suicide." This scenario, in which a patient's testing of the clinician's commitment results in that clinician's overinvolvement, is common.

After two weeks, Anne is still despondent. She attends her sessions and calls Dr. B every other day, but her ruminations keep her up at night. "Dr. B is no different from any of my previous therapists. She can't understand what I am going through, and no one can," she thinks, as her idealization of Dr. B turns into disappointment. "I don't know what your experience is with treating depression, but your therapy is not working," Anne tells her doctor. Dr. B starts feeling angry. She thinks, "I am not charging her, she is calling me at all hours, and she is not even grateful." Being a professional, Dr. B tries not to show her anger, but she cannot fully control it. "I have been working in this field for 10 years. I am very experienced," she says, not realizing how defensive she sounds.

Anne is 30 minutes late for her next appointment and does not answer her phone. Dr. B's heart sinks, and she assumes the worst. She leaves an anxious message: "Anne, please call me back as soon as you can, I am worried about you." Anne calls back at 9 p.m.: "I have been having suicidal thoughts," she says, "but I am not going to do anything." Dr. B is relieved but very angry.

She dreads the next session. This time, Anne arrives 10 minutes late. "I forgot and fell asleep," she says, "but these sessions are not helping. My bad thoughts are still there. You don't understand what I am going through, and you never will."

Dr. B is livid. "No wonder you have no friends," she thinks, and, "If this is how you treat people who help you, who could stand being with you?" "We have been making progress," she says out loud, "I have been trying very hard to help you, but if you feel that we are not connecting, I can refer you to one of my colleagues." "Yes, maybe next time," says Anne, sarcastically. "I will find you somebody who is more experienced than I am," says Dr. B, thinking that she sounds concerned, and not realizing she also comes across as sarcastic. "She can't wait to get rid of me," thinks Anne as she leaves the session.

Dr. B felt relieved. She knew exactly to whom she wanted to refer Anne. However, her relief was short-lived. She could not put the troublesome patient out of her mind. When the phone rang at 5 a.m., Dr. B thought "Anne," and she was right: Anne was in the medical intensive care unit after she had overdosed on Tylenol. She died two days later of liver failure.

When discussing Anne's case, the root cause analysis concluded that Dr. B did everything correctly: The patient was not suicidal, she had promised to come to the next appointment, and Dr. B had no grounds to hospitalize her. Dr. B, however, was very distressed by Anne's suicide and particularly the fact that, in retrospect, she "knew" that the intensity of her initial positive response to Anne was unique, as was the rapidity with which these feelings changed to dread. If/when she has a similar reaction to a patient in the future, she may recognize this as a sign of high imminent suicidal risk.

This vignette describes the evolution of a therapeutic relationship between a suicidal patient and an experienced therapist from hope for a cure on both sides to an increasingly intense negative emotional response on the part of the doctor and despair and suicide by the patient. The doctor initially had the somewhat unrealistic belief that she had a unique rapport with Anne, and she felt affection for her new patient. As treatment progressed, that affection changed to increasingly intense anger, anxiety, and dread before their meetings, as well as unrecognized hostility with resulting rejecting behavior.

There may be many reasons for Dr. B's insensitivity to Anne's increasing despair, which resulted in the deterioration of their therapeutic relationship. Volumes have been written about the psychotherapeutic process and about therapists' emotional responses to their patients (Varghese & Kelly, 1999). Research ties the psychotherapeutic outcome to therapists' ability to recognize and repair ruptures in therapeutic relationships (Eubanks-Carter et al., 2015; Lombardo et al., 2009). The latter in part depends on their ability to assess their own emotions as their emotions change during their work with patients.

Correspondingly, in working with suicidal individuals, clinicians able to distinguish the unique emotions aroused in them by those patients' suicidal narratives and crises are better at assessing their patients' risk for near-term suicide. Both the positive and the negative emotions felt by Dr. B were responses to Anne's feelings of despair and to her suicidal urges. The fact that Anne was her first thought when the phone rang at 5 a.m. shows that Dr. B had some awareness that her reaction to Anne was different from her reaction to other suicidal patients. However, she was not able to identify it as such during their last session.

Dr. B's emotional response to Anne had two distinct phases: the initial positivity and unrealistic expectation of saving Anne, and later, anxiety, hostility, and dread. In other real-life clinical scenarios, paradoxical hopefulness and dread before seeing the patient can happen in isolation, at the same time, or fluctuate from session to session. However, the previously discussed characteristic mixture of feelings about the suicidal patient is unique and can be recognized and used as a diagnostic tool.

Countertransference Love

When clinicians minimize a patient's suicide risk factors, believe that they have a unique relationship, and become overinvolved with, or fantasize about saving, the patient, they allow their affection for the patient to cloud their judgment. This countertransference love, and the resulting optimism, is a complex emotional response to the patient's suicidal narrative or suicide crisis and is also a predictor of near-term suicide risk (Maltsberger & Buie, 1974; Marcinko et al., 2008; Nivoli et al., 2011). In our retrospective study, optimism was one of the emotions clinicians felt in the last session before a suicide attempt or completed suicide (Yaseen et al., 2013). Prospectively, optimism was, paradoxically, associated with near-term suicidal behavior (Hawes et al., 2017).

The psychological mechanisms underlying countertransference love may involve reaction formation (discussed above). Clinicians who suddenly believe that their suicidal patient is no longer suicidal need to ask themselves if the patient's history supports their sudden optimism. What are the chronic risk factors? Does the patient's life fit into the suicidal narrative? Does the patient have symptoms and signs of a suicidal crisis? An affirmative answer to any of these questions calls for suicide risk reassessment.

If the answer to any of the previous questions is Yes, then the clinician must ask whether he or she has a unique understanding of the patient being evaluated and if it can be attributed to a common social or cultural background or to a feeling of being connected for no particular reason. The sense of having a unique bond with a suicidal patient is a sign of unrecognized countertransference love; this calls for a rational reassessment of one's emotions.

Case 50

Dr. A, a postgraduate year 2 (PGY-2) resident of Albanian descent, was assigned a suicidal Albanian patient, Edith, because of their common background and language. Dr. A felt like he was put on the spot but also felt flattered that the team trusted his judgment and his clinical skills. He eagerly started working with Edith, a 60-year-old recent immigrant, who reminded him of his mother. Edith had been hospitalized twice in Albania with depression. Currently, she was living with her son, a building superintendent, and felt like a burden to him. She told Dr. A that she had no friends and no job. Dr. A could relate to this because he remembered his family's difficult time after their immigration. Hopeful about the patient's future, he spent a lot of time daily helping her understand American society. Edith's mood improved. No longer suicidal, she told Dr. A that he was better than her son, who was too busy to visit her in the hospital. Dr. A was relieved and thought that the patient could be discharged with a follow-up in one of the local clinics, which had an interpreting service. On the day of discharge, Edith was very disappointed that Dr. A would not be her outpatient doctor. She thanked him profusely, and he felt good about his work with her. She denied SI, but she jumped off the roof of her son's building three hours after her discharge.

This case illustrates unrecognized countertransference love. Because of his own family's immigrant experience, Dr. A overidentified with Edith and did not fully appreciate her psychopathology and the intensity of her suicidal narrative. Her narrative included burdensomeness (to her son), alienation (from her past and culture), and entrapment (seeing no good options). Dr. A's "rejection" of her as an outpatient further contributed to her narrative.

In this case, the clinician's belief that he had a special relationship with this patient was unwittingly created by the treatment team, which put an inexperienced doctor in a position of responsibility without supervision by more experienced clinicians. He thus did not properly assess the patient's stresses or the intensity of her suicidal crisis.

Countertransference Hate

In 1974, Maltsberger and Buie described countertransference hate as simultaneous feelings of aversion and malice that suicidal patients invoke in psychotherapists. The authors suggested that therapists manage this negative countertransference through full awareness, self-restraint, and appreciation of their defense mechanisms. The term *countertransference* implies knowledge of the exact psychological mechanism of therapists' emotional responses, which have never been proven experimentally. This term is accepted in psychoanalytic literature but not in clinical literature, which is evidence-based. The descriptive term *emotional response* is more suited for clinical work. However, the term *countertransference hate* is so widely known and accepted that it is used interchangeably with *negative emotional response*, which does not relay the full emotionality of clinicians' reactions to acutely suicidal individuals.

Of the two components of countertransference hate, aversion is more problematic. Aversion may result in (conscious or unconscious) abandonment of the patient, which in turn may precipitate suicidal action. Malice is less dangerous (although more painful to tolerate) because it is almost always conscious and therefore easier to manage.

Countertransference hate may develop when patients test the clinician's commitment to them in the course of a long-term therapeutic relationship, during an ED one-time suicide risk assessment, or prior to discharge from the acute psychiatric unit. Testing of the clinician by suicidal patients often manifests as a provocation, such as direct disparagement of the clinician's appearance, occupation, experience, and training—for example: "You are too young to understand," "I would like a female psychiatrist," or "Which medical school did you go to?" The direct provocations most difficult to handle are threats of suicide.

Indirect provocations (e.g., persistent evasiveness, lack of eye contact, and disturbing silences) are more subtle and more difficult to detect. These tend to create a sense of seemingly unfounded unease, discomfort, anger, or irritation directed either at the patient or inward. Other indirect provocations include sudden unexpected cheerfulness, optimism, and minimization of stressors that only minutes ago seemed overwhelming. Finally, there may be continuing expectations of the therapist to "know" what the patient is thinking or to develop a miracle cure. These unreachable expectations can make the clinician feel like a failure. Furthermore, the different meanings that patients and clinicians attribute to death increase the communication gap, which worsens the state of unease state experienced by the therapist.

Regardless of how experienced a clinician may be, he or she will always respond to this testing with some degree of irritation or other negative emotions, which are often too uncomfortable to experience in their raw form. These responses are managed through well-known psychological defenses (i.e., turning against the self or projection), which reduce discomfort but also obscure its source, creating the possibility that a clinician would unknowingly act out his negative emotion, to the patient's detriment. Finally, other factors, such as lack of hope, confusion, and undervaluing the patient's life, seem to take part in countertransference hate (Michaud et al., 2020). Fortunately, these defenses can be brought into consciousness and used diagnostically to identify patients at imminent suicide risk.

Clinicians' Conflicting Emotional Responses in the Prediction of Imminent Suicide

A suicidal patient' thwarting of the clinician's attempts at connection may result in countertransference hate (Maltsberger & Buie, 1974), and such a reaction may, in turn, elicit in a clinician a variety of compensatory defense mechanisms aimed to neutralize unacceptable emotional states threatening a positive view of the clinician's self (Baumeister et al., 1998; Maltsberger & Buie, 1974). Our research shows that these defenses are primarily reaction formation and denial (Hawes et al., 2017; Yaseen et al., 2017).

Reaction formation to countertransfernce hate, not dissimilar to countertransference love, may result in hopeful rescue fantasies, with anxious urgency to cure (Rycroft, 2010). Likewise, interventions driven by clinicians' reaction formation against countertransference hate may take the form of overinvolvement or inappropriate optimism (Maltsberger & Buie, 1974).

Such actions are most problematic during hospital discharge and the unavoidable withdrawal of inpatient care; "inappropriately optimistic" premature discharge of a suicidal patient may result in the patient's feelings of abandonment and despair (Schechter et al., 2016), increasing suicide risk.

Alternatively, denial of countertransference hate, in which the clinician is unaware of negative feelings toward the acutely suicidal patient, may result in hopelessness and feelings of indifference. Inappropriately acted upon clinician's indifference may result in an early hospital discharge. Such discharge will indicate clinician's acting out their negative countertranseference to a suicidal patient as overt rejection and abandonment (Maltsberger & Buie, 1974), which will be accurately perceived as such by the patient.

Our research has shown that in clinicians taking care of high-risk suicidal patients, the combination of hopefulness and distress was the emotional reaction most consistent with the rescue fantasy and countertransference love (Yaseen et al., 2016). We termed this mixed emotion "anxious overinvovlment" and described it as paradoxical because hopefulness typically brings calm rather than distress. Further, our research has also shown that the paradoxical combination of hopefulness and distress in a clinician was predictive of a patient's near-term suicide death.

On the other end of the countertransference spectrum, in the same group of clincians the combination of hopelessness and calm was the emotional reaction most consistent with the denial of countertransference hate (Yaseen et al., 2016). We termed this mixed emotion "collusion-abandonment or distancing" and described it as paradoxical because hopelessness about the patient's preventable suicide would bring distress rather than calm. As with anxious overinvolement, our research has also shown that the paradoxical combination of hopelessness and calm in a clinician was predictive of a patient's near-term suicide death.

In summary, our research has demonstrated that for high-risk inpatients, clinicians' conflicting combinations of distress and hope, consistent with a reaction formation and countertransference love, and of nondistress and hopelessness, consistent with denial and countertransference hate, were predictive of suicide outcomes after discharge. Moreover, these two conflicting emotional responses by clinicians were predictive above and beyond other risk factors, such as depression, entrapment, and SI. This result underscores the value of, and the need for, attention to patient–clinician relational factors in work with patients at risk for suicide (Yaseen et al., 2016).

Relevance of Clinician Emotional Response in Clinical Practice

A Predictive Factor in Suicide Risk Assessment

Self-assessment of emotional response seems to have potential clinical utility in the treatment of suicidal patients. Alternatively, poorly managed emotional responses to suicidal patients can result in harm. Research suggests that negative emotional responses correlate with negative patient outcomes (Marcinko et al., 2008), and clinician failure to control hostility, hate, and aggressiveness may even help push patients to suicide (Varghese & Kelly, 1999).

Clinical judgment, relying on both intuitive and rational processes, has been shown to hold predictive value in the assessment of near-term suicidal behavior (Barzilay et al., 2020). Of note, clinicians' negative emotional responses to suicidal patients, assessed with the Therapist Response Questionnaire–Suicide Form (TRQ-SF), were predictive of patients' suicidal thoughts and behaviors at one-month follow-up (Barzilay et al., 2019, 2018). Furthermore the association between clinicians' negative emotional responses and patients' prospective SI was shown to be partly mediated by patients' perception of a poor therapeutic alliance (Barzilay et al., 2020). Qualitative findings from Soulié et al. (2020) suggested that clinicians' positive attitudes toward patients at risk for suicide were associated with enhanced treatment outcomes, as the degree of clinician-perceived connectedness to the patient was found to be inversely correlated with patients' suicidality.

Taken together, these results suggest that awareness and management of emotional responses may be a useful skill for clinicians who encounter suicidal patients. Specifically, effective management and awareness of clinicians' emotional responses may enhance diagnostic judgments, strengthen the therapeutic relationship, and help guide clinicians in determining appropriate courses of treatment and intervention. In other words, clinicians' negative emotional response would appear to be directly correlated with the intensity of suicidality and thus could be predictive of high-risk conditions. However, since current research design can only establish associations but not the directionality of the findings, it is also possible that clinicians' negative emotional responses to suicidal patients may *lead* to increased suicide risk. Hence the challenge for e front-line clinicians lies not only in how to experience and utilize their emotional responses as a diagnostic tool but also in how to manage their negative emotional responses without revealing them to their suicidal patients.

Recent research conducted by Barzilay and colleagues (2022) examined the relationship between clinicians' ability to manage their emotions when working with suicidal patients, their treatment recommendations, and patients' prospective SI outcomes. The results showed that, among clinicians who exercised greater regulation of negative emotional responses to suicidal patients, such negative emotional responses were associated with intensified treatment decisions and were predictive of lower levels of SI at one-month follow-up. On the other hand, for clinicians who demonstrated lower emotional regulation abilities, the joint impact of negative emotional responses and treatment intensification plans predicted an increase in patients' SI one month later. The authors suggested that these results highlight the potential role of clinicians' emotional response regulation in the reduction of short-term SI (Barzilay et al., 2022). The same study highlighted that intensification of treatment was mediated by clinicians' negative emotional experience rather than directly affected by a patient's severity of SI. In light of these results, Barzilay and colleagues (2022) posited that the ability of clinicians to recognize and manage negative emotions may buffer against the adverse effects of such emotions on the therapeutic relationship. These findings align with a large body of psychotherapy research investigating the role of clinician countertransference in patient outcomes and treatment decisions (Abramovitz et al., 1976; Carlson, 2009).

How to Appraise the Emotional Response

Emotion Differentiation

To use our emotions as tools in the assessment of patients' risk for imminent suicide, we must be able to identify them. Emotions are essential to the human experience and have a tremendous influence over our behavior. We seek positive emotions (e.g., happiness, fulfillment, and satisfaction) and avoid negative ones (e.g., shame, humiliation, and abandonment). The ability to recognize and identify one's emotions is not a skill that we are born with, but a complex learned task that requires near-continuous conscious and unconscious judgments. This task is most complicated when one's profession requires one to ignore emotions; in medicine, clinicians must care for patients regardless of their feelings about the patients.

Emotional experiences are life's essential sources of information (Farmer & Kashdan, 2013; Keltner & Kring, 1998), which may be both clear (e.g., feeling saddened by a loss) or confusing (e.g., a general sense of unease). The ability to classify felt experiences into discrete categories is termed *emotion differentiation* (Barrett et al., 2001; Tugade et al., 2004). People's capacity to differentiate emotions varies widely (Kashdan et al., 2010; Tugade et al., 2004). Those skilled at emotion differentiation are able to feel and identify dozens of emotions and are capable of experiencing and naming several emotions simultaneously. At the opposite end of the spectrum are those whose descriptions of their emotional states are broad and nonspecific, often limited to feeling "good" or "bad."

The capacity to differentiate emotions from thoughts also differs from person to person. People often say, "I feel" when they mean "I think." For example, when clinicians say, "I feel that this person is going to recover because the treatment is working," they are expressing a thought and an opinion rather than an emotion. One may think that the thoughts versus feeling distinction is only semantic and carries no consequences, but in medicine in general, and in the assessment of imminent suicide risk in particular, distinguishing thoughts from emotions is the first essential step toward emotion differentiation.

Those who are better able to differentiate their emotions are more skilled in using them to guide their behavior (Barrett et al., 2001). The identification of negative emotions may be particularly important for clinicians who are trained to behave positively regardless of what they feel. Psychiatrists' emotions toward their patients may change dramatically both from encounter to encounter and within each session. Clinicians who are able to differentiate negative emotions may also be able to employ emotion regulation strategies to their advantage (Barrett et al., 2001), rather than suppressing these emotions them (Tugade et al., 2004). This ability is essential for using one's emotions as a tool to identify those at risk for imminent suicide.

Mindfulness

Mindfulness is the skill of gauging one's emotional response to a suicidal patient, which requires the ability to attend to one's inner experiences, such as thoughts and emotions, without judgment and with acceptance (Baer et al., 2006; Bishop et al., 2004; Brown & Ryan, 2003; Germer et al., 2005; Hill & Updegraff, 2012). Mindfulness has gained popularity during the past two decades in therapies that reduce emotional distress, such as DBT (Linehan,

1993a, 1993b), mindfulness-based stress reduction (Kabat-Zinn, 1990), and MBCT (Segal et al., 2002). These are particularly useful in treating depression, anger, anxiety, and the like in individuals with borderline personality traits.

However, in addition to its use in therapy, mindfulness is also a skill that is useful in developing an awareness of subtle differences in one's emotional experiences (Bishop et al., 2004). The idea of emotional awareness, which is defined as "the extent to which people are aware of emotions in both themselves and others" (Ciarrochi et al., 2003, p. 1478), is not new. Buddhist meditation seeks to improve emotional awareness by teaching its followers to focus attention on specifics of emotional responses (Goleman, 2003; Nielsen & Kaszniak, 2006).

The capacity for mindfulness is associated with emotional intelligence, including emotional clarity and recognition (Baer et al., 2004; Brown & Ryan, 2003). In order to be mindful, one must view emotions as mental states not demanding an immediate reaction. The reality of psychiatric work, which requires rapid decision-making in time-sensitive situations, rarely allows for emotional self-examination. Yet precisely under these circumstances, inner observation without action is necessary to moderate the urge to preemptively label the experienced emotions. Such rapid labeling may cause clinicians to rely on past emotional experiences instead of recognizing the distinguishing features of the present moment.

Incorporating Clinicians' Emotional Responses in Patient Suicide Risk Assessment—A Quantitative Measure

Developing a systematic assessment of clinicians' emotional responses has the potential to meaningfully inform clinical judgment of patient suicide risk. To illustrate the promising implications of the inclusion of clinician emotional response in assessment of near-term suicide, a recently developed multi-informant instrument, titled the Modular Assessment of Risk for Imminent Suicide (MARIS), was shown to be predictive of short-term suicidal behavior among high-risk psychiatric inpatients (Hawes et al., 2017). Aimed at detecting patients' near-term suicide risk, MARIS consists of four modules, two of which are patient-reported modules, one assessing patients' state-focused suicidal symptoms (Module 1) and the other assessing patient attitudes toward suicide (Module 2). The other two modules are clinician-rated; one evaluates traditional patient risk factors (Module 3), and the other assesses clinicians' own emotional responses to the patient (Module 4;

Hawes et al., 2017). In particular, the patient-reported component evaluating acute suicidal states (Module 1) and the clinician-reported module assessing clinicians' emotional responses (Module 4) performed notably well in a recent validation study of MARIS (Calati et al., 2020). Module 4 consists of the Therapeutic Response Questionnaire-Suicide Form (TRQ-SF), a validated measure that has 10 items rated on a 5-point Likert scale (see Chapter 9, Appendix B) and is aimed at capturing clinicians' emotional responses to their patients (Barzilay et al., 2018; Yaseen et al., 2017). Extending prior explorations of multi-informant approaches to suicide risk, recent research has demonstrated that the combination of SCS diagnostic criteria with the TRQ-SF scores significantly predicted suicidal attempts and plans in psychiatric outpatients at one month follow-up and even outperformed traditional suicide assessment measures in predicting suicidality in the patient sample (Ying et al., 2020). Such results highlight the potential value of combining these two measures in guiding clinical judgment of patient suicide risk and merit further investigation into the incorporation of multi-informant approaches in suicide risk assessment practices.

A Practical Method for Assessing One's Emotional Response

To summarize, clinicians working with imminently suicidal patients often feel countertransference love, but more often they feel countertransference hate. Frequently, these two emotions are consciously experienced as vague positive or negative feelings, respectively. Because both countertransference love and, particularly, countertransference hate can be viewed as "unprofessional" or unethical, clinicians use common psychological defenses to modify these unacceptable emotional states.

The previously discussed conceptual framework is invaluable in understanding clinicians' interactions with suicidal individuals. Clinicians high in emotional intelligence may use mindfulness to directly assess to what extent they may be experiencing countertransference love and/or hate and to identify the conflicting emotions consistent with various defense mechanisms.

Examining one's psychological defenses is another technique. Some defense mechanisms, such as rationalization or turning against self, are relatively easy to identify. Others may be more difficult, even for clinicians of high emotional intelligence. Even those skilled in emotional differentiation may not be able to recognize their denial, repression, and projection.

Clinicians can decipher their emotional responses by identifying the related emotions and behaviors, which are either more acceptable or more obvious. With high-risk inpatients, a number of clinicians' emotions/behaviors have been shown to predict patients' postdischarge suicidal behavior. Clinicians can identify such emotions/behaviors by asking themselves direct questions and giving honest answers. This technique can be used by all; it requires no special talent for emotional differentiation—just internal honesty.

A clinician can use the following five questions to probe reaction formation, in order of increasing emotional intensity:

1. Do I see him/her more frequently, or for longer sessions, than other patients?
2. Does he/she make me feel good about myself?
3. Do I like him/her very much?
4. Do I look forward to seeing him/her all day?
5. Do I feel sexually attracted to him/her?

An affirmative answer to one or more of these questions regarding a high-risk patient suggests the reaction formation defense, which is associated with increased risk for a patient's suicide attempt shortly. Whereas clinicians are likely to perceive the first two questions as routine, they may be threatened by the fifth question. Although sexual attraction per se is not unethical, any action resulting from it is unethical. Many clinicians would find being attracted to a patient so threatening that they may use every possible defense mechanism to protect themselves from it. In imminent risk assessment, sexual attraction to a patient is a diagnostic sign that needs to be noted and processed rationally. In doing so, being nonjudgmental toward oneself is essential and can be made easier through mindfulness.

The five questions to probe denial, manifested as distancing from the patient, are the following, also in order of increasing emotional intensity:

1. Do I return his/her phone calls less promptly than I should?
2. Does he/she make me feel like my hands are tied?
3. Do I feel dismissed or devalued?

4. Do I wish I had never treated him/her and/or do I dread seeing him/her?
5. Does he/she give me chills or make my skin crawl?

An affirmative answer to one of these questions suggests a distancing emotional response, consistent with the denial defense and indicative of increased risk for the patient's suicide attempt in the near future. Countertransference hate is often easier for clinicians to uncover because dislike of a patient is farther away from possible ethical misconduct than sexual attraction and may be easier to admit to oneself. For the same reason, denial may be easier to identify than reaction formation.

When asking the previous questions, it saves time to go in reverse order and to ask the most emotionally loaded question first. If the answer is positive, there is no need to ask the other, less charged questions.

An eleventh question, "Do I feel guilty about my feelings toward him/her?" applies to both positive and negative emotional responses. Many clinicians feel guilty when admitting both extremes of feelings. This question should be asked last, as a reality check. Guilt is a diagnostically valuable emotional response. Feeling guilt in the absence of a positive or negative response should indicate that the true response may not have been uncovered and may warrant a re-examination for a defense mechanism other than reaction formation and denial.

Furthermore, feeling positive emotions does not preclude feeling negative emotions: Both are often felt at the same time, creating a confusion of undifferentiated and unpleasant tension mixing excitement and anxiety. This confused state is exactly when the probing questions are most helpful in teasing out more differentiated and diagnostic emotions. The following case is an example of an internal dialog probing mixed countertransference.

Case 51

Stanley, a 55-year-old highly accomplished male without a psychiatric history, was admitted to an inpatient unit following a drug overdose. He overdosed after a fight with his wife when she told him that she was filing for divorce. The wife visited the unit and reconciled with the patient, who was then set for discharge. The intern felt intensely anxious about it: "On the negative side, this patient makes my skin crawl," she thought, "He is putting me in an impossible bind: I think that if his wife leaves him, he will kill himself. And yet I need to discharge him because he says he is not suicidal. On the positive side, I think I could help him. I really understand him, and he appreciates me. He makes me feel good about myself. Do I feel a special bond?"

Case Examples

Case 52: High Risk for Imminent Suicide— Reaction Formation

Christie was referred to Dr. E by his residency training director, who told him, "She has chronic SI and two serious past attempts, one of them very recently. Wealthy parents who are overinvolved. You are a strong resident, and if anybody can work with her, you can." Dr. E felt put on the spot and became very anxious. "Bad luck," he thought. "I am now under the microscope with a high-risk. This is all I need."

Dr. E was dreading meeting Christie. When he finally did, he was pleasantly surprised. Christie was a very attractive 21-year-old Chinese woman dressed in skin-tight jeans and a T-shirt. She seemed exceptionally bright and motivated to be in treatment. With her, she brought a neatly organized folder with pictures and notes. "These are all the men in my life I had relations with and crushes on," she said, "My middle school tennis coach, my high school English teacher, and my college Spanish professor. You need to know everything about me."

The session went very well. Dr. E felt an instant rapport with Christie, as if he had known her for a long time. She was cooperative, open, insightful, and ready to change. "You are very different from my previous therapists," she said at the end of the session, "When is our next session?"

Instead of a weekly visit, Dr. E scheduled Christie for two days later. His distress diminished. Moreover, he felt elated and looked forward to their next session so he could implement a strategy he had designed to treat her suicidality, which he was sure would be successful. In supervision, however, the attending alerted him to a discrepancy between his exuberant and hopeful response to Christie and the severity of her illness, as well as her chronic risk for suicide.

Dr. E asked himself the 11 questions to probe his emotions and gave the following answers:

Question	Answer
1. Did I (plan to) see her more frequently?	Yes
2. Does she make me feel good about myself?	Yes
3. Do I like her very much?	Yes
4. Do I look forward to seeing her all day?	Don't know
5. Do I feel sexually attracted to her?	Yes
6. Do I return her phone calls less promptly than I do with my other patients?	Don't know
7. Does she make me feel like I was put in an impossible bind?	Yes
8. Do I feel dismissed or devalued?	No
9. Do I wish I had never taken her on as a patient?	Yes
10. Does she give me chills or make my skin crawl?	No/no
11. Do I feel guilty about my feelings toward her?	Yes

When analyzing the answers to the probing questions, Dr. E was able to identify his unusually positive response to Christie, his uncharacteristic scheduling of her, and even his attraction to her. He was then able to identify his developing overinvolvement with Christy. Furthermore, recognizing early distress and subsequent hopefulness in himself made him realize his reaction formation defense, which reduced the anxiety he initially felt about the case. He then assessed Christie as having an elevated risk for imminent suicide.

Case 53: High Risk for Imminent Suicide—Repression and Denial

Leo was admitted to an inpatient psychiatric unit with the chief complaint, "I am desperate, and I need to be admitted to the psychiatric unit, because I do not want to repeat what I did in April." In April, Leo attempted suicide by overdose on benzodiazepines and alcohol, and he drank a detergent. Prior to the attempt, he posted a long suicide note on his Facebook page. His suicide attempt was interrupted by the police; somebody who read the Facebook page had called 911. Leo was then admitted first to the intensive care unit and later for two weeks on an inpatient psychiatric unit. Leo did not follow up with his postdischarge outpatient treatment.

During his assessment, Leo told the resident, Dr. N, that his most recent stressor was a comment at work about his hair loss—it made him think that he was going to become bald like his father, whom he detested. His April attempt followed a comment by his date that she could not understand him because of his accent. Leo was a Bulgarian immigrant who left Bulgaria at age 16, and he was very proud of his English.

Dr. N initially liked talkative Leo. However, as the interview dragged on, he became increasingly irritated and angry because Leo was talking only about his hair and his looks, and he was difficult to understand, just like his date had told him. Leo was turning out to be a self-absorbed, entitled individual. Whatever question he was asked, his response was about either his receding hair or his being overweight, both of which made him feel excluded.

"I am weird," said Leo, "and I like weird girls. But even they don't go out with me. It is my hair. Also, I am not athletic, I am overweight, and I am Bulgarian." Dr. N thought that Leo's whining was completely unfounded. He was a tall, attractive, muscular guy, with regular dark hair. "What a wimp," thought Dr. N, "He will never be happy."

Dr. N started Leo on an SSRI for his depression. On the unit, Leo was intrusive, and in groups, he continued to perseverate on his appearance. The staff disliked him, and Dr. N always saw him last. On Friday, Leo denied SI and a suicide plan. Mindful of the need to shorten the length of Leo's hospital stay, Dr. N discharged him from the unit with a Monday follow-up appointment. He was relieved: Dr. N was very aware that he had disliked Leo, but he thought he had provided good care.

Leo was readmitted on Sunday night after another overdose. A different admitting team decided that Leo was delusional and put him on an antipsychotic. Dr. N realized that he had not recognized Leo's first episode of schizophrenia and felt guilty about his anger at the patient. His answers to the 11 questions would have been as follows:

Question	Answer
1. Do I see him more frequently or for longer sessions than other patients?	No
2. Does he make me feel good about myself?	No

Question	Answer
3. Do I like him very much?	No
4. Do I look forward to seeing him all day?	Definitely no
5. Do I feel sexually attracted to him?	No
6. Do I return his phone calls less promptly than I do with my other patients?	N/A
7. Does he make me feel like my hands are tied?	No
8. Do I feel dismissed or devalued?	No
9. Do I wish I had never taken him on as a patient and do I dread seeing him?	Yes/yes
10. Does he give me chills or make my skin crawl?	Yes/yes
11. Do I feel guilty about my feelings toward him?	Yes

Dr. N's emotional response to Leo was fairly characteristic of repression and denial defenses against countertransference hate. He repressed his hate toward the patient, and his conscious experience was anger and irritation. He used denial to distance himself from the patient. As a result, his superficial mental status examination misinterpreted Leo's delusional perception of his appearance as self-absorption. In reality, Leo's desperation was a sign of entrapment in his delusional world, with both emotions being symptoms of the suicidal crisis. If Dr. N had asked himself the countertransference questions, he would have realized that his emotional responses to the patient indicated a high risk for the patient's imminent suicide.

Case 54: Low Risk for Imminent Suicide

Dr. K was asked to assess Rosette, a 23-year-old mother of three and a clinical trial participant, because she was having suicidal thoughts and wanted to be admitted to the hospital for protection, as she had been "last time." She had one recent hospitalization after a suicide attempt when she took 18 pills of lorazepam and cut her left wrist because she felt overwhelmed taking care of her children. She agreed to be in the study at that time.

The resident assistant called the study clinician, Dr. K, to assess Rosette's suicide risk. Rosette was a slim, neatly dressed Latina who seemed to be bewildered by Dr. K's sudden appearance. She explained to Dr. K that she was on her way to be admitted to the hospital she was at previously, but she decided to stop at the research office for a follow-up assessment on the way. Her boyfriend was waiting for her outside in the car with their daughters to drive her to the ED.

Upon further questioning, Rosette told Dr. K that she had difficulty staying home with her children for long periods of time. Her oldest daughter was oppositional, and the baby was colicky. Rosette was always exhausted, and she had difficulty controlling her anger and thought that she must be a bad mother. The previous night, she had inflicted superficial cuts on her thighs because seeing blood made her feel good. She said that something needed to change, or she would kill herself.

Dr. K had a dilemma: A suicidal patient with a history of a suicidal attempt felt unsafe and wanted to be admitted, but to a different hospital. Should he walk her to his hospital's ED or trust her to go to the other ED? As the study's principal investigator, he was responsible for Rosette's safety. Dr. K felt irritated by the patient's manipulative behavior with regard to her boyfriend. "Manipulative patients do kill themselves," he thought, "particularly those with borderline personality disorder, which she probably has."

Dr K asked Rosette, "Do you feel trapped in your situation?" Next, he proceeded to assess her for suicidal narrative and suicidal crisis. Neither was present. Dr. K then walked to the patient's car, confirmed that her boyfriend was driving Rosette to the other hospital's ED and instructed the boyfriend to call him if there was a problem. Although he did not need to ask himself the probing questions, his answers would have been as follows:

Question	Answer
1. Do I see her more frequently or for longer sessions than other patients?	N/A
2. Does she make me feel good about myself?	No
3. Do I like her very much?	No
4. Do I look forward to seeing her all day?	N/A
5. Do I feel sexually attracted to her?	No
6. Do I return her phone calls less promptly than I do with my other patients?	N/A
7. Does she make me feel like my hands are tied or that I am put in an impossible bind?	Yes

Question	Answer
8. Do I feel dismissed or devalued?	No
9. Do I wish I had never taken her on as a patient and/or do I dread seeing her?	No
10. Does she give me chills or make my skin crawl?	No
11. Do I feel guilty about my feelings toward her?	No

Despite Rosette's determination to be admitted to a psychiatric unit and her history of suicidal behavior, Dr. K's emotional response to Rosette indicates a low risk for imminent suicide. He diffuses his anger with rationalization and then calmly assesses her suicide risk. Despite his negative response to Rosette, his walking her down to the car and speaking to the boyfriend is perceived as caring.

Conclusion

Suicide is devastating for the relatives of its victims. Death of a spouse, a parent, or a child is at the top of the life stressors severity list (Holmes & Rahe, 1967; Rahe & Arthur, 1978), but death by suicide is even more dreadful because it is viewed as preventable (Feigelman et al., 2009; Hendin et al., 2000). In addition to grieving, survivors of a significant other's suicide often blame themselves for missing the warning signs, for being absent in the time of crisis, and for acting in a way that could have pushed their loved one toward suicide.

Furthermore, working with suicidal patients has been recognized as one of the most stressful occupational roles (American Association of Suicidiology, 2002), and psychiatrists who lose a patient to suicide also feel a devastating sense of loss (Hendin et al., 2000). They often second-guess their actions prior to the patient's suicide, identifying signs of the catastrophe that they may have missed. The literature is full of reports describing the anguish and guilt clinicians experience after a patient's suicide (Hendin et al., 2000, 2004; Veilleux, 2011). These emotions are compounded by doubts about one's professional skills, perceived treatment mistakes, and fears of lawsuits, with potential career-ending consequences (Maltsberger, 1993).

The flood of disturbing emotions that clinicians experience after a patient's suicide is often accompanied by the memories of negative or uncomfortable feelings toward the patient prior to their death. Prominent among these may be anger, hostility, anxiety, frustration, and helplessness (Hendin et al., 2000, 2004; Veilleux, 2011). Also common are negative emotions related to the clinician's reluctance to treat such patients, delays in answering their phone calls, or attempts to discharge them prematurely from the caseload.

Maltsberger and Buie (1974) noted that the dysphoria during an encounter with a suicidal patient may be too intense to be experienced consciously. As discussed previously, clinicians employ unconscious defenses to transform these responses into more acceptable emotions and thoughts, which then may be brought into consciousness. However, clinicians need to be aware that they may still act out their emotional responses, either through overinvolvement with patients or through distancing and rejection.

Suicidal patients, who often feel alienated and lonely, are exquisitely sensitive to their clinicians' feelings toward them. During the evaluation or treatment, they try to guess their clinicians' "real" emotions. They search for and see the subtle signs of irritation, frustration, or dislike that clinicians may be unaware of. Unfortunately, suicidal patients' perception of their clinicians' dislike may be the final evidence they need to convince themselves that they are a burden to others and that not one person in the world, including their psychiatrist, cares if they live or die. Under these circumstances, a clinician's perceived indifference or dislike may be one of many factors triggering a suicidal act.

The pressure clinicians feel when deciding whether to discharge or hospitalize suicidal patients weighs heavily on their shoulders. Whether conscious or subconscious, this pressure makes clinicians' emotions even more apparent to the patients—a fact that clinicians are often aware of but powerless to change. Ultimately, left untreated, the SCS leaves individuals in a precarious state of risk. Often, illnesses inhibit individuals' capacity to maintain a clear vision of their state of health, often impairing the ability to articulate feelings, needs, and experiences. Hence it is paradoxical that, to date, self-reported SI is the determining factor in guiding suicide risk assessment. A method for assessing imminent suicide risk without relying on patient-reported ideation will both improve the chances of averting suicide and reduce clinicians' negative responses to suicidal patients. This perspective underscores our efforts to improve the assessment and awareness of clinicians' emotional response.

References

Abramowitz, S. I., Abramowitz, C. V., Roback, H. B., Corney, R. T., & McKee, E. (1976). Sex-role related countertransference in psychotherapy. *Archives of General Psychiatry*, *33*(1), 71–73.

Ægisdóttir, S., White, M., Spengler, P., Maugherman, A., Anderson, L., Cook, R. S., Nichols, C. N., Lampropoulos, G. K., Walker, B. S., Cohen, G., & Rush, J. D. (2006). The meta-analysis of clinical judgment project: Fifty-six years of accumulated research on clinical versus statistical prediction. *The Counseling Psychologist*, *34*(3), 341–382.

American Association of Suicidology, Clinician Survivor Task Force. (2002). *Therapists as survivors of suicide: Basic information.* http://www.iusb.edu/~jmcintos/basicinfo.html

Baer, R. A., Hopkins, J., Krietemeyer, J., Smith, G. T., & Toney, L. (2006). Using self-report assessment methods to explore facets of mindfulness. *Assessment*, *13*(1), 27–45.

Baer, R. A., Smith, G. T., & Allen, K. B. (2004). Assessment of mindfulness by self-report: The Kentucky Inventory of Mindfulness Skills. *Assessment*, *11*(3), 191–206.

Bagge, C., Littlefield, A., Wiegand, T., Hawkins, E., Trim, R., Schumacher, J., Simmons, K., & Conner, K. (2022). A controlled examination of acute warning signs for suicide attempts among hospitalized patients. *Psychological Medicine*, 1–9.

Banja J. (2004). Back to basics. *The Case Manager*, *15*(5), 16–18. https://doi.org/10.1016/j.casemgr.2004.07.00

Barrett, L. F., Gross, J., Christensen, T. C., & Benvenuto, M. (2001). Knowing what you're feeling and knowing what to do about it: Mapping the relation between emotion differentiation and emotion regulation. *Cognition & Emotion*, *15*(6), 713–724.

Bartel, C. A., & Saavedra, R. (2000). The collective construction of work group moods. *Administrative Science Quarterly*, *45*(2), 197.

Barzilay, S., Gagnon, A., Yaseen, Z. S., Chennapragada, L., Lloveras, L., Bloch-Elkouby, S., & Galynker, I. (2022). Associations between clinicians' emotion regulation, treatment recommendations, and patient suicidal ideation. *Suicide & Life-Threatening Behavior*, *52*(2), 329–340. https://doi.org/10.1111/sltb.12824

Barzilay, S., Schuck, A., Bloch-Elkouby, S., Yaseen, Z. S., Hawes, M., Rosenfield, P., Foster, A., & Galynker, I. (2020). Associations between clinicians' emotional responses, therapeutic alliance, and patient suicidal ideation. *Depression and Anxiety*, *37*(3), 214–223.

Barzilay, S., Yaseen, Z. S., Hawes, M., Gorman, B., Altman, R., Foster, A., Apter, A., Rosenfield, P., & Galynker, I. (2018). Emotional responses to suicidal patients: Factor structure, construct, and predictive validity of the Therapist Response Questionnaire–Suicide Form. *Frontiers in Psychiatry*, *9*, 104.

Barzilay, S., Yaseen, Z. S., Hawes, M., Kopeykina, I., Ardalan, F., Rosenfield, P., Murrough, J., & Galynker, I. (2019). Determinants and predictive value of clinician assessment of short-term suicide risk. *Suicide and Life-Threatening Behavior*, *49*(2), 614–626.

Baumeister, R. F., Bratslavsky, E., Muraven, M., & Tice, D. M. (1998). Ego depletion: Is the active self a limited resource? *Journal of Personality and Social Psychology*, *74*(5), 1252.

Berman, A. L. (2018). Risk factors proximate to suicide and suicide risk assessment in the context of denied suicide ideation. *Suicide and Life-Threatening Behavior*, *48*(3), 340–352.

Birtchnell, J. (1983). Psychotherapeutic considerations in the management of the suicidal patient. *American Journal of Psychotherapy*, *37*(1), 24–36.

Bishop, S. R., Lau, M., Shapiro, S., Carlson, L., Anderson, N. D., Carmody, J., Segal, Z. V., Abbey, S., Speca, M., Velting, D., & Devins, G. (2004). Mindfulness: A proposed operational definition. *Clinical Psychology, 11*(3), 230–241.
Brewe, A. M., Mazefsky, C. A., & White, S. W. (2021). Therapeutic alliance formation for adolescents and young adults with autism: Relation to treatment outcomes and client characteristics. *Journal of Autism and Developmental Disorders, 51*(5), 1446–1457.
Brown, K. W., & Ryan, R. M. (2003). The benefits of being present: Mindfulness and its role in psychological well-being. *Journal of Personality and Social Psychology, 84*(4), 822–848.
Calati, R., Cohen, L. J., Schuck, A., Levy, D., Bloch-Elkouby, S., Barzilay, S., Rosenfield, P. J., & Galynker, I. (2020). The Modular Assessment of Risk for Imminent Suicide (MARIS): A validation study of a novel tool for suicide risk assessment. *Journal of Affective Disorders, 263*, 121–128.
Carlson, S. N. (2009). Whose hate is it? Encountering emotional turbulence in the crosscurrents of projective identification and countertransference experience. *Psychoanalytic Review, 96*(6), 895–915.
Ciarrochi, J., Caputi, P., & Mayer, J. D. (2003). The distinctiveness and utility of a measure of trait emotional awareness. *Personality and Individual Differences, 34*(8), 1477–1490.
Cohen, L. J., Gorman, B., Briggs, J., Jeon, M. E., Ginsburg, T., & Galynker, I. (2019). The suicidal narrative and its relationship to the suicide crisis syndrome and recent suicidal behavior. *Suicide & Life-Threatening Behavior, 49*(2), 413–422. https://doi.org/10.1111/sltb.12439
Cohen, L. J., Mokhtar, R., Richards, J., Hernandez, M., Bloch-Elkouby, S., & Galynker, I. (2022). The narrative-crisis model of suicide and its prediction of near-term suicide risk. *Suicide & Life-Threatening Behavior, 52*(2), 231–243.
Cramer, P. (2015). Understanding defense mechanisms. *Psychodynamic Psychiatry, 43*(4), 523–552.
Deisenhammer, E. A., Ing, C. M., Strauss, R., Kemmler, G., Hinterhuber, H., & Weiss, E. M. (2009). The duration of the suicidal process: How much time is left for intervention between consideration and accomplishment of a suicide attempt? *Journal of Clinical Psychiatry, 70*, 19–24.
Eubanks-Carter, C., Muran, J. C., & Safran, J. D. (2015). Alliance-focused training. *Psychotherapy, 52*(2), 169–173.
Farmer, A. S., & Kashdan, T. B. (2013). Affective and self-esteem instability in the daily lives of people with generalized social anxiety disorder. *Clinical Psychological Science, 2*(2), 187–201.
Feigelman, W., Gorman, B. S., & Jordan, J. R. (2009). Stigmatization and suicide bereavement. *Death Studies, 33*(7), 591–608.
Galynker, I., Yaseen, Z. S., Cohen, A., Benhamou, O., Hawes, M., & Briggs, J. (2017). Prediction of suicidal behavior in high risk psychiatric patients using an assessment of acute suicidal state: The Suicide Crisis Inventory. *Depression and Anxiety, 34*(2), 147–158.
Germer, C. K., Siegel, R. D., & Fulton, P. R. (2005). *Mindfulness and psychotherapy.* Guilford
Glenn, C. R., & Nock, M. K. (2014). Improving the short-term prediction of suicidal behavior. *American Journal of Preventive Medicine, 47*(3), S176–S180.
Goleman, D. (2003). Maxed emotions. *Business Strategy Review, 14*(2), 26–32.

Groenewoud, J. H., van der Maas, P. J., van der Wal, G., Hengeveld, M. W., Tholen, A. J., Schudel, W. J., & van der Heide, A. (1997). Physician-assisted death in psychiatric practice in the Netherlands. *New England Journal of Medicine, 336*(25), 1795–1801.

Hatfield, E., Cacioppo, J., & Rapson, R. (1993). Emotional contagion. *Current Directions in Psychological Sciences, 2*, 96–99.

Hawes, M., Yaseen, Z., Briggs, J., & Galynker, I. (2017). The Modular Assessment of Risk for Imminent Suicide (MARIS): A proof of concept for a multi-informant tool for evaluation of short-term suicide risk. *Comprehensive Psychiatry, 72*, 88–96.

Hendin, H., Lipschitz, A., Maltsberger, J. T., Haas, A. P., & Wynecoop, S. (2000). Therapists' reactions to patients' suicides. *American Journal of Psychiatry, 157*(12), 2022–2027.

Hendin, H., Maltsberger, J. T., Haas, A. P., Szanto, K., & Rabinowicz, H. (2004). Desperation and other affective states in suicidal patients. *Suicide and Life-Threatening Behavior, 34*(4), 386–394.

Hill, C. L., & Updegraff, J. A. (2012). Mindfulness and its relationship to emotional regulation. *Emotion, 12*(1), 81–90.

Holmes, T. H., & Rahe, R. H. (1967). The social readjustment rating scale. *Journal of Psychosomatic Research, 11*(2), 213–218.

Kabat-Zinn, J. (1990). *Full catastrophe living: Using the wisdom of your body and mind to face stress, pain and illness*. Delacorte.

Kashdan, T. B., Ferssizidis, P., Collins, R. L., & Muraven, M. (2010). Emotion differentiation as resilience against excessive alcohol use: An ecological momentary assessment in underage social drinkers. *Psychological Science, 21*(9), 1341–1347.

Keltner, D., & Kring, A. M. (1998). Emotion, social function, and psychopathology. *Review of General Psychology, 2*(3), 320–342.

Kramer, A. D. I., Guillory, J. E., & Hancock, J. T. (2014). Experimental evidence of massive-scale emotional contagion through social networks. *Proceedings of the National Academy of Sciences, 111*(24), 8788–8790.

Kim, E., Zeppenfeld, V., & Cohen, D. (2013). Sublimation, culture, and creativity. *Journal of Personality and Social Psychology, 105*(4), 639–666.

Laconi, S., Cailhol, L., Pourcel, L., Thalamas, C., Lapeyre-Mestre, M., & Chabrol, H. (2014). Relationship between defense mechanism and therapeutic alliance. *L'encephale, 41*(5), 429–434.

Linehan, M. M. (1993a). *Cognitive–behavioral treatment of borderline personality disorder*. Guilford.

Linehan, M. M. (1993b). *Skills training manual for treating borderline personality disorder*. Guilford.

Lombardo, C., Milne, D., & Proctor, R. (2009). Getting to the heart of clinical supervision: A theoretical review of the role of emotions in professional development. *Behavioural and Cognitive Psychotherapy, 37*(02), 207.

Machado, D. D. B., Teche, S. P., Lapolli, C., Tavares, B. F., Almeida, L. S. P. D., Silva, G. B. D., Magalhães, P. V., & Eizirik, C. L. (2015). Countertransference and therapeutic alliance in the early stage of adult psychodynamic psychotherapy. *Trends in Psychiatry and Psychotherapy, 37*, 133–142.

Maltsberger, J. T. (1993). A career plundered. *Suicide and Life-Threatening Behavior, 23*(4), 285–291.

Maltsberger, J. T., & Buie, D. H. (1974). Countertransference hate in the treatment of suicidal patients. *Archives of General Psychiatry, 30*(5), 625–633.

Marcinko, D., Skocic, M., Popovic-Knapic, V., & Tentor, B. (2008). Countertransference in the therapy of suicidal patients—An important part of integrative treatment. *Psychiatria Danubina, 20*, 402–405.

Michaud, L., Ligier, F., Bourquin, C., Corbeil, S., Saraga, M., Stiefel, F., Seguin, M., Turecki, G., & Richard-Devantoy, S. (2020). Differences and similarities in instant countertransference towards patients with suicidal ideation and personality disorders. *Journal of Affective Disorders, 265*, 669–678.

Michel, K., Maltsberger, J. T., Jobes, D. A., Leenaars, A. A., Orbach, I., Stadler, K., Dey, P., Young, R. A., & Valach, L. (2002). Discovering the truth in attempted suicide. *American Journal of Psychotherapy, 56*(3), 424–437.

Nielsen, L., & Kaszniak, A. W. (2006). Awareness of subtle emotional feelings: A comparison of long-term meditators and nonmeditators. *Emotion, 6*(3), 392–405.

Nivoli, A., Nivoli, F., Nivoli, G., & Lorettu, L. (2011). Therapist's reactions on the treatment of suicidal patients. *Rivista di Psichiatria, 46*(1), 57–65.

Nummenmaa, L., Hirvonen, J., Parkkola, R., & Hietanen, J. K. (2008). Is emotional contagion special? An fMRI study on neural systems for affective and cognitive empathy. *Neuroimage, 43*(3), 571–580.

Prasko, J., Diveky, T., Grambal, A., Kamaradova, D., Mozny, P., Sigmundova, Z., Slepecky, M., & Vyskocilova, J. (2010). Transference and countertransference in cognitive behavioral therapy. *Biomedical Papers, 154*(3), 189–197.

Rahe, R. H., & Arthur, R. J. (1978). Life change and illness studies: Past history and future directions. *Journal of Human Stress, 4*(1), 3–15.

Ribeiro, J. D., Bender, T. W., & Buchman, J. M. (2015). An investigation of the interactive effects of the capability for suicide and acute agitation on suicidality in a military sample. *Depression and Anxiety, 32*(1), 25–31.

Rogers, M. L., Galynker, I., Yaseen, Z., Defazio, K., & Joiner, T. E. (2017). An overview and comparison of two proposed suicide-specific diagnoses: Acute suicidal affective disturbance (ASAD) and suicide crisis syndrome (SCS). *Psychiatric Annals, 47*, 416–420.

Rogers, M. L., Bafna, A., & Galynker, I. (2022). Comparative clinical utility of screening for suicide crisis syndrome versus suicidal ideation in relation to suicidal ideation and attempts at one-month follow-up. *Suicide and Life-Threatening Behavior*, https://doi.org/10.1111/sltb.12870

Rycroft C. (2010). Why analysts need their patients' transferences. 1993. *American Journal of Psychoanalysis, 70*(2), 112–118. https://doi.org/10.1057/ajp.2010.2

Schechter, M., Goldblatt, M. J., Ronningstam, E., Herbstman, B., & Maltsberger, J. T. (2016). Post discharge suicide: A psychodynamic understanding of subjective experience and its importance in suicide prevention. *Bulletin of the Menninger Clinic, 80*(1), 80–96.

Schein, M. (2016). Thinking forbidden thoughts: The Oedipus Complex as a complex of knowing. *The Psychoanalytic Review, 103*(2), 251–263.

Schuck, A., Calati, R., Barzilay, S., Bloch-Elkouby, S., & Galynker, I. (2019). Suicide crisis syndrome: A review of supporting evidence for a new suicide-specific diagnosis. *Behavioral Sciences & The Law, 37*(3), 223–239.

Segal, Z. V., Williams, J. M. G., & Teasdale, J. D. (2002). *Mindfulness-based cognitive therapy for depression: A new approach to preventing relapse.* Guilford.

Soulié, T., Bell, E., Jenkin, G., Sim, D., & Collings, S. (2018). Systematic exploration of countertransference phenomena in the treatment of patients at risk for suicide. *Archives of Suicide Research.*

Soulié, T., Levack, W., Jenkin, G., Collings, S., & Bell, E. (2020). Learning from clinicians' positive inclination to suicidal patients: A grounded theory model. *Death Studies*, 46(2), 485–494.

Stefana, A. (2017). *History of countertransference: From Freud to the British object relations school*. Routledge.

Stone, D. M., Simon, T. R., Fowler, K. A., Kegler, S. R., Holland, K. M., Ivey-Stephenson, A. Z., & Crosby, A. E. (2018). Vital signs: Trends in state suicide rates—United States, 1999–2016 and circumstances contributing to suicide—27 states, 2015. *Morbidity Mortality Weekly Report*, 67, 617–624.

Sy, T., Côté, S., & Saavedra, R. (2005). The contagious leader: Impact of the leader's mood on the mood of group members, group affective tone, and group processes. *Journal of Applied Psychology*, 90(2), 295–305.

Tucker, R. P., Crowley, K. J., Davidson, C. L., & Gutierrez, P. M. (2015). Risk factors, warning signs, and drivers of suicide: What are they, how do they differ, and why does it matter?. *Suicide and Life-Threatening Behavior*, 45(6), 679–689. https://doi.org/10.1111/sltb.12161

Tugade, M. M., Fredrickson, B. L., & Barrett, L. F. (2004). Psychological resilience and positive emotional granularity: Examining the benefits of positive emotions on coping and health. *Journal of Personality*, 72(6), 1161–1190.

Van Wagoner, S. L., Gelso, C. J., Hayes, J. A., & Diemer, R. A. (1991). Countertransference and the reputedly excellent therapist. *Psychotherapy*, 28(3), 411–421.

Varghese, F., & Kelly, B. (1999). Countertransference and assisted suicide. In G. Gabbard (Ed.), *Countertransference issues in psychiatric treatment* (pp. 85–116). American Psychiatric Press.

Veilleux, J. C. (2011). Coping with client death: Using a case study to discuss the effects of accidental, undetermined, and suicidal deaths on therapists. *Professional Psychology*, 42(3), 222–228.

Werner, E. R., & Korsch, B. M. (1976). The vulnerability of the medical student: Posthumous presentation of LL Stephens' ideas. *Pediatrics*, 57(3), 321–328.

Yaseen, Z. S., Briggs, J., Kopeykina, I., Orchard, K. M., Silberlicht, J., Bhingradia, H., & Galynker, I. I. (2013). Distinctive emotional responses of clinicians to suicide-attempting patients: A comparative study. *BMC Psychiatry*, 13, 230.

Yaseen, Z. S., Chartrand, H., Mojtabai, R., Bolton, J., & Galynker, I. I. (2013). Fear of dying in panic attacks predicts suicide attempt in comorbid depressive illness: Prospective evidence from the National Epidemiological Survey on Alcohol and Related Conditions. *Depression and Anxiety*, 30(10), 930–939.

Yaseen, Z. S., Galynker, I. I., Briggs, J., Freed, R. D., & Gabbay, V. (2016). Functional domains as correlates of suicidality among psychiatric inpatients. *Journal of Affective Disorders*, 203, 7–83.

Yaseen, Z. S., Galynker, I. I., Cohen, L. J., & Briggs, J. (2017). Clinicians' conflicting emotional responses to high suicide-risk patients—Association with short-term suicide behaviors: A prospective pilot study. *Comprehensive Psychiatry*, 76, 69–78.

Ying, G., Chennapragada, L., Musser, E. D., & Galynker, I. (2021). Behind therapists' emotional responses to suicidal patients: A study of the narrative crisis model of suicide and clinicians' emotions. *Suicide and Life-Threatening Behavior*, 51(4), 684–695.

Ying, G., Cohen, L. J., Lloveras, L., Barzilay, S., & Galynker, I. (2020). Multi-informant prediction of near-term suicidal behavior independent of suicidal ideation. *Psychiatry Research*, 291, e1131169.

9

Conducting Short-Term Risk
Assessment Interviews

The preceding chapters have discussed the theoretical and historical frameworks for the narrative-crisis model of suicidal behavior (NCM; Chapters 2 and 3), followed by a detailed discussion of the key constructs used for the assessment of short-term suicide risk (Chapters 4 through 8). This chapter describes several ways to integrate all the constructs into assessment interviews that can be used in different clinical settings.

To recap, the first construct is trait vulnerability, which creates fertile ground for the possibility of suicide (Chapter 4). The second is stressful life events (Chapter 5), which could be interpreted in terms of a suicidal narrative (SN). The third construct is the SN (Chapter 6), which reduces one's perception of one's life to a series of failures, a perception that makes the present unacceptable and the future unfathomable. The fourth construct is the suicide crisis syndrome (SCS), which, if intense enough, could culminate in suicide as a solution to an unbearable life situation (Chapter 7). The fifth construct is the clinician's emotional response to suicidal patients, which may affect the assessment of short-term risk and could also be used to refine and finalize the assessment.

This chapter has five sections. The first section combines the all the key constructs of the short-term risk assessment into one comprehensive risk assessment outline, while staying within the theoretical framework of the NCM. The second section addresses the real-world challenges of risk assessment, with specific focus on the limitations of patients' self-report of suicidal ideation (SI) and intent and strategies for minimizing the interview bias. The third section is devoted to the potential advantages and pitfalls of the short-term risk assessment instruments. The fourth section describes three risk assessment interview strategies and gives examples of each. The fifth section describes a frequent clinical scenario, as a reminder that the clinician's negative emotional responses (NER) are a critical part of suicide risk assessment.

Comprehensive Short-Term Risk Assessment Outline

The comprehensive outline below includes all demographic and clinical information that could be used for short-term suicide risk assessments in any clinical setting. The information is organized within the NCM framework.

Long-Term Risk Factors

Demographics
- Age, race, ethnicity: How old is the patient? What is their ethnicity? In the United States, men and women 35 to 64 years old are at the highest risk for suicide, but the picture is complex (see Chapter 3). Caucasians and Native Americans have the highest suicide rate among all ethnicities.
- Gender and sexual orientation: What are the patient's biological sex and gender, and does the patient identify with the LGBT community? In the United States, suicide rates are higher for men than for women, with the highest differential being 5.8 in the 10- to 24-year-old group. Suicide rates are higher in the LGBT community than in heterosexual patients.

History of Mental Illness and of Suicide Attempts
- History of mental illness: Was the patient ever given a psychiatric diagnosis? How early? How consistent was the diagnosis over their lifetime? Over 90% of individuals who die by suicide have been diagnosed with a mental illness, such as an affective disorder, schizophrenia, alcohol or drug use disorder, or personality disorder.
- History of suicide attempt(s): Has the patient ever attempted suicide? Past suicide attempt with intent to die increases lifetime risk of death by suicide thirtyfold.

Childhood History
- Childhood trauma: Was there a history of childhood adversity and/or childhood trauma, including sexual abuse? Both childhood adversity and trauma are independently associated with increased suicide risk; the highest increase (10 to 14 times the risk) is seen in adult males who were sexually abused as boys.
- Parenting style: Were the patient's parents neglectful, authoritarian and overbearing, or distant and controlling? Children of mothers with an

"affectionless control" parenting style are at higher risk for suicide as adults.

- Attachment style: How comfortable is the patient being emotionally close to others and do they seek emotional intimacy? Individuals with insecure and anxious attachment styles have increased suicide rates.

Traits
- Impulsivity: How impulsive (versus premeditated) is the patient in their actions? Impulsivity may be associated with increased short-term suicide risk in crisis-driven suicide attempters (see Chapter 2).
- Hopelessness and pessimism: Does the patient have a pessimistic and negative outlook on life in general? In the United States, although not in some Eastern European cultures, trait hopelessness and pessimism are associated with higher lifetime suicide risk.
- Perfectionism: Does the patient consider themself a perfectionist? Do others? Perfectionism is strongly associated with higher long-term suicide risk and can form a foundation for the first stages of the SN: setting up unrealistic life goals and failure to redirect.
- Fearlessness and pain insensitivity (capability): Is the patient anxious or fearless? Afraid of the pain of dying or pain in general? Patients who have lower anxiety rates, such as those with externalizing and antisocial traits, are at higher lifetime risk.

Cultural Acceptability
- Cultural attitudes: Is suicide accepted or honored in the patient's culture? In certain cultures, suicide is still sanctioned following family dishonor.
- Immigration status: Is the person a recent immigrant? From where? Recent immigrants tend to have lower suicide rates, which increase with time and often exceed the suicide rates of those born in the United States.
- Moral, philosophical, and religious objections: Does the patient have a moral or religious objection to suicide? Faith and strong religious affiliation are some of the strongest protective factors against suicidal behavior.
- Regional affiliation: Does the patient live in one of the U.S. "honor" states? Were they born in one of those states? Do they feel an emotional and cultural kinship to one of those states? In the United States, suicide rates are highest in the West and the lowest on the Eastern Seaboard.

- <u>Suicide in the family</u>: Has anybody in the patient's family died by suicide? A mother's suicide, in particular, is associated with a significant increase in her child's lifetime risk of suicide.
- <u>Suicide clusters</u>: Have any of the patient's relatives, friends, or acquaintances recently died by suicide? Suicides are likely to occur in temporal and geographic clusters, and recent suicides by close others or even celebrities increase short-term suicide risk.
- <u>Suicide exposure and practicing</u>: Has the patient been discussing suicide in online chat rooms, or researching and discussing methods, even in relation to others? All these behaviors signify increased short-term risk.

Stressful Life Events

Work and Career
- <u>Economic hardship</u>: Does the patient have enough money to support him- or herself and his or her family? Are they in debt? Has there been a recent deterioration in socioeconomic status? Is the patient recently unemployed? Economic hardship is one of the two stressful life events (the other being a relationship failure) associated most strongly with increased short-term suicide risk.
- <u>Business or work failure</u>: Has there been a recent business or work failure? Was it public? Was it humiliating? Was the patient fired from his or her job? Was his or her project terminated? All the above may feed into the later stages of the SN, increasing short-term risk dramatically.
- <u>Loss of home</u>: Has the patient recently lost their home? Are they about to be evicted, or is the family facing foreclosure? Recent and particularly impending loss of home increases short-term risk of suicide; foreclosure carries a higher risk than eviction.

Relationship Conflict
- <u>Romantic rejection</u>: Has the patient suffered a romantic rejection or the breakup of an intimate relationship? The ending of a marriage or long-term relationship, particularly due to infidelity, sharply increases imminent risk for suicide, with most deaths occurring within 24 hours of the event. Recent separation and divorce are also strong short-term risk factors, as is romantic rejection in adolescents and young adults.

- Intimate relationship conflict: Was the patient in an abusive relationship and was there intimate partner violence? Poor relationship quality is a suicide risk factor for women, while domestic violence is a risk factor for both men and women. Further, men tend to underreport physical abuse due to the shame associated with appearing "weak."
- Parents in conflict with children: Was a parent recently made to feel like they are a burden to their children? In some cultures, being a burden to one's children may feel like a disgrace and may be a short-term risk factor for suicide.
- Children in conflict with parents: Did a child or adolescent report a recent, shameful conflict with parents, even one that was seemingly trivial? Was a young adult in recent conflict with their parents, particularly over a being a burden to them? Conflict with parents is the most frequent reason for suicide in children and adolescents. Feeling like a burden feeds directly into the SN.
- Ongoing childhood and adolescent abuse and neglect: Is the child or adolescent patient a victim of ongoing sexual or physical abuse? Ongoing abuse is strongly associated with childhood and adolescent suicide attempts. Does the adult patient have a history of sexual abuse? (See also "Childhood trauma" above.)
- Bullying: Is the patient being bullied at school or at work? Bullying is associated with increased suicide risk, particularly in adolescent girls. Workplace bullying by supervisors is more common than is typically acknowledged.

Serious Medical Illness

- Recent diagnosis: Was the patient recently diagnosed with a serious medical illness with a poor prognosis? Such a diagnosis significantly reconfigures one's life narrative and can increase suicide risk. In middle-aged adults, short-term risk is highest in the first month after the diagnosis (6-fold increase in risk), and then it decreases, although risk remains high for the first year.
- Prolonged and debilitating illness: Has the patient been suffering painful setbacks while in treatment for an illness, such as cancer or COPD? Has the patient recently developed additional comorbid illnesses? Suicide risk is higher for patients with prolonged and debilitating illnesses, particularly when there are other comorbid conditions.

- Acute and chronic pain: Is the patient in pain? Is the painful condition chronic? Suicide rates are higher for patients with chronic back pain and chronic headaches. These symptoms also increase the danger of death from unintended opiate overdose.

Serious Mental Illness
- Recent diagnosis: Was the patient recently diagnosed with a serious psychiatric illness, such as schizophrenia, bipolar disorder, or major depressive disorder (MDD)? In the first three months after being given one of these diagnoses, the short-term risk for suicide increases 20-fold for schizophrenia and 10-fold for bipolar disorder and MDD.
- Recent hospitalization: Was the patient recently discharged from an inpatient psychiatric unit? In the first week after discharge, suicide risk is 250 times higher for women and 100 times higher for men compared to those never admitted, regardless of diagnosis. The risk remains very high (20-fold) in the first month after discharge.
- Recent suicide attempts: Has the patient attempted suicide in the last year? How recently? How many times? Short-term suicide risk is higher in patients with a history of recent suicide attempts, particularly the elderly. Risk is higher in those with multiple attempts, which may indicate practicing or rehearsing. Additionally, risk is higher with unsuccessful completed attempts (e.g., survival after an overdose with a bottle of pills) compared to aborted attempts (e.g., changing one's mind after ingesting a few pills and going to the hospital) or interrupted attempts (e.g., someone or something interfered with pill ingestion).
- Attempt lethality: What was the method chosen in each of the attempt(s), and did the more recent attempts use more lethal methods? (See Chapter 5.) Recent failed attempts by hanging confer a 50% risk of death by suicide within the next six months. Failed attempts by drowning and shooting also signify very high short-term risk. Risk is lowest with failed attempts by cutting.
- Exacerbation and acute episodes: Is the patient in the midst of a psychotic, depressive, or mixed manic episode? For any diagnosis, an acute episode increases short-term risk by an order of magnitude. The short-term risk is highest for mixed mania (38-fold), followed by MDD (> 20-fold).
- Medication changes: initiation, discontinuation, or noncompliance: Was the patient recently started on any medications, particularly

SSRIs, which may cause anxiety, agitation, panic attack, insomnia, irritability, hostility, aggressiveness, impulsivity, akathisia (psychomotor restlessness), and/or hypomania/mania? (See Chapter 5.) Has the patient recently stopped taking any psychoactive drugs, in particular benzodiazepines, sedating antipsychotics (such as quetiapine, clozapine, or chlorpromazine), hypnotics or sedating mood stabilizers, and SNRIs? Were the doses of any of the above medications recently reduced? Any changes in medications can contribute to the affective disturbance of the SCS (Chapter 7).

Recent Substance Misuse
- <u>Drug and alcohol use disorder</u>: Does the patient have a history of Alcohol or Drug Use Disorder (AUD)? Suicide rates in patients with AUD and substance use disorder are much higher than in those without these disorders.
- <u>Acute alcohol intoxication and recent drug use</u>: Is the patient under the influence of drugs or alcohol at the time of the interview (determined by observation and inquiry)? Was there any intent to use alcohol or drugs as a suicide facilitator or method? One-third to one-half of suicide deaths are preceded by acute use of alcohol (AUA) and/or drugs.
- <u>Drug or alcohol withdrawal</u>: Has the patient used alcohol or drugs in the last 24 hours? Could they be in withdrawal either currently or imminently (determined by observation and inquiry)? Withdrawal from alcohol and most illicit or prescription drugs of abuse is associated with affective disturbance and changes in arousal, which may exacerbate the suicide crisis. The symptoms of cannabis withdrawal are delayed and peak in the second week after the last use.

Suicidal Narrative

Stages of the Narrative
- <u>Stage 1: Unrealistic life goals</u> Has the patient set unreachable life goals or do others (family, significant others, clinician) perceive their goals as unreachable given their abilities and background? Life goals that are either objectively unreachable or perceived as unreachable often form the foundation and first stage of the SN. Life goals (both realistic and unrealistic) may include career success, such as becoming a celebrity or CEO at 25,

having a high-income, secure job (doctor, lawyer, developer), or simply having a job and an income. Alternatively, life goals may refer to personal success, such as looks, material possessions, lifestyle, or attachments and relationships.

- Stage 2: Entitlement to happiness Does the patient believe that their goals are attainable due to their hard work, or due to special talents and personal qualities? Was the patient expecting to be much happier than they are, and is that because of a belief that the world has failed to deliver on its promise of success and happiness? Was this happiness contingent on an unrealistic goal set in Stage 1?

- Stage 3: Failure to disengage and redirect to more realistic goals Is the patient able to appreciate that their goals have either always been unachievable or have become unachievable due to changing life circumstances? When asked about alternatives, is the patient able to formulate alternative, more realistic goals and/or accept alternative goals when the clinician suggests them? Does the patient continue to insist that only the achievement of the original goal (Stage 1) can bring them fulfillment and happiness (Stage 2)?

- Stage 4: Humiliating personal or social defeat Has the patient recently suffered, or are they about to suffer, a defeat that is perceived as catastrophic, demeaning, or humiliating? Such a defeat could be real, perceived, or imaginary, and involve a loss or impending loss of self, status, or attachment. The loss of self could involve the body or the soul, such as a terminal medical illness or serious mental illness. The defeat or loss in status could involve a humiliating failure at work or school, as well as real or relative financial hardship or loss of home. Rejection by a romantic partner could involve unrequited love, a break-up, or infidelity. Was the humiliation public or was it perceived as public? Can the patient see themself living with such a defeat? Has the defeat come as a result of failed pursuit of the unrealistic life goal (Stages 1 and 2) and failure to adjust (Stage 3)?

- Stage 5: Perceived burdensomeness Does the patient believe that they are a burden to others, particularly loved ones, such as parents, children, romantic partners, and close friends? Does the patient think that these people would be better off if the patient were gone? Is the burdensomeness financial or emotional? Is it real (i.e., explicitly stated by others), perceived, or imagined? Does the patient believe they are a burden as a result of the humiliating failure in Stage 4?

- Stage 6: Thwarted belongingness Does the patient feel alienated and disconnected from others? Do they feel isolated and lonely? Does the patient feel they have no one to turn to, because they are sure to be rejected? Does the patient's alienation and fear of reaching out stem from the humiliating personal or social defeat (Stage 4) and from the guilt and shame of facing others after suffering this real or perceived setback? Is the patient's alienation a result of their feeling like a burden to others (Stage 5)?
- Stage 7: Perception of no future Does the patient believe that their life situation is unacceptable, intolerable, and inescapable? Can the patient imagine their future going forward? Can the patient see any good solutions or good options to resolve the situation or to find an acceptable alternative? Is the patient capable of communicating a need for help?

Constructing the Suicidal Narrative
Does the patient's life narrative, as described in the course of the assessment, fit the seven stages of the SN? Which stages fit well, and which do not? Has the patient's predicament resulted from the failure to reach unrealistic life goals and an inability to adjust to more manageable ones? Did this lead to a shameful defeat (Stage 4), causing the patient to be a real or perceived burden on others (Stage 5) and to consider themselves out of options and without a future? If the patient does not volunteer this interpretation during the assessment, how readily do they agree with it?

Suicide Crisis Syndrome

Criterion A: Frantic hopelessness/entrapment
- Entrapment: A core feature of the SCS is a persistent and desperate feeling of entrapment. Does the patient feel trapped in their unbearable life situation? Does the patient see no good options or solutions to relieve the pain they are in? Does death appear to be the only solution to the unbearable pain?
- Desperation: Another core feature of the SCS is the urgency to escape or avoid an unbearable life situation when escape is perceived as impossible. Can the patient wait for relief? How long? Does the patient feel desperate to escape the situation right now? Does the promise of relief in the future seem irrelevant because the patient can no longer bear it?

Criterion B1: Affective disturbance
- <u>Emotional pain</u>: Does the patient feel a sense of inner pain that is too much to bear and needs to be stopped? Is the pain severe and relentless?
- <u>Rapid spikes of negative emotions</u>: Has the patient been experiencing rapid changes in emotion or extreme mood swings? Does the patient have rapid switches in mood from anxiety to depression to anger? Do these changes involve aggressiveness, frustration, anger, and irritation? Do these emotions come in waves? Are they too confusing and intense to distinguish and differentiate? Are there any surges or decreases in drive or motivation?
- <u>Extreme anxiety that may be accompanied by dissociation or sensory disturbances</u>: Is the patient experiencing waves of extreme anxiety? Does the patient feel so vulnerable and defenseless before the outside world that a minor slight is immensely painful? Do they feel or appear frenzied, tense, or on edge? Is the patient having panic attacks? Are there any dissociative symptoms (during or independent of panic attacks)? Does the patient perceive the world around them as looking and feeling different? Do ordinary things look strange or distorted? Does the ground feel solid or rubbery? Do they feel steady on their feet? Does the patient feel strange sensations in their body or skin? Do they feel that something is wrong with them physically? Are these sensations new, something they have never felt before, or that they cannot describe? Is there any mention of burning on the skin, feeling blood rushing in their veins, eyelids burning, or ringing in the ears? During a panic attack, is the patient afraid that something is wrong with them physically? Are they afraid of suddenly dying or being killed? Are they afraid that something indescribably bad might happen?
- <u>Acute anhedonia</u>: Does the patient express an inability to experience, remember, or imagine experiencing things as enjoyable?

Criterion B2: Loss of cognitive control
- <u>Ruminations</u>: Does the patient have intense and persistent ruminations about their own distress and its possible causes and consequences? Does the patient also ruminate about the life events and actions that brought on the distress? Do they ruminate about possible solutions to these problems (reflective pondering)?
- <u>Cognitive rigidity</u>: Can the patient deviate from this repetitive negative pattern of thought (i.e., is there cognitive flexibility)? Can the patient offer alternatives to these negativistic ruminations? Can the patient

accept alternative explanations offered by the clinician, or acknowledge them as a possibility? Does the patient exhibit any flexibility in thinking about any subject?

- Ruminative flooding: Does the patient feel that they have lost control over their thinking, and that changing these thoughts is impossible even with extreme mental effort? Does the patient experience pain or pressure in the head stemming from loss of control over negative thoughts? Does the patient feel that their head may explode from all the negative thinking?
- Failed thought suppression: What happens when the patient tries to suppress repetitive negative or disturbing thoughts? What happens when the patient tries with conscious effort not to think suicidal thoughts? Are the efforts successful or do the unpleasant thoughts, including those about suicide, come back with even more frequency and intensity?

Criterion B3: Hyperarousal

- Agitation: Is the patient agitated or restless during the assessment? Have the patient's significant others noticed them to be in a state of extreme arousal or agitation and being more anxious than usual? Does the patient feel agitated inside? Are they aware of increased difficulty with staying in control and with anger management?
- Hypervigilance: Is the patient in a state of excessive arousal? Scanning the room during the session? Overinterpreting stimuli seen with peripheral vision (e.g., somebody moving in a window across the street)? Excessively sensitive to sounds, smells, or colors (e.g., voices outside the window or in the waiting area)? Making comments about people's thoughts and motives (e.g., a vendor on the street or a receptionist)?
- Irritability: Do you feel that the patient is unusually sensitive and that you need to choose your words more carefully than usual, like "walking on eggshells"? Do the patient's significant others have similar feelings? Do you or patient's family/friends feel that regardless of what they say they are in the wrong or "can't win"? Does the patient say that they are irritable and that they are getting annoyed by every little thing?
- Insomnia: Is the patient having difficulty falling asleep, particularly because of ruminative thinking about the situation they feel trapped in? Do they wake up repeatedly at night, sometimes even every hour? Is the patient bothered by dreams, nightmares, or night terrors? (This can

indicate nocturnal panic attacks.) Does the patient feel exhausted and drained in the morning?

Criterion B4: Acute social withdrawal
- Withdrawal from or reduction in scope of social activity: Has the patient been less social than usual? Have they avoided social engagements and cancelled plans with their friends?
- Evasive communication with close others: Has the patient told anybody that they are in a situation with no good solutions (Criterion A)? About their emotional pain (Criterion B1)? About the thoughts that keep them up at night (Criterion B3)? Has the patient been giving vague answers about their immediate and remote plans?

Suicidal Ideation, Intent, and Plan

- This assessment is to be done last. Because some patients who intend to die would want to hide their suicidal intent, this explicit assessment of suicidality may elicit biased responses. For that reason, it is preferable to perform the explicit assessment of SI and intent at the very end of the interview.
- SI: Does the patient have persistent thoughts of wanting to die or to kill themself as a way to escape an unacceptable life situation that is perceived as intolerable and inescapable? Is there explicit SI (i.e., the desire to die or be dead)? How frequent and painful is the thought and how strongly is it associated with the perception of no exit, affective disturbance, and ruminative flooding?
- Suicidal intent: Is there current intent? Does the patient set conditions to be met as a reason to live or die? For example: "If I get evicted next week, I am not going to survive;" "I am hoarding pills because if my mother dies, I have no reason to live;" "If my wife gets the custody of the kids, I will kill myself;" "I cannot live without her;" "If I don't get the job, I have no hope." Has the patient "put his affairs in order" and given away any belongings?
- Suicidal plan: Has the patient chosen a method? Have there been any preparatory actions for suicide? Has the patient researched the method online? Bought the pills? Gone to the bridge or train tracks? Has the

patient sent or posted any explicit or cryptic messages revealing their suicidal intent?

Preliminary Risk Assessment

- In the preliminary risk assessment, the clinician integrates all the clinical material, with the exception of the clinician's emotional response component, which is assessed separately. The patient information could be summarized in tables and analyzed as described in the corresponding chapters of this book.

Clinician's Emotional Response

- <u>Reaction formation or countertransference love</u>: Does the clinician performing the assessment have an unusually positive emotional response to the patient? This would cause the clinician to express feelings of liking, admiration, and attachment, and behave in a way that would maximize their contact with the patient. Does the clinician feel compelled to see the patient more frequently or for longer sessions than for other patients? The following questions probe for the clinician's unfounded optimism about the patient's safety: Does the patient make me feel good about myself? Do I like the patient very much? Do I look forward to seeing the patient all day? Do I feel sexually attracted to the patient? Positive answers to these questions, particularly when the clinician's feelings are otherwise distressing, conflicted, or induce guilt, indicate reaction formation. The use of this defense is consistent with an increase in the patient's short-term suicide risk.
- <u>Denial of countertransference hate</u>: Does the clinician have an unusually negative emotional response to the patient? Is the patient at such high risk for suicide long term that the case may seem hopeless? These two clinical aspects would cause the clinician to try to minimize their expressed anger, irritation, or frustration, and may lead to attempts to minimize their contact with the patient. Does the clinician postpone seeing the patient until the very end of the day, or return the patient's phone calls less promptly than they return those of other patients? The

following questions probe for countertransference hate: Does the patient make me feel like my hands are tied or like I am in an impossible bind? Do I feel dismissed or devalued by the patient? Do I wish I had never met the patient and/or do I dread seeing the patient? Does the patient give me chills or make my skin crawl? Positive answers to these questions, particularly when the clinician's feelings are conflicted or induce guilt, indicate the use of the denial defense with countertransference hate. Like reaction formation, this indicates an increase in the patient's short-term suicide risk.

Final Risk Assessment

- In the final risk assessment, the clinician integrates the preliminary risk assessment with the information obtained through the analysis of their emotional responses and introduces corrections for their potential biases due to either reaction formation or denial.

Suicidal Ideation and Intent: Self-Report and Its Limitations

The leading sentence in the proposed DSM criteria for the SCS describes "persistent thoughts of wanting to die or kill oneself" as a way to escape an unacceptable life situation, which is perceived as simultaneously painfully intolerable and inescapable. Typical situations include a loss or impending loss of self-worth, status, or attachment, such as terminal illness, humiliating failure at work, or rejection by a romantic partner, respectively. Therefore, one of the key items of short-term suicide risk is the assessment of the intensity of the SI and suicide intent.

Although in theory any clinician can assess any patient for suicide risk, such assessments are predominantly conducted by mental health professionals. Sixty-five percent of them ask questions about suicide risk factors during routine visits, compared to 13% of primary care providers and 10% of medical specialists (Smith et al., 2013).

Traditionally, in our clinical assessments of risk for imminent suicide, we overwhelmingly rely on suicidal patients' truthful reporting of their SI, intent, and plan. Indeed, both the clinical assessment of risk and the psychometric

risk assessment instruments depend on patients' accurate answers to three
direct questions:

1. Have you been thinking about suicide?
2. Do you have an intention to commit suicide?
3. What is your plan?

Unfortunately, although patients' SI, intent, and plan are the key components
of the acute suicidal crisis, patients' self-report of these factors during the
risk assessment interview is a poor predictor of imminent suicidal behavior.
The main reasons for the poor predictive validity of self-report in explicit suicide risk assessment are the patient's hiding their suicidal intent, the patient's
lack of conscious awareness of suicidal intent, the patient's inability to communicate a need for help, and the fleeting nature of the suicidal crisis.

Many acutely suicidal individuals who think about suicide are intent on
ending their lives and have a plan, and they will deny or minimize their SI, as
well as their intent and the plan. Thus, a patient who has made up their mind to
end their life may not tell the truth to the evaluating clinician. Suicidal people
determined to die are aware that their admission of having a suicidal plan will
result in their plan's being disrupted by involuntary hospitalization. Of patients
who die by suicide, 85% deny SI when assessed, and 75% deny SI within seven
days of death by suicide. They know how the game is played, so to speak.

There may be other reasons for the high denial rates that are unconscious.
Our ability to accurately assess suicidal risk through patents' self-report is
further complicated by some patients' inability to recognize their own suicidal feelings and thoughts due to poor emotional differentiation or their
use of psychological defenses (such as denial). Moreover, inability to ask for
help by expressing feelings of despair and suicidal thoughts to people close
to oneself is associated with increased suicide risk (Gvion et al., 2014; Levi-
Belz et al., 2014). Thus, low self-disclosure in and of itself may be a risk factor
for suicidal behavior. Moreover, while mental pain and depression predicted
the presence of suicidal behavior, communication difficulties (e.g., self-
disclosure) are related to the lethality and seriousness of the suicide attempts
(Gvion et al., 2014; Levi-Belz et al., 2014).

This effect is so strong that difficulty in communication differentiates lethal suicide attempters from nonlethal suicide attempters, underscoring that
a combination of intense mental pain with inability to communicate this pain
to others significantly enhances the risk of more lethal suicidal behaviors

(Levi-Belz et al., 2014). Interestingly, the degree of aggression and impulsivity in lethal and nonlethal attempters appears to be the same (Gvion et al., 2014). Thus, it appears that problems with sharing feelings is an important risk factor for near-lethal suicide, above and beyond the contribution of psychiatric illness and mental pain (Busch et al., 2003; Horesh et al., 2004; Levi et al., 2008).

Another complicating factor is that the patient's suicidal intent or their awareness of it can change sharply over a short period of time (Diesenhammer et al., 2009). For half of patients attempting suicide, the period between the initial thought of suicide and the actual attempt can be as short as 10 minutes. Patients for whom this process takes longer have a higher suicidal intent; impulsivity is not associated with the duration of the suicidal process. The very short window of time for identifying suicidal intent may explain why these patients do not communicate their suicidal feelings to others despite often being in close personal contact with them.

Self-report of past and current suicidal behavior can be as unreliable as self-report of current ideation and intent. Some acutely suicidal individuals may hide their past suicidal behavior because they understand that revealing either recent or past attempts will increase the likelihood of their involuntary admission to the hospital. Others may be deeply ashamed of their past behavior, either because they had failed or because they attempted in the first place. Moreover, others may simply "forget" that they attempted suicide or may not consider their past suicidal behavior an attempt (e.g., "I just took some pills. It was a long time ago.")

In sum, although patients' SI, intent, and plan are central to the suicidal process, the accurate assessment of these factors is extremely challenging and often unreliable. Specifically, patients' denial of their SI and intent should be considered in the context of their other SCS symptoms and in relation to the strength of their SN.

Development and Use of Suicide Risk Assessment Instruments

Short-Term Risk Assessment Instruments

Under the ideal circumstance with no time constraints, clinicians using the comprehensive assessment described in the preceding sections would obtain all the necessary information to make the best possible clinical decisions regarding their patient's short-term suicide risk. Yet, due to limited time and resources, or due to explicit administrative policies, very few clinicians will have this time available to them and will have to make their decisions based on short interviews and on concise risk assessment questionnaires with fixed cutoff scores. Although the use of these questionnaires may make clinicians feel secure about their assessments, this security is not supported by the research data.

To date, over 20 suicide risk assessment questionnaires and other tools have been developed for prediction of future suicide attempts and completed suicide (Roos et al., 2013). Surprisingly, predictive validity for future suicide attempts for some of them have never been tested in prospective studies, while others, such as the Beck Depression Inventory (BDI), Beck Hopelessness Scale (BHS), and Scale for Suicidal Ideation (SSI), were only effective in predicting long-term suicidal behavior (Beck et al., 1985, 1988; Beck & Weishaar, 1990; Beck & Steer, 1989; Brown et al., 2000; Stefanson et al., 2012).

The SAD PERSONS Scale
The oldest and, until the emergence of the C-SSRS, most well-known among short-term risk assessment scale is the SAD PERSONS scale, which was developed in 1983 as a simple suicide risk assessment tool based on 10 risk factors, taken from published literature reports (Patterson et al., 1983).

The acronym SAD PERSONS stands for:

S, male Sex; A, old Age; D, Depression; P, Previous attempt; E, Excess alcohol or substance use; R, Rational thinking loss; S, Social support lacking; O, Organized plan; N, No spouse; and S, Sickness. Each affirmative answer is given one point, and this score is then mapped onto a risk assessment scale as follows:

- 0–4: Low
- 5–6: Medium
- 7–10: High

Remarkably, the SAD PERSONS scale was implemented nationally and internationally and has been widely used for years without ever being tested to see if it can predict suicidal behavior prospectively. When very recently the ability of SAD PERSONS to predict future suicide attempts was assessed among a large group of general psychiatric referrals ($N = 4,019$; Bolton et al.,

2012), the scale as a whole had a predictive value of no better than chance. Only several individual items from the scale, such as moderate alcohol abuse and SI with intent, were associated with suicide attempts in the near future.

In 1996, the scale was modified into the Modified SAD PERSONS scale (MSPS), which had the same acronym but somewhat different questions. The Yes/No questions were weighted either 1 or 2, as below:

- S: Male sex → 1
- A: Age 15–25 or 59 + years → 1
- D: Depression or hopelessness → 2
- P: Previous suicidal attempts or psychiatric care → 1
- E: Excessive ethanol or drug use → 1
- R: Rational thinking loss (psychotic or organic illness) → 2
- S: Single, widowed, or divorced → 1
- O: Organized or serious attempt → 2
- N: No social support → 1
- S: Stated future intent (determined to repeat or ambivalent) → 2

As in the original version, this score is then mapped onto a risk assessment scale, also modified as follows:

- 0–5: May be safe to discharge (depending upon circumstances)
- 6–8: Probably requires psychiatric consultation
- > 8: Probably requires hospital admission.

As was the case for the original scale, the MSPS was implemented without its validity being assessed to predict future suicidal behavior, imminent or not, in prospective studies. When such testing was done, the MSPS proved to be no more predictive of future suicidal behavior than the original SPS. Most recently, the SPS proved less effective in predicting suicide attempts and suicides over a period of six months than the clinician's "best guess" mapped onto a 10-point Likert scale (Roos et al., 2013; Wang et al., 2016).

Thus, at this time, the risk factors for suicide must be assessed individually, and it is up to the clinician to establish how they fit into the overall picture of the assessment, which includes the evaluation of trait vulnerability, stressful life events, the SN, acute suicidal state, and, finally, the clinician's own emotional response. The overall presentation should be assessed according to the NCM, at which point the clinician should be able to make the best possible clinical decision about the patient's risk for imminent suicide and act accordingly.

Other relatively short assessment scales (Lecrubier et al., 1997; Oquendo, 2015; Sheehan et al., 2014; Sheehan, Giddens, & Sheehan, 2014; Youngstrom et al., 2015) are no better in predicting suicide attempts or completed suicide short term than the SPS and the MSPS. Thus, while having an easy algorithm that would produce a score allowing the clinician to act (and relieve them of the burden of personal and legal responsibility for consequences of their action), would be both desirable and comforting, at present no such scale is available. The skepticism about the use of the short-term risk assessment scales was underscored by British guidelines for suicide risk assessment (Harding, 2016; Morriss et al., 2013):

> Assessing the risk of suicide in a person expressing suicidal thoughts or presenting with self-harm or a suicide attempt is crucial in attempting to prevent deaths. There are a number of risk-predicting score systems for determining suicidal intent. However, none have good predictive ability, and National Institute for Health and Care Excellence (NICE) guidelines advise these should NOT be used. Instead, a comprehensive clinical interview should be used for assessment.

Classification and Assessment of Suicide in Clinical Drug Trials
In 2012, the United States Food and Drug Administration (FDA) introduced the latest version of the Columbia Classification Algorithm of Suicide Assessment (C-CASA), a classification algorithm developed for the detection of potential treatment-induced increases in suicide risk among participants in clinical drug trials. The FDA requires that participants involved in clinical pharmacological studies be evaluated on 11 categories of suicidal thoughts and behaviors (FDA, 2012). Thus, by extension, any suicide risk instrument used in clinical trials must map onto the 2012 FDA-approved C-CASA categories for monitoring ideation and behavior.

The Columbia Suicide Severity Rating Scale
One instrument that has been theorized to map onto each of the 11 C-CASA categories is the Columbia Suicide Severity Rating Scale (C-SSRS; Posner et al., 2011), a structured clinical interview assessing lifetime and current SI and behavior. In fact, shortly after the publication of the first C-SSRS validity

studies, the FDA designated the C-SSRS as the gold standard for measuring SI and suicidal behavior in clinical trials. This conferral appears to have been shaped by the role of the C-SSRS in guiding the development of the most recent FDA classification categories for prospective assessment of suicidal thoughts and behaviors in clinical drug trials. As a result, the C-SSRS has since become one of the most widely used suicide risk assessments in clinical research.

According to the authors of the scale, the C-SSRS aims to provide a standardized language for screening, identifying, and categorizing suicide risk (Posner et al., 2011). The measure is organized into four subscales, corresponding to four constructs: (1) severity of ideation, divided into five types of suicidal thoughts of increasing in severity; (2) intensity of ideation, assessing frequency, duration, controllability, deterrents, and reasons for ideation; (3) suicidal behavior, assessing the presence/absence of nonsuicidal self-injury, actual, interrupted, and aborted attempts, as well as preparatory acts; and (4) lethality, measuring the extent to which medical damage is incurred as a result of a suicidal attempt.

Since the FDA designated the C-SSRS as the gold standard in 2012, concerns have been raised about the psychometric properties and utility of the C-SSRS, including its lack of rigorous empirical testing at the time of its conferral as the preferred instrument by the FDA, as well as its propensity to underidentify, overidentify, or entirely fail to detect combinations of suicidal thoughts and behaviors (Giddens et al., 2014). Moreover, because the C-SSRS was not designed to be sensitive to rapid changes in suicidal thoughts and behavior, some authors (e.g., Alphs et al., 2016) have argued that the scale may not be well suited to detect potential fluctuations in suicidality that may arise in a clinical drug trial.

The Sheehan Suicidality Tracking Scale
In response to these mounting concerns, other research groups have since developed alternative instruments to assess suicidal thoughts and behaviors in agreement with the C-CASA categories. One notable measure is the Sheehan Suicidality Tracking Scale (S-STS; Sheehan et al., 2014), a brief (16-item), prospective patient self-report or clinician-administered assessment developed to assess and monitor spontaneous and treatment-emergent SI and behavior. The most recent formulation of the S-STS has been adapted to map onto the C-CASA and has been subject to extensive empirical testing in diverse samples. The standard version of S-STS evaluates the seriousness,

frequency, and duration of time spent engaging in SI and suicidal behavior, using a Likert-scale response (0–4) ranging from "not at all" (0) to "extremely" (4). Unlike the C-SSRS, the S-STS can be easily adapted to cover a wide range of time frames, such as "since the last visit," "in the past month," or "in the past hour," allowing clinicians to capture the more acute features of SI and suicidal behavior.

Reliability and validity studies to date lend support for the improved psychometric properties of the S-STS in comparison to the C-SSRS and other similar scales that map onto the C-CASA algorithm. One study found that the S-STS and the InterSePT Scale for Suicidal Thinking Plus (ISST-P; Lindenmayber et al., 2003) showed acceptable agreement with the C-SSRS on only half of the categories delineated in the C-CASA algorithm, although the former two scales agreed closely on all categories (Sheehan et al., 2014). In another study, the S-STS and C-SSRS showed good accuracy for broad categories of SI and behavior, and S-STS interrater agreement and internal consistency statistics were both strong. On the other hand, interrater agreement among the more granular C-SSRS categories (e.g., ideation with method and intent but no plan) varied widely, and internal consistency scores were adequate for C-SSRS ideation scales (Youngstrom et al., 2015). These results likely reflect the different scoring algorithms: the S-STS attempts to classify each patient into a single category of ideation based on severity, whereas the C-SSRS may assign the same patient to more than one domain of ideation. Thus, it remains unclear if the more granular SI categories included in the C-SSRS offer more clinical value than a simple index of SI severity, as provided by the S-STS.

Nevertheless, despite general dissatisfaction with its complexity (Sheehan et al., 2014) and psychometric properties (Giddens et al., 2014), the C-SSRS has been used widely in the United States and internationally, including its use in tracking SI and for predicting suicide risk (The Columbia Lighthouse Project, 2020). The scale is owned by The Columbia Lighthouse Project, which has its own training institute, and its use is proprietary for institutions and organizations (The Columbia Lighthouse Project, 2016).

The Suicide Crisis Inventory

Many existing suicide risk assessment tools, including those discussed in the previous paragraphs, attempt to detect suicide risk by gathering information about long-term risk factors, such as history of mental illness and past suicide attempts. As mentioned in Chapter 1, although this information is important for identifying who is at risk for suicide, these factors do not help identify when an individual might engage in suicidal behavior. Thus, in response to an urgent need for valid and clinically useful tools to improve our ability to predict near-term suicide risk, our research group has developed and tested several iterations of the Suicide Crisis Inventory (SCI), which assesses the presence and severity of symptoms that comprise the SCS.

The first Suicide Crisis Inventory (SCI-1 or simply SCI) is a 49-item patient-report questionnaire developed by our research group to assess the symptom dimensions of the first formulation of the SCS (Galynker et al., 2017), primarily as a clinical research tool. The SCI evolved out of our earliest research assessment for short-term suicide risk, the Suicide Trigger Scale (STS; Galynker, Yaseen, & Briggs, 2014; Yaseen et al., 2010, 2012). The SCI measured five symptomatic dimensions: frantic hopelessness/entrapment, ruminative flooding, fear of dying, panic-dissociation, and emotional pain. The SCI has demonstrated good convergent and discriminant validity (Barzilay et al., 2020), good predictive validity for near-term suicidal behavior in psychiatric inpatients (Parghi et al., 2020), and incremental validity above and beyond self-reported SI and other validated measures for predicting suicidal behaviors (Barzilay et al., 2020). Because the 49-item SCI takes 20 to 30 minutes to complete, making its outpatient and emergency department (ED) use impractical, we have created the eight-item SCI Short Form (SCI-SF), which is suited for both research and clinical work (Hawes et al., 2017). The SCI-SF was validated as one of the Modular Assessment of Risk for Imminent Suicide (MARIS) modules (see MARIS section below) and was used both in research (Hawes et al., 2017) and clinically (Mitelman et al., under review).

Since the initial formulation of the SCI in 2017, emerging lines of evidence have established other important predictors of imminent suicide risk. Among these other predictors are rapid spikes of emotion dysregulation (Bagge et al., 2017; Kleiman et al., 2017), social withdrawal (Kleiman et al., 2017; Yaseen et al., 2019), acute anhedonia (Ballard et al., 2016; Ducasse et al., 2018), and arousal-related disturbances, such as insomnia (Chu et al., 2017). In light of these findings, SCS was updated to its current formulation (discussed in Chapter 7). Reflecting this change, SCI was updated to Suicide Crisis Inventory–2 (SCI-2; Bloch-Elkouby et al., 2021). Comprised of 61 items and rated on a five-point Likert scale ranging from 0 (*Not at all*) to 4 (*Extremely*), the SCI-2 assesses the presence of five dimensions of the SCS: entrapment, affective disturbance, loss of cognitive control, hyperarousal, and social withdrawal. The full version of the SCI-2 can be found in Appendix A at the end of this chapter.

Focusing on the state factors comprising the acute suicidal crisis, the SCI-2 asks patients to rate each item based on the way they "were feeling over the last several days," when they "were feeling their worst." The SCI-2 demonstrated excellent internal consistency, as well as good discriminant, convergent, and current criterion validity with other similar measures of suicide risk. Moreover, the SCI-2 significantly predicted SI, suicide attempts, and preparatory acts at one-month follow-up in a large sample of psychiatric inpatients and outpatients. In the same study, the SCI-2 was the only significant predictor of suicide attempts at follow-up, outperforming risk factors like lifetime and current SI and lifetime and recent suicide attempts (Bloch-Elkouby et al., 2021). At the time this book is being written, the development of the SCI-2 Short Form (SCI-2-SF), designed for fast-paced clinical use, is ongoing.

The Suicide Crisis Syndrome Checklist

Although SCI-2 is a powerful clinical and research tool, it does not sufficiently address the need for a categorical measure optimized for use by front-line clinicians, who are required to use categorical DSM criteria to determine the presence or absence of a psychiatric diagnosis. In response to this need, our research team piloted the Suicide Crisis Syndrome Checklist (SCS-C), a brief clinician-administered diagnostic tool assessing the DSM-format SCS diagnostic criteria (Bafna et al., under review; Yaseen et al., 2019). Similar to the SCI-2, the SCS-C is designed to assess risk for imminent suicidal behavior without relying on patient report of SI, and it measures the presence or absence of the five SCS symptom criteria: entrapment, affective disturbance, loss of cognitive control, hyperarousal, and social withdrawal. However, unlike the patient-reported SCI-2, which is scored ordinally as an index of SCS severity, the SCS-C is completed by clinicians during or following conversational patient interviews, with the goal being to formulate an SCS diagnosis (for the SCS-C, see Appendix C).

Evidence to date supports the clinical utility of the SCS-C in diverse clinical settings. A pilot validation study demonstrated that the SCS-C, constructed from other validated scales and proxy variables into a categorical checklist format, was strongly predictive of imminent suicidal behavior above and beyond self-reported SI or suicide attempt history (Yaseen et al., 2019). This finding was successfully replicated in the recent sample of 903 inpatients and outpatients recruited from three Mount Sinai Health System hospitals between 2016 and 2019 (Bafna et al., under review), and the SCS-C was also predictive of near-term suicidal behavior in adolescents (Apter et al., 2021). Preliminary evidence also lends support for the utility and validity of the SCS-C in hospitals cross-nationally, including in Korea (Park et al., under review), Russia (Chistopolskay et al., 2020), and India (Menon et al., 2022).

More recently the SCS-C was used to develop an Abbreviated SCS Checklist (A-SCS-C), which enables clinicians to formulate an SCS diagnosis through a two-step screening process (Karsen et al., under review). Part A1 of the A-SCS-C contains two screening questions, to which patients respond either Yes or No: "Do you feel trapped with no good options left?" and "Are you overwhelmed or have you lost control by negative thoughts filling your head?" The former question measures the presence of the SCS criterion of entrapment, and the latter question assesses the presence of the SCS criterion loss of cognitive control. A positive response to either of the questions prompts further assessment of additional SCS diagnostic criteria using the A-SCS-C. Specifically, patients respond to a series of Yes/No questions measuring symptoms of entrapment (SCS Criterion A), affective disturbance, loss of cognitive control, hyperarousal, and social withdrawal (SCS Criteria B). Following the completion of the checklist questions, clinicians score patients' responses on each criterion as either Yes, No, or Extreme: patient endorsement of one or two symptoms within a criterion warrants a Yes, while patient endorsement of three or four symptoms within a criterion is rated as Extreme. A positive score (both items are rated as Yes) and an Extreme score (both items are scored Extreme) indicate a positive SCS diagnosis.

Implemented in the EDs of six hospitals in the NorthShore University Health System in Illinois, the A-SCS-C demonstrated high clinical utility in guiding admit/discharge clinical decision-making over reports of SI, resulting in the reduction of postdischarge suicidal outcomes (Karsen et al., under review). Thus, the A-SCS-C represents a powerful clinician-administered diagnostic tool for accessing patients with or without SI who are at high risk of imminent postdischarge suicide.

The Modular Assessment of Risk for Imminent Suicide,
Version 2.0 (MARIS-2)
Aiming to design a theoretically sound, practical tool specifically for prospective assessment of short-term suicide risk, we have recently developed MARIS (Hawes et al., 2017), which, in its current form, MARIS-2 (Appendix B; Rogers et al., 2021), combines the SCI-SF and the Therapist Response

Questionnaire–Suicide Form (TRQ-SF; Barzilay et al., 2018; Yaseen et al., 2017) into one instrument. As shown by De Los Reyes and others, having more than one informant improves the diagnostic accuracy of psychiatric assessment, including assessment of suicide risk (De Los Reyes et al., 2015; Ohannessian & De Los Reyes, 2014). Like the MARIS interviews, MARIS-2 utilizes the clinician's emotional responses as a diagnostic tool, making the evaluating clinician the second informant.

MARIS is a two-part, two-informant modular short assessment measure that takes under two minutes to administer. Because MARIS was designed to be a brief and practical tool for potential use by frontline clinicians everywhere, the scale includes only selected aspects of the comprehensive interview. In initial studies in high-risk psychiatric inpatients, MARIS was predictive of suicidal behavior over the initial four to eight weeks after discharge, with an odds ratio = 19 in comparison to those with no suicidal behaviors (Hawes et al., 2017).

Initially, Part One of MARIS contained two self-report patient modules assessing the SCS intensity and the acceptability of suicide as a solution to life's problems and Part Two consisted of two clinician-rated modules assessing the explicit suicide intent and attempt history as well as the clinician's emotional response to the patient. However, in replication studies, the shorter version of MARIS, with just the SCI-SF and TRQ-SF, had the same predictive validity as the MARIS. Hence, this shorter scale was named MARIS-2 and is our preferred tool for both clinical and research use.

At the time of this writing, MARIS is strictly a research tool. More studies with diverse patient populations and different clinical settings are needed to establish if a validated scoring system with clear cutoff scores could be developed to guide clinical decision-making. Most importantly, for the potential implementation of MARIS for clinical use, studies are needed on the proper documentation of the TRQ-SF. At present, even a conceptual framework for such documentation is lacking. Until such studies are conducted, clinicians may use MARIS as an efficient interview guide for obtaining important clinical material on suicide and their own emotional response to the patient.

Risk Assessment Interview Strategies

The Comprehensive Short-Term Risk Assessment Outline delineates all the information an evaluating clinician needs to have at their disposal to assess the risk and formulate the clinical plan. There is more than one interviewing strategy for obtaining this clinical material, of which three are suggested below. The strategy choice would depend primarily on the amount of time a clinician has at their disposal, the patient's awareness of their suicidal intent, and their willingness to be forthcoming with the interview.

The three interview strategies described differ in duration and in the order of questions, but all are intended as conversational interviews rather than fixed checklists. In a conversational interview, the clinician also may take questions from a list but will ask them in an order guided in part by the patient's answers. While, ultimately, all the questions are asked, the patient does have some control over the interview, which feels like a dialog rather than an interrogation.

The comprehensive risk assessment interview covers a wide range of subjects, which could be confusing to the patient and, occasionally, to the interviewing clinician. To maintain conceptual clarity, we recommend conducting the interview in modules reflecting the NCM components, as delineated in the interview outline, regardless of the chosen strategy. These modules, the long-term risk factors, the stressful life events, the SN, and the SCS, are sufficient to make a preliminary risk assessment. The interview should conclude with the clinician's self-assessment of their emotional response to the patient, followed by the final risk assessment.

The three interview strategies are the Comprehensive Interview, the Brief MARIS Interview, and the Expanded MARIS Interview. Their main features and intended use are as follows:

- The Comprehensive Interview follows the exact Comprehensive Assessment Outline. This strategy is best suited for routine clinical intake of patients who either actively seek help or who were brought in by their concerned family members. The Comprehensive Interview differs from the Comprehensive Assessment Outline in that all the explicit suicide-related questions (i.e., acceptability, family history and suicide clusters, attempt history, recent attempt history, SI, intent, and plan) are asked at the end. The estimated assessment time is 90 minutes.
- The Brief MARIS Interview works best in inpatient and emergency settings, when time is a factor. The MARIS interview has just four modules: the SCS, the acceptability of suicide, the explicit risk assessment, and the clinician's emotional response. The interview should take 20 minutes if the suicide risk is present and obvious. If no clinical

judgment can be made after the MARIS interview, it must be expanded with two additional modules, to the Extended MARIS interview.

- The Extended MARIS Interview includes the MARIS Interview with additional stressful life events and SN modules. It is almost always an extension of the MARIS Interview when more information is needed for the risk assessment than was provided during the very concise MARIS Interview. The Extended MARIS Interview takes 30 to 40 minutes.

Comprehensive Interview

The Comprehensive Interview strategy is based on the exact Comprehensive Assessment Outline with one significant exception: all the explicit suicide-related questions (i.e., acceptability, family history and suicide clusters, attempt history, recent attempt history, SI, intent, and plan) are asked at the end. This adjustment is made to improve the reliability of the patient's self-report. Otherwise, the clinician conducts a modular assessment interview in the same order as in the outline.

Suicidal individuals who have decided to die and know that they are being assessed for suicide risk have reasons to deny, minimize, or misrepresent their current, recent, and past SI and behavior. Consequently, an interviewer who asks explicit and direct questions about a patient's suicidality may make the patient aware of the interviewer's intention to assess imminent suicide risk and to prevent suicide; the interviewer then runs the risk of being misled by denials and nonreport of psychopathology by the patient in an effort to minimize his or her risk of hospitalization. Yet, in patients who want clinicians' help in staying alive, which are the majority, this is the most important part of the assessment for clinical, medical, and legal reasons. Moreover, a suicidal patient may perceive a lack of explicit assessment as callous and rejecting, adding to this experience of the SN.

One possible solution to this clinical dilemma is for the clinician to begin the assessment interview with less obvious aspects of the imminent risk evaluation, such as assessing the patient's past history and long-term factors, then their more recent stressors, and finally their mental state for the signs and symptoms of SCS other than SI. Questions about history and symptoms are usually perceived as caring rather than threatening and may help the clinician build rapport as well as receive genuine answers, unaffected by the patient's possible desire to conceal their SI, plan, or intent. The

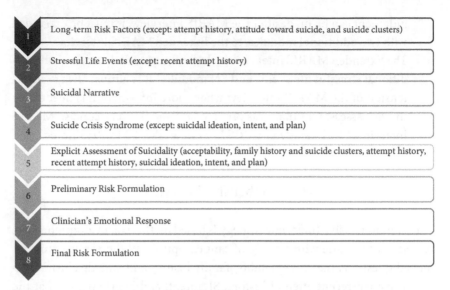

Figure 9.1 Comprehensive Short-Term Risk Assessment Interview.

bulk of the assessment thus consists of a conversational interview about what stressful life events and personal history play the most important role in the patient's life narrative. The explicit direct and detailed questions about the patient's past and present suicidal behavior are not asked until the very end.

The Comprehensive Interview Strategy (see Figure 9.1).

- The clinician starts the interview by greeting the patient and establishing rapport, then moves on to obtaining the clinical history. If the patient spontaneously brings up suicide, the clinician should acknowledge it but then indicate that he would come back to the issue later in the interview.
- The first module of the interview focuses on the history and long-term risk factors, such as perfectionism, impulsivity, fearlessness, and childhood trauma. Questions about past attempts, family history of suicide, or suicide clusters are saved for the fifth module.
- The second module consists of the conversational interview about the patient's life events and possible recent stressors.
- The third module is composed of a discussion about the patient's perception of their life stressors in terms of the stages of the SN. The

clinician should attempt to construct the SN and obtain the patient's feedback on it.

- The fourth module consists of the mental status assessment aimed at eliciting possible symptoms of SCS, such as frantic hopelessness/entrapment, affective disturbance, ruminative flooding, and social withdrawal. No questions about SI or intent should be asked at this stage.
- The fifth module is a direct and explicit assessment of all suicide-related clinical material listed in the Comprehensive Assessment, including a family history of suicide, suicide clusters, attitudes toward suicide, recent and remote past suicidal behavior, and current ideation, intent, and plan.
- The sixth module is the clinician's formulation of short-term risk based on objective clinical material and preliminary clinical decisions regarding the immediate treatment, disposition, and follow-up.
- The seventh module involves the clinician's assessment of their emotional reaction to the patient, with emphasis on the clinican's distress as well as possible countertransference love and countertransference hate, which should be factored into the final decision-making process.
- The eighth module is the synthesis of all clinical material into the final formulation of risk and the final decision regarding treatment, disposition, and follow-up.

Case 55: Comprehensive Short-term Risk Assessment Interview Example

Location: Outpatient office

Patient: Hans is a 30-year-old man with a history of bipolar disorder and alcohol use.

Circumstances/Chief Complaint: Patient was brought in for a reassessment of his diagnosis and medication regimen and because he said he was going to kill himself.

History of the Present Illness: Hans is jobless and is living with his parents on their full financial support. His parents recently refused to give him money to start a new marijuana-growing business.

Building Rapport

DR: Hello Hans, how are you feeling today?

HANS: I am fine.

DR: I understand that you are looking for a psychiatrist to help you with your bipolar disorder. Is that so?

HANS: Yes.

DR: Let's start, then. I will do my usual interview, which may be a little longer than you are accustomed to, but bear with me. OK?

HANS: OK.

Long-term Risk Factors

DR: How old are you?

HANS: 30.

DR: Interesting. . . . You came here with your parents; what's your relationship like with them?

HANS: You don't fool around . . . go straight to the point, don't you? It is not good.

DR: Sorry to hear that. Why?

HANS: All they do is criticize me. I can never do a thing right.

DR: Are you close with them?

HANS: I am closer than I want to be.

DR: Sounds like your relationship with them is too close for your comfort. Are they strict? Authoritarian?

HANS: I told you I can't seem to do anything right.

DR: Are they abusive?

HANS: They never beat me or anything, but you can call it emotional abuse.

DR: Any sexual abuse?

HANS: No.

DR: Was there any history of mental illness in the family?

HANS: My grandfather was mentally ill. He killed himself when I was little.

DR: I am sorry to hear that. I will come back to that later if you do not mind. Did you have any traumatic experiences as a child? With your parents or otherwise?

HANS: I was bullied in school.

DR: It must have been pretty bad for you to bring it up now. Why were you bullied?

HANS: I was fat, and I did not do well in sports.

DR: Is this when you first saw a psychiatrist?

HANS: No, I was diagnosed with ADHD when I was in elementary school. I was on Ritalin and Seroquel and on all kinds of other stuff.

DR: Did you have any friends in elementary school?

HANS: Yeah.

DR: And in high school?

HANS: I had a few friends.

DR: Girlfriends?

HANS: Not in high school.

DR: What is your sexual orientation?

HANS: I am very straight.

DR: I see. Do you have a girlfriend now?

HANS: Yeah! But don't tell my parents. They do not approve.

DR: It seems that your care about your parents' approval. Are you a sensitive person?

HANS: I am pretty thin-skinned. Things get to me more than they should.

DR: When things get to you, are you the kind of person who fights, or who avoids the conflict?

HANS: It depends. I fight with my parents a lot.

DR: How about street fights? Did you get into fights as a kid?

HANS: Not really. I am pretty laid back.

DR: Is it fair to say that you are not a perfectionist?

HANS: Yeah.

DR: Just a couple of more questions about you as a person: Do you generally see a glass as half-full or half-empty? Are you an optimist or a pessimist?

HANS: A pessimist. People tell me I complain a lot.

DR: OK. Finally, are you a spontaneous person or a planner?

HANS: I am not a planner. I can be pretty impulsive.

Trait Vulnerability Summary: Hans is a 30-year-old White male with a long history of mood disorder and anxiety disorder, as well as a history of childhood bullying. His attachment style appears to be anxious and fearful. Hans acknowledges his own impulsivity and notable lack of perfectionism. Hans shows signs of dependent personality disorder.

Stressful Life Events

DR: Are you currently working?

HANS: No, but I want to start a business.

DR: Want kind of business?

HANS: Growing medical marijuana.

DR: Do you know how to start a business?

HANS: No, but I have a friend who does. I just need my parents to put up some money.

DR: Are they willing?

HANS: No. That's one of the reasons we have been fighting.

DR: How does the fighting make you feel?

HANS: I feel that they owe me. I have had a mental illness since I was a little kid. I graduated from high school. I finished college. I worked before. I have been trying to live a productive life. And now that I have a real opportunity "to grow up" (their words) and to be independent, they are not giving me the money. I am not asking for much, and they can afford it.

DR: I see. As far as their wanting you "to grow up," are they threatening to kick you out of the house?

HANS: No. They say I can live in the basement as long as I want.

DR: What do they mean by "growing up," then?

HANS: Get a job and find my own place. They don't care if I flip hamburgers.

DR: When was the last time you worked, and what did you do?

HANS: Two years ago. I worked for my dad.

DR: And?

HANS: I left because I was treated like a little kid. My brother is only two years older than me, and he is a manager! They wanted me to make copies and stuff.

DR: It sounds like you think that your parents are unfair to you.

HANS: They have always been. Since I can remember.

DR: And what does your girlfriend think about all this?

HANS: She thinks that I am crazy, but she also thinks they should be more supportive.

DR: Why don't your parents approve of her?

HANS: They don't know her, and they think she drinks and does drugs. The also think she is not very smart.

DR: Does she use drugs? Is she smart?

HANS: She smokes pot, and she drinks, like everybody else. And hangs out with me, though I am crazy. And she laughs at my jokes.

DR: It sounds like things are OK with your girlfriend. Is this long-term?

HANS: No (*smiles*), but she does not know it.

DR: Noted (*smiles*). And how does all this affect your depression?

HANS: I have been very depressed, and I have been drinking more. I am 30 years old. I am living with my parents, and my life is not going anywhere. Here I have an opportunity to make something of myself, and they are not supportive.

DR: Is your depression worse than usual? Can you work and study with your symptoms?

HANS: I can work. I just need the money to start my business.

DR: What medications are you taking?

HANS: I have been taking the same meds for years. They just don't help. I am taking Seroquel, Lamictal, Lexapro, and Adderall.

DR: Have the doses been changed recently?

HANS: No. Same old, same old.

DR: How much have you been drinking?

HANS: Two to three beers a day. I just drink beer.

DR: What about on weekends?

HANS: Ooh, more on weekends when I get together with my buddies . . . maybe five beers.

DR: Do you black out?

HANS: Occasionally (*smiles*).

DR: How much worse is this than, let's say, about a year ago?

HANS: Well . . . not that much more, now that you asked.

Stressful Life Events Summary: Hans reports no recent intimate relationship or health-related stressors and no recent increase in alcohol use. He reports an ongoing conflict with his parents and a possible upcoming change in his financial status, depending on how this conflict is resolved. He shows signs of severe externalizing traits (narcissistic and antisocial).

Suicidal Narrative

DR: So, Hans, let me ask you: What are your life goals?

HANS: A big question . . . I want what everybody else wants. I want to be happy. I would like to have a business, a family, and a house with a back yard. The American Dream.

DR: Do you think your goals are realistic? You are 30, you are living with your parents, and you are depressed, and I presume that your parents are paying for this appointment.

HANS: Are you trying to tell me that I am a failure?

DR: No, not at all, I didn't mean to sound like that. I have just repeated some facts that you told me earlier. Do you think your goals are achievable?

HANS: Yes they are. I want to start this business with my friend.

DR: OK. Let's say your parents would not put up the money and the business does not happen. Will you be able to adjust your life goal of the American Dream? Maybe scale it down a little? A job, maybe, a smaller house?

HANS: I am not giving up yet. I do not work well in the corporate environment.

DR: Are you where you thought you would be at this point in your life? Are you getting the share of happiness you think you deserve given what you have been through?

HANS: Nobody understands how hard life has been for me. I have been struggling since I can remember. And I have been trying really hard. I have been looking for opportunities. The medical marijuana business is a once-in-a-lifetime opportunity. The window will close soon.

DR: Let me ask you a hypothetical question. Let's say your parents will not finance your MJ adventure. What would this mean for you?

HANS: I would be very angry. I have been trying so hard to find this opportunity!

DR: Would this be a crushing defeat for you?

HANS: It would be a defeat, all right. It would take a while to get over it. . . . My depression would get worse.

DR: Will you be able to get over it?

HANS: I have doctors, I have friends . . . I hope so.

DR: What if your parents stop supporting you altogether?

HANS: They would need to support me a while, until I get on my feet. They can't just cut me off. They won't . . . they never mentioned it.

DR: Do they make you feel like you are a burden to them, financially or emotionally?

HANS: They are critical. They tell me I am not making use of my talents, but they promised they would support me until I find my calling, something that makes me happy.

DR: You said at one point that you were bullied in high school. From what you are saying, you were bullied for being different, really. Do you still feel like that sometimes . . . that you are different and that you do not belong?

HANS: Definitely. I am not good at playing the corporate game. I tried hard enough when I worked for my father.

DR: Do you want to belong? Maybe giving it another try if the MJ business does not work out?

HANS: That's just too painful. I don't think I can.

DR: So, your future hinges on the marijuana business. Can you see your future without it? Are there other options?

HANS: Not working for somebody. Maybe another business. I want this one, though.

DR: So, let me see if I understand: It sounds like your life goal is to be happy and to be like everybody else, but that because of your mental illness you think you don't belong in a corporate environment. The marijuana business seems like a perfect opportunity but there may be other options. You feel that although your parents are supportive, they also do not understand how hard life is for you. Given how hard you were trying and the resources they have, it is only fair that they support you until you find what you are looking for. Is this a reasonable summary?

HANS: Yes, except, if they don't fund the business, I am going to kill myself.

Suicidal Narrative Summary: With the exception of entitlement to happiness, Hans's perception of his life is not consistent with a compelling SN. His goals are achievable, he can redirect to lesser goals, he feels entitled rather than burdensome, and he feels connected rather alienated and withdrawn. He has a sense of a future.

Suicide Crisis Syndrome

DR: I will come back to your suicidal thoughts very shortly; we are almost there. But first, please tell me more about your current state of mind. Do you feel trapped in your current life situation?

HANS: What do you mean?

DR: I mean: is your life situation unbearable and do you want to escape it?

HANS: No, I am depressed and feel mistreated by my parents, but I want to work on it.

DR: Do you think you have enough patience to work through this situation with your family?

HANS: I would like to have it resolved sooner rather than later.

DR: Is your situation causing you emotional pain?

HANS: Of course, it does.

DR: Is your emotional pain there all the time and is it so intense it must be stopped?

HANS: It comes and goes, but I want it to stop. Enough is enough.

DR: Have you been more moody lately? Have you had intense mood swings? When you feel so bad you can't even tell what you are feeling?

HANS: It happens sometimes, but mostly I know what I am feeling.

DR: You told me that you are an anxious person. Have you recently been feeling so vulnerable and defenseless before the outside world that even a minor slight is immensely painful? Like your parents' criticism?

HANS: It's not minor, doc. They know where it hurts the most.

DR: Do you have panic attacks, and do you feel strange sensations in your body and skin?

HANS: No, that's weird.

DR: Are you able to enjoy things you usually enjoy? Like food, sex, watching TV?

HANS: Not as much as I wish.

DR: Do you have intense and persistent thoughts about your problems, and what may have brought them on?

HANS: I think about this all the time. Are you kidding me? I am 30, living in my parents' basement.

DR: Do you ruminate about possible solutions to your problems?

HANS: Yeah, I need to start a business!

DR: When you think about it, can you consider other options, or is your thinking circular, always coming back to the same thing?

HANS: Always the same thing.

DR: Do you feel that you can change your thoughts with a lot of effort? Or have you lost control of your thought process?

HANS: When I think about this stuff, I cannot shut it down.

DR: What happens when you try? Do your unpleasant thoughts come back with even more frequency and intensity?

HANS: They come back with more intensity.

DR: You seem restless. How do you sleep?

HANS: Not well. Too many things to think about.

Suicide Crisis Syndrome Summary: Although Hans complains of severe emotional pain and some anhedonia, he does not acknowledge any symptoms of entrapment. He acknowledges ruminations and thought suppression and shows signs of cognitive rigidity, which add up to significant loss of cognitive control. His insomnia reveals disturbance in arousal.

Explicit Suicide Risk Assessment

DR: I understand that when your parents told you they would not give you money for your marijuana business, you told them you would kill yourself.

HANS: I did, and I meant it.

DR: Your grandfather killed himself. Do you remember him?

HANS: I do. We were buddies. I was seven when he died. He was a drinker and he shot himself.

DR: Did you know at the time that he killed himself?

HANS: No, I only learned when I was in high school. It was a blow. Made me think.

DR: What do you mean?

HANS: It made me think about suicide. Taking your own life.

DR: And what are your thoughts about suicide.

HANS: It's an option. When things get really tough.

DR: Do you think a suicide is a reasonable solution to life's problems?

HANS: If the pain is too much, and there are no others.

DR: Did you know anybody else, besides your grandfather, who died by suicide?

HANS: I had two friends who died from a heroin overdose. They were pretty miserable.

DR: Were those suicides?

HANS: They did not leave notes or anything. . . . Robin Williams killed himself.

DR: What did his suicide mean to you?

HANS: He had depression or bipolar disorder or something like that. If nobody could help him, then some cases are just beyond hope. Maybe my grandfather was one of those who couldn't be helped.

DR: What about you? Can you be helped?

HANS: I need that money for my business; it's simple enough.

DR: But what if your parents stick to their guns so to speak and refuse to fund your business?

HANS: Then I will kill myself.

DR: How would you do it?

HANS: With a gun, like my grandfather.

DR: Do you have a gun?

HANS: I don't, but I know how to get one.

DR: How?

HANS: I have friends. I am not going to tell you.

DR: Have you attempted suicide in the past?

HANS: I tried once.

DR: What did you do?

HANS: I took a bunch of pills when I was in high school.

DR: And what happened?

HANS: Just went to sleep.

DR: And?

HANS: Woke up the next day and decided to go on.

DR: Do you remember what pills?

HANS: No, it was 15 years ago.

DR: Do you have an intention to end your life now?

HANS: If my parents don't support me . . .

DR: What would be you plan?

HANS: I told you, I would shoot myself.

DR: I hope it won't come to that. I hope we'll find a better medication for your depression and that you are able to negotiate your business plans with your parents. I would like to speak to them now if you don't mind. Is that OK?

HANS: Yeah, that's OK. Keep me posted.

Explicit Risk Assessment Summary: Hans reveals remote history of one suicide attempt, acceptance of suicide as a solution to the life's problems and no moral objections to it, as well as awareness of a celebrity suicide. He has clear SI and conditional intent with a high-lethality plan.

Preliminary Risk Formulation

Hans is a 30-year-old single White male with a long history of mood disorder and likely severe mixed personality disorder, with dependent, narcissistic, antisocial, and borderline traits, who was brought in by his parents because he had threatened suicide. His long-term risk factors are his acceptance of suicide as a solution to life's problems, his anxious attachment style, his grandfather's suicide, and his own remote impulsive suicide attempt of low lethality. His stressful life events are his parents' refusal to fund his unrealistic business plans and their general frustration with his dependency on them.

Hans's perception of his life is not consistent with the SN. Hans reports some symptoms of SCS, which include SI, intent, and a plan of high lethality; emotional pain; mild anhedonia; loss of cognitive control; and insomnia. Of note, the indirect risk assessment indicates low suicide risk, but this contradicts his self-report during the explicit risk assessment, which indicates high risk. The doctor's opinion is that Hans's self-report was both dramatic and vague, casting doubt on his sincerity.

Because of the conflict between the clinical information obtained in the direct and the indirect parts of an interview, and the presumed better reliability of the information obtained indirectly, the doctor's preliminary formulation was that Hans was at low risk for short-term suicidal behavior.

Doctor's Emotional Response
The doctor's self-examination of his emotional response revealed some distress due to strong feelings of anger and disdain for the patient. The doctor became aware of his negative emotional response early during the interview, when Hans noticed his disdain and responded to it, in the following exchange:

DR: You are 30, you are living with your parents, and you are depressed, and
    I presume that your parents are paying for this appointment.
HANS: Are you trying to tell me that I am a failure?

The doctor thought that the patient was entitled, exploitative, and manipulative toward his parents and that the patient tried to manipulate the interview by exaggerating his suicidal risk. The doctor further noticed his own guilt feelings about allowing his negative emotional response to the patient to affect his behavior and concluded that his preliminary risk formulation may have been affected by his negative view of the patient and his desire to minimize his further involvement in this troubling case. The doctor then assessed his own emotional response as countertransference hate and his defense mechanism as denial, which he knew were indicative of higher risk; he then factored his response into his revised final risk assessment.

Final Risk Formulation
Hans is a 30-year-old male with a long history of mood disorder, alcohol use disorder, and a history of a suicide attempt in high school who was brought in by his parents for suicidal threat. Hans's trait vulnerability is due to his

age, race, history of mental illness, history of suicide attempt, his acceptance of suicide as a solution to life's problems, his anxious and fearful attachment style, and his impulsivity. His stressful life events include potential personal defeat (if his parents refuse to support his marijuana business), which could become crushing with the threat of loss of his parents' financial support and his home. His SN is fragmented and noted primarily for entitlement to happiness, but it could become coherent with the loss of his parents' financial support and his home. His SCS includes SI and a suicide plan, emotional pain, and loss of cognitive control. The revised overall risk formulation was that, at the time of the assessment, despite significant SCS, Hans is at low risk for short-term suicidal behavior because of his lack of SN. However, the doctor's opinion was that there was a potential for the risk to increase sharply with the threat of loss of home and financial support, which may result in the SN.

The above comprehensive interview is typical of an assessment of short-term risk performed during consultations and intakes in outpatient psychiatric clinics and private offices. The interview illustrates a modular assessment technique in accordance with the NCM model of suicidal behavior that can bring conceptual clarity to the complex clinical material. The interview also demonstrates how holding back the explicit risk assessment until the end of the interview allows most of the interview to be unaffected by possible self-report bias. Finally, the interview illustrates how the clinician's ignoring their own distress and a denial defense (against a strong countertransference hate response to a manipulative patient) can both bias the risk assessment and be factored into adjustment of risk by a shrewd clinician. The revised risk formulation correctly identified potential high risk in the near future, which depended on the resolution of the parental conflict, and included the family meeting in the treatment plan.

The Brief MARIS Interview

The MARIS Interview is a concise interview to be used primarily in ongoing inpatient and outpatient assessments. MARIS is a self-report questionnaire, and its items are worded differently from the language a clinician may use during a face-to-face conversational interview. Still, the MARIS structure and content provide a useful framework for an abbreviated assessment of

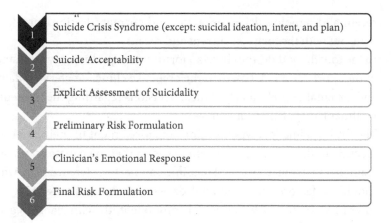

1 Suicide Crisis Syndrome (except: suicidal ideation, intent, and plan)

2 Suicide Acceptability

3 Explicit Assessment of Suicidality

4 Preliminary Risk Formulation

5 Clinician's Emotional Response

6 Final Risk Formulation

Figure 9.2 The MARIS Interview.

short-term risk. MARIS modules provide a useful assessment algorithm for a focused bare-bones interview when the clinician is either short on time or already knows the history, making the comprehensive interview unnecessary (see Figure 9.2).

The MARIS Interview Strategy

- As in the Comprehensive Interview, the clinician first builds rapport, but rather than following the Comprehensive Assessment outline, quickly transitions to the first SCS module—the mental status examination aimed at eliciting possible symptoms of entrapment, affective disturbance, loss of cognitive control, and social withdrawal. As in the Comprehensive Interview, no questions about SI or intent are asked until the end.
- The second module assesses a patient's attitudes toward suicide as a solution to life's problems. Both permissive and prohibitive attitudes should be assessed, with an emphasis on faith and culture. Although this module does not contain direct questions about the patient's suicidality, its purpose as a suicide risk assessment tool is more transparent than that of Module One.
- The third module is an abbreviated explicit assessment of suicide-related clinical material, as in the Comprehensive Assessment, including a family history of suicide, suicide clusters, attitudes toward suicide, past

recent and remote suicidal behavior, and current ideation, intent, and plan, but with the focus on current and recent.

- In the fourth module, the clinician formulates a preliminary assessment of the short-term risk based on the objective clinical material obtained and also makes preliminary clinical decisions regarding the immediate treatment, disposition, and follow-up.
- The fifth module involves the clinician's assessment of their emotional reaction to the patient, with an emphasis on their own distress, possible countertransference love, and possible countertransference hate, which should be factored into the final decision-making process. Since the Brief MARIS Interview has no SN component, the clinicians' Negative Emotional Responses (NERs), which are typically correlated with it, also serve as a SN proxy (Ying et al., 2021).
- The sixth and the final module involves the synthesis of all the clinical material into the final formulation of risk and the decision regarding treatment, disposition, and follow-up.

The MARIS Interview strategy is particularly useful when working with high-risk patients on inpatient psychiatric units.

Case 56: Brief MARIS Interview Example

Location: Inpatient psychiatric unit.

Patient: Karen is a 37-year-old woman with a history of MDD and generalized anxiety disorder being assessed prior to her planned discharge from an inpatient psychiatric hospitalization.

Circumstances/Chief Complaint: Karen was admitted after a suicide attempt by asphyxiation (using a plastic bag) after her boyfriend told her he wanted to break up.

Hospital Course: The patient was treated with antidepressants, and her depression and anxiety appeared to have improved somewhat. Although her boyfriend still wanted to break up, he agreed to start couples counseling. Karen's affect had brightened. She was attending groups, making future plans (with and without her boyfriend), and was waiting impatiently for discharge.

Suicide Crisis Syndrome

DR: How are you feeling this morning?

KAREN: Better, much calmer than before.

DR: Very good, what has been on your mind?

KAREN: I have a lot to think about. Why does Alex want to break up? Why I did what I did. Why was I feeling so bad? How can I avoid feeling like I did again?

DR: Sounds like you still have too many thoughts in your head . . .

KAREN: Yes, but they are different thoughts, positive thoughts, constructive thoughts.

DR: Do you still feel pressure in your head from thinking too much?

KAREN: Sometimes, but it is OK, I need to think.

DR: Do you feel pain in your head from having too many thoughts?

KAREN: Just one or two times.

DR: Are your thoughts confused?

KAREN: A little. It is confusing, isn't it? He was leaving, then he was staying, then he was leaving again, the couple's sessions make you think. . . . But it's all good.

DR: Are you scared that something bad may happen?

KAREN: Not as much as before. I feel much better.

DR: Is your fear coming in waves, unpredictably?

KAREN: Yes, it's kind of hard to know how you are going to feel the next moment.

DR: Are you able to enjoy things?

KAREN: It is hard to enjoy things on the unit. It feels like jail, to tell you the truth, but maybe when I leave.

DR: Do you feel trapped?

KAREN: Being locked up does not help.

DR: Do you feel like there is no exit from your life situation?

KAREN: I don't see any yet, but I will work on them with Alex and the therapist after I am discharged. When am I going home?

Suicide Crisis Syndrome Summary: Karen still has some residual symptoms of SCS, such as entrapment, ruminative flooding, and anhedonia, but the content of her thinking is more positive.

Acceptability

DR: Do you still feel that suicide is a possible solution to one's problems?

KAREN: It would certainly end the suffering for some people. I thought it would end mine, but I was wrong.

DR: Do you think that suicide is immoral?

KAREN: I don't think it's immoral. In my case it was premature. I can see the future now.

DR: And from a moral or religious point of view?

KAREN: I am not religious.

DR: What about how it affects others?

KAREN: I don't want to hurt other people. But I felt I was a burden to Alex, and maybe I still am. I hope not.

Acceptability Summary: Patient continues to accept suicide as a solution to life's problems, although she states that hers was a mistake.

Explicit Assessment

DR: And in your case?

KAREN: Alex says that he loves me. I would never do this to him again.

DR: How were you able to hurt him the first time?

KAREN: I just told you. I thought I was a burden and I would always be a burden. Time heals.

DR: Are you still having thoughts about suicide?

KAREN: No, they went away. Therapy helps, and the antidepressants. I am looking forward to seeing Alex. He is coming in the evening.

DR: Are you planning to kill yourself?

KAREN: Not anymore. I am working on alternatives. Even if things with Alex do not work out. I should be strong enough to be on my own. The therapy here is helping me figure things out.

DR: What do you mean?

KAREN: I mean that I am feeling better. I am not in the dark place I was in before. I understand I need to work on my problems.

DR: And what will you do if you again find yourself in a dark place as before?

KAREN: I will call my therapist, my parents, I will go to the emergency department.

DR: How many times have you attempted suicide in the past?

KAREN: Two. But the first time was many years ago.

DR: What were your attempts?

KAREN: When I was young, I took some pills.

DR: And recently?

KAREN: I put a bag over my head.

DR: And what happened?

KAREN: Alex found me unconscious and brought me to the hospital.

DR: If you feel bad, would you attempt suicide on the unit?

KAREN: How? Everybody is watching you all the time.

DR: I see. I hope you feel better. I will talk to the team about your discharge.

Explicit Assessment Summary: Karen has had two attempts of increasing lethality but currently denies SI and intent and commits to safety.

Preliminary Risk Formulation

Karen is a 37-year-old woman with history of chronic mental illness and two suicide attempts. Her most recent attempt was by asphyxiation and of high lethality, an attempt made when she was experiencing severe symptoms of SCS. She has no moral prohibitions against suicide, which puts her at a higher risk. However, at the time of the assessment, her SCS has resolved. She has no SI or intent, does not feel entrapment, sees options, and has future plans. Her mood symptoms have improved significantly with treatment. The preliminary conclusion based on this information is that Karen is at a high short-term suicide risk and should remain hospitalized.

Doctor's Emotional Response

The doctor's self-assessment of his emotional responses revealed that he liked the patient, felt a lot of empathy for her, and was somewhat attracted to her. The doctor noted that he was looking forward to seeing the patient every day, and that Karen's neediness made him feel powerful and confident, as well as proud that she improved so much under his care and was no longer suicidal. The doctor noted that he felt a little guilty about his attraction to Karen and distressed at his own guilt. He noted the distress and concluded that he was using the reaction formation defense to a suicidal patient, which may have resulted in seeing the patient as being healthier than she was and may have biased his risk assessment toward lower risk. He then reassessed his interview and revised the formulation.

Final Risk Formulation

Karen is a 37-year-old woman with a history of chronic mental illness and two suicide attempts, the most recent of which was of high lethality—by asphyxiation. Karen denies SI and intent but continues to experience significant SCS symptoms, both affective disturbance (depressive turmoil and anhedonia) and loss of cognitive control (ruminations, reflective pondering, ruminative flooding). Her sense of entrapment has improved, and she can see a future, but her future is primarily contingent on her therapy's helping her keep Alex, her boyfriend. She has no moral prohibitions against suicide, and her commitment to safety on the unit is actually due to means restriction ("How? Everybody is watching me all the time."). Given Karen's intense residual SCS symptoms, if, after discharge, Karen feels betrayed by Alex again and she has suicide means available, she would be at very high risk. Moreover, she is at high risk on the unit, subject to Alex's intention to stay or leave. The doctor's revised conclusion is that the patient is still at high short-term risk for suicide.

Following the clinician's assessment, a room search was done, and a plastic bag was discovered under Karen's mattress. Karen admitted to a conditional plan to use the bag in a suicide attempt if Alex made it clear he would leave. She was placed on close observation and a meeting with Alex was scheduled.

The above MARIS Interview was limited in scope but sufficiently detailed to reveal Karen's continuing suicidal crisis and the acceptability of suicide. The interview also revealed the clinician's use of the reaction formation defense, which was an indicator of higher risk than the patient would have otherwise. No additional interviewing was necessary to make the correct clinical decision to do a room search, which revealed Karen's preparatory actions for suicide on the unit, and to place the patient on close observation afterward.

Karen's case illustrates a frequent clinical situation in which a recently suicidal patient denies SI and intent, wanting to convince the clinical team that they are no longer suicidal and are safe for discharge. In Karen's case, both the residual SCS symptoms (particularly in the cognitive domain) and the clinician's intense emotional response allowed the clinician to diagnose high suicide risk. (This is not always the case, however. For another, more difficult example of a sudden improvement in mood and SCS symptoms after a high-lethality suicide attempt, see the section "The Case of Eerie Calm" at the end of this chapter.)

Expanded MARIS Interview

Due to its intended use as a brief assessment and screening tool, MARIS focuses primarily on SCS, as does the MARIS Interview. Still, the MARIS format allows clinicians to detect the signs and symptoms of the suicidal crisis and to identify individuals with no moral prohibitions against taking their own lives and with high trait vulnerability to suicide due to past history. Further, the MARIS Interview alerts clinicians to their strong emotional responses, which are related to the SN glimpsed in the interview (Ying et al., 2021), and gives clinicians an opportunity to factor their emotional responses into clinical decision-making,

The strength of the MARIS Interview is that it provides the clinician with an efficient strategy for detection of a suicide crisis and crisis-driven short-term suicide risk. However, the MARIS Interview is less sensitive to the narrative-driven risk and may not identify the patient with high risk due to strong SN. For that reason, in cases when no SCS is elicited during the MARIS Interview, the clinician needs to continue the interview using the Expanded MARIS Interview format (Figure 9.3), which adds the missing modules from the Comprehensive Assessment that target recent life stressors and the SN.

Time permitting, the Expanded MARIS Interview may also include a more detailed assessment of trait suicidality. Whether it does or does not, after completing the additional modules, the clinician would need to reassess their emotional response to the patient, which may change as a result

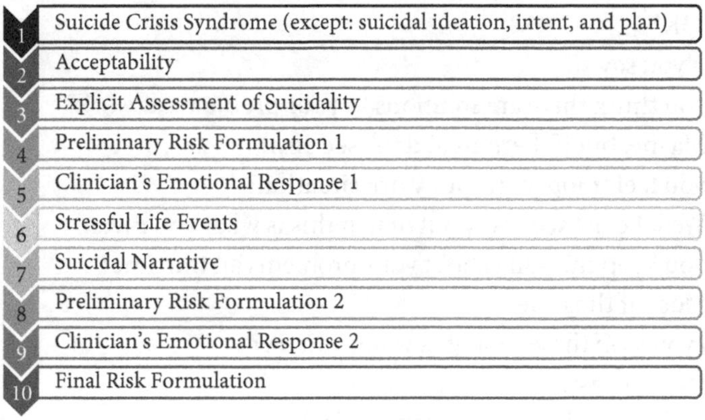

1	Suicide Crisis Syndrome (except: suicidal ideation, intent, and plan)
2	Acceptability
3	Explicit Assessment of Suicidality
4	Preliminary Risk Formulation 1
5	Clinician's Emotional Response 1
6	Stressful Life Events
7	Suicidal Narrative
8	Preliminary Risk Formulation 2
9	Clinician's Emotional Response 2
10	Final Risk Formulation

Figure 9.3 The Expanded MARIS Interview.

of the additional information. Overall, the Expanded MARIS Interview could be as thorough as the Comprehensive Assessment but differently organized, with the explicit part of the assessment moved to the beginning of the interview.

Case 57: Expanded MARIS Interview Example

Location: Emergency Department

Patient: Ellen is a 47-year-old woman with a long history of depression being assessed in the psychiatric ED.

Circumstances/Chief Complaint: Ellen's husband brought her in for an evaluation of her depression.

History of the Present Illness: Patient's husband has been very concerned that Ellen's new antidepressant is making her worse. He thinks this is the worst she has ever been.

Suicide Crisis Syndrome

DR: Good evening, Ellen. How are you feeling?

ELLEN: I feel depressed.

DR: What is making you depressed?

ELLEN: I have been having problems at work.

DR: I may ask you more about your work situation a little later, but for now, I need to focus on how these problems make you feel and think. Is that OK?

ELLEN: If you say so.

DR: Do you think there are solutions to your problems at work?

ELLEN: Maybe, but if there are, I don't see any.

DR: Do you feel trapped in your work situation?

ELLEN: Well, I can't see a way out of it, if this is what you mean.

DR: Do you keep thinking about your problems all the time?

ELLEN: Most of the time.

DR: Can you stop these thoughts when you try?

ELLEN: It is not easy.

DR: Does all this thinking give you headaches?

ELLEN: Sometimes.

DR: Do these thoughts make you feel pressure in your head?

ELLEN: (*smiles*) Not right now.

DR: It sounds like sometimes you do, though. When you feel your worst, do you get scared you will die?

ELLEN: Not really.

DR: When you feel your worst, are you afraid that something horrible may happen, like a heart attack, and kill you?

ELLEN: No.

DR: Have you been experiencing mental pain?

ELLEN: Yes, I have been in terrible pain.

DR: Does this pain come in waves?

ELLEN: More like in shocks.

Suicide Crisis Syndrome Summary: Ellen has strong sense of entrapment, significant loss of cognitive control, and affective disturbance.

Acceptability

DR: Some people, and I am not saying that you are one of them, believe that when things are really bad in life, suicide may be the only escape.

ELLEN: I can see some situations where this would be the case.

DR: Do you think other people can tell when somebody is suicidal?

ELLEN: Not if the person chooses not to tell them about their plans.

DR: Do you think that suicide is an evil act?

ELLEN: Evil is a strong word. I think it is up to the individual. Sometimes, life may just be too painful to bear.

DR: Are you religious?

ELLEN: I am Jewish, but I am not observant.

Attitude Summary: Ellen accepts suicide as a solution and has no objection to some people hiding the intent.

Explicit Assessment

DR: Is this the case for you?

ELLEN: You said this is not about me. I am depressed.

DR: Have you ever attempted suicide in the past?

ELLEN: No, but I thought about it.

DR: Recently?

ELLEN: Not recently. Years back, when I was going through a rough patch in life.

DR: Worse than now?

ELLEN: No. Now is actually tougher.

DR: At the time, did you have a plan?

ELLEN: I had an idea of what I would do.

DR: What was it?

ELLEN: I would jump off something high. So there would be no chance of surviving and becoming a vegetable.

DR: You seem very clear-headed about this. Do you still have this plan?

ELLEN: No. I said it was in the past.

DR: Any thoughts about suicide now?

ELLEN: No. I am depressed but not suicidal.

DR: If discharged and feeling suicidal, would you be able to ask for help?

ELLEN: Yes, I am here, aren't I?

EXPLICIT RISK SUMMARY: Ellen denies SI and intent and commits to safety.

Preliminary Risk Formulation

Ellen is a 47-year-old woman with a history of depression and past SI with a high-lethality plan she did not enact, who currently has significant symptoms of SCS, accepts suicide as a solution to problems, but denies SI and intent and commits to safety. The information is contradictory in two ways: first, although both the patient and the husband state that this is the worst she ever felt, she is less suicidal than during the previous, less severe episode. Second, her self-report of no SI is inconsistent with high intensity of her SCS. The preliminary conclusion is that no conclusion regarding risk can be made, and the conflicting information requires conducting the expanded interview.

Doctor's Emotional Response 1

The doctor's self-assessment of her emotional responses revealed sympathy and liking for Ellen as well as confidence in her ability to help the patient. The doctor also felt deep concern for Ellen and a sense of unease about not having a clear understanding of her suicide risk. The doctor concluded that she was experiencing neither countertransference love nor countertransference hate, and that she was not using either the reaction formation or the denial defense. She then proceeded with the Expanded MARIS Interview.

Stressful Life Events

DR: Now please tell me about your problems at work. What is it that makes you feel trapped at work?

ELLEN: I don't think I am getting my grant renewed.

DR: What does that mean for you?

ELLEN: This means I cannot continue my research. I have had this grant for 15 years. This may be the end of my academic career.

DR: Does this mean you may lose your job?

ELLEN: Almost certainly. They are not going to give me enough bridge money to write another grant, I don't have tenure. Nobody has tenure anymore. You are expected to bring in your own research money.

DR: And if you can't?

ELLEN: I will have to tell my research team that they need to look for jobs and look for one myself.

DR: What kind of job would you look for?

ELLEN: I can work in the pharmaceutical industry. . . . I never thought I would end up like this.

DR: What is wrong with the pharmaceutical industry?

ELLEN: Everything. It's all about profit. I worked there before I got my PhD. I hated it.

DR: Is there a way for you to continue your academic career?

ELLEN: I could teach in some community college, if you can call that academia (*laughs sarcastically*).

DR: How are things financially?

ELLEN: My husband has a good job. Finances are not the issue.

DR: Are things OK with your husband?

ELLEN: As OK as they will ever be. He is limited in what he understands.

DR: What are his limitations?

ELLEN: He is in construction. He never understood science.

DR: Are you having any medical problems?

ELLEN: I am fine.

STRESSFUL LIFE EVENTS SUMMARY: Ellen is facing the acute stress of a job loss, which could be career-ending. She also feels isolated and misunderstood at home, but that stress is chronic.

Suicidal Narrative

DR: It sounds like you have set very high goals for yourself. Are you a perfectionist?

ELLEN: Yes, one cannot be a scientist and do sloppy work.

DR: Do you set high goals for yourself?

ELLEN: You can't be a medical scientist and be otherwise. It takes five years to do anything in science, and you might as well make it consequential. I wanted to find a cure for cancer. And we were getting closer. Our results were incredible.

DR: Would you say you are an overachiever?

ELLEN: I am a very hard worker, and I don't cut corners.

DR: Were you expecting to be in a better place at this time in your life? Do you think that life has treated you fairly?

ELLEN: What do you think? I brought in $15,000,000 of grant money over the years and $10,000,000 in overhead that went to the school and didn't get a penny of it. Don't you think I deserve better?

DR: I certainly do, and it sounds like you did amazing work. But it is not up to me, unfortunately. If the school does not give you the bridge money, will you be able to adjust and maybe reset your aims? Let's call it plan B. Maybe in industry, or even in teaching?

ELLEN: I can't even think about this right now. This would be so incredibly humiliating. What will I tell my colleagues? I won't even be able to go to ACS meetings! I will have nothing to present . . .

DR: I am sure other people you know did not get their grants renewed.

ELLEN: And they are pitied or avoided at meetings.

DR: Are you afraid that you will be one of them?

ELLEN: I can't see how I won't be. I will be too humiliated to look people in the eye. I will be hiding in my apartment.

DR: But life can be so unpredictable. People understand. It sounds like your life is not turning out the way you have imagined. Can you imagine a different future for yourself? As project leader in industry, or star teacher?

ELLEN: I can't. You are suggesting that my whole life was a failure.

DR: Not really, but is this how you see your life? A failure with no future? (*Patient nods.*)

DR: Now I understand why you feel trapped. Please tell me:that one time that you were suicidal in the past, and you thought of ending your life by jumping, so you would not end up "being a vegetable," was it also related to work?

ELLEN: Yes, somebody could not reproduce my results and questioned my scientific integrity. It was political.

DR: And what happened?

ELLEN: My mentor stepped in, and they backed off.

DR: I see. Let me stop for now. I would like to speak to your husband if you do not mind.

SUICIDAL NARRATIVE SUMMARY: Ellen's perception of her life includes most stages of the SN, including perfectionism, failure to disengage from what has become an unreachable goal (continuing her research), humiliating failure, alienation, and a sense of no future. Her SN is so clear that the doctor does not see the need to reprise it for the patient with a formulation.

Preliminary Risk Formulation 2

Ellen is a 47-year-old woman with a history of depression, past SI, and a past high-lethality plan she did not enact. She has no moral prohibitions against suicide, and therefore has a strong trait vulnerability for suicide. Her stress due to imminent career-ending job loss is overwhelming. At present, Ellen perceives herself as being in an unacceptable life situation due to humiliating failure at work. The future she imagines is painful and unacceptable to her, and she perceives her life in terms of a clear SN. She cannot imagine a future and sees her situation as simultaneously painfully intolerable and inescapable. The patient had a high-lethality plan in the past under less stressful circumstances, and she currently has many symptoms of SCS. Other than subjective denial of her SI and intent, all other clinical information points toward a very high risk for a narrative-driven suicide.

Clinician's Emotional Response 2

The doctor's second self-assessment of her emotional responses was less sympathetic toward the patient than her first, and she felt some irritation at Ellen's lack of flexibility. The doctor continued to feel deep concern for the patient, while her initial unease about not having a clear understanding of Ellen's suicide risk changed to concern that, if discharged, Ellen may kill herself by jumping off a building or by some other very lethal means. The doctor concluded that she was experiencing neither countertransference love nor countertransference hate and that she was not using either the reaction formation or the denial defense. She then proceeded to meet with the husband to discuss the treatment plan.

Final Risk Formulation
Same as Preliminary Risk Formulation 2.

The Case of Eerie Calm

The criteria for SCS, which precedes suicide, describe a state of frantic hopelessness/entrapment dominated by an urgency to escape an unbearable life situation when escape is perceived as impossible. Thus, death appears as the only achievable solution to unbearable pain. SCS also involves at least one symptom of affective disturbance, loss of cognitive control, hyperarousal, and social withdrawal. Many patients in the midst of SCS project a feeling of unnerving intensity, which could make a clinician feel uncomfortable, and yet some individuals prior to their suicide are remembered to have appeared calm, composed, and even placid, giving a clinician a sense of unease.

There are several reasons why suicidal individuals may appear calm and content in the hours or even minutes preceding suicide. First, the symptoms of SCS (e.g., frantic hopelessness/entrapment, anxiety, ruminations) describe subjective inner experiences that are not always visible to an outside observer, particularly if the patient is careful not to reveal their inner state. Only agitation, insomnia, and evasive communication with others are readily observable, but the patient may not always be agitated, and insomnia and evasiveness are not specific to suicidal individuals. Thus, even patients with severe SCS may appear calm outwardly.

Second, in individuals with narrative-driven suicides, the SCS severity may be lower than in those with crisis-driven suicides. For example, an elderly person with ALS or advancing malignancy and poor pain control may be more distressed by the pain and the prospect of imminent death than by SCS symptoms. For these individuals, death as the only perceived solution to the unbearable pain may even appear to be a respite, and after they have planned their suicide, they may appear calmer than before.

Third, in some individuals, SCS may be of sudden onset and of very short duration, lasting only hours or even minutes (Deisenhammer et al., 2009). When assessed by a clinician prior to the onset of their suicide crises, these individuals may not feel entrapped and may experience or exhibit no symptoms of affective disturbance or loss of cognitive control. They may also appear calm or, if not, they may look and behave like their usual selves to their loved ones and outsiders.

Clinicians can encounter any of the above scenarios when taking care of recently suicidal individuals. The calm—or at times the upbeat mood and even elation—exhibited by those who were agitated and desperate just a day earlier can have an eerie, unreal quality that makes clinicians feel a deep sense of unease. The abrupt change in affect can be confusing for both the patients' loved ones and their clinicians. The eeriness and confusion come from the difficulty in reconciling the patient's sudden change of affect, mood, and thought process with their unchanged or almost unchanged suicidal life narrative, which had just recently brought on their suicide attempt.

On the one hand, the patient's relatives and clinicians are relieved by the patient's change; they want to believe that the patient is no longer suicidal, that they see life differently and can therefore be discharged from the hospital. This sudden, incongruent, "exemplary" mental state of somebody who has just survived a suicide attempt and who may have been recently saying that they had no reason to live often makes the clinician anxious and insecure.

Clinicians most frequently experience this unease when treating psychiatric patients who have been admitted to psychiatric inpatient units for safety because of their explicit suicidal intent or after a suicide attempt. Some patients may have already planned their next and more lethal suicide attempt and want to be discharged so they can accomplish their goal. Others may be so deeply embarrassed by the failure of their attempt, their subsequent hospitalization, and the new need to rely on the family in a "sick role," that they are in denial that the circumstances that brought on their suicide attempt have not really changed. In either case, such patients explicitly deny suicidal intent, follow the unit routine, and promise to comply with any discharge treatment plan.

Because on the surface these patients are no longer suicidal, exhibit "insight" into their behavior, and agree to the outpatient follow-up, their psychiatrists can no longer justify their hospital stay to the bed utilization review or the managed care companies. Some of these patients leave the hospital accompanied by a family member and with a proper follow-up plan and after "warm hand-off" to outpatient clinicians with a safety plan, but go on to kill themselves, sometimes within hours of discharge.

In their first postdischarge week, previously hospitalized patients have the highest risk of death by suicide, which in comparison with those never hospitalized is 252:1 for women and 108:1 for men (Qin & Nordentoft, 2005). One of the prospective short-term risk studies (Yaseen et al., 2014) showed that both ultra-high and ultra-low scorers on the STS-3 risk assessment scale were likely to attempt suicide within the first two months after discharge. In fact, the majority were ultra-low scorers, who very quickly after their admission denied having any traces of the ruminative flooding and feelings of anxiety, dread, and desperation that brought them to the hospital in the first place.

What can the clinician do to justify continuing hospitalization of a patient who has exhibited insight into their behavior, has agreed to treatment follow-up, and has "committed" to safety when the clinician's intuition and inner discomfort indicate that the patient is at acute risk? One option is to forcefully explore the patient's understanding of the abrupt changes in mood and the possibility of the patient's seeing their life in terms of the SN or feeling SCS symptoms.

> You seem so calm to me, is this how you feel inside?
>
> Are you able to see your future more clearly now? What are your options?
>
> Your change in mood is a little unexpected, you wanted to die just last week. What changed?
>
> Please tell me about the anguish you were feeling.
>
> You felt so trapped last week—what happened to those feelings?
>
> Please tell me, how is your thinking? What were your thoughts like last night?

Answers revealing the patient's continuing perception of their life's having reached a dead end with no good options for the future or the continuing SCS symptoms would indicate high short-term risk for suicide. These findings need to be carefully documented in the mental status exam and need to be followed by an assessment that the patient remains suicidal and requires further inpatient hospital stay for safety and treatment. Vague or guarded answers indicate the patient's reluctance to be open with the clinician and should raise a concern about how genuine the patient's insight is, which also should be documented as a justification for the extended hospital stay.

The following is a representative case of an eerie calm exhibited by a patient after high-lethality suicidal behavior.

Case 58

Michael, a 55-year-old single man, was transferred to an inpatient psychiatric unit from the hospital ICU, where he was admitted after a failed suicide attempt by hanging on a door handle. He was found unconscious but breathing and, as a result of his attempt, suffered subclavian steal syndrome but no anoxic brain injury. Prior to his suicide attempt, Michael, who was gay, worked as a manager and rug salesman in a store owned by his friend John, with whom he may have been involved in a long-term love affair. John was married and had two adult children. One month prior to Michael's suicide attempt, John suddenly told Michael that he was retiring and moving to Florida. He then left town to look for a new house and delegated Michael to close the store and let go of the long-term employees, who Michael felt were like a family to him. Feeling betrayed and devastated, Michael did as he was told, but the night after the last person left the premises and he closed the store for good, he tried to hang himself. He passed out and would have died, but the handle he had tied the rope to broke off.

After a week-long stay in the MICU, Michael was transferred to an inpatient psychiatric unit, where he was given an antidepressant. On his first day on the inpatient unit, Michael was withdrawn and quiet. However, on the second day, his affect brightened, and on the third day, Michael was seen smiling and even joking. In groups and sessions with his doctor, he was cooperative and remorseful about his attempt, which he called stupid. He participated in all groups and activities, where he exhibited superficial insight and avoided questions about his personal life and about his future plans. His general plan was to get out of the hospital, to take medications, and to get some therapy to "sort things out" and "to figure out how he could be so stupid." Michael's affect was bright, he was future-oriented, and he denied suicidal intent. However, Michael's improvement made his doctor and the nursing staff feel uneasy. His change in mood seemed sudden and unjustified. He did not want to discuss his relationship with John and his anger at John for both leaving for Florida and for leaving him to do the dirty work of laying people off and closing the store.

Still, after a weeklong hospital stay, Michael maintained his improvement in mood and affect, and the team discussed the patient's progress and discharge plans. Most staff members felt uneasy about discharging him and thought that his progress was "too good to be true" and that nobody really knew what was "inside his head." However, the staff could not justify a longer hospital stay because Michael was "saying and doing all the right things."

The next day, Michael was given outpatient appointments with a psychiatrist and a psychotherapist and was discharged to the care of a friend. When leaving, Michael said good-bye and thanked the psychiatrists and the nurses for taking good care of him. The friend picked him up, drove Michael home, and left him in the living room of his eighteenth-floor apartment. He and Michael agreed to meet for lunch the next day and do something afterward. However, tragically, two hours after his friend left, Michael jumped to his death off his apartment balcony.

Michael's case is an illustration of a patient's eerie calm after a high-lethality attempt, which made clinicians feel anxious and uneasy, because the changes in mood and affect were not justified by the changes in the patient's life narrative and stressors. At least two scenarios are possible. The first scenario is that on the unit Michael sincerely believed that his attempt was in the past, and that the future looked brighter with medications and therapy. However, something did not go as planned when he got home: for instance, John refused to talk to him. Such a refusal might have precipitated his second suicidal crisis and his suicide. The second scenario is that Michael planned his suicide soon after admission to the unit and was actively hiding his intent. In either case, the sudden change in mood and the lack of detail in the patient's description of his mental state to justify such a change gave his calm affect an eerie quality and made the staff uneasy.

Appendix A: The Suicide Crisis Inventory-2 (SCI-2)

Please answer the following questions about the way you were feeling over the last several days.

During this time when you were feeling your worst:

1. Did you feel a sense of inner pain that had to be stopped?
   0 = Not at all
   1 = A little
   2 = Somewhat
   3 = Quite a bit
   4 = Extremely

2. Did you feel there was no exit?
   0 = Not at all
   1 = A little

2 = Somewhat
3 = Quite a bit
4 = Extremely

3. Did you enjoy being with your family or close friends?
   0 = Not at all
   1 = A little
   2 = Somewhat
   3 = Quite a bit
   4 = Extremely

4. Did you feel yourself thinking that things would never change?
   0 = Not at all
   1 = A little
   2 = Somewhat
   3 = Quite a bit
   4 = Extremely

5. Did you have a decreased ability to think, concentrate, or make decisions, due to too many thoughts?
   0 = Not at all
   1 = A little
   2 = Somewhat
   3 = Quite a bit
   4 = Extremely

6. Did you feel suddenly frightened to such an extent that you developed physical symptoms or had a panic attack?
   0 = Not at all
   1 = A little
   2 = Somewhat
   3 = Quite a bit
   4 = Extremely

7. Did you feel you were constantly watching for signs of trouble?
   0 = Not at all
   1 = A little
   2 = Somewhat
   3 = Quite a bit
   4 = Extremely

8. Did you feel any unusually intense or deep negative feelings or mood swings directed toward someone else?
   0 = Not at all
   1 = A little
   2 = Somewhat
   3 = Quite a bit
   4 = Extremely

9. Did you feel your views were very consistent over time?
   0 = Not at all
   1 = A little

2 = Somewhat
3 = Quite a bit
4 = Extremely

10. Did you feel you had lost your interest in other people?
    0 = Not at all
    1 = A little
    2 = Somewhat
    3 = Quite a bit
    4 = Extremely

11. Did you feel bothered by thoughts that did not make sense?
    0 = Not at all
    1 = A little
    2 = Somewhat
    3 = Quite a bit
    4 = Extremely

12. Did you feel blood rushing through your veins?
    0 = Not at all
    1 = A little
    2 = Somewhat
    3 = Quite a bit
    4 = Extremely

13. Did you feel nervousness or shakiness inside?
    0 = Not at all
    1 = A little
    2 = Somewhat
    3 = Quite a bit
    4 = Extremely

14. Did you feel pressure in your head from thinking too much?
    0 = Not at all
    1 = A little
    2 = Somewhat
    3 = Quite a bit
    4 = Extremely

15. Did you feel trapped?
    0 = Not at all
    1 = A little
    2 = Somewhat
    3 = Quite a bit
    4 = Extremely

16. Did you feel you wanted to crawl out of your skin?
    0 = Not at all
    1 = A little
    2 = Somewhat
    3 = Quite a bit
    4 = Extremely

17. Did you feel that it was hard for you to stop worrying?
    0 = Not at all
    1 = A little
    2 = Somewhat
    3 = Quite a bit
    4 = Extremely

18. Did you become afraid that you would die?
    0 = Not at all
    1 = A little
    2 = Somewhat
    3 = Quite a bit
    4 = Extremely

19. Did you feel that there were no good solutions to your problems?
    0 = Not at all
    1 = A little
    2 = Somewhat
    3 = Quite a bit
    4 = Extremely

20. Did you feel that most people could not be trusted?
    0 = Not at all
    1 = A little
    2 = Somewhat
    3 = Quite a bit
    4 = Extremely

21. Did you wake up from sleep tired and not refreshed?
    0 = Not at all
    1 = A little
    2 = Somewhat
    3 = Quite a bit
    4 = Extremely

22. Did you have strange sensations in your body or on your skin?
    0 = Not at all
    1 = A little
    2 = Somewhat
    3 = Quite a bit
    4 = Extremely

23. Did you feel isolated from others?
    0 = Not at all
    1 = A little
    2 = Somewhat
    3 = Quite a bit
    4 = Extremely

24. Did you often change your mind?
    0 = Not at all
    1 = A little

2 = Somewhat
3 = Quite a bit
4 = Extremely

25. Did you feel helpless to change?
0 = Not at all
1 = A little
2 = Somewhat
3 = Quite a bit
4 = Extremely

26. Did you want your troubling thoughts to go away but they wouldn't?
0 = Not at all
1 = A little
2 = Somewhat
3 = Quite a bit
4 = Extremely

27. Did you feel doomed?
0 = Not at all
1 = A little
2 = Somewhat
3 = Quite a bit
4 = Extremely

28. Did you find pleasure in your hobbies and pastimes?
0 = Not at all
1 = A little
2 = Somewhat
3 = Quite a bit
4 = Extremely

29. Did you have trouble falling asleep because you were having thoughts that you could not control?
0 = Not at all
1 = A little
2 = Somewhat
3 = Quite a bit
4 = Extremely

30. Did you feel that ordinary things looked strange or distorted?
0 = Not at all
1 = A little
2 = Somewhat
3 = Quite a bit
4 = Extremely

31. Did you feel you did not open up to members of your family/friends?
0 = Not at all
1 = A little
2 = Somewhat
3 = Quite a bit

4 = Extremely

32. Did you feel that if you didn't stay alert and watchful, something bad would happen?
    0 = Not at all
    1 = A little
    2 = Somewhat
    3 = Quite a bit
    4 = Extremely

33. Did you feel that ideas kept turning over and over in your mind and they wouldn't go away?
    0 = Not at all
    1 = A little
    2 = Somewhat
    3 = Quite a bit
    4 = Extremely

34. Did you feel you could change your mind once you've come to a conclusion?
    0 = Not at all
    1 = A little
    2 = Somewhat
    3 = Quite a bit
    4 = Extremely

35. Did you feel hopeless?
    0 = Not at all
    1 = A little
    2 = Somewhat
    3 = Quite a bit
    4 = Extremely

36. Did you feel a lot of emotional turmoil in your gut?
    0 = Not at all
    1 = A little
    2 = Somewhat
    3 = Quite a bit
    4 = Extremely

37. Did you feel you could easily change your mind over things that bother you?
    0 = Not at all
    1 = A little
    2 = Somewhat
    3 = Quite a bit
    4 = Extremely

38. Did you feel dissatisfied or bored with everything?
    0 = Not at all
    1 = A little
    2 = Somewhat
    3 = Quite a bit
    4 = Extremely

39. Did you feel that there was no way out?
    0 = Not at all
    1 = A little
    2 = Somewhat
    3 = Quite a bit
    4 = Extremely

40. Did you push away people who care about you?
    0 = Not at all
    1 = A little
    2 = Somewhat
    3 = Quite a bit
    4 = Extremely

41. Did you have temper outbursts that you could not control?
    0 = Not at all
    1 = A little
    2 = Somewhat
    3 = Quite a bit
    4 = Extremely

42. Did you get into frequent arguments?
    0 = Not at all
    1 = A little
    2 = Somewhat
    3 = Quite a bit
    4 = Extremely

43. Did you feel that the urge to escape the pain was very hard to control?
    0 = Not at all
    1 = A little
    2 = Somewhat
    3 = Quite a bit
    4 = Extremely

44. Did you have a sense of inner pain that was too much to bear?
    0 = Not at all
    1 = A little
    2 = Somewhat
    3 = Quite a bit
    4 = Extremely

45. Did you feel any unusually intense or deep negative feelings or mood swings directed toward yourself?
    0 = Not at all
    1 = A little
    2 = Somewhat
    3 = Quite a bit
    4 = Extremely

46. Did you feel relentless, agonizing emotional pain?
    0 = Not at all
    1 = A little
    2 = Somewhat
    3 = Quite a bit
    4 = Extremely

47. Did you feel tense or keyed up?
    0 = Not at all
    1 = A little
    2 = Somewhat
    3 = Quite a bit
    4 = Extremely

48. Did you feel powerless to stop thoughts that were upsetting you?
    0 = Not at all
    1 = A little
    2 = Somewhat
    3 = Quite a bit
    4 = Extremely

49. Did you feel so restless you could not sit still?
    0 = Not at all
    1 = A little
    2 = Somewhat
    3 = Quite a bit
    4 = Extremely

50. Did you feel unusual physical sensations that you have never felt before?
    0 = Not at all
    1 = A little
    2 = Somewhat
    3 = Quite a bit
    4 = Extremely

51. Did you feel your thoughts were racing?
    0 = Not at all
    1 = A little
    2 = Somewhat
    3 = Quite a bit
    4 = Extremely

52. Did you interact less with people who care about you?
    0 = Not at all
    1 = A little
    2 = Somewhat
    3 = Quite a bit
    4 = Extremely

53. Did you feel easily annoyed or irritated?
    0 = Not at all
    1 = A little
    2 = Somewhat
    3 = Quite a bit
    4 = Extremely

54. Did you feel that your emotional pain was unbearable?
    0 = Not at all
    1 = A little
    2 = Somewhat
    3 = Quite a bit
    4 = Extremely

55. Did you evade communications with people who care about you?
    0 = Not at all
    1 = A little
    2 = Somewhat
    3 = Quite a bit
    4 = Extremely

56. Did you feel there is no escape?
    0 = Not at all
    1 = A little
    2 = Somewhat
    3 = Quite a bit
    4 = Extremely

57. Did you feel like you were getting a headache from too many thoughts in your head?
    0 = Not at all
    1 = A little
    2 = Somewhat
    3 = Quite a bit
    4 = Extremely

58. Did you feel that the world was closing in on you?
    0 = Not at all
    1 = A little
    2 = Somewhat
    3 = Quite a bit
    4 = Extremely

59. Did you feel that your head could explode from too many thoughts?
    0 = Not at all
    1 = A little
    2 = Somewhat
    3 = Quite a bit
    4 = Extremely

60. Did you feel so stirred up inside you wanted to scream?
    0 = Not at all
    1 = A little
    2 = Somewhat
    3 = Quite a bit
    4 = Extremely

61. Did you have many thoughts in your head?
    0 = Not at all
    1 = A little
    2 = Somewhat
    3 = Quite a bit
    4 = Extremely

Subscales (Dimensions)

Entrapment: 2, 35, 39, 58, 25, 15, 27, 4, 56, 19
Affective disturbance: 43, 44, 46, 1, 54, 45, 8, 18, 50, 30, 6, 22, 12, 13, 38, 10, 28R, 3R
Loss of cognitive control: 61, 51, 33, 11, 24R, 37R, 34R, 9, 59, 5, 14, 57, 26, 48, 17
Hyperarousal: 47, 49, 16, 60, 36, 32, 7, 20, 41, 42, 53, 29, 21
Social withdrawal: 52, 31, 23, 55, 40
Numbers represent items of SCI. R represents reverse score.

Appendix B: The Modular Assessment of Risk for Imminent Suicide (MARIS-2)

Part 1: Self-Report SCI-SF

Please rate how much each of the following applies to you by writing the appropriate number on the line following each question. Follow the scale below:
0 = Not at all
1 = A little
2 = Somewhat
3 = Quite a bit
4 = Extremely
In the past couple of days, when you felt your worst . . .

1. Did you become afraid that you would die? _____
2. Did you think something, such as a heart attack or accident, would suddenly kill you? _____
3. Did you feel your thoughts are confused? _____
4. Did you feel there is no exit? _____
5. Did you feel that your head could explode from too many thoughts? _____

6. Did you feel bothered by thoughts that did not make sense? _____
7. Did you feel trapped? _____
8. Did you feel like you were getting a headache from too many thoughts in your head? _____

   Subtotal: _____

Part 2: Clinician Assessment TRQ-SF

Rate how much each of the following is true regarding how you felt with/about this patient by writing the appropriate number on the line following each item. Follow the scale below:

0 = Not at all
1 = A little
2 = Somewhat
3 = Quite a bit
4 = Extremely

1. S/he made me feel good about myself. _____
2. I liked him/her very much. _____
3. I felt like my hands were tied or that I was put in an impossible bind. _____
4. I felt dismissed or devalued. _____
5. I felt guilty about my feelings toward him/her. _____
6. I thought life really might not be worth living for him/her. _____
7. This patient gave me chills. _____
8. I had to force myself to connect with him/her. _____
9. I feel confident in my ability to help him/her. _____
10. We trust one another. _____

Subtotal: _____
Grand Total: _____

Appendix C: Suicide Crisis Syndrome Checklist (SCS-C)

Diagnostic Criteria for the Suicide Crisis Syndrome Checklist (SCS-C):

A. Entrapment: Patient presents with a problem that *they perceive* as intolerable and unsolvable (they may describe themselves as 'trapped', 'having no exit' or 'having reached a dead end'):
□no   □yes   □extreme [Patient screens "extreme" if the symptom is overwhelmingly distressful]

B. Associated disturbances: [Patient screens positive (yes) if any of the symptoms below are marked "yes", meets extreme if more than half of the symptoms in each domain are present.]
□no   □yes   □extreme

(B1) Affective disturbance: □no   □yes   □extreme [For (a), (b), (c), (d) criteria patient screens positive (yes) if any of the symptoms below are marked "yes", meets "extreme" if more than half of the symptoms in each domain are present.]

Manifested self- or collateral-report or observation of any of:
(1) emotional pain
□no   □yes
(2) rapid spikes of negative emotions or extreme mood swings
□no   □yes
(3) extreme anxiety that may be accompanied by dissociation or sensory disturbances
□no   □yes
(4) acute anhedonia (i.e., a new or increased inability to experience interest or pleasure or imagine future experience of interest or pleasure)
□no   □yes

(B2) Loss of cognitive control: □no   □yes   □extreme

Manifested by self- or collateral-report or observation of any of:
(1) intense or persistent rumination about one's own distress and the life events that brought on distress
□no   □yes
(2) an inability to deviate from a repetitive negative pattern of thought (cognitive rigidity)
□no   □yes
(3) an experience of an overwhelming profusion of negative thoughts accompanied by a sensation of pressure or pain in one's head, impairing ability to process information or make a decision (ruminative flooding)
□no   □yes
(4) repeated unsuccessful attempts to suppress negative or disturbing thoughts
□no   □yes

(B3) Disturbance in arousal: □no   □yes   □extreme

Manifested by self- or collateral-report or observation of any of:
(1) agitation   □no   □yes
(2) hypervigilance   □no   □yes
(3) irritability   □no   □yes
(4) global insomnia □no   □yes

(B4) Social withdrawal: □no   □yes   □extreme

Manifested by self- or collateral-report or observation of any of:
(1) withdrawal from or reduction in scope of social activity   □no   □yes
(2) evasive communication with close others   □no   □yes

© 2018 Igor I. Galynker

References

Alphs, L., Brashear, H. R., Chappell, P., Conwell, Y., Dubrava, S., Khin, N. A., Kozauer, N., Hartley, D. M., Miller, D. S., Schindler, R. J., Siemers, E. R., Stewart, M., & Yaffe, K. (2016). Considerations for the assessment of suicidal ideation and behavior in older adults with cognitive decline and dementia. *Alzheimer's & Dementia, 2*(1), 48–59. https://doi.org/10.1016/j.trci.2016.02.001

Apter, A., Barzilay, S., & Levy-Betz, Y. (2021). *Assessment and intervention for suicide crisis syndrome in youth* [Paper presentation]. *International Summit for Suicide Research. Virtual.*

Bafna, A., Rogers, M. L., Richards, J., Lloveras, L., & Galynker, I. (under review). Development and validation of a clinician-administered interview to assess suicide crisis syndrome: The Suicide Crisis Syndrome Checklist. *Acta Psychiatrica Scandinavica.*

Bagge, C. L., Littlefield, A. K., & Glenn, C. R. (2017). Trajectories of affective response as warning signs for suicide attempts: An examination of the 48 hours prior to a recent suicide attempt. *Clinical Psychological Science, 5*(2), 259–271. https://doi.org/10.1177/2167702616681628

Ballard, E. D., Vande Voort, J. L., Luckenbaugh, D. A., Machado-Vieira, R., Tohen, M., & Zarae, C. A. (2016). Acute risk factors for suicide attempts and death: Prospective findings from the STEP-BD study. *Bipolar Disorder, 18*(4), 363–372. https://doi.org/10.1111/bdi.12397

Barzilay, S., Assounga, K., Veras, J., Beaubian, C., Bloch-Elkouby, S., & Galynker, I. (2020). Assessment of near-term risk for suicide attempts using the Suicide Crisis Inventory. *Journal of Affective Disorders, 276,* 183–190. https://doi.org/10.1016/j.jad.2020.06.053

Barzilay, S., Yaseen, Z. S., Hawes, M., Gorman, B., Altman, R., Foster, A., Apter, A., Rosenfield, P., & Galynker, I. (2018). Emotional responses to suicidal patients: Factor structure, construct, and predictive validity of the Therapist Response Questionnaire–Suicide Form. *Frontiers in Psychiatry, 9,* 104. https://doi.org/10.3389/fpsyt.2018.00104

Beck, A. T., & Steer, R. A. (1989). Clinical predictors of eventual suicide: A 5- to 10-year prospective study of suicide attempters. *Journal of Affective Disorders, 17*(3), 203–209. https://doi.org/10.1016/0165-0327(89)90001-3

Beck, A. T., Steer, R. A., Kovacs, M., & Garrison, B. (1985). Hopelessness and eventual suicide: a 10-year prospective study of patients hospitalized with suicidal ideation. *The American Journal of Psychiatry, 142*(5), 559–563. https://doi.org/10.1176/ajp.142.5.559

Beck, A. T., Steer, R. A., & Ranieri, W. F. (1988). Scale for Suicide Ideation: Psychometric properties of a self-report version. *Journal of Clinical Psychology, 44*(4), 499–505. https://doi.org/10.1002/1097-4679(198807)44:4<499::aid-jclp2270440404>3.0.co;2-6

Beck, A. T., & Weishaar, M. E. (1990). Suicide risk assessment and prediction. *Crisis, 11*(2), 22–30.

Bloch-Elkouby, S., Barzilay, S., Gorman, B., Lawrence, O., Rogers, M. L., Richards, J., Cohen, L., Johnson, B. N., & Galynker, I. (2021). The revised Suicide Crisis Inventory (SCI-2): Validation and assessment of prospective suicidal outcomes at one month follow-up. *Journal of Affective Disorder, 295,* 1280–1291.

Bolton, J. M., Spiwak, R., & Sareen, J. (2012). Predicting suicide attempts with the SAD PERSONS scale: A longitudinal analysis. *The Journal of Clinical Psychiatry, 73*(6), e735–e741. https://doi.org/10.4088/JCP.11m07362

Brown, G. K., Beck, A. T., Steer, R. A., & Grisham, J. R. (2000). Risk factors for suicide in psychiatric outpatients: A 20-year prospective study. *Journal of Consulting and Clinical Psychology, 68*(3), 371–377.

Busch, K. A., Fawcett, J., & Jacobs, D. G. (2003). Clinical correlates of inpatient suicide. *Journal of Clinical Psychiatry, 64*, 14–19.

Chistopolskaya, K. A., Rogers, M. L., Cao, E., Galynker, I., Richards, J., Enikolopov, S. N., Nikolaev, E. L., Sadovnichaya, V. S., & Drovosekov, S. E. (2020). Adaptation of the Suicidal Narrative Inventory in a Russian sample. *Suicidology, 11*(4), 76–90. https://doi. org/10.32878/suiciderus.20-11-04(41)-76-90

Chu, C., Buchman-Schmitt, J. M., Stanley, I. H., Hom, M. A., Tucker, R. P., Hagan, C. R., Rogers, M. L., Podlogar, M. C., Chiurliza, B., Ringer, F. B., Michaels, M. S., Patros, C., & Joiner, T. E. (2017). The interpersonal theory of suicide: A systematic review and meta-analysis of a decade of cross-national research. *Psychological Bulletin, 143*(12), 1313–1345. https://doi.org/10.1037/bul0000123

Deisenhammer, E. A., Ing, C. M., Strauss, R., Kemmler, G., Hinterhuber, H., & Weiss, E. M. (2009). The duration of the suicidal process: How much time is left for intervention between consideration and accomplishment of a suicide attempt? *The Journal of Clinical Psychiatry, 70*(1), 19–24.

De Los Reyes, A., Augenstein, T. M., Wang, M., Thomas, S. A., Drabick, D., Burgers, D. E., & Rabinowitz, J. (2015). The validity of the multi-informant approach to assessing child and adolescent mental health. *Psychological Bulletin, 141*(4), 858–900. https://doi. org/10.1037/a0038498

Ducasse, D., Loas, G., Dassa, D., Gramaglia, C., Zeppegno, P., Guillame, S., Olié, E., & Courtet, P. (2018). Anhedonia is associated with suicidal ideation independently of depression: A meta-analysis. *Depression and Anxiety, 35*(5), 382–392. https://doi.org/10.1002/da.22709

Galynker, I., Yaseen, Z. S., Cohen, A., Benhamou, O., Hawes, M., & Briggs, J. (2017). Prediction of suicidal behavior in high risk psychiatric patients using an assessment of acute suicidal state: The Suicide Crisis Inventory. *Depression and Anxiety, 34*(2), 147–158. https://doi.org/10.1002/da.22559

Galynker, I., Yaseen, Z., & Briggs, J. (2014). Assessing risk for imminent suicide. *Psychiatric Annals, 44*(9), 431–436. https://doi.org/10.3928/00485713-20140908-071

Giddens, J. M., Sheehan, K. H., & Sheehan, D. V. (2014). The Columbia-Suicide Severity Rating Scale (C-SSRS): Has the "gold standard" become a liability? *Innovations in Clinical Neuroscience, 11*(9-10), 66–80.

Gvion, Y., Horresh, N., Levi-Belz, Y., Fischel, T., Treves, I., Weiser, M., David, H. S., Stein-Reizer, O., & Apter, A. (2014). Aggression–impulsivity, mental pain, and communication difficulties in medically serious and medically non-serious suicide attempters. *Comprehensive Psychiatry, 55*(1), 40–50. https://doi.org/10.1016/j.comppsych.2013.09.003

Harding, M. (2016, August 1). *Suicide risk assessment and threats of suicide.* http://patient. info/doctor/suicide-risk-assessment-and-threats-of-suicide

Hawes, M., Yaseen, Z., Briggs, J., & Galynker, I. (2017). The Modular Assessment of Risk for Imminent Suicide (MARIS): A proof of concept for a multi-informant tool for evaluation of short-term suicide risk. *Comprehensive Psychiatry, 72*, 88–96. https://doi.org/10.1016/j.comppsych.2016.10.002

Horesh, N., Zalsman, G., & Apter, A. (2004). Suicidal behavior and self-disclosure in adolescent psychiatric inpatients. *Journal of Nervous and Mental Disease, 192*(12), 837–842. https://doi.org/10.1097/01.nmd.0000146738.78222.e5

Karsen, E., Cohen, L., Miller, F., De Luca, G., & White, B. (under review). Impact of the Abbreviated Suicide Crisis Syndrome assessment on clinical decision making in the emergency department. *Acta Psychiatrica Scandinavica*.

Kleiman, E. M., Turner, B. J., Fedor, S., Beale, E. E., Huffman, J. C., & Nock, M. K. (2017). Examination of real-time fluctuations in suicidal ideation and its risk factors: Results from two ecological momentary assessment studies. *Journal of Abnormal Psychology, 126*(6), 726–738. https://doi.org/10.1037/abn0000273

Lecrubier, Y., Sheehan, D. V., Weiller, E., Amorim, P., Bonora, I., Sheehan, K. H., Janavs, J., & Dunbar, G. C. (1997). The Mini International Neuropsychiatric Interview (MINI): A short diagnostic structured interview—Reliability and validity according to the CIDI. *European Psychiatry, 12*(5), 224–231. https://doi.org/10.1016/S0924-9338(97)83296-8

Levi, Y., Horesh, N., Fischel, T., Treves, I., Or, E., & Apter, A. (2008). Mental pain and its communication in medically serious suicide attempts: An "impossible situation." *Journal of Affective Disorders, 111*(2-3), 244–250. https://doi.org/10.1016/j.jad.2008.02.022

Levi-Belz, Y., Gvion, Y., Horesh, N., Fischel, T., Treves, I., Or, E., Stein-Reisner, O., Weiser, M., David, H. S., & Apter, A. (2014). Mental pain, communication difficulties, and medically serious suicide attempts: A case-control study. *Archives of Suicide Research, 18*(1), 74–87. https://doi.org/10.1080/13811118.2013.809041

Lindenmayer, J. P., Czobor, P., Alphs, L., Nathan, A. M., Anand, R., Islam, Z., Chou, J. C., & InterSePT Study Group. (2003). The InterSePT scale for suicidal thinking reliability and validity. *Schizophrenia Research, 63*(1-2), 161–170. https://doi.org/10.1016/s0920-9964(02)00335-3

Menon, V., Bafna, A. R., Rogers, M. L., Richards, J., & Galynker, I. (2022). Factor structure and validity of the Revised Suicide Crisis Inventory (SCI-2) among Indian adults. *Asian Journal of Psychiatry, 73*, 103119. https://doi.org/10.1016/j.ajp.2022.103119

Morriss, R., Kapur, N., & Byng, R. (2013). Assessing risk of suicide or self harm in adults. *BMJ Clinical Research, 347*, f4572. https://doi.org/10.1136/bmj.f4572

Ohannessian, C. M., & De Los Reyes, A. (2014). Discrepancies in adolescents' and their mothers' perceptions of the family and adolescent anxiety symptomatology. *Parenting, Science and Practice, 14*(1), 1–18. https://doi.org/10.1080/15295192.2014.870009

Oquendo, M. A. (2015). Suicidal behavior: Measurement and mechanisms. *The Journal of Clinical Psychiatry, 76*(12), 1675. https://doi.org/10.4088/JCP.15f10520

Parghi, N., Chennapragada, L., Barzilay, S., Newkirk, S., Ahmedani, B., Lok, B., & Galynker, I. (2020). Assessing the predictive ability of the Suicide Crisis Inventory for near-term suicidal behavior using machine learning approaches. *International Journal of Methods in Psychiatric Research, 30*(1), e1863. https://doi.org/10.1002/mpr.1863

Park, J., Rogers, M. L., Bloch-Elkouby, S., Richards, J. A., Lee, S., Galynker, I., & You, S. (under review). Factor structure and validation of the revised Suicide Crisis Inventory (SCI-2) in a Korean population.

Patterson, W. M., Dohn, H. H., Bird, J., & Patterson, G. A. (1983). Evaluation of suicidal patients: The SAD PERSONS scale. *Psychosomatics, 24*(4), 343–349. https://doi.org/10.1016/S0033-3182(83)73213-5

Posner, K., Brown, G. K., Stanley, B., Brent, D. A., Yershova, K. V., Oquendo, M. A., Currier, G. W., Melvin, G. A., Greenhill, L., Shen, S., & Mann, J. J. (2011). The Columbia–Suicide Severity Rating Scale: Initial validity and internal consistency findings from three multisite studies with adolescents and adults. *American Journal of Psychiatry, 168*(12), 1266–1277. https://doi.org/10.1176/appi.ajp.2011.10111704

Qin, P., & Nordentoft, M. (2005). Suicide risk in relation to psychiatric hospitalization: Evidence based on longitudinal registers. *Archives of General Psychiatry, 62*(4), 427–432. https://doi.org/10.1001/archpsyc.62.4.427

Rogers, M. L., Vespa, A., Bloch-Elkouby, S., & Galynker, I. (2021). Validity of the modular assessment of risk for imminent suicide in predicting short-term suicidality. *Acta Psychiatrica Scandinavica, 144*(6), 563–577. https://doi.org/10.1111/acps.13354

Roos, L., Sareen, J., & Bolton, J. M. (2013). Suicide risk assessment tools, predictive validity findings and utility today: time for a revamp? *Neuropsychiatry, 3*(5), 483–495.

Sheehan, D. V., Alphs, L. D., Mao, L., Li, Q., May, R. S., Bruer, E. H., Mccullumsmith, C. B., Gray, C. R., Li, X., & Williamson, D. J. (2014). Comparative validation of the S-STS, the ISST-Plus, and the C-SSRS for assessing the suicidal thinking and behavior FDA 2012 suicidality categories. *Innovations in Clinical Neuroscience, 11*(9-10), 32–46.

Sheehan, D. V., Giddens, J. M., & Sheehan, K. H. (2014). Current assessment and classification of suicidal phenomena using the FDA 2012 Draft Guidance Document on suicide assessment: A critical review. *Innovations in Clinical Neuroscience, 11*(9-10), 54–65.

Smith, E. G., Kim, H. M., Ganoczy, D., Stano, C., Pfeiffer, P. N., & Valenstein, M. (2013). Suicide risk assessment received prior to suicide death by Veterans Health Administration patients with a history of depression. *The Journal of Clinical Psychiatry, 74*(3), 226–232. https://doi.org/10.4088/JCP.12m07853

Stefansson, J., Nordström, P., & Jokinen, J. (2012). Suicide Intent Scale in the prediction of suicide. *Journal of Affective Disorders, 136*(1-2), 167–171. https://doi.org/10.1016/j.jad.2010.11.016

The Columbia Lighthouse Project. (2020). *The Columbia Suicide Severity Rating Scale (C-SSRS) supporting evidence.* https://cssrs.columbia.edu/wp-content/uploads/CSSRS_Supporting-Evidence_Book_2020-01-14.pdf

United States Food and Drug Administration, United States Department of Health and Human Services. (2012). *Guidance for industry: Suicidality—Prospective assessment of occurrence in clinical trials, draft guidance.* http://www.fda.gov/downloads/Drugs/Guidances/UCM225130.pdf

Wang, Y., Bhaskaran, J., Sareen, J., Bolton, S.-L., Chateau, D., & Bolton, J. M. (2016). Clinician prediction of future suicide attempts: A Longitudinal Study. *The Canadian Journal of Psychiatry, 61*(7), 428–432. https://doi.org/10.1177/0706743716645287

Yaseen, Z. S., Galynker, I. I., Cohen, L. J., & Briggs, J. (2017). Clinicians' conflicting emotional responses to high suicide-risk patients—Association with short-term suicide behaviors: A prospective pilot study. *Comprehensive Psychiatry, 76*, 69–78. https://doi.org/10.1016/j.comppsych.2017.03.013

Yaseen, Z. S., Gilmer, E., Modi, J., Cohen, L. J., & Galynker, I. I. (2012). Emergency room validation of the revised Suicide Trigger Scale (STS-3): A measure of a hypothesized suicide trigger state. *PLOS One, 7*(9), e45157. https://doi.org/10.1371/journal.pone.0045157

Yaseen, Z. S., Hawes, M., Barzilay, S., & Galynker, I. (2019). Predictive validity of proposed diagnostic criteria for the suicide crisis syndrome: An acute presuicidal state. *Suicide and Life-Threatening Behavior, 49*(4), 1124–1135. https://doi.org/10.1111/sltb.12495

Yaseen, Z. S., Katz, C., Johnson, M. S., Eisenberg, D., Cohen, L. J., & Galynker, I. (2010). Construct development: The Suicide Trigger Scale (STS-2), a measure of a hypothesized suicide trigger state. *BMC Psychiatry, 10*, 110. https://doi.org/10.1186/1471-244X-10-110

Yaseen, Z. S., Kopeykina, I., Gutkovich, Z., Bassirnia, A., Cohen, L. J., & Galynker, I. I. (2014). Predictive validity of the Suicide Trigger Scale (STS-3) for post-discharge suicide attempt in high-risk psychiatric inpatients. *PLOS One, 9*(1), e86768. https://doi.org/10.1371/journal.pone.0086768

Ying, G., Chennapragada, L., Musser, E. D., & Galynker, I. (2021). Behind therapists' emotional responses to suicidal patients: A study of the narrative crisis model of suicide and clinicians' emotions. *Suicide and Life-Threatening Behavior, 51*(4), 684–695. https://doi.org/10.1111/sltb.12730

Youngstrom, E. A., Hameed, A., Mitchell, M. A., Van Meter, A. R., Freeman, A. J., Algorta, G. P., White, A. M., Clayton, P. J., Gelenberg, A. J., & Meyer, R. E. (2015). Direct comparison of the psychometric properties of multiple interview and patient-rated assessments of suicidal ideation and behavior in an adult psychiatric inpatient sample. *The Journal of Clinical Psychiatry, 76*(12), 1676–1682. https://doi.org/10.4088/JCP.14m09353

10

The Narrative-Crisis Model of Suicide as a Framework for Suicide Prevention

With Inna Goncearenco, Lakshmi Chennapragada, and Megan L. Rogers

Introduction

As described in Chapters 4 and 5, researchers have identified multiple correlates and risk factors for suicidal thoughts, suicide attempts, and death by suicide. However, the majority of factors have been studied in isolation and cross-sectionally (Franklin et al., 2017), limiting their clinical utility in preventing suicidal thoughts and behaviors, particularly in the short term (Glenn & Nock, 2014). Up to half of suicide decedents made contact with a healthcare provider within a month of their death (Luoma et al., 2002), and up to 80% made contact within a year (Stene-Larsen & Reneflot, 2017), presenting multiple opportunities for suicide prevention. This chapter describes a theoretical framework for a coherent approach to suicide prevention that may aid in better understanding, assessing, and intervening to forestall suicide (see Klonsky, 2020).

The narrative-crisis model (NCM) introduced in Chapter 3 serves as a comprehensive, empirically supported, and clinically relevant framework for identifying individuals at risk, for intervening, and ultimately for preventing suicide. This chapter begins with an overview of the NCM, its distinct stages, and empirical support. Next, applicable treatment modalities that target each stage of the NCM are discussed. Finally, the chapter concludes with relevant clinical and research implications, as well as future directions for both clinical practice and research.

Overview of the Narrative-Crisis Model

As described in Chapter 3, the NCM (see Figure 3.1) is a three-stage, dynamic, diathesis-stress model that incorporates chronic (long-term), subacute (proximal), and acute (short-term) suicide risk factors. The NCM postulates that after exposure to stressful life events, individuals with heightened baseline vulnerability to suicide (i.e., those with long-term/chronic risk factors) may develop distorted views of themselves and/or society that are consistent with a suicidal narrative. As part of this narrative, individuals struggle to disengage from unrealistic life goals, which, if achieved, would have entitled them to happiness. Feeling like a burden on others and society, defeated, humiliated, and incapable of belonging, these individuals eventually start to perceive themselves as having no future, whereby suicide becomes a viable option (Cohen et al., 2019). In some individuals, this state may trigger an acute suicidal crisis state—the suicide crisis syndrome (SCS)—that precedes imminent suicide risk (Galynker, 2017).

A wide range of long-term factors, otherwise known as trait vulnerabilities or distal factors, influence a person's baseline propensity for suicide. Key long-term risk factors include genetics (Smith et al., 2012), childhood abuse or other traumatic experiences (Angelakis et al., 2020; Ásgeirsdóttir et al., 2018), psychiatric disorders (Harris & Barraclough, 1997), previous suicide attempts (Ribeiro et al., 2016), insecure attachment (Palitsky et al., 2013), perfectionism (O'Connor, 2007), a lack of moral objections to suicide (Dervic et al., 2006), and deficits in executive functioning (e.g., impulsivity or problem-solving deficits; Saffer & Klonsky, 2017; Wenzel & Beck, 2008; see Chapter 4 for a more comprehensive list). Ultimately, the combination of long-term risk factors or trait vulnerabilities describes the individual's baseline level of suicide risk.

Exposure to a stressful life event, especially to one matching an individual's predisposing vulnerabilities, may activate a suicidal narrative characterized by distorted self-representation schemas and leading to increased emotional distress and risk for suicide (Chistopolskaya et al., 2020; Cohen et al., 2019; Menon et al., under review). The suicidal narrative was originally adapted from the work on life narratives, which posits that individuals form their identity by incorporating their life experiences into an internalized and evolving narrative that includes the past, present, and imagined future (McAdams et al., 2001). In contrast to the life narrative, the suicidal narrative is a coherent (although distorted) narrative that leads to no acceptable future. As described in Chapters 3 and 6, the suicidal narrative has seven stages: failure to disengage from unrealistic life goals, entitlement to happiness, failure to redirect to realistic life goals, humiliating personal or social defeat, perceived burdensomeness, thwarted belongingness, and perception of no future. Goal disengagement theory posits that the ability to disengage from unrealistic or unattainable goals and to re-engage with more achievable ones is a crucial aspect of well-being and health (Wrosch et al., 2003, 2007). Difficulties disengaging from old goals and re-engaging with new ones have been linked to suicidal ideation and behaviors (O'Connor et al., 2009, 2012). Entitlement to happiness, in turn, may exacerbate difficulties in engaging with more adaptive goals (Grubbs & Exline, 2016). Humiliating personal or social defeat is a feeling of defeat (i.e., the belief that one is socially trapped, coupled with a strong desire for escape) accompanied by a fear of humiliation (i.e., feeling disparaged, scorned, or ridiculed for one's identity, rather than one's actions). Both defeat and fear of humiliation have been emphasized as proximal predictors of suicidal ideation by the integrated motivational-volitional model of suicidal behavior (O'Connor & Kirtley, 2018) and have accumulated empirical support in the literature (Klein, 1991; Siddaway et al., 2015; Taylor et al., 2011). Thwarted belongingness (i.e., loneliness, social disconnection, the perceived absence of reciprocal care) and perceived burdensomeness (i.e., feeling as though one is a burden on others and/or society) are two core concepts of the interpersonal theory of suicide (see Chapter 2; Joiner, 2005; Van Orden et al., 2010). Their simultaneous presence and interaction have multiplicative influences on suicidal desire (Chu et al., 2017). Additionally, the simultaneous presence of thwarted belongingness and perceived burdensomeness (and hopelessness about these states) trigger a person's perception of having no future (Hirsch et al., 2006), with suicide as the only viable option for escape.

The final stage of the NCM is the SCS, an acute, primarily affective suicidal state that precipitates imminent suicidal behavior (Galynker et al., 2017; Rogers et al., 2017). As described in Chapter 7, the SCS is characterized by five empirically based and empirically supported symptom domains that cohere as a unidimensional syndrome (Schuck et al., 2019). The SCS core diagnostic symptom (Criterion A) is a persistent, intense, desperate, and recurrent feeling of frantic hopelessness or entrapment, which is an urgency to escape or avoid a life situation perceived as unacceptable, intolerable, and unsolvable (Galynker et al., 2017; Yaseen et al., 2014). Additionally, SCS includes four affective, cognitive, physiological, and social/behavioral symptom domains (Criterion B): affective disturbances (B1), loss of cognitive control (B2), hyperarousal (B3), and social withdrawal (B4; Rogers et al., 2017; Schuck et al., 2019). Notably, diagnostic criteria for SCS do not include any conscious suicidal ideation, which allows clinicians to diagnose individuals unwilling to disclose their suicidal thoughts and behaviors.

An accumulating body of research has demonstrated the coherence and unidimensionality of the SCS (Barzilay et al., 2020; Bloch-Elkouby, Gorman, Lloveras, et al., 2020; Bloch-Elkouby et al., 2021; Galynker et al., 2017), its convergent and discriminant validity in relation to other symptoms of psychopathology and the suicidal narrative (Barzilay et al., 2020; Calati, Cohen, et al., 2020; Galynker et al., 2017; Otte et al., 2020), its concurrent validity in relation to concurrent and lifetime suicidality (Barzilay et al., 2020; Calati, Cohen, et al., 2020; Cohen et al., 2018; Galynker et al., 2017), and its predictive utility in relation to short-term suicidal behavior (i.e., within one month; Bloch-Elkouby, Gorman, Lloveras, et al., 2020; Parghi et al., 2020; Ying et al., 2020), above and beyond suicidal ideation and other validated indicators of risk (Barzilay et al., 2020; Galynker et al., 2017; Rogers, Vespa, et al., 2021; Rogers et al., 2021; Yaseen et al., 2019). Additionally, the SCS has demonstrated strong clinical utility when implemented in the emergency department setting of a large urban hospital, guiding over 85% of clinical discharge versus admission decisions (Karsen et al., under review). Together, these findings provide strong evidence for the existence of an acute suicidal crisis state that indicates imminent suicide risk.

Empirical Support for the Narrative-Crisis Model

Accumulating research provides empirical support for components of the NCM as a relevant theoretical framework for understanding and preventing suicide, with two tests of the full model to date (Bloch-Elkouby, Gorman, Lloveras, et al., 2020; Cohen et al., 2022). The first study demonstrated the statistical significance of direct pathways from trait vulnerabilities to the suicidal narrative to the SCS and suicidal thoughts and behaviors at one-month follow-up among a small sample of psychiatric inpatients, explaining approximately 10% of the variance in future suicidal ideation and 40% of the variance in future suicide attempts (Bloch-Elkouby, Gorman, Lloveras, et al., 2020). The second study, conducted with a large sample of psychiatric inpatients and outpatients, showed that chronic risk factors were indirectly associated with suicidal thoughts and behaviors through stressful life events, the suicidal narrative, and the SCS in a serial mediation model, both concurrently and at one-month follow-up (Cohen et al., 2022). Limitations of these studies included the small number of suicide-related outcomes (i.e., four to eight suicide attempts at one-month follow-up). Thus, replication and extension of these findings with a larger number and proportion of suicide-related outcomes are needed.

Moreover, a number of studies have tested associations between various components of the NCM (Cohen et al., 2018, 2019; Li et al., 2017; Pia ct al., 2020; Rogers, Cao, et al., 2021). Among a sample of psychiatric inpatients, the SCS accounted for the relationship between several trait vulnerability/long-term risk factors (perfectionism, impulsivity, chronic substance abuse, insecure attachment, poor social support, childhood trauma) and lifetime suicidal thoughts and behaviors, with reverse pathways largely unsupported (Cohen et al., 2018). Although this study did not provide evidence for the temporal relationship between trait vulnerabilities, the SCS, and suicide-related outcomes, it demonstrated preliminary, clinically relevant associations between two components of the NCM. Additionally, Cohen et al. (2019) conducted a study among psychiatric outpatients, investigating relations between interpersonal and goal-orientation facets of the suicidal narrative, the SCS, and lifetime and past-month suicidal thoughts and behaviors. The SCS accounted for the relationship between the interpersonal (social defeat, thwarted belongingness, humiliation, perceived burdensomeness) suicidal narrative and past-month suicidal thoughts and behaviors, providing evidence for the specificity—although not temporality—of these pathways in relation to near-term suicide risk (Cohen et al., 2019).

Finally, several studies tested some of the individual components of the NCM. A serial mediation model found indirect effects leading from socially prescribed perfectionism (trait vulnerability) to fear of humiliation (suicidal narrative), from fear of humiliation to the SCS, and from the SCS to suicidal thoughts and behaviors at one-month follow-up (Pia et al., 2020). Ruminative flooding (SCS) accounted for the relationship between goal orientation (suicidal narrative) and suicidal thoughts and behaviors at one-month follow-up in a large sample of psychiatric outpatients (Rogers, Cao, et al., 2021). Likewise, fearful attachment styles (trait vulnerability) were linked to postdischarge suicidal behavior via perception of entrapment (SCS) among psychiatric inpatients (Li et al., 2017). Moreover, thwarted belongingness and perceived burdensomeness have been repeatedly identified as proximal risk factors for suicidal ideation and behavior, accounting for links between more distal vulnerabilities (e.g., minority stress, childhood trauma) and suicide-related outcomes (see Chu et al., 2017, for meta-analysis).

Overall, while future research is needed to confirm the temporality and directionality of these effects, several studies now provide empirical support for the use of the NCM as a framework for understanding and assessing short-term risk for suicide.

Utilizing the Narrative-Crisis Model as a Framework for Clinical Intervention

The NCM highlights ample opportunities for intervention through all stages of the suicidal process, from long-term baseline vulnerabilities to acute suicidal crises. It guides clinicians' assessments of their patients' short-term and potential long-term suicide risks, as well as their clinical decision-making. The subsequent sections of this chapter highlight specific empirically supported interventions that have demonstrated promise in mitigating suicide risk at each stage of the suicidal process, including lethal means counseling, psychopharmacology, crisis management, psychotherapy, and skills coaching.

This NCM-driven comprehensive treatment approach for suicide prevention addresses symptoms arising over the course of a suicidal episode and across the three NCM stages in reverse order, from most to least acute (see Figure 10.1). After the safety of the patient's environment is ensured through lethal means counseling (e.g., removing suicidal patients' access to firearms), the acute symptoms of a suicidal mental state (i.e., the SCS) should be targeted via pharmacological or somatic intervention, followed by safety planning initiatives. Once SCS symptoms are treated and resolved (or at least reduced substantially), clinicians are then able to initiate psychotherapeutic modalities to manage the subacute symptoms of the suicidal narrative. Finally, after the suicidal narrative is restructured to a viable life narrative (i.e., after acute and subacute suicidal episodes abate), long-term treatment for chronic symptoms (i.e., trait vulnerabilities) is warranted. Although we believe these treatment modalities should be utilized sequentially, this hypothesis should ultimately be tested empirically through clinical trials.

Lethal Means Counseling

Lethal means counseling is critical for ensuring the safety of the patient's environment during an acute suicidal crisis to minimize the possibility of

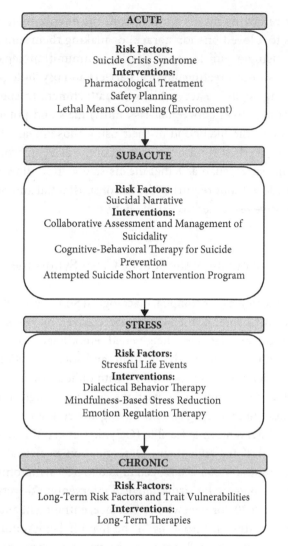

Figure 10.1 Clinical intervention framework based on the narrative-crisis model of suicide.

attempted suicide. Suicide risk is exponentially magnified when patients report a suicide plan involving readily accessible and potentially lethal means (Joiner et al., 2003). Lethal means counseling aims to restrict access to, or reduce the lethality of, means for suicide (Barber & Miller, 2014; Khazem et al., 2016) in order to mitigate the risk of suicidal behavior, both in general and within the context of suicidal crises. These strategies may involve removing means entirely from the environment (e.g., giving medications to a loved one for storage) or making them more difficult to access (e.g., using a gun lock and storing ammunition separately from firearms). In essence, creating physical barriers and psychological distance (i.e., decreasing cognitive accessibility and attachment to specific means; see Rogers et al., 2019) between at-risk individuals and potential suicide methods reduces the likelihood of their using those means for a suicide attempt during a crisis. Within the context of the SCS, environmental and contextual measures, such as lethal means safety, may allow time for the crisis to subside without requiring the use of substantial and possibly unavailable cognitive resources to ensure safety.

Treatment of the Suicide Crisis Syndrome

Step 1: Pharmacological or Nonpharmacological Somatic Treatment

As described in Chapter 6, the SCS is characterized by perceptions of entrapment/frantic hopelessness, heightened emotional and physiological arousal and lability, cognitive dysfunction, and social isolation. Given the near-psychotic nature of its presentation, with difficulties in cognitive functioning and unusual somatic sensations, pharmacological intervention may be essential in managing and improving an acute suicidal crisis before psychological intervention is feasible (Galynker et al., 2017), analogous to the treatment of status epilepticus. Dysregulation in neural, neuroendocrine, and autonomic systems has been linked to SCS symptoms, suggesting these systems as potential pharmacological intervention targets (see Calati, Nemeroff, et al., 2020, for review). For instance, entrapment and severe anxiety may be linked to disturbances in the hypothalamic-pituitary-adrenal (HPA) axis, with dysregulated corticotropin-releasing hormone and cortisol levels. Affective disturbances may, in part, relate to alterations in dopaminergic circuits that are involved in reward and antireward systems. Loss of cognitive control could be considered a form of thought disorder and may be associated with disrupted neurocognitive functioning, including deficits in executive functioning, attention, and decision-making. Hyperarousal may be linked to autonomic dysregulation, characterized by reductions in both heart rate variability and electrodermal activity, as well as amygdala hyperactivity. Acute social withdrawal may be associated with HPA axis activation, alterations in endogenous opioid and cannabinoid systems, and low oxytocin availability. Finally, inflammation and inflammatory processes may play a contributory role across each of these symptoms.

Accordingly, targeting these implicated biological underpinnings with medications or neuromodulation strategies may improve a suicidal crisis state, mitigating acute suicide risk. For example, the frantic aspect of entrapment/frantic hopelessness (Criterion A of the SCS), as well as hyperarousal (Criterion B3) and panic-somatization aspect of affective disturbances (Criterion B1), could be treated with long-acting benzodiazepines, positive allosteric modulators (PAMs) of the GABA A receptor, some of the sedating second-generation antipsychotics, and/or corticotropin-releasing hormone receptor 1 antagonists. Emotional pain (B1) could be targeted with a pulse treatment of ketamine-related agents or exogenous opiates, the latter with or without adjunct naloxone, although abuse liability is obviously a concern. It is important to note that naltrexone pretreatment completely blocked the antisuicidal effects of IV ketamine (Williams et al., 2019). Loss of cognitive control (B2), and its most severe form of ruminative flooding, can be treated acutely with small doses of potent first-, second-, and third-generation antipsychotics. Acute social withdrawal (B4) and possibly anhedonia (B1) may be responsive to oxytocin receptor agonists, although such treatments are not available currently. Alternatively, advances in neuromodulation, mainly with accelerated theta-burst transcranial magnetic stimulation (TMS), have shown promise (Cole et al., 2020), and focused ultrasound (FUS) has the potential to, for example, reduce amygdala hyperactivity.

Moreover, medications like clozapine, lithium, and ketamine, which have been shown to alleviate suicidality long term, may be efficacious in the acute management of the SCS.

Clozapine

Clozapine, an FDA-approved atypical antipsychotic, is used to treat patients with treatment-resistant schizophrenia, meaning they have shown no or partial clinical response to at least two different antipsychotic medications (Mayall & Banerjee, 2014). In the InterSept (International Suicide Prevention Trial), a multicenter, randomized study comparing suicidal behavior in patients with schizophrenia and schizoaffective disorders at high risk for suicide, patients taking clozapine showed a significantly higher reduction in suicide attempts than those taking olanzapine, a more widely prescribed antipsychotic (Meltzer et al., 2003). Other research findings later supported these positive results (Taipale et al., 2021; Thomas et al., 2015). The mechanism by which clozapine may directly alleviate suicidality, apart from the indirect effects of reducing psychotic symptoms, is yet unknown and requires further research. While clozapine is highly effective, adverse effects associated with the drug include agranulocytosis, cardiovascular events, dementia, hypotension, and seizures, which require appropriate management (De Berardis et al., 2018; De Fazio et al., 2015; Miller, 2000).

Lithium

Lithium is a well-researched mood stabilizer and a commonly prescribed treatment for bipolar disorder. Cipriani and colleagues (2005) found that suicidal behavior and mortality decreased significantly in patients with mood disorders who received lithium treatment. A follow-up study found that lithium was statistically more effective than a placebo and same class drugs in reducing suicide deaths (Cipriani et al., 2013). The antisuicidal effects of lithium treatment were also supported by a recent meta-analysis of literature spanning 40 years (Smith & Cipriani, 2017). Although the mechanism behind these findings is yet to be discovered, it is posited that lithium decreases suicidal behavior through reduction of patients' impulsivity (Müller-Oerlinghausen & Lewitzka, 2010). An important concern with the continued use of lithium is its toxicity profile, particularly with long-term use. Its potential long-term side effects include diabetes insipidus, thyroid dysfunction, kidney dysfunction, and neurotoxicity (Gonzalez et al., 2008).

Ketamine (Anesthetic Agent)

Anesthetic agents are garnering attention and support as therapeutics for suicidal patients. Ketamine has been widely used by clinicians as a general anesthetic and short-acting analgesic agent. Recent evidence indicates that ketamine at low levels may also have antidepressant properties, which can last three to seven days, as quickly as 40 minutes after an intravenous infusion (Murrough et al., 2013). Ketamine has also demonstrated promise in reducing acute suicidal ideation (Al Jurdi et al., 2015; Dadiomov & Lee, 2019; Witt et al., 2020). A recent randomized, double-blind, placebo-controlled study demonstrated a rapid remission of severe suicidal ideation in adults treated with ketamine (Abbar et al., 2022). However, the rates of suicide attempts during follow-up were similar between the ketamine-treated group and a placebo group. More evidence is needed to establish the scope and efficacy of ketamine treatment for suicidal ideation and behavior. In the interim, Lee et al. (2016) proposed that the antidepressant and antisuicidal effects reported with ketamine administration are mediated, in part, by targeting neural circuits relevant to executive function and cognitive-emotional processing.

The major concern regarding ketamine and ketamine-like compounds is their potential for recreational use and abuse and their current classification as controlled substances (Newport et al., 2016). Ketamine is an opiate mu-receptor agonist and is ineffective after naloxone pretreatment (Williams et al., 2019). This suggests that ketamine's effectiveness for reducing suicidal ideation could be due to transient mood elevation or analgesia, not unlike that induced by opiates, such as oxycontin or buprenorphine (Ballard et al., 2014). Indeed, in preliminary studies, buprenorphine was effective in reducing suicidal ideation (Yovell et al., 2016). However, given that ketamine and opiate analgesics are fast-acting, these drugs may be used short term with extreme care in an emergency department setting or otherwise for those in a crisis or waiting for traditional medication to take effect. With further research into their effectiveness and additional potential, ketamine and opiate analgesics may become an acute intervention to mitigate immediate suicide concerns (Newport et al., 2015).

Altogether, although the mechanisms of many of these medications in reducing suicidality are unclear, we posit that the use of pharmacological intervention should be considered as a frontline treatment for the management of the SCS. The interventions must be effective enough to fully treat or substantially reduce the SCS intensity within the three- to seven-day timeframe of the Comprehensive Psychiatric Emergency Program or inpatient hospitalization (Galynker et al., 2017).

Step 2: Safety Planning

Following fast-acting pharmacological or somatic interventions aimed at stabilizing a patient for engagement in subsequent treatment, brief psychosocial interventions that require few cognitive resources may be helpful in managing patients' acute periods of arousal, suicidal thoughts, and urges. In particular, crisis response planning (Rudd et al., 2004) and safety planning intervention (Stanley & Brown, 2012) represent two comparable, validated, brief (completed in 20 to 45 minutes) single-session interventions that involve the development of a written safety plan. Safety planning intervention results in the creation of written individualized steps for patients to follow during moments of intense emotional distress and/or suicidal crises when their cognitive control is impaired. An effective safety plan includes six primary components: (1) recognizing warning signs (e.g., thoughts, images, physiological sensations, affects/moods, behaviors) that typically precede a suicidal crisis, (2) using self-directed or internal coping strategies as an intentional form of distraction from suicidal urges and intense affects, (3) engaging with social contacts for distraction (i.e., without explicitly focusing on one's distress) and/or support (i.e., discussing one's emotions and experiences with the goal of receiving support), (4) connecting with mental health professionals or agencies if the aforementioned steps do not help mitigate the crisis, (5) identifying patients' individualized reasons for living, and (6) safety planning to reduce environmental risk for suicidal behavior.

Patient use of safety plans is high (Bryan, May, et al., 2018), and patients and staff each perceive safety plans to be highly useful in increasing safety, preventing suicidal behavior, and increasing treatment engagement (Chesin et al., 2017; Stanley et al., 2016). Consistent with these perceptions, safety planning interventions have demonstrated efficacy in reducing suicidal ideation (Bryan, Mintz, et al., 2018; Rozek et al., 2019) and decreasing engagement in suicidal behavior (Bryan et al., 2017; Stanley et al., 2018) among emergency department patients and active-duty military service members. Although not yet empirically examined, several factors may explain the efficacy of safety planning: providing a distraction, increasing connection, promoting autonomy, building competence, reducing engagement in impulsive urges, hindering engagement in suicidal behavior, and reducing patients' cognitive load (see Rogers, Gai, et al., 2022, for an overview).

Treatment of the Suicidal Narrative

After the management of an acute suicidal crisis (SCS), short-term psychotherapies aiming to restructure the suicidal narrative into an acceptable life narrative (McAdams et al., 2001) and to address individual components of the suicidal narrative (i.e., thwarted belongingness, perceived burdensomeness, defeat, fear of humiliation, difficulties with goal disengagement and reorientation) are relevant to prevent the onset of future crises and to diminish an identity-based connection with suicide-related beliefs and cognitions.

Several psychosocial interventions specifically intended to treat suicidality have been developed and validated. The most widely utilized and empirically supported psychosocial interventions include the Collaborative

Assessment and Management of Suicidality (CAMS; Jobes, 2006), Cognitive-Behavioral Therapy for Suicide Prevention (CBT-SP; Stanley et al., 2009), and the Attempted Suicide Short Intervention Program (ASSIP; Michel & Gysin-Maillart, 2015), among others. Within the NCM framework, the above methods are slated for the treatment of the suicidal narrative. Whether this sequential approach yields superior results to utilizing psychosocial interventions concurrently with or prior to the psychopharmacological treatment of the SCS requires a direct comparison in prospective randomized clinical trials.

Collaborative Assessment and Management of Suicide

The Collaborative Assessment and Management of Suicide (CAMS; Jobes, 2006) is an empirically supported framework for suicide risk assessment and intervention designed to manage suicidal thoughts and behaviors through a time-limited, flexible approach. Originally developed for use in university counseling centers and with outpatients experiencing suicidal ideation (Jobes, 1995; Jobes et al., 1997), CAMS has since been implemented virtually in emergency departments (Dimeff et al., 2020), with active-duty military/veteran samples (Jobes et al., 2017; Johnson et al., 2019), and in inpatient settings (Ellis et al., 2017; Ryberg et al., 2019). The unique approach of CAMS emphasizes collaboration and transparency, alongside an empathetic, nonjudgmental stance, throughout the consent, assessment, intervention, and termination processes (Jobes, 2006). It is agnostic about theoretical orientations and thus can be administered by psychotherapists from various theoretical and practice backgrounds. Treatment continues until suicidality resolves and typically lasts approximately 12 sessions (Comtois et al., 2011).

Treatment is guided by the Suicide Status Form (SSF; Jobes, 2016) completed at the start of each session. The first-session version of the SSF contains three sections. Section A assesses several empirically derived risk factors for suicide, such as psychological pain, stress, agitation, hopelessness, self-hatred, and perceived suicide risk, using both quantitative ratings and open-ended qualitative responses. Section B identifies and describes other proximal risk factors related to the patient's lifetime suicide attempts, substance abuse, and relationship problems, among others. The third section of the SSF (Section C) guides the treatment planning, focusing on addressing self-harm, creating a stabilization plan, and reducing patients' individual suicidal risk factors (identified in Section A). Subsequent sessions utilize tracking versions of the SSF to assess suicidal thoughts and revise treatment planning as needed. Hence, CAMS can be flexibly tailored to factors driving a patient's suicidal narrative (e.g., perceived burdensomeness, defeat), thereby mitigating the risk of subsequent episodes of the SCS. The treatment concludes after three consecutive sessions of low suicide risk (i.e., no or manageable suicidal ideation, no self-injurious behaviors). Overall, a meta-analysis of nine studies indicated that CAMS results in significantly lower suicidal ideation, general distress, and hopelessness, as well as significantly higher treatment acceptability, than other commonly used interventions (Swift et al., 2021).

Cognitive Behavioral Therapy for Suicide Prevention

Cognitive Behavioral Therapy for Suicide Prevention (CBT-SP) is a manualized cognitive-behavioral therapy for individuals with suicidal ideation and behaviors. Although this intervention was originally developed for adolescents with recent (i.e., < 90 days) suicide attempts, it can also be applied to individuals with acute suicidal ideation in which precipitating factors can be identified (Stanley et al., 2009). The primary objectives of CBT-SP are to identify and reduce suicide risk factors, improve coping, and develop cognitive, behavioral, emotional, and interpersonal skills that aid in preventing suicidal behavior. Like the NCM, CBT-SP is based on the principles of diathesis-stress models, in which interaction between trait vulnerabilities and stressors triggers suicidal behaviors in individuals who possess vulnerabilities yet lack appropriate skills for regulating emotions, solving problems, tolerating distress, and/or addressing negative thoughts or beliefs (e.g., hopelessness, worthlessness). Treatment usually consists of approximately 10 to 12 sessions (Stanley et al., 2009) and involves a chain analysis of the events leading up to a suicide attempt, developing a safety plan for future suicidal crises, psychoeducation, building reasons for living and hope, improving individual skills (e.g., behavioral activation, emotion regulation, distress tolerance, cognitive restructuring, goal-setting), enhancing family support and communication, and various other strategies to mitigate future suicide risk. The suicidal narrative component of the NCM can be utilized to guide treatment planning and tailoring, as deficits in social support (i.e., thwarted belongingness), cognitive restructuring (i.e., perceived burdensomeness, defeat, fear of humiliation), and goal-setting (i.e., goal disengagement and reorientation) can be identified and explicitly targeted through CBT-SP. Notably, CBT-SP components are recommended as part of standard empirically supported care with suicidal patients (Bryan, 2019; Stanley et al., 2009).

Attempted Suicide Short Intervention Program

The Attempted Suicide Short Intervention Program (ASSIP) is a manualized brief psychotherapy designed for patients who recently attempted suicide (Michel & Gysin-Maillart, 2015), as previous suicide attempts are often cited as strong risk factors for future suicide attempts (Bostwick et al., 2016; cf. Ribeiro et al., 2016). Consisting of only three to four sessions, ASSIP focuses on the development of an early therapeutic alliance, in conjunction with psychoeducation, a cognitive case conceptualization, safety planning, and continued long-term outreach contact via personalized letters over a two-year period (every three months in the first year, followed by every six months in the second year; Gysin-Maillart et al., 2016). Consistent with the principles of the NCM's suicidal narrative, the first session involves a narrative interview, providing biographical context to the recent suicide attempt. Then, in the following session, clinicians and patients jointly review a video recording of the first session to reactivate the patient's suicidal crisis in a safe environment. Emotional, cognitive, physiological, and behavioral changes that occurred during the transition from psychological pain to suicidal actions are identified. Additionally, a psychoeducational handout is provided during this session. In the final session, patients' long-term goals, individual warning signs, triggers, and safety strategies are discussed and formulated in a written safety plan. ASSIP helps to reduce suicidal behaviors (Gysin-Maillart et al., 2016), is cost-effective (Park et al., 2018), and can be adapted to address related substance use problems in hospital settings (Conner et al., 2021).

Stress Management

Stressful life events often act as precipitating factors for suicidal behavior (see Chapter 4 for a detailed overview). Associated with the SCS and the suicidal narrative (Cohen et al., 2022) stressful life events serve a moderating role in the NCM. Stress management techniques address the propensity to react strongly to stressful life events and/or negative emotions, mitigating their associations with the SCS and the suicidal narrative and, ultimately, preventing the onset or relapse of a suicidal narrative or crisis among individuals at risk. Although not explicitly focused on suicidality, several existing, empirically supported psychosocial interventions are designed to address reactivity to stressors and enhance stress management more generally, focusing on building skills in tolerating distress, mindfulness, and emotion regulation.

Dialectical Behavior Therapy

Dialectical behavior therapy (DBT; Linehan, 1993, 2014) is a cognitive-behavioral treatment designed to manage the symptoms of borderline personality disorder, including chronic suicidality and self-injury. According to the Linehan's biosocial model, a borderline personality disorder is primarily a disorder of emotional and behavioral self-dysregulation that emerges from a dynamic interaction between biological/trait vulnerabilities and certain dysfunctional environments (Linehan, 1993). Individuals with borderline personality disorder experience heightened emotional sensitivity, an inability to regulate intense emotions, and a gradual return to emotional baseline. Stressful life events may exacerbate these symptoms and lead to suicidal behavior as a response to unbearable emotional experiences (Linehan, 2014). Thus, DBT is an ideal mechanism to intervene in processes that exacerbate the impact of stressful experiences on baseline vulnerabilities.

DBT components include weekly individual therapy, skills training in a group setting, and phone-based coaching between therapy sessions. Four modules encompass DBT: core mindfulness (i.e., focusing on the present moment, both internally and externally, in a nonjudgmental manner), interpersonal effectiveness (i.e., communicating more effectively and dealing with challenging people, while balancing desires to maintain a relationship and one's self-respect), emotion regulation (i.e., identify emotions, change unwanted emotions, and build more positive emotions), and distress tolerance (i.e., accept oneself and the current situation through both crisis management and radical acceptance). Several formats of DBT, especially those that include skills training (Linehan et al., 2015), have demonstrated efficacy in reducing nonsuicidal and suicidal behaviors (DeCou et al., 2019; Kliem et al., 2010), possibly through reductions in emergency department visits (Coyle et al., 2018). Overall, DBT fits the NCM model well because it can target suicide risk through managing suicidal crises, addressing the suicidal narrative, and reducing vulnerability to stressful life events (see DeCou & Carmel, 2020, for examples).

Mindfulness-Based Stress Reduction

Mindfulness-based stress reduction (MBSR; Kabat-Zinn & Hanh, 2009) is a structured program of mindfulness training that emphasizes both focused attention (i.e., object-based selective attention in the present moment) and open monitoring (i.e., settling attention into observation or monitoring of the present moment without any explicit focus on an object or any given experience; Lutz et al., 2008). Altogether, MBSR aims to enhance the ability to observe the immediate experience, particularly the transient nature of thoughts, emotions, memories, mental images, and physical sensations. Coinciding with the goal of improving responses to stressful life events within the framework of the NCM, MBSR diminishes emotional reactivity and ruminative thinking in response to transient thoughts and sensations (Ramel et al., 2004), enhances emotional and behavioral self-regulation (Goldin & Gross, 2010; Lykins & Baer, 2009), modifies distorted views of oneself (Goldin et al., 2009), and subsequently reduces symptoms of stress, depression, and anxiety (Chiesa & Serretti, 2009; Evans et al., 2008; Segal et al., 2018).

Emotion Regulation Therapy

Emotion regulation therapy (ERT) is a psychosocial intervention designed to target mechanisms underlying distress-based disorders, including self-referential thinking (e.g., rumination, worry, self-criticism), behavioral responses (e.g., avoidance, reassurance-seeking), and contextual learning consequences (Mennin & Fresco, 2013). It consists of 16 manualized weekly sessions that focus first on cultivating mindful emotion regulation skills through the promotion of intentional and flexible responses to intense emotional experiences. Activities in this phase include psychoeducation, self-monitoring of one's emotional experiences, gaining competency in mindful emotion regulation skills, and practicing actions opposite to the current feelings and urges to restore emotional equilibrium. Then, in the next phase of treatment, behavioral proactivity through identification of one's values and taking actions reflective of these values and their meaning is emphasized (Renna et al., 2017). This phase involves applying one's emotion regulation skills to activities that reflect a meaningful and rewarding life, imaginal exposures that focus on specific actions, perceiving obstacles to action, and practicing valued actions between sessions. Preliminary evidence supports the efficacy of ERT in reducing symptoms of anxiety, worry, rumination, depression, and functional impairment, as well as in increasing patients' quality of life (Mennin et al., 2015, 2018).

Attachment-Based Family Therapy

Attachment-based family therapy (ABFT) is an empirically supported treatment that focuses on restoration of healthy family interaction and function (Diamond et al., 2016). Family relationships have been identified as powerful risk and protective factors for adolescents at risk of suicide (see Wagner et al., 2003, for review). Negative parenting and family environment have been linked to adolescent suicidality and depression (Diamond et al., 2021: Wagner et al., 2003; see also Chapter 4 of this book). Conflicts with family precede 20% of suicide deaths and 50% of nonfatal suicidal acts by adolescents (Diamond et al., 2010). Although several family studies have shown promising results in treating suicidal youth, ABFT is one of the first manualized family therapies tailored to address severely depressed and su- icidal patients (Ewing et al., 2015; Shpigel et al., 2012). The ABFT includes five distinct therapeutic tasks. Task 1, the relational reframe, aims to shift the focus from the patient's symptoms to the improvement of the relationship between parents and adolescent. Task 2, the adolescent alliance-building, involves individual sessions with the adolescent aimed at identifying the patient's strength, interests, and perceived attachment ruptures. Task 3 is to create an alliance with caregivers by exploring how their life stressors and intergenerational attachment issues may have affected their parenting practices. Once the therapeutic alliances are built, in Task 4 the patient and caregivers are brought together, so that the patient can share their thoughts, feelings, and grievances and receive empathy from caregivers. This mutu- ally respectful conversation provides a "corrective attachment experience" that restores trust between adolescent and caregivers. Finally, Task 5, the autonomy-promoting task, focuses on practicing new relationship skills. The adolescent is encouraged to take developmentally appropriate responsibility for their behavior and choices while the parents create a safe "nest" for the adolescent to mature in.

Attachment-based therapy may be applied to address long-term suicide risk factors, such as maladaptive attachment styles. Indeed, research shows that fearful attachment is a significant predictor of suicide risk behavior following hospital discharge (Li et al., 2017). Therefore, attachment-based interventions may be required to prevent suicide.

Digital Interventions

While efficacious treatments for suicidality exist, there are many structural and attitudinal barriers to seeking professional help, such as stigma, shame, negative prior experience with mental health professionals, financial diffi- culties, low perceived need, and preference for self-management (Bruffaerts et al., 2011; Czyz et al., 2013; Goldsmith et al., 2002). Easily accessible from everywhere, digital interventions may help address some of these barriers and serve as vital connectors between the treatment of acute episodes and long-term maintenance.

Digital interventions can be delivered over Internet websites, apps, wearable devices, virtual reality, and video games (Mohr et al., 2013) and vary from self-guided tools to those incorporating human support (Kruzan et al., 2021). A recent comprehensive meta-analysis of 16 randomized controlled studies, with a total of over 4,300 participants, demonstrated that self-guided digital interventions directly targeting suicidal ideation are effective immediately after treatment (Torok et al., 2020). However, this effect was not sustained over the long term, highlighting the need for more research on ways to maintain treatment effects.

Various approaches are used in self-guided digital interventions targeting suicidality: DBT (iDBT-ST), therapeutic evaluative conditioning (TEC), acceptance and commitment therapy (iBobbly app), CBT (Virtual Hope Box), and mixed methods (ThinkLife, Living with Deadly Thoughts; Torok et al., 2020), providing ample opportunities for choosing the right treatment approach.

Low adherence remains a significant drawback of self-guided digital interventions. A meta-analysis by Witt et al. (2017) identified that in the studies that reported information on adherence, up to one-half of participants allocated to the intervention group did not complete all treatment modules. Torok et al. (2020) found similarly poor levels of adherence: almost two-thirds of studies reported that participants completed less than 50% of the treatment.

Human support may help overcome participants' engagement and dropout issues (Rosenberg et al., 2022). Indeed, guided digital interventions have greater efficacy than self-guided ones (Fairburn & Patel, 2017; Musiat et al., 2022), potentially due to the better treatment adherence in the presence of support (Mohr et al., 2011). A meta-analysis by Musiat et al. (2022) demonstrated that guidance in digital mental health interventions increases adherence. However, evidence for the guidance impact on adherence is limited, and more research is required for better understanding of the specific interactions between guidance, adherence, and outcomes.

Virtual reality (VR) therapeutic interventions have been recognized as a promising innovation for treating mental disorders like acrophobia (Donker et al., 2019); delusions, hallucinations, cognitive and social challenges associated with the schizophrenia spectrum (Bisso et al., 2020); posttraumatic stress disorder (PTSD; Best et al., 2020); anxiety and depression (Baghaei et al., 2021). However, future research needs to investigate the transferability of the VR interventions to suicidality.

Although promising, digital interventions come with a complex range of privacy, confidentiality, security, and accountability concerns, which require the development of evidence-based policies (Balcombe & De Leo, 2021).

Long-Term Risk Factors/Trait Vulnerabilities

After acute (i.e., SCS) and subacute (i.e., suicidal narrative) risk for suicide has been managed, and patients have developed coping skills for responding to stressful life events, psychotherapy and pharmacology are relevant to address long-term risk factors and trait vulnerabilities. Given the multitude of long-term risk factors for suicide and since many of these factors are not modifiable (e.g., sociodemographic characteristics), a comprehensive overview of all applicable interventions is not provided in this section. Rather, the reader is directed to consider empirically supported interventions for each particular risk factor. For instance, trauma resulting in symptoms of posttraumatic stress may be treated through gold-standard psychosocial interventions: cognitive processing therapy (Resick et al., 2016; Resick & Schnicke, 1992) and prolonged exposure (Foa, 2011; Foa et al., 2007). Problematic alcohol and/or substance use may be addressed through a variety of psychosocial interventions, such as contingency management (Davis et al., 2016), motivational interviewing/enhancement (DiClemente et al., 2017), and other cognitive-behavioral approaches (see Dutra et al., 2008, for meta-analysis). Perfectionism and other maladaptive cognitive processes may be addressed through a variety of therapeutic approaches (e.g., cognitive-behavioral therapies). Overall, clinicians should assess the spectrum of long-term risk factors for suicide collaboratively with patients and address those that are most distressing, impairing, and/or modifiable.

Cultural Considerations

Research demonstrates that suicide rates and behavior vary substantially across racial and ethnic groups, from adolescence into adulthood (CDC,

2020; Nock et al., 2008). The highest U.S. suicide rate is in the American Indian/Alaskan Native population (Curtin et al., 2021; SPRC, 2020). While the overall suicide rates for African American adolescents have been lower than those for other racial groups, suicide attempts have increased drastically among African American youth (Lindsey et al., 2019), resulting in suicide's becoming the third leading cause of death for African American adolescents (Robinson et al., 2021). Although historically, Hispanics have been at a lower risk for suicide compared to other racial or ethnic groups in the United States, recent research demonstrates a significant increase in suicide rates among Hispanics, particularly among females, with a 50% suicide rate increase from 2000 to 2015 (Silva & Van Orden, 2018).

There is, therefore, a significant need for the development of culturally adapted treatments for suicide that would consider and account for the sociocultural and socioeconomic factors contributing to disparities (SAMHSA, 2020). However, despite this glaring need, there has been limited research examining the efficacy of suicidality treatment for racial and ethnic minorities (Meza & Bath, 2021). A meta-analysis of 158 studies demonstrated that racial and ethnic groups were underrepresented in suicide research (Cha et al., 2018). Research also suggests that findings based on predominantly White-majority samples may have limited generalizability to racial/ethnic minoritized groups (Choi et al., 2009; Meza & Bath, 2021). Hence, understanding of the efficacy of suicide treatment among racial and ethnic minorities is incomplete, and future research focused on racial and ethnic minorities is required.

African Americans

ABFT showed promising results in the randomized controlled study of predominantly African American adolescents at risk of suicide. Adolescents treated with ABFT demonstrated greater improvement on self-reported suicidal ideation than those who received enhanced usual care, which included referral to a therapist, weekly tracking of depression and suicidal ideation, and access to a 24/7 crisis line (Diamond et al., 2010). However, since this study did not report any effects by race, the efficacy of this intervention for African American adolescents is undetermined (Robinson et al., 2021a). Another promising culturally grounded suicide intervention for African American adolescents is the Adapted-Coping with Stress Course (A-CWS;

Robinson et al., 2021b). The A-CWS is a 15-session, group-based, cognitive-behavioral intervention designed to enhance African American adolescents' coping skills and reduce suicidal ideation. The A-CWS emphasizes unique stressors associated with African American suicide risk, such as systemic racism, and provides culturally adapted strategies to counter these stressors. Two randomized controlled trials supported the efficacy of the A-CWS in reducing suicide risk and ideation among African American adolescents (Robinson et al., 2021a).

The Grady Nia intervention, a manualized, culturally informed, and empowerment-focused 10-week psychoeducational group intervention, was developed to reduce suicidal ideation, depressive symptoms, PTSD, and general psychological distress in low-income African American women with a recent history of intimate partner violence and a suicide attempt (Kaslow et al., 2010). A randomized controlled trial of the Nia intervention demonstrated that the women receiving the intervention showed lower levels of depressive symptoms and general distress initially and at the follow-up than the women assigned to a treatment as usual group. Although the Nia intervention did not result in a greater reduction in suicidal ideation, after the intervention, the women from the Nia intervention group experienced less severe suicidal ideation when exposed to intimate partner violence than the women in the control group (Kaslow et al., 2010).

Hispanics

While there has been some research providing evidence for the efficacy of CBT, problem-solving therapy (PST), interpersonal therapy (IPT), and behavioral activation (BA) in treating depression among Hispanic groups (Cardemil et al., 2020), there is still a lack of research exploring culturally tailored suicidality interventions designed for the Hispanic population (Silva & Van Orden, 2018; Villarreal-Otálora et al., 2019). Overall, it has been suggested that family-based interventions promoting cultural engagement and values may be a promising avenue for suicide risk management and prevention among the Hispanic population (Silva & Van Orden, 2018). Familias Unidas, a family-based, culturally specific intervention, was developed to prevent and decrease risky behaviors in Hispanic adolescents, such as substance use and risky sexual behavior, by improving family functioning (Prado et al., 2007). Although Familias Unidas was not designed to target suicidal behavior specifically, the effectiveness trial findings suggest that, indirectly, it significantly reduced suicidal behaviors among Hispanic adolescents with low levels of parent–adolescent communication (Vidot et al., 2016). DBT has been culturally adapted for Hispanic female adolescents at risk of suicide and their parents by suggesting specific treatment targets for extreme behavioral patterns, such as old school versus new school and overprotecting versus underprotecting (German et al., 2015). However, the efficacy of this culturally adapted intervention has not been tested yet.

American Indians/Alaskan Natives

In a recent systematic review examining the outcomes of suicide interventions for American Indian and Alaska Native populations, Pham et al. (2021) reported significant research limitations in this area. Only eleven studies included assessments that measured changes in direct suicide outcomes. Moreover, only three of the studies employed randomized or nonrandomized controlled trials. Additionally, only one of the 23 reviewed interventions demonstrated statistically significant improvement of suicide factors. Particularly, the Zuni Life Skills Development intervention, a curriculum program that engages adolescents with interactive scenarios describing problematic life events typical for American Indian adolescents, demonstrated statistically significant improvement on the Suicide Probability Scale, an assessment that was used to measure suicide potential and its subscale measures of suicidal ideation, hopelessness, and hostility (LaFromboise & Howard-Pitney, 1994).

Asian Americans

There is a lack of research exploring the effectiveness of suicidality treatments for the Asian American population. Existing therapies, such as DBT and acceptance and commitment therapy, while based on the mindfulness and acceptance principles of Asian philosophies, still tend to reflect the Western majority's views and experiences, such as the conceptualization of self versus others (Hahm & Yasui, 2019). The effectiveness of culturally adapted CBT for the Asian American population may be a promising avenue for future research. Thus, a randomized controlled trial demonstrated a slight advantage of the culturally adapted version of CBT in reducing depressive symptoms in Chinese Americans compared to the standard version of CBT (Hwang et al., 2015). Additionally, the AWARE intervention, a culturally and gender-specific psychotherapy program, was developed to treat Asian American females of East Asian descent (Hahm et al., 2019). The AWARE intervention consists of eight in-person weekly psychotherapy sessions and daily text messages to participants that address Asian American women's personal stories related to their mental and sexual health. The intervention targets identified culturally specific suicide risk factors among Asian American women by focusing on reducing perfectionism, building up emotional distress tolerance, alleviating conflicts within families, fostering a sense of belonging and connectedness to one's racial and ethnic group, and overcoming the stigma associated with mental health problems and help-seeking. A randomized clinical trial of the AWARE intervention suggested that it may effectively reduce suicidal outcomes (Hahm et al., 2019). Moreover, CAMS may be a potentially useful tool for culturally sensitive work with Asian American college students. The collaborative approach and flexibility of CAMS allow for the identification of vital and relevant cultural factors related to suicidality, and CAMS could potentially help Asian Americans to be more verbally active in the counseling process (Choi et al., 2009).

Cultural Competence

Overall, considering the limited research examining the effectiveness of treatments for suicidality among racial and ethnic minority groups, the cultural competence of the clinician becomes an essential therapeutic skill (Cardemil et al., 2020). The meta-analysis by Soto et al. (2018) suggested that the client's perception of the therapist's ability to successfully work with people of various cultural backgrounds is associated with treatment outcomes, a finding emphasizing the importance of the cultural competence of the therapist. Indeed, awareness of the culturally specific context and patterns of suicidal behavior, including culture-specific suicide risks and protective factors, as well as culture's impact on help-seeking behaviors, is one of the vital skills of culturally competent therapists (Goldston et al., 2008). The Cultural Theory and Model of Suicide developed by Chu et al. (2010) suggested that four factors encompass 95% of culturally specific suicide risk literature: (1) cultural sanctions (acceptability of suicide within one's cultural context), (2) idioms of distress (the way suicide symptoms are expressed and means for engaging in suicidal behavior), (3) minority stress (the added stress that cultural minorities experience because of their identity, including acculturation, discrimination-related strain, and social disadvantages) and (4) social discord (lack of integration or alienation from family, community, and friends). A culturally competent therapist should be aware of culturally relevant beliefs and attitudes about life, death, and acceptability of suicide as an option (Wong et al., 2014).

Moreover, it is essential to keep in mind that individuals from different cultural backgrounds may have various ways of expressing emotional distress (Chu et al., 2010; Goldston et al., 2008). The use of intersectionality as a practice lens can help clinicians to examine how systems of privilege and oppression may impact suicide risk factors. Indeed, cultural minorities may experience heightened stress because of their social identity and position (Chu et al., 2010; Goldston et al., 2008; Leong & Leach, 2008). Furthermore, the intersection of multiple marginalized identities (e.g., ethnic minority and sexual/gender minority) may increase the likelihood of discrimination (Opara et al., 2020; Shadick et al., 2015), leading to an increased risk of suicide behavior (Oh et al., 2019). However, clinicians should also consider exploring strengths developed by racial and ethnic minorities due to oppression and marginalization (Cardemil et al., 2020). Finally, lack of integration into the community and alienation from family and friends may serve as suicide risk factors among ethnic and racial minorities (Chu et al., 2010; Goldston et al., 2008).

In addition to recognizing culture's impact on the suicidal behavior of patients, clinicians should also be aware of their own assumptions, biases, and values and their potential influence on the assessment and treatment of patients (Sue & Sue, 2003).

In conclusion, to address existing disparities, cultural consideration should be implemented on multiple levels, such as cultural adaptation of suicide interventions, cultural competence of clinicians, and finally, a culturally informed comprehensive public health approach targeting structural inequality, privilege, and oppression systems.

Implications for Future Research and Clinical Practice

The NCM provides a comprehensive framework for understanding, assessing, and intervening in suicide risk across its chronic, subacute, and acute stages. Given the potential to reduce suicidal thoughts and behaviors, implementing the full NCM framework in clinical practice across various settings (e.g., hospitals, community mental health centers, Veterans Affairs medical centers) and unique populations (e.g., across the lifespan, among racial/ethnic/sexual/gender minority individuals, among those with military service, among those with chronic illness, cross-culturally) may be a promising avenue for future work. In particular, future work should assess the generalizability, clinical utility, acceptability, adoption, appropriateness, and feasibility of the NCM across a variety of settings and populations.

First and foremost, however, randomized clinical trials are needed to establish optimal pharmacological or neuromodulation treatment for the SCS. These should include single-drug or neuromodulation trials targeting individual categories of symptoms included in SCS criteria. For example, benzodiazepines, PAMs of the GABA A receptor, and sedating low-potency first- and second-generation antipsychotics should be studied for the treatment of extreme anxiety and disturbances in arousal, as well as emotional pain. Third-generation antipsychotics should be tested to treat the loss of cognitive control. Long-acting opiates could be considered for treatment of emotional pain and entrapment, not necessarily as a solution but to determine the role opiate systems may play in this syndrome. Combination treatments targeting all or most symptoms of the SCS also need to be studied so that both optimal combinations and doses can be found.

Second, as alluded to previously in this chapter, the sequential nature of interventions, spanning from psychopharmacological treatment of acute suicidal crises (SCS) to psychosocial treatment of subacute risk (suicidal narrative), stressful life events, and long-term risk factors, has not yet been established. Specifically, although it is posited that psychosocial interventions may be ineffective until the SCS is treated and resolved through medications, this has not yet been empirically tested.

Finally, future innovations in treatment may potentially benefit from the NCM framework. For instance, examination of real-time risk for suicidal thoughts and behaviors utilizing intensive longitudinal methods, such as ecological momentary assessment (Kleiman & Nock, 2018), created new opportunities for suicide research. Intervening in real time may be similarly useful. In particular, the development and implementation of strategies that target subacute and acute risk (i.e., the suicidal narrative and SCS) as they occur in real life, including just-in-time (Nahum-Shani et al., 2018) or ecological momentary interventions (Armey, 2012), may mitigate the risk of suicidal behavior occurring in those moments. Preliminary evidence examining a DBT coaching mobile application has indicated that these types of interventions may reduce distress and self-injurious behaviors (Rizvi et al., 2011, 2016). However, few suicide-specific just-in-time or real-time interventions have been developed or evaluated, highlighting an area in need of future work. Altogether, should the NCM be used to guide innovations in intervention research, it may have impactful results on clinical practice and patient outcomes.

Conclusions

Empirically supported frameworks are essential to the understanding, assessment, and treatment of suicidal thoughts, urges, and behaviors. The NCM provides a comprehensive framework through which suicidal behavior can be understood and prevented, with specific guidance and applicable interventions at each distinct stage of the model. Utilization of this framework, as well as future research and clinical efforts to further refine the NCM, have the potential to save lives and reduce rates of death by suicide.

References

Abbar, M., Demattei, C., El-Hage, W., Llorca, P. M., Samalin, L., Demaricourt, P., Gaillard, R., Courtet, P., Vaiva, G., Gorwood, P., Fabbro, P., & Jollant, F. (2022). Ketamine for the acute treatment of severe suicidal ideation: Double blind, randomised placebo-controlled trial. *BMJ Clinical Research*, *376*, e067194. https://doi.org/10.1136/bmj-2021-067194

Al Jurdi, R. K., Swann, A., & Mathew, S. J. (2015). Psychopharmacological agents and suicide risk reduction: Ketamine and other approaches. *Current Psychiatry Reports*, *17*(10), 81. https://doi.org/10.1007/s11920-015-0614-9

Angelakis, I., Austin, J. L., & Gooding, P. (2020). Association of childhood maltreatment with suicide behaviors among young people: A systematic review and meta-analysis. *JAMA Network Open*, *3*, e2012563–e2012563. https://doi.org/10.1001/jamanetworkopen.2020.12563

Armey, M. F. (2012). Ecological momentary assessment and intervention in nonsuicidal self-injury: A novel approach to treatment. *Journal of Cognitive Psychotherapy*, *26*, 299–317. https://doi.org/10.1891/0889-8391.26.4.299

Ásgeirsdóttir, H. G., Valdimarsdóttir, U. A., Þorsteinsdóttir, Þ. K., Lund, S. H., Tomasson, G., Nyberg, U., Ásgeirsdóttir, T. L., & Hauksdóttir, A. (2018). The association between different traumatic life events and suicidality. *European Journal of Psychotraumatology*, *9*(1), 1510279. https://doi.org/10.1080/20008198.2018.1510279

Baghaei, N., Chitale, V., Hlasnik, A., Stemmet, L., Liang, H., & Porter, R. (2021). Virtual reality for supporting the treatment of depression and anxiety: Scoping review. *JMIR Mental Health, 8*(9), e29681. https://doi.org/10.2196/29681

Balcombe, L., & De Leo, D. (2021). Digital mental health challenges and the horizon ahead for solutions. *JMIR Mental Health, 8*(3), e26811. https://doi.org/10.2196/26811

Ballard, E. D., Ionescu, D. F., Vande Voort, J. L., Niciu, M. J., Richards, E. M., Luckenbaugh, D. A., Brutsché, N. E., Ameli, R., Furey, M. L., & Zarate, C. A., Jr. (2014). Improvement in suicidal ideation after ketamine infusion: Relationship to reductions in depression and anxiety. *Journal of Psychiatric Research, 58,* 161–166. https://doi.org/10.1016/j.jps ychires.2014.07.027

Barber, C. W., & Miller, M. J. (2014). Reducing a suicidal person's access to lethal means of suicide: A research agenda. *American Journal of Preventive Medicine, 47,* S264–S272. https://doi.org/10.1016/j.amepre.2014.05.028

Barzilay, S., Assounga, K., Veras, J., Beaubian, C., Bloch-Elkouby, S., & Galynker, I. (2020). Assessment of near-term risk for suicide attempts using the Suicide Crisis Inventory. *Journal of Affective Disorders, 276,* 183–190. https://doi.org/10.1016/j.jad.2020.06.053

Best, P., McKenna, A., Quinn, P., Duffy, M., & Van Daele, T. (2020). Can virtual reality ever be implemented in routine clinical settings? A systematic narrative review of clinical procedures contained within case reports for the treatment of PTSD. *Frontiers in Virtual Reality, 1,* 563739. https://doi.org/10.3389/frvir.2020.563739

Bisso, E., Signorelli, M. S., Milazzo, M., Maglia, M., Polosa, R., Aguglia, E., & Caponnetto, P. (2020). Immersive virtual reality applications in schizophrenia spectrum therapy: A systematic review. *International Journal of Environmental Research and Public Health, 17*(17), 6111. https://doi.org/10.3390/ijerph17176111

Bloch-Elkouby, S., Barzilay, S., Gorman, B., Lawrence, O., Rogers, M. L., Richards, J., Cohen, L., Johnson, B. N., & Galynker, I. (2021). The revised Suicide Crisis Inventory (SCI-2): Validation and assessment of near-term suicidal ideation and attempts. *Journal of Affective Disorders, 1*(295), 1280–1291.

Bloch-Elkouby, S., Gorman, B., Lloveras, L., Wilkerson, T., Schuck, A., Barzilay, S., Calati, R., Schnur, D., & Galynker, I. (2020). How do distal and proximal risk factors combine to predict suicidal ideation and behaviors? A prospective study of the narrative crisis model of suicide. *Journal of Affective Disorders, 277,* 914–926. https://doi.org/10.1016/j.jad.2020.08.088

Bloch-Elkouby, S., Gorman, B., Schuck, A., Barzilay, S., Calati, R., Cohen, L. J., Begum, F., & Galynker, I. (2020). The suicide crisis syndrome: A network analysis. *Journal of Counseling Psychology, 67*(5), 595–607. https://doi.org/10.1037/cou0000423

Bostwick, J. M., Pabbati, C., Geske, J. R., & McKean, A. J. (2016). Suicide attempt as a risk factor for completed suicide: Even more lethal than we knew. *The American Journal of Psychiatry, 173,* 1094–1100. https://doi.org/10.1176/appi.ajp.2016.15070854

Bruffaerts, R., Demyttenaere, K., Hwang, I., Chiu, W. T., Sampson, N., Kessler, R. C., Alonso, J., Borges, G., de Girolamo, G., de Graaf, R., Florescu, S., Gureje, O., Hu, C., Karam, E. G., Kawakami, N., Kostyuchenko, S., Kovess-Masfety, V., Lee, S., Levinson, D., . . . Nock, M. K. (2011). Treatment of suicidal people around the world. *The British Journal of Psychiatry, 199*(1), 64–70. https://doi.org/10.1192/bjp.bp.110.084129

Bryan, C. J. (2019). Cognitive behavioral therapy for suicide prevention (CBT-SP): Implications for meeting standard of care expectations with suicidal patients. *Behavioral Sciences & the Law, 37,* 247–258. https://doi.org/10.1002/bsl.2411

Bryan, C. J., May, A. M., Rozek, D. C., Williams, S. R., Clemans, T. A., Mintz, J., Leeson, B., & Burch, T. S. (2018). Use of crisis management interventions among suicidal patients: Results of a randomized controlled trial. *Depression and Anxiety, 35*, 619–628. https://doi.org/10.1002/da.22753

Bryan, C. J., Mintz, J., Clemans, T. A., Burch, T. S., Leeson, B., Williams, S., & Rudd, M. D. (2018). Effect of crisis response planning on patient mood and clinician decision making: A clinical trial with suicidal U.S. soldiers. *Psychiatric Services, 69*, 108–111. https://doi.org/10.1176/appi.ps.201700157

Bryan, C. J., Mintz, J., Clemans, T. A., Leeson, B., Burch, T. S., Williams, S. R., Maney, E., & Rudd, M. D. (2017). Effect of crisis response planning vs. contracts for safety on suicide risk in U.S. Army soldiers: A randomized clinical trial. *Journal of Affective Disorders, 212*, 64–72. https://doi.org/10.1016/j.jad.2017.01.028

Calati, R., Cohen, L. J., Schuck, A., Levy, D., Bloch-Elkouby, S., Barzilay, S., Rosenfield, P. J., & Galynker, I. (2020). The Modular Assessment of Risk for Imminent Suicide (MARIS): A validation study of a novel tool for suicide risk assessment. *Journal of Affective Disorders, 263*, 121–128. https://doi.org/10.1016/j.jad.2019.12.001

Calati, R., Nemeroff, C. B., Lopez-Castroman, J., Cohen, L. J., & Galynker, I. (2020). Candidate biomarkers of suicide crisis syndrome: What to test next? A concept paper. *International Journal of Neuropsychopharmacology, 23*, 192–205. https://doi.org/10.1093/ijnp/pyz063

Cardemil, E. V., Noyola, N., & He, E. (2020). Cultural considerations in treating depression. In L. T. Benuto, F. R. Gonzalez, & J. Singer (Eds.), *Handbook of Cultural Factors in Behavioral Health* (pp. 309–321). Springer, Cham. https://doi.org/10.1007/978-3-030-32229-8_22

Centers for Disease Control and Prevention [CDC]. (2020). *Web-based Injury Statistics Query and Reporting System (WISQARS).* https://www.cdc.gov/injury/wisqars/index.html

Cha, C. B., Tezanos, K. M., Peros, O. M., Ng, M. Y., Ribeiro, J. D., Nock, M. K., & Franklin, J. C. (2018). Accounting for diversity in suicide research: Sampling and sample reporting practices in the United States. *Suicide and Life-Threatening Behavior, 48*(2), 131–139. https://doi.org/10.1111/sltb.12344

Chesin, M. S., Stanley, B., Haigh, E. A. P., Chaudhury, S. R., Pontoski, K., Knox, K. L., & Brown, G. K. (2017). Staff views of an emergency department intervention using safety planning and structured follow-up with suicidal veterans. *Archives of Suicide Research, 21*, 127–137. https://doi.org/10.1080/13811118.2016.1164642

Chiesa, A., & Serretti, A. (2009). Mindfulness-based stress reduction for stress management in healthy people: A review and meta-analysis. *Journal of Alternative and Complementary Medicine, 15*, 593–600. https://doi.org/10.1089/acm.2008.0495

Chistopolskaya, K. A., Rogers, M. L., Cao, E., Galynker, I., Richards, J., Enikolopov, S. N., Nikolaev, E. L., Sadovni- Chaya, V. S., & Drovosekov, S. E. (2020). Adaptation of the Suicidal Narrative Inventory in a Russian sample [In Russian]. *Suicidology, 11*(4), 76–90. doi.org/10.32878/suiciderus.20-11-04(41)-76-90

Choi, J. L., Rogers, J. R., & Werth, J. L., Jr. (2009). Suicide risk assessment with Asian American college students: A culturally informed perspective. *The Counseling Psychologist, 37*(2), 186–218. https://doi.org/10.1177/0011000006292256

Chu, C., Buchman-Schmitt, J. M., Stanley, I. H., Hom, M. A., Tucker, R. P., Hagan, C. R., Rogers, M. L., Podlogar, M. C., Chiurliza, B., Ringer, F. B., Michaels, M. S., Patros, C. H. G., & Joiner, T. E. (2017). The interpersonal theory of suicide: A systematic review and meta-analysis of a decade of cross-national research. *Psychological Bulletin, 143*, 1313–1345. https://doi.org/10.1037/bul0000123

Chu, J. P., Goldblum, P., Floyd, R., & Bongar, B. (2010). The cultural theory and model of suicide. *Applied and Preventive Psychology, 14*(1–4), 25–40.

Cipriani, A., Hawton, K., Stockton, S., & Geddes, J. R. (2013). Lithium in the prevention of suicide in mood disorders: Updated systematic review and meta-analysis. *BMJ Clinical Research, 346*, f3646. https://doi.org/10.1136/bmj.f3646

Cipriani, A., Pretty, H., Hawton, K., & Geddes, J. R. (2005). Lithium in the prevention of suicidal behavior and all-cause mortality in patients with mood disorders: A systematic review of randomized trials. *The American Journal of Psychiatry, 162*(10), 1805–1819. https://doi.org/10.1176/appi.ajp.162.10.1805

Cohen, L. J., Ardalan, F., Yaseen, Z., & Galynker, I. (2018). Suicide crisis syndrome mediates the relationship between long-term risk factors and lifetime suicidal phenomena. *Suicide and Life-Threatening Behavior, 48*, 613–623. https://doi.org/10.1111/sltb.12387

Cohen, L. J., Gorman, B., Briggs, J., Jeon, M., Ginsburg, T., & Galynker, I. (2019). The suicidal narrative and its relationship to the suicide crisis syndrome and recent suicidal behavior. *Suicide and Life-Threatening Behavior, 49*, 413–422. https://doi.org/10.1111/sltb.12439

Cohen, L. J., Mokhtar, R., Richards, J., Hernandez, M., Bloch-Elkouby, S., & Galynker, I. (i2022). The narrative-crisis model of suicide and its prediction of near-term suicide risk. *Suicide and Life-Threatening Behavior, 52*(2), 231–243. https://doi.org/10.1111/sltb.12816

Cole, E. J., Stimpson, K. H., Bentzley, B. S., Gulser, M., Cherian, K., Tischler, C., Nejad, R., Pankow, H., Choi, E., Aaron, H., Espil, F. M., Pannu, J., Xiao, X., Duvio, D., Solvason, H. B., Hawkins, J., Guerra, A., Jo, B., Raj, K. S., . . . Williams, N. R. (2020). Stanford Accelerated Intelligent Neuromodulation Therapy for treatment-resistant depression. *The American Journal of Psychiatry, 177*, 716–726. https://doi.org/10.1176/appi.ajp.2019.19070720

Comtois, K. A., Jobes, D. A., O'Connor, S. S., Atkins, D. C., Janis, K., Chessen, C. E., Landes, S. J., Holen, A., & Yuodelis-Flores, C. (2011). Collaborative Assessment and Management of Suicidality (CAMS): Feasibility trial for next-day appointment services. *Depression and Anxiety, 28*, 963–972. https://doi.org/10.1002/da.20895

Conner, K. R., Kearns, J. C., Esposito, E. C., Pizzarello, E., Wiegand, T. J., Britton, P. C., Michel, K., Gysin-Maillart, A. C., & Goldston, D. B. (2021). Pilot RCT of the Attempted Suicide Short Intervention Program (ASSIP) adapted for rapid delivery during hospitalization to adult suicide attempt patients with substance use problems. *General Hospital Psychiatry, 72*, 66–72. https://doi.org/10.1016/j.genhosppsych.2021.07.002

Coyle, T. N., Shaver, J. A., & Linehan, M. M. (2018). On the potential for iatrogenic effects of psychiatric crisis services: The example of dialectical behavior therapy for adult women with borderline personality disorder. *Journal of Consulting and Clinical Psychology, 86*, 116–124. https://doi.org/10.1037/ccp0000275

Curtin, S. C., Hedegaard, H., & Ahmad, F. B. (2021). *Provisional numbers and rates of suicide by month and demographic characteristics: United States, 2020*. National Center for Health Statistics. https://www.cdc.gov/nchs/data/vsrr/VSRR016.pdf

Czyz, E. K., Horwitz, A. G., Eisenberg, D., Kramer, A., & King, C. A. (2013). Self-reported barriers to professional help seeking among college students at elevated risk for suicide.

Journal of American College Health, 61(7), 398–406. https://doi.org/10.1080/07448 481.2013.820731

Dadiomov, D., & Lee, K. (2019). The effects of ketamine on suicidality across various formulations and study settings. *The Mental Health Clinician, 9*, 48–60. https://doi.org/10.9740/mhc.2019.01.048

Davis, D. R., Kurti, A. N., Skelly, J. M., Redner, R., White, T. J., & Higgins, S. T. (2016). A review of the literature on contingency management in the treatment of substance use disorders, 2009–2014. *Preventive Medicine, 92*, 36–46. https://doi.org/10.1016/j.ypmed.2016.08.008

De Berardis, D., Rapini, G., Olivieri, L., Di Nicola, D., Tomasetti, C., Valchera, A., Fornaro, M., Di Fabio, F., Perna, G., Di Nicola, M., Serafini, G., Carano, A., Pompili, M., Vellante, F., Orsolini, L., Martinotti, G., & Di Giannantonio, M. (2018). Safety of antipsychotics for the treatment of schizophrenia: A focus on the adverse effects of clozapine. *Therapeutic Advances in Drug Safety, 9*(5), 237–256. https://doi.org/10.1177/2042098618756261

DeCou, C. R., & Carmel, A. (2020). Efficacy of dialectical behavior therapy in the treatment of suicidal behavior. In J. Bedics (Ed.), *The handbook of dialectical behavior therapy* (pp. 97–112). Academic Press. https://doi.org/10.1016/B978-0-12-816384-9.00005-1

DeCou, C. R., Comtois, K. A., & Landes, S. J. (2019). Dialectical behavior therapy is effective for the treatment of suicidal behavior: A meta-analysis. *Behavior Therapy, 50*, 60–72. https://doi.org/10.1016/j.beth.2018.03.009

De Fazio, P., Gaetano, R., Caroleo, M., Cerminara, G., Maida, F., Bruno, A., Muscatello, M. R., Moreno, M. J., Russo, E., & Segura-García, C. (2015). Rare and very rare adverse effects of clozapine. *Neuropsychiatric Disease and Treatment, 11*, 1995–2003. https://doi.org/10.2147/NDT.S83989

Dervic, K., Oquendo, M. A., Currier, D., Grunebaum, M. F., Burke, A. K., & Mann, J. J. (2006). Moral objections to suicide: Can they counteract suicidality in patients with cluster B psychopathology? *The Journal of Clinical Psychiatry, 67*, 620–625.

Diamond, G., Kodish, T., Ewing, E. S. K., Hunt, Q., & Russon, J. (2021). Family processes: Risk, protective and treatment factors for youth at risk for suicide. *Aggression and Violent Behavior, 64*, 101586. https://doi.org/10.1016/j.avb.2021.101586

Diamond, G., Russon, J., & Levy, S. (2016). Attachment-based family therapy: A review of the empirical support. *Family Process, 55*(3), 595–610. https://doi.org/10.1111/famp.12241

Diamond, G. S., Wintersteen, M. B., Brown, G. K., Diamond, G. M., Gallop, R., Shelef, K., & Levy, S. (2010). Attachment-based family therapy for adolescents with suicidal ideation: A randomized controlled trial. *Journal of the American Academy of Child and Adolescent Psychiatry, 49*(2), 122–131. https://doi.org/10.1097/00004583-201002000-00006

DiClemente, C. C., Corno, C. M., Graydon, M. M., Wiprovnick, A. E., & Knoblach, D. J. (2017). Motivational interviewing, enhancement, and brief interventions over the last decade: A review of reviews of efficacy and effectiveness. *Psychology of Addictive Behaviors, 31*, 862–887. https://doi.org/10.1037/adb0000318

Dimeff, L. A., Jobes, D. A., Chalker, S. A., Piehl, B. M., Duvivier, L. L., Lok, B. C., Zalake, M. S., Chung, J., & Koerner, K. (2020). A novel engagement of suicidality in the emergency department: Virtual Collaborative Assessment and Management of Suicidality. *General Hospital Psychiatry, 63*, 119–126. https://doi.org/10.1016/j.genhosppsych.2018.05.005

Donker, T., Cornelisz, I., van Klaveren, C., van Straten, A., Carlbring, P., Cuijpers, P., & van Gelder, J. L. (2019). Effectiveness of self-guided app-based virtual reality cognitive behavior therapy for acrophobia: A randomized clinical trial. *JAMA Psychiatry, 76*(7), 682–690. https://doi.org/10.1001/jamapsychiatry.2019.0219

Dutra, L., Stathopoulou, G., Basden, S. L., Leyro, T. M., Powers, M. B., & Otto, M. W. (2008). A meta-analytic review of psychosocial interventions for substance use disorders. *The American Journal of Psychiatry, 165*, 179–187. https://doi.org/10.1176/appi.ajp.2007.06111851

Ellis, T. E., Rufino, K. A., & Allen, J. G. (2017). A controlled comparison trial of the Collaborative Assessment and Management of Suicidality (CAMS) in an inpatient setting: Outcomes at discharge and six-month follow-up. *Psychiatry Research, 249*, 252–260. https://doi.org/10.1016/j.psychres.2017.01.032

Evans, S., Ferrando, S., Findler, M., Stowell, C., Smart, C., & Haglin, D. (2008). Mindfulness-based cognitive therapy for generalized anxiety disorder. *Journal of Anxiety Disorders, 22*, 716–721. https://doi.org/10.1016/j.janxdis.2007.07.005

Ewing, E. S. K., Diamond, G., & Levy, S. (2015). Attachment-based family therapy for depressed and suicidal adolescents: Theory, clinical model and empirical support. *Attachment & Human Development, 17*(2), 136–156. https://doi.org/10.1080/14616734.2015.1006384

Fairburn, C. G., & Patel, V. (2017). The impact of digital technology on psychological treatments and their dissemination. *Behaviour Research and Therapy, 88*, 19–25. https://doi.org/10.1016/j.brat.2016.08.012

Foa, E. B. (2011). Prolonged exposure therapy: Past, present, and future. *Depression and Anxiety, 28*, 1043–1047. https://doi.org/10.1002/da.20907

Foa, E. B., Hembree, E., & Rothbaum, B. (2007). *Prolonged Exposure Therapy for PTSD: Therapist guide—Emotional processing of traumatic experiences.* Oxford University Press.

Franklin, J. C., Ribeiro, J. D., Fox, K. R., Bentley, K. H., Kleiman, E. M., Jaroszewski, A. C., Chang, B. P., & Nock, M. K. (2017). Risk factors for suicidal thoughts and behaviors: A meta-analysis of 50 years of research. *Psychological Bulletin, 143*, 187–232.

Galynker, I. (2017). *The suicidal crisis: Clinical guide to the assessment of imminent suicide risk.* Oxford University Press.

Galynker, I., Yaseen, Z. S., Cohen, A., Benhamou, O., Hawes, M., & Briggs, J. (2017). Prediction of suicidal behavior in high risk psychiatric patients using an assessment of acute suicidal state: The Suicide Crisis Inventory. *Depression and Anxiety, 34*(2), 147–158. https://doi.org/10.1002/da.22559

Germán, M., Smith, H. L., Rivera-Morales, C., González, G., Haliczer, L. A., Haaz, C., & Miller, A. L. (2015). Dialectical behavior therapy for suicidal Latina adolescents: Supplemental dialectical corollaries and treatment targets. *American Journal of Psychotherapy, 69*(2), 179–197. https://doi.org/10.1176/appi.psychotherapy.2015.69.2.179

Glenn, C. R., & Nock, M. K. (2014). Improving the short-term prediction of suicidal behavior. *American Journal of Preventive Medicine, 47*, S176–S180. https://doi.org/10.1016/j.amepre.2014.06.004

Goldin, P. R., & Gross, J. J. (2010). Effects of mindfulness-based stress reduction (MBSR) on emotion regulation in social anxiety disorder. *Emotion, 10*, 83–91. https://doi.org/10.1037/a0018441

Goldin, P. R., Manber-Ball, T., Werner, K., Heimberg, R., & Gross, J. J. (2009). Neural mechanisms of cognitive reappraisal of negative self-beliefs in social anxiety disorder. *Biological Psychiatry, 66*, 1091–1099. https://doi.org/10.1016/j.biopsych.2009.07.014

Goldsmith, S. K., Pellmar, T. C., Kleinman, A. M., & Bunney, W. E. (Eds.). (2002). Barriers to effective treatment and intervention. In: *Reducing suicide: A national imperative.* National Academies Press. https://www.ncbi.nlm.nih.gov/books/NBK220944/

Goldston, D. B., Molock, S. D., Whitbeck, L. B., Murakami, J. L., Zayas, L. H., & Hall, G. C. (2008). Cultural considerations in adolescent suicide prevention and psycho social treatment. *The American Psychologist, 63*(1), 14–31. https://doi.org/10.1037/0003-066X.63.1.14

Gonzalez, R., Bernstein, I., & Suppes, T. (2008). An investigation of water lithium concentrations and rates of violent acts in 11 Texas counties. *Journal of Clinical Psychiatry, 69*(2), 325–326. https://doi.org/10.4088/jcp.v69n0221a

Grubbs, J. B., & Exline, J. J. (2016). Trait entitlement: A cognitive-personality source of vulnerability to psychological distress. *Psychological Bulletin, 142*, 1204–1226. https://doi.org/10.1037/bul0000063

Gysin-Maillart, A., Schwab, S., Soravia, L., Megert, M., & Michel, K. (2016). A novel brief therapy for patients who attempt suicide: A 24-months follow-up randomized controlled study of the Attempted Suicide Short Intervention Program (ASSIP). *PLOS Medicine, 13*, e1001968. https://doi.org/10.1371/journal.pmed.1001968

Hahm, H. C., & Yasui, M. (2019). Guest editors' introduction to the special section: Cultural adaptation of mental health interventions for Americans of East Asian descent. *American Journal of Orthopsychiatry, 89*(4), 458–461. http://dx.doi.org.tc.idm.oclc.org/10.1037/ort0000421

Hahm, H. C., Zhou, L., Lee, C., Maru, M., Petersen, J. M., & Kolaczyk, E. D. (2019). Feasibility, preliminary efficacy, and safety of a randomized clinical trial for Asian Women's Action for Resilience and Empowerment (AWARE) intervention. *The American Journal of Orthopsychiatry, 89*(4), 462–474. https://doi.org/10.1037/ort0000383

Harris, E. C., & Barraclough, B. (1997). Suicide as an outcome for mental disorders: A meta-analysis. *The British Journal of Psychiatry, 170*, 205–228. https://doi.org/10.1192/bjp.170.3.205

Hirsch, J. K., Duberstein, P. R., Conner, K. R., Heisel, M. J., Beckman, A., Franus, N., & Conwell, Y. (2006). Future orientation and suicide ideation and attempts in depressed adults ages 50 and over. *The American Journal of Geriatric Psychiatry, 14*, 752–757. https://doi.org/10.1097/01.JGP.0000209219.06017.62

Hwang, W. C., Myers, H. F., Chiu, E., Mak, E., Butner, J. E., Fujimoto, K., Wood, J. J., & Miranda, J. (2015). Culturally adapted cognitive-behavioral therapy for Chinese Americans with depression: A randomized controlled trial. *Psychiatric Services (Washington, D.C.), 66*(10), 1035–1042. https://doi.org/10.1176/appi.ps.201400358

Jobes, D. A. (1995). The challenge and the promise of clinical suicidology. *Suicide and Life-Threatening Behavior, 25*, 437–449. https://doi.org/10.1111/j.1943-278X.1995.tb00237.x

Jobes, D. A. (2006). *Managing suicidal risk: A collaborative approach.* Guilford. http://search.proquest.com.proxy.lib.fsu.edu/psycinfo/docview/621443927/FB473999A32E4B25PQ/5?accountid=4840

Jobes, D. A. (2016). *Managing suicidal risk: A collaborative approach* (2nd ed.). Guilford.

Jobes, D. A., Comtois, K. A., Gutierrez, P. M., Brenner, L. A., Huh, D., Chalker, S. A., Ruhe, G., Kerbrat, A. H., Atkins, D. C., Jennings, K., Crumlish, J., Corona, C. D., O'Connor, S., Hendricks, K. E., Schembari, B., Singer, B., & Crow, B. (2017). A randomized controlled trial of the Collaborative Assessment and Management of Suicidality versus enhanced care as usual with suicidal soldiers. *Psychiatry, 80*, 339–356. https://doi.org/10.1080/00332747.2017.1354607

Jobes, D. A., Jacoby, A. M., Cimbolic, P., & Hustead, L. A. T. (1997). Assessment and treatment of suicidal clients in a university counseling center. *Journal of Counseling Psychology, 44*, 368–377.

Johnson, L. L., O'Connor, S. S., Kaminer, B., Gutierrez, P. M., Carney, E., Groh, B., & Jobes, D. A. (2019). Evaluation of structured assessment and mediating factors of suicide-focused group therapy for veterans recently discharged from inpatient psychiatry. *Archives of Suicide Research, 23*, 15–33. https://doi.org/10.1080/13811118.2017.1402722

Joiner, T. E. (2005). *Why people die by suicide*. Harvard University Press.

Joiner, T. E., Steer, R. A., Brown, G., Beck, A. T., Pettit, J. W., & Rudd, M. D. (2003). Worst-point suicidal plans: A dimension of suicidality predictive of past suicide attempts and eventual death by suicide. *Behaviour Research and Therapy, 41*, 1469–1480. https://doi.org/10.1016/S0005-7967(03)00070-6

Kabat-Zinn, J., & Hanh, T. N. (2009). *Full catastrophe living: Using the wisdom of your body and mind to face stress, pain, and illness*. Random House.

Kaslow, N. J., Leiner, A. S., Reviere, S., Jackson, E., Bethea, K., Bhaju, J., Rhodes, M., Gantt, M. J., Senter, H., & Thompson, M. P. (2010). Suicidal, abused African American women's response to a culturally informed intervention. *Journal of Consulting and Clinical Psychology, 78*(4), 449–458. https://doi.org/10.1037/a0019692

Khazem, L. R., Houtsma, C., Gratz, K. L., Tull, M. T., Green, B. A., & Anestis, M. D. (2016). Firearms matter: The moderating role of firearm storage in the association between current suicidal ideation and likelihood of future suicide attempts among United States military personnel. *Military Psychology, 28*, 25–33. https://doi.org/10.1037/mil0000099

Kleiman, E. M., & Nock, M. K. (2018). Real-time assessment of suicidal thoughts and behaviors. *Current Opinion in Psychology, 22*, 33–37. https://doi.org/10.1016/j.copsyc.2017.07.026

Klein, D. C. (1991). The humiliation dynamic: An overview. *Journal of Primary Prevention, 12*, 93–121. https://doi.org/10.1007/BF02015214

Kliem, S., Kröger, C., & Kosfelder, J. (2010). Dialectical behavior therapy for borderline personality disorder: A meta-analysis using mixed-effects modeling. *Journal of Consulting and Clinical Psychology, 78*, 936–951. https://doi.org/10.1037/a0021015

Klonsky, E. D. (2020). The role of theory for understanding and preventing suicide (but not predicting it): A commentary on Hjelmeland and Knizek. *Death Studies, 44*, 459–462. https://doi.org/10.1080/07481187.2019.1594005

Kruzan, K. P., Meyerhoff, J., Biernesser, C., Goldstein, T., Reddy, M., & Mohr, D. C. (2021). Centering lived experience in developing digital interventions for suicide and self-injurious behaviors: User-centered design approach. *JMIR Mental Health, 8*(12), e31367. https://doi.org/10.2196/31367

LaFromboise, T. D., & Howard-Pitney, B. (1994). The Zuni Life Skills Development curriculum: A collaborative approach to curriculum development. *American Indian and*

Alaska Native Mental Health Research, 4(Mono), 98–121. https://doi.org/10.5820/aian. mono04.1994.98

Lee, Y., Syeda, K., Maruschak, N. A., Cha, D. S., Mansur, R. B., Wium-Andersen, I. K., Woldeyohannes, H. O., Rosenblat, J. D., & McIntyre, R. S. (2016). A new perspective on the anti-suicide effects with ketamine treatment: A procognitive effect. *Journal of Clinical Psychopharmacology, 36*(1), 50–56. https://doi.org/10.1097/JCP.000000000 0000441

Leong, F. T. L., & Leach, M. M. (Eds.). (2008). *Suicide among racial and ethnic minority groups: Theory, research, and practice.* Routledge/Taylor & Francis Group.

Li, S., Galynker, I. I., Briggs, J., Duffy, M., Frechette-Hagan, A., Kim, H., Cohen, L. J., & Yaseen, Z. S. (2017). Attachment style and suicide behaviors in high risk psychiatric inpatients following hospital discharge: The mediating role of entrapment. *Psychiatry Research, 257*, 309–314. https://doi.org/10.1016/j.psychres.2017.07.072

Lindsey, M., Sheftall, A., Xiao, Y., Joe, S. (2019). Trends of suicidal behaviors among high school students in the United States: 1991–2017. *Pediatrics, 144*(5), e20191187. https://doi.org/10.1542/peds.2019-1187

Linehan, M. M. (1993). *Cognitive-behavioral treatment of borderline personality disorder.* Guilford. http://search.proquest.com.proxy.lib.fsu.edu/psycinfo/docview/618396253/A2265652FA7347E8PQ/2?accountid=4840

Linehan, M. M. (2014). *DBT skills training manual* (2nd ed.). Guilford.

Linehan, M. M., Korslund, K. E., Harned, M. S., Gallop, R. J., Lungu, A., Neacsiu, A. D., McDavid, J., Comtois, K. A., & Murray-Gregory, A. M. (2015). Dialectical behavior therapy for high suicide risk in individuals with borderline personality disorder: A randomized clinical trial and component analysis. *JAMA Psychiatry, 72*, 475–482. https://doi.org/10.1001/jamapsychiatry.2014.3039

Luoma, J. B., Martin, C. E., & Pearson, J. L. (2002). Contact with mental health and primary care providers before suicide: A review of the evidence. *The American Journal of Psychiatry, 159*, 909–916. https://doi.org/10.1176/appi.ajp.159.6.909

Lutz, A., Slagter, H. A., Dunne, J. D., & Davidson, R. J. (2008). Attention regulation and monitoring in meditation. *Trends in Cognitive Sciences, 12*, 163–169. https://doi.org/10.1016/j.tics.2008.01.005

Lykins, E. L. B., & Baer, R. A. (2009). Psychological functioning in a sample of long-term practitioners of mindfulness meditation. *Journal of Cognitive Psychotherapy, 23*, 226–241. https://doi.org/10.1891/0889-8391.23.3.226

Mayall, S. J., & Banerjee, A. K. (2014). *Therapeutic risk management of medicines.* Woodhead Publishing.

McAdams, D. P., Josselson, R., & Lieblich, A. (2001). *Turns in the road: Narrative studies of lives in transition* (pp. xxi, 310). American Psychological Association. https://doi.org/10.1037/10410-000

Meltzer, H. Y., Alphs, L., Green, A. I., Altamura, A. C., Anand, R., Bertoldi, A., Bourgeois, M., Chouinard, G., Islam, M. Z., Kane, J., Krishnan, R., Lindenmayer, J. P., Potkin, S., & International Suicide Prevention Trial Study Group. (2003). Clozapine treatment for suicidality in schizophrenia: International Suicide Prevention Trial (InterSePT). *Archives of General Psychiatry, 60*, 82–91. https://doi.org/10.1001/archpsyc.60.1.82

Mennin, D. S., & Fresco, D. M. (2013). What, me worry and ruminate about DSM-5 and RDoC? The importance of targeting negative self-referential processing. *Clinical Psychology, 20*, 258–267. https://doi.org/10.1111/cpsp.12038

Mennin, D. S., Fresco, D. M., O'Toole, M. S., & Heimberg, R. G. (2018). A randomized controlled trial of emotion regulation therapy for generalized anxiety disorder with and without co-occurring depression. *Journal of Consulting and Clinical Psychology*, 86(3), 268–281. https://doi.org/10.1037/ccp0000289

Mennin, D. S., Fresco, D. M., Ritter, M., & Heimberg, R. G. (2015). An open trial of emotion regulation therapy for generalized anxiety disorder and co-occurring depression. *Depression and Anxiety*, 32, 614–623. https://doi.org/10.1002/da.22377

Meza, J. I., & Bath, E. (2021). One size does not fit all: Making suicide prevention and interventions equitable for our increasingly diverse communities. *Journal of the American Academy of Child and Adolescent Psychiatry*, 60(2), 209–212. https://doi.org/10.1016/j.jaac.2020.09.019

Michel, K., & Gysin-Maillart, A. (2015). *ASSIP—Attempted Suicide Short Intervention Program: A manual for clinicians* (pp. x, 113). Hogrefe Publishing. https://doi.org/10.1027/00476-000

Miller, D. D. (2000). Review and management of clozapine side effects. *The Journal of Clinical Psychiatry*, 61(Suppl. 8), 14–17.

Mohr, D. C., Burns, M. N., Schueller, S. M., Clarke, G., & Klinkman, M. (2013). Behavioral intervention technologies: Evidence review and recommendations for future research in mental health. *General Hospital Psychiatry*, 35(4), 332–338.

Mohr, D. C., Cuijpers, P., & Lehman, K. (2011). Supportive accountability: A model for providing human support to enhance adherence to eHealth interventions. *Journal of Medical Internet Research*, 13(1), e30. https://doi.org/10.2196/jmir.1602

Müller-Oerlinghausen, B., & Lewitzka, U. (2010). Lithium reduces pathological aggression and suicidality: A mini-review. *Neuropsychobiology*, 62, 43–49. https://doi.org/10.1159/000314309

Murrough, J. W., Iosifescu, D. V., Chang, L. C., Al Jurdi, R. K., Green, C. E., Perez, A. M., Iqbal, S., Pillemer, S., Foulkes, A., Shah, A., Charney, D. S., & Mathew, S. J. (2013). Antidepressant efficacy of ketamine in treatment-resistant major depression: A two-site randomized controlled trial. *The American Journal of Psychiatry*, 170(10), 1134–1142. https://doi.org/10.1176/appi.ajp.2013.13030392

Musiat, P., Johnson, C., Atkinson, M., Wilksch, S., & Wade, T. (2022). Impact of guidance on intervention adherence in computerised interventions for mental health problems: A meta-analysis. *Psychological Medicine*, 52(2), 229–240. https://doi.org/10.1017/S0033291721004621

Nahum-Shani, I., Smith, S. N., Spring, B. J., Collins, L. M., Witkiewitz, K., Tewari, A., & Murphy, S. A. (2018). Just-in-time adaptive interventions (JITAIs) in mobile health: Key components and design principles for ongoing health behavior support. *Annals of Behavioral Medicine*, 52, 446–462. https://doi.org/10.1007/s12160-016-9830-8

Newport, D. J., Carpenter, L. L., McDonald, W. M., Potash, J. B., Tohen, M., Nemeroff, C. B., & APA Council of Research Task Force on Novel Biomarkers and Treatments. (2015). Ketamine and other NMDA antagonists: Early clinical trials and possible mechanisms in depression. *The American Journal of Psychiatry*, 172(10), 950–966. https://doi.org/10.1176/appi.ajp.2015.15040465

Newport, D. J., Schatzberg, A. F., & Nemeroff, C. B. (2016). Whither ketamine as an antidepressant: Panacea or toxin? *Depression and Anxiety*, 33(8), 685–688. https://doi.org/10.1002/da.22535

Nock, M. K., Borges, G., Bromet, E. J., Cha, C. B., Kessler, R. C., & Lee, S. (2008). Suicide and suicidal behavior. *Epidemiologic Reviews*, 30(1), 133–154. https://doi.org/10.1093/epirev/mxn002

FRAMEWORK FOR SUICIDE PREVENTION 501

O'Connor, R. C. (2007). The relations between perfectionism and suicidality: A systematic review. *Suicide and Life-Threatening Behavior, 37*, 698–714. https://doi.org/10.1521/suli.2007.37.6.698

O'Connor, R. C., Fraser, L., Whyte, M., MacHale, S., & Masterton, G. (2009). Self-regulation of unattainable goals in suicide attempters: The relationship between goal disengagement, goal reengagement and suicidal ideation. *Behaviour Research and Therapy, 47*, 164–169. https://doi.org/10.1016/j.brat.2008.11.001

O'Connor, R. C., & Kirtley, O. J. (2018). The integrated motivational volitional model of suicidal behaviour. *Philosophical Transactions of the Royal Society B, 373*(1754), 20170268. https://doi.org/10.1098/rstb.2017.0268

O'Connor, R. C., O'Carroll, R. E., Ryan, C., & Smyth, R. (2012). Self-regulation of unattainable goals in suicide attempters: A two year prospective study. *Journal of Affective Disorders, 142*, 248–255. https://doi.org/10.1016/j.jad.2012.04.035

Oh, H., Stickley, A., Koyanagi, A., Yau, R., & DeVylder, J. E. (2019). Discrimination and suicidality among racial and ethnic minorities in the United States. *Journal of Affective Disorders, 245*, 517–523. https://doi.org/10.1016/j.jad.2018.11.059

Opara, I., Assan, M. A., Pierre, K., Gunn, J. F., 3rd, Metzger, I., Hamilton, J., & Arugu, E. (2020). Suicide among Black children: An integrated model of the interpersonal-psychological theory of suicide and intersectionality theory for researchers and clinicians. *Journal of Black Studies, 51*(6), 611–631. https://doi.org/10.1177/0021934720935641

Otte, S., Lutz, M., Streb, J., Cohen, L. J., Galynker, I., Dudeck, M., & Büsselmann, M. (2020). Analyzing suicidality in German forensic patients by means of the German version of the Suicide Crisis Inventory (SCI-G). *The Journal of Forensic Psychiatry & Psychology, 31*(5), 731–746. https://doi.org/10.1080/14789949.2020.1787487

Palitsky, D., Mota, N., Afifi, T. O., Downs, A. C., & Sareen, J. (2013). The association between adult attachment style, mental disorders, and suicidality: Findings from a population-based study. *The Journal of Nervous and Mental Disease, 201*, 579–586. https://doi.org/10.1097/NMD.0b013e31829829ab

Parghi, N., Chennapragada, L., Barzilay, S., Newkirk, S., Ahmedani, B., Lok, B., & Galynker, I. (2020). Assessing the predictive ability of the Suicide Crisis Inventory for near-term suicidal behavior using machine learning approaches. *International Journal of Methods in Psychiatric Research, 30*(1), e1863. https://doi.org/10.1002/mpr.1863

Park, A., Gysin-Maillart, A., Müller, T. J., Exadaktylos, A., & Michel, K. (2018). Cost-effectiveness of a brief structured intervention program aimed at preventing repeat suicide attempts among those who previously attempted suicide: A secondary analysis of the ASSIP randomized clinical trial. *JAMA Network Open, 1*, e183680–e183680. https://doi.org/10.1001/jamanetworkopen.2018.3680

Pham, T. V., Fetter, A. K., Wiglesworth, A., Rey, L. F., Prairie Chicken, M. L., Azarani, M., Riegelman, A., & Gone, J. P. (2021). Suicide interventions for American Indian and Alaska Native populations: A systematic review of outcomes. *SSM - Mental Health, 1*, 100029. https://doi.org/10.1016/j.ssmmh.2021.100029

Pia, T., Galynker, I., Schuck, A., Sinclair, C., Ying, G., & Calati, R. (2020). Perfectionism and prospective near-term suicidal thoughts and behaviors: The mediation of fear of humiliation and suicide crisis syndrome. *International Journal of Environmental Research and Public Health, 17*, 1424. https://doi.org/10.3390/ijerph17041424

Prado, G., Pantin, H., Briones, E., Schwartz, S. J., Feaster, D. J., & Huang, S. (2007). A randomized controlled trial of Familias Unidas in preventing substance use and HIV risk behaviors in Hispanic adolescents. *Journal of Consulting and Clinical Psychology, 75,* 914–926.

Ramel, W., Goldin, P. R., Carmona, P. E., & McQuaid, J. R. (2004). The effects of mindfulness meditation on cognitive processes and affect in patients with past depression. *Cognitive Therapy and Research, 28,* 433–455. https://doi.org/10.1023/B:COTR.000 0045557.15923.96

Renna, M. E., Quintero, J. M., Fresco, D. M., & Mennin, D. S. (2017). Emotion regulation therapy: A mechanism-targeted treatment for disorders of distress. *Frontiers in Psychology, 8,* 98. https://doi.org/10.3389/fpsyg.2017.00098

Resick, P. A., Monson, C. M., & Chard, K. M. (2016). *Cognitive processing therapy for PTSD: A comprehensive manual.* Guilford.

Resick, P. A., & Schnicke, M. K. (1992). Cognitive processing therapy for sexual assault victims. *Journal of Consulting and Clinical Psychology, 60,* 748–756. https://doi.org/ 10.1037/0022-006X.60.5.748

Ribeiro, J. D., Franklin, J. C., Fox, K. R., Bentley, K. H., Kleiman, E. M., Chang, B. P., & Nock, M. K. (2016). Self-injurious thoughts and behaviors as risk factors for future suicide ideation, attempts, and death: A meta-analysis of longitudinal studies. *Psychological Medicine, 46,* 225–236. https://doi.org/10.1017/S0033291715001804

Rizvi, S. L., Dimeff, L. A., Skutch, J., Carroll, D., & Linehan, M. M. (2011). A pilot study of the DBT Coach: An interactive mobile phone application for individuals with borderline personality disorder and substance use disorder. *Behavior Therapy, 42,* 589–600. https://doi.org/10.1016/j.beth.2011.01.003

Rizvi, S. L., Hughes, C. D., & Thomas, M. C. (2016). The DBT Coach mobile application as an adjunct to treatment for suicidal and self-injuring individuals with borderline personality disorder: A preliminary evaluation and challenges to client utilization. *Psychological Services, 13,* 380–388. https://doi.org/10.1037/ser0000100

Robinson, W. L., Whipple, C. R., Jason, L. A., & Flack, C. E. (2021b). African American adolescent suicidal ideation and behavior: The role of racism and prevention. *Journal of Community Psychology, 49*(5), 1282–1295. https://doi.org/10.1002/jcop.22543

Robinson, W. L., Whipple, C. R., Keenan, K., Flack, C. E., & Wingate, L. (2021a). Suicide in African American adolescents: Understanding risk by studying resilience. *Annual Review of Clinical Psychology, 9*(18), 359–385. https://doi.org/10.1146/annurev-clin psy-072220-021819

Rogers, M. L., Bafna, A., & Galynker, I. (2022). Comparative clinical utility of screening for suicide crisis syndrome versus suicidal ideation in relation to suicidal ideation and attempts at one-month follow-up. *Suicide and Life-Threatening Behavior, 52*(5), 866–875. https://doi.org/10.1111/sltb.12870

Rogers, M. L., Cao, E., Sinclair, C., & Galynker, I. (2021). Associations between goal orientation and suicidal thoughts and behaviors at one-month follow-up: Indirect effects through ruminative flooding. *Behaviour Research and Therapy, 145,* 103945. https:// doi.org/10.1016/j.brat.2021.103945

Rogers, M. L., Gai, A. R., Lieberman, A., Musacchio Schafer, K., & Joiner, T. E. (2021). Why does safety planning prevent suicidal behavior? *Professional Psychology: Research and Practice, 53*(1), 33–41. https://doi.org/10.1037/pro0000427

Rogers, M. L., Galynker, I., Yaseen, Z., Defazio, K., & Joiner, T. E. (2017). An overview and comparison of two proposed suicide-specific diagnoses: Acute suicidal affective disturbance (ASAD) and suicide crisis syndrome (SCS). *Psychiatric Annals, 47,* 416–420.

Rogers, M. L., Hom, M. A., Stanley, I. H., & Joiner, T. E. (2019). Brief measures of phys-ical and psychological distance to suicide methods as correlates and predictors of sui-cide risk: A multi-study prospective investigation. *Behaviour Research and Therapy*, *20*, 103330. https://doi.org/10.1016/j.brat.2018.11.001

Rogers, M. L., Vespa, A., Bloch-Elkouby, S., & Galynker, I. (2021). Validity of the Modular Assessment of Risk for Imminent Suicide in predicting short-term suicidality. *Acta Psychiatrica Scandinavica*, *144*(6), 563–577. https://doi.org/10.1111/acps.13354

Rosenberg, B. M., Kodish, T., Cohen, Z. D., Gong-Guy, F., & Craske, M. G. (2022). A novel peer-to-peer coaching program to support digital mental health: Design and im-plementation. *JMIR Mental Health*, *9*(1), e32430. https://doi.org/10.2196/32430

Rozek, D. C., Keane, C., Sippel, L. M., Stein, J. Y., Rollo-Carlson, C., & Bryan, C. J. (2019). Short-term effects of crisis response planning on optimism in a U.S. Army sample. *Early Intervention in Psychiatry*, *13*, 682–685. https://doi.org/10.1111/eip.12699

Rudd, M. D., Joiner, T. E., & Rajab, M. H. (2004). *Treating suicidal behavior: An effective, time-limited approach* (1st ed.). Guilford.

Ryberg, W., Zahl, P., Diep, L. M., Landrø, N. I., & Fosse, R. (2019). Managing suicidality within specialized care: A randomized controlled trial. *Journal of Affective Disorders*, *249*, 112–120. https://doi.org/10.1016/j.jad.2019.02.022

Saffer, B. Y., & Klonsky, E. D. (2017). The relationship of self-reported executive func-tioning to suicide ideation and attempts: Findings from a large U.S.-based online sample. *Archives of Suicide Research*, *21*, 577–594. https://doi.org/10.1080/13811 118.2016.1211042

Schuck, A., Calati, R., Barzilay, S., Bloch-Elkouby, S., & Galynker, I. (2019). Suicide crisis syndrome: A review of supporting evidence for a new suicide-specific diagnosis. *Behavioral Sciences and the Law*, *37*, 223–239.

Segal, Z. V., Williams, M., & Teasdale, J. (2018). *Mindfulness-based cognitive therapy for depression* (2nd ed.). Guilford.

Shadick, R., Backus Dagirmanjian, F., & Barbot, B. (2015). Suicide risk among college students: The intersection of sexual orientation and race. *Crisis*, *36*(6), 416–423. https://doi.org/10.1027/0227-5910/a000340

Shpigel, M. S., Diamond, G. M., & Diamond, G. S. (2012). Changes in parenting behaviors, attachment, depressive symptoms, and suicidal ideation in attachment-based family therapy for depressive and suicidal adolescents. *Journal of Marital and Family Therapy*, *38*(Suppl. 1), 271–283. https://doi.org/10.1111/j.1752-0606.2012.00295.x

Siddaway, A. P., Taylor, P. J., Wood, A. M., & Schulz, J. (2015). A meta-analysis of perceptions of defeat and entrapment in depression, anxiety problems, posttraumatic stress disorder, and suicidality. *Journal of Affective Disorders*, *184*, 149–159. https://doi.org/10.1016/j.jad.2015.05.046

Silva, C., & Van Orden, K. A. (2018). Suicide among Hispanics in the United States. *Current Opinion in Psychology*, *22*, 44–49. https://doi.org/10.1016/j.copsyc.2017.07.013

Smith, A. R., Ribeiro, J., Mikolajewski, A., Taylor, J., Joiner, T., & Iacono, W. G. (2012). An examination of environmental and genetic contributions to the determinants of suicidal behavior among male twins. *Psychiatry Research*, *197*, 60–65. https://doi.org/10.1016/j.psychres.2012.01.010

Smith, K. A., & Cipriani, A. (2017). Lithium and suicide in mood disorders: Updated meta-review of the scientific literature. *Bipolar Disorders*, *19*, 575–586. https://doi.org/10.1111/bdi.12543

Soto, A., Smith, T. B., Griner, D., Rodríguez, M. D., & Bernal, G. (2018). Cultural adaptations and therapist multicultural competence: Two meta-analytic reviews. *Journal of Clinical Psychology, 74*(11), 1907–1923.https:/doi.org/10.1002/jclp.22679

Stanley, B., & Brown, G. K. (2012). Safety planning intervention: A brief intervention to mitigate suicide risk. *Cognitive and Behavioral Practice, 19,* 256–264. https://doi.org/10.1016/j.cbpra.2011.01.001

Stanley, B., Brown, G. K., Brenner, L. A., Galfalvy, H. C., Currier, G. W., Knox, K. L., Chaudhury, S. R., Bush, A. L., & Green, K. L. (2018). Comparison of the safety planning intervention with follow-up vs usual care of suicidal patients treated in the emergency department. *JAMA Psychiatry, 75,* 894–900. https://doi.org/10.1001/jamapsychiatry.2018.1776

Stanley, B., Brown, G., Brent, D., Wells, K., Poling, K., Curry, J., Kennard, B. D., Wagner, A., Cwik, M., Klomek, A. B., Goldstein, T., Vitiello, B., Barnett, S., Daniel, S., & Hughes, J. (2009). Cognitive behavior therapy for suicide prevention (CBT-SP): Treatment model, feasibility and acceptability. *Journal of the American Academy of Child and Adolescent Psychiatry, 48,* 1005–1013. https://doi.org/10.1097/CHI.0b013e3181b5dbfe

Stanley, B., Chaudhury, S. R., Chesin, M., Pontoski, K., Bush, A. M., Knox, K. L., & Brown, G. K. (2016). An emergency department intervention and follow-up to reduce suicide risk in the VA: Acceptability and effectiveness. *Psychiatric Services, 67,* 680–683. https://doi.org/10.1176/appi.ps.201500082

Stene-Larsen, K., & Reneflot, A. (2017). Contact with primary and mental health care prior to suicide: A systematic review of the literature from 2000 to 2017. *Scandinavian Journal of Public Health, 47*(1), 9–17. https://doi.org/10.1177/1403494817746274

Substance Abuse and Mental Health Services Administration [SAMHSA]. (2020). *Treatment for suicidal ideation, self-harm, and suicide attempts among youth.* https://store.samhsa.gov/sites/default/files/SAMHSA_Digital_Download/PEP20-06-01-002.pdf

Sue, D. W., & Sue, D. (2003). *Counseling the culturally diverse: Theory and practice* (4th ed.). John Wiley & Sons.

Suicide Prevention Resource Center [SPRC]. (2020). *American Indian and Alaskan Native populations.* https://www.sprc.org/scope/racial-ethnic-disparities/american-indian-alaska-native-populations

Swift, J. K., Trusty, W. T., & Penix, E. A. (2021). The effectiveness of the Collaborative Assessment and Management of Suicidality (CAMS) compared to alternative treatment conditions: A meta-analysis. *Suicide and Life-Threatening Behavior, 51*(5), 882–896. https://doi.org/10.1111/sltb.12765

Taipale, H., Lähteenvuo, M., Tanskanen, A., Mittendorfer-Rutz, E., & Tiihonen, J. (2021). Comparative effectiveness of antipsychotics for risk of attempted or completed suicide among persons with schizophrenia. *Schizophrenia Bulletin, 47*(1), 23–30. https://doi.org/10.1093/schbul/sbaa111

Taylor, P. J., Gooding, P., Wood, A. M., & Tarrier, N. (2011). The role of defeat and entrapment in depression, anxiety, and suicide. *Psychological Bulletin, 137,* 391–420. https://doi.org/10.1037/a0022935

Thomas, K., Jiang, Y., & Mccombs, J. (2015). Clozapine revisited: Impact of clozapine vs olanzapine on health care use by schizophrenia patients on Medicaid. *Annals of Clinical Psychiatry, 27,* 90–99.

Torok, M., Han, J., Baker, S., Werner-Seidler, A., Wong, I., Larsen, M. E., & Christensen, H. (2020). Suicide prevention using self-guided digital interventions: A systematic review and meta-analysis of randomised controlled trials. *The Lancet Digital Health*, 2(1), e25–e36. https://doi.org/10.1016/S2589-7500(19)30199-2

Van Orden, K. A., Witte, T. K., Cukrowicz, K. C., Braithwaite, S. R., Selby, E. A., & Joiner, T. E. (2010). The interpersonal theory of suicide. *Psychological Review, 117,* 575–600. https://doi.org/10.1037/a0018697

Vidot, D. C., Huang, S., Poma, S., Estrada, Y., Lee, T. K., & Prado, G. (2016). Familias Unidas' Crossover Effects on Suicidal Behaviors among Hispanic Adolescents: Results from an Effectiveness Trial. *Suicide & Life-Threatening Behavior, 46*(S1), S8–S14.

Villarreal-Otálora, T., Jennings, P., & Mowbray, O. (2019). Clinical interventions to reduce suicidal behaviors in Hispanic adolescents: A scoping review. *Research on Social Work Practice, 29*(8), 924–938. https://doi.org/10.1177/1049731519832100

Wagner, B. M., Silverman, M. A. C., & Martin, C. E. (2003). Family factors in youth suicidal behaviors. *American Behavioral Scientist, 46* (9), 1171–1191.

Wenzel, A., & Beck, A. T. (2008). A cognitive model of suicidal behavior: Theory and treatment. *Applied and Preventive Psychology, 12,* 189–201. https://doi.org/10.1016/j.appsy.2008.05.001

Williams, N. R., Heifets, B. D., Bentzley, B. S., Blasey, C., Sudheimer, K. D., Hawkins, J., Lyons, D. M., & Schatzberg, A. F. (2019). Attenuation of antidepressant and antisuicidal effects of ketamine by opioid receptor antagonism. *Molecular Psychiatry, 24,* 1779–1786. https://doi.org/10.1038/s41380-019-0503-4

Witt, K., Potts, J., Hubers, A., Grunebaum, M. F., Murrough, J. W., Loo, C., Cipriani, A., & Hawton, K. (2020). Ketamine for suicidal ideation in adults with psychiatric disorders: A systematic review and meta-analysis of treatment trials. *The Australian and New Zealand Journal of Psychiatry, 54,* 29–45. https://doi.org/10.1177/000486741 9883341

Witt, K., Spittal, M. J., Carter, G. et al. (2017). Effectiveness of online and mobile telephone applications ('apps') for the self-management of suicidal ideation and self-harm: A systematic review and meta-analysis. *BMC Psychiatry, 17,* 297. https://doi.org/10.1186/s12888-017-1458-0

Wong, Y. J., Maffini, C. S., & Shin, M. (2014). The racial-cultural framework: A framework for addressing suicide-related outcomes in communities of color. *The Counseling Psychologist, 42*(1), 13–54. https://doi.org/10.1177/0011000012470568

World Health Organization [WHO]. (2014). *Preventing suicide: A global imperative.*

Wrosch, C., Miller, G. E., Scheier, M. F., & de Pontet, S. B. (2007). Giving up on unattainable goals: Benefits for health? *Personality & Social Psychology Bulletin, 33,* 251–265. https://doi.org/10.1177/0146167206294905

Wrosch, C., Scheier, M. F., Miller, G. E., Schulz, R., & Carver, C. S. (2003). Adaptive self-regulation of unattainable goals: Goal disengagement, goal reengagement, and subjective well-being. *Personality and Social Psychology Bulletin, 29,* 1494–1508. https://doi.org/10.1177/0146167203256921

Yaseen, Z. S., Hawes, M., Barzilay, S., & Galynker, I. (2019). Predictive validity of proposed diagnostic criteria for the suicide crisis syndrome: An acute presuicidal state. *Suicide and Life-Threatening Behavior, 49,* 1124–1135. https://doi.org/10.1111/sltb.12495

Yaseen, Z. S., Kopeykina, I., Gutkovich, Z., Bassirnia, A., Cohen, L. J., & Galynker, I. I. (2014). Predictive validity of the Suicide Trigger Scale (STS-3) for post-discharge suicide attempt in high-risk psychiatric inpatients. *PLOS One, 9*(1), e86768. https://doi.org/10.1371/journal.pone.0086768

Ying, G., Cohen, L. J., Lloveras, L., Barzilay, S., & Galynker, I. (2020). Multi-informant prediction of near-term suicidal behavior independent of suicidal ideation. *Psychiatry Research*, *291*, 113169. https://doi.org/10.1016/j.psychres.2020.113169

Yovell, Y., Bar, G., Mashiah, M., Baruch, Y., Briskman, I., Asherov, J., Lotan, A., Rigbi, A., & Panksepp, J. (2016). Ultra-low-dose buprenorphine as a time-limited treatment for severe suicidal ideation: A randomized controlled trial. *The American Journal of Psychiatry*, *173*(5), 491–498. https://doi.org/10.1176/appi.ajp.2015.15040535

Index

For the benefit of digital users, indexed terms that span two pages (e.g., 52–53) may, on occasion, appear on only one of those pages.

Note: Tables and figures are indicated by *t* and *f* following the page number